Vitamin K Metabolism and Vitamin K-Dependent Proteins

Proceedings of the 8th Steenbock Symposium held at the University of Wisconsin-Madison, June 10–13, 1979

Vitamin K Metabolism and Vitamin K–Dependent Proteins

Edited by

J. W. Suttie, Ph.D.
Department of Biochemistry
University of Wisconsin
Madison, Wisconsin

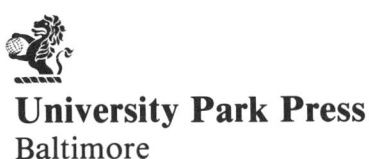

University Park Press
Baltimore

UNIVERSITY PARK PRESS
International Publishers in Science, Medicine, and Education
233 East Redwood Street
Baltimore, Maryland 21202

Copyright ©1980 by University Park Press

Manufactured in the United States of America by
The Maple Press Company.

All rights, including that of translation into other languages, reserved. Photomechanical reproduction (photocopy, microcopy) of this book or parts thereof without special permission of the publisher is prohibited.

Library of Congress Cataloging in Publication Data

Harry Steenbock Symposium, 8th, University of Wisconsin, Madison, 1979.
   Vitamin K metabolism and vitamin K-dependent protein.

   Includes index.
   1. Vitamin K—Metabolism—Congresses. 2. Vitamin K—Physiological effect—Congresses. 3. Prothrombin—Congresses. 4. Protein—Congresses. I. Suttie, John W., 1934–   II. Title.
QP772.V55H37   1979   291.1'33   79-21274
ISBN 0-8391-1540-7

Contents

Preface xi

CHEMISTRY AND FUNCTIONING OF VITAMIN K-DEPENDENT PLASMA PROTEINS 1

Structural Properties of Vitamin K-Dependent Plasma Proteins
 E. W. Davie 3
Crystallographic Investigation of the A-Fragment (Fragment-1) from Bovine Prothrombin
 Gustav Olsson, Oliver Lindqvist, Torben E. Petersen, Staffan Magnusson, and Lars Sottrup-Jensen 8
Protein Substrates for γ-Carboxylation: Evidence for Alanine Hydroxylation to Serine in Vitamin K-Dependent Enzymes
 Karl J. Matthes 13
Cooperativity of Calcium Ion Binding to Bovine Prothrombin, Prothrombin Fragment-1 and Factor X
An Alternative to Conformational Changes for Explaining Such Behavior
 Craig M. Jackson 16
Prothrombin Fragment 1 Modifications: Effects on Protein-Membrane Interaction
 G. L. Nelsestuen, R. M. Resnick, C. S. Kim, and C. Pletcher 28
Correlation of Metal Ion-Induced Fluorescence Transitions With Conformational Changes in Prothrombin Fragment 1
 F. G. Prendergast, J. Bloom, M. R. Downing, and K. G. Mann 39
Calcium-Induced Conformational Change in Human Prothrombin
 Richard Benarous, Gérard Gacon, Marie-Josèphe Rabiet, and Dominique Labie 49
Calcium Binding to Prothrombin Fragment-1 by Ultraviolet Difference Spectroscopy
 G. M. Brenckle, C. W. Peng, and C. M. Jackson 54
Gla-Region Secondary Structure in Prothrombin and Factor X
 T. L. Carlisle, T. Morita, and C. M. Jackson 58
Effect of γ-Carboxyglutamic Acids on Properties of Prothrombins and Their Fragments
 O. P. Malhotra 62
Conformation-Specific Antibodies to Abnormal Prothrombin and Prothrombin
 R. A. Blanchard, B. Furie, and B. C. Furie 66
Functions for Protein C
 C. T. Esmon, P. C. Comp, and F. J. Walker 72
Amino Acid Sequence of Bovine Protein C
 Per Fernlund and Johan Stenflo 84
Interaction Between Prothrombin and the Platelet Receptor for Factor Xa
Inhibitory Effect of Protein C
 Johan Stenflo and Bjorn Dahlbäck 89

Function of Previously Unrecognized Plasma Protein M in Thrombin
Generation
    Walter H. Seegers, Abha Ghosh, and Van-Yu Wu 96
Purification of Protein S from Bovine Plasma
    Johan Stenflo 102
Activation of Human Prothrombin: Kinetics and Regulation
    Carolyn L. Orthner, Sam Morris, Frank Robey, and David P. Kosow 106
The Influence of Bovine Coagulation Factor V and Va on the Function
of "Prothrombinase"
    *Michael E. Nesheim, James W. Bloom, Paula Tracy, and
Kenneth G. Mann*..110
Human Prothrombin Activation: Radioimmunoassay of Fragment 3
    Daniel A. Walz and Thomas R. Brown 116
Bovine Factors X_1 and X_2: Activation Peptide Based Chromatographic
Differences
    Takashi Morita and Craig M. Jackson................................120
Structural and Functional Characteristics of a Proteolytically Modified
"Gla Domain-Less" Bovine Factor X and Xa (des Light Chain
Residues 1-44)
    Takashi Morita and Craig M. Jackson................................124
C Reactive Protein: A Fruitless Search for Gla
    R. M. Iammarino, G. Blank and W. Diven 129

CHEMISTRY OF γ-CARBOXYGLUTAMIC ACID 135

Chemistry of Peptides Containing γ-Carboxyglutamic Acid Residues
    *H. C. Marsh, N. T. Boggs III, P. Robertson Jr., M. M. Sarasua,
M. E. Scott, P. B. W. Ten Kortenaar, J. A. Helpern, L. G. Pedersen,
K. A. Koehler, and R. G. Hiskey* 137
Detection of γ-Carboxyglutamic Acid by Dansylation
    Margaret Low, John J. Van Buskirk, and Wolff M. Kirsch 150
A New Method for the Detection of γ-Carboxyglutamic Acid at the
Nanomole Level
    C. M. Gundberg, J. B. Lian, and P. M. Gallop 153
A New Synthesis of γ-Carboxyglutamic Acid and Its Derivatives
    Robert K. Y. Zee-Cheng, and Robert E. Olson.........................157
Identification of γ-carboxyglutamic Acid During Automated Sequenator
Degradation of Proteins
    Per Fernlund and Johan Stenflo.....................................161
β-Carboxyglutamic Acid: An Internal Standard for the Quantitation of
Free γ-Carboxyglutamic Acid in Urine Fluids
    Per Fernlund...166
Qualitative Identification of Gla by Two-Dimensional High Voltage
Paper Electrophoresis. Purification and Amino Acid Composition
of Protein Z, a Gla-Containing Plasma Protein
    *Torben E. Petersen, Hans C. Thøgersen, Staffan Magnusson,
and Lars Sottrup-Jensen* 171

NON-MAMMALIAN VITAMIN K METABOLISM 175

Functions of Vitamin K_2 in Microorganisms
    H. Taber...177

Enzymes Involved in Vitamin K Biosynthesis
  R. Meganathan, T. Folger, and R. Bentley 188
The Specificity of Quinones for Restoration of Active Transport of
  Amino Acids and Oxidative Phosphorylation
    A. F. Brodie, T. O. Sutherland, and S. H. Lee 193
Vitamin K-Dependent Sphingolipid Synthesis in *Bacteroides
  melaninogenicus*
    Meir Lev and Albert Milford 203
Biosynthesis and Metabolism of Vitamin K in Invertebrates
    J. F. Pennock and V. T. Burt 208

NON-PLASMA VITAMIN K–DEPENDENT PROTEINS 217

Structure and Function of the Vitamin K-Dependent Protein of Bone
  Paul A. Price, David J. Epstein, Joseph W. Lothringer,
  Satoru K. Nishimoto, James W. Poser, and Matthew K. Williamson 219
Osteocalcin in Developing Bone Systems
  Peter V. Hauschka 227
Osteocalcin Content in Normal, Rachitic and Vitamin K Antagonized
  Bone
    Jane B. Lian, Barry Reit, Albert H. Roufosse, Melvin J. Glimcher,
    and Paul M. Gallop 237
In Vitro Studies of Osteocalcin Biosynthesis in Embryonic Chick Bone
  Cultures
    J. B. Lian and K. M. Heroux 245
Possible Physiological Role of the Vitamin K-Dependent Bone Protein
    S. Reddy and J. W. Suttie 255
Macromolecular Inhibitors of Calcium Phosphate Precipitation in Bone
    Austin G. Diamond and William F. Neuman 259
The Occurrence of γ-Carboxyglutamic Acid in Elasmobranch
  Endoskeleton
    J. B. Lian, J. A. Glowacki, and M. J. Glimcher 263
γ-Carboxyglutamic Acid and Atherosclerotic Plaque
    Robert J. Levy, Jane B. Lian, and Paul M. Gallop 269
Growth Related Changes in the Carboxylation of *E. coli* Ribosomes
    John J. Van Buskirk, Margaret Low, and Wolff M. Kirsch 274
The Presence of γ-Carboxyglutamic Acid in Nascent Polypeptides and
  Ribosomal Proteins From Rat Liver
    J. Scheinbuks 279
Vitamin K-Dependent Carboxylation in Lung Microsomes
    Robert G. Bell 286
Requirement of Egg Shell for Expression of Vitamin K-Dependent
  Calcium-Binding Protein in the Chick Embryonic Chorioallantoic
  Membrane
    Rocky S. Tuan 294
Vitamin K-Dependent Carboxylation in Spleen and Kidney
    Steven D. Buchthal and Robert G. Bell 299
Isolation of a Vitamin K-Dependent Protein Containing
  γ-Carboxyglutamic Acid from Chicken Kidney Microsomes
    Hector P. Traverso, Peter V. Hauschka, and Paul M. Gallop 303
Purification of a Protein Containing γ-Carboxyglutamic Acid From
  Bovine Kidney
    Anne E. Griep and Paul A. Friedman 307

Vitamin K-Dependent Carboxylation in Microsomal Preparations
Derived from Cultured Kidney Cells, Chick Embryo Fiberblasts and
Pancreas
    Hector P. Traverso, Peter V. Hauschka, and Paul M. Gallop 311

MAMMALIAN VITAMIN K METABOLISM AND ANTICOAGULANT ACTION 315

Nutritional Aspects of Vitamin K in the Human
    M. J. Shearer, V. Allan, Y. Haroon, and P. Barkhan 317
Disposition and Turnover of Vitamin K_1 in Man
    *Thorir D. Bjornsson, Peter J. Meffin, Sarah E. Swezey, and
Terrence F. Blaschke* 328
Effect of the Choro Analog of Vitamin K on Phylloquinone Metabolism
in Liver Mitochondria
    *M. J. Thierry-Palmer, M. S. Stern, C. A. Kost, and
J. C. Montgomery* 333
Fetal/Maternal Vitamin K-Dependent Reactions: Some Hormonal
Effects
    D. W. Jolly, R. McBride, S. Seibert, B. Kadis, and T. E. Nelson Jr. 337
Clinical Responses to Vitamin K_1
    R. G. Malia, F. E. Preston, and C. D. Holdsworth 342
Investigation of Anticoagulants and Vitamin K_1 in the Rabbit
    B. K. Park, J. B. Leck, A. Wilson, and A. Breckenridge 348
Studies of the Vitamin K Epoxide Reductase System
    Charles M. Siegfried 354
Studies on the *in vitro* Reduction of Vitamin K_1 Epoxide
    Michael G. Townsend, Edward M. Odam, and Allan K. Nadian 361
R and S Warfarin and Metabolites as Probes of Vitamin K_1 Epoxide
Reductase
    M. J. Fasco and L. S. Kaminsky 366
Possible Phenylbutazone Potentiation of Warfarin by Inhibition of
Vitamin K-Dependent Carboxylation
    Linda J. Kelly and Robert G. Bell 370
γ-Carboxyglutamate Excretion and Vitamin K Metabolism
    Robert J. Levy, Jane B. Lian, Caren Gundberg, and Paul M. Gallop 375
Antithrombotic Actions of Warfarin
    Sanford N. Gitel and Stanford Wessler 380
Chromogenic Assays for the Determination of Prothrombin-Related
Material in Microsomal Fractions
    Linda J. Beecroft and J. H. Sanderson 384
Isolation of Multiple Forms of Dicoumarol-Induced Prothrombins
From Bovine Liver
    Joyce Cassen and Om P. Malhotra 388
Present Distribution of Anticoagulant Resistance in the United States
    William B. Jackson and A. D. Ashton 392

THE VITAMIN K-DEPENDENT CARBOXYLASE 399

Dissociation of Vitamin K-Dependent γ-Carbon-Hydrogen Bond
Cleavage From Carboxylation of Peptide-Bound Glutamic Acid
Residues
    Paul A. Friedman 401

A Radical-Radical C-Carboxylation Reaction as a Model Related to
the Vitamin K-Dependent Carboxylation
  Paul M. Gallop, Paul A. Friedman, and Edward Henson 408
Investigations of the Role of Oxygen in the Vitamin K-Dependent
Carboxylase Reaction
  A. E. Larson, J. J. McTigue, and J. W. Suttie 413
The Role of Superoxide in the Carboxylation of Glutamyl Residues
  *M. P. Esnouf, A. I. Burgess, S. J. Walter, M. R. Green,
  H. A. O. Hill, and M. J. Okolow-Zubkowska* 422
Vitamin K-Dependent Carboxylase for Peptide-Bound Glutamate
  *Anne L. Hall, Paul M. Turner, Barbara F. Dunkle, David A. Wing,
  and Robert E. Olson* 433
Species Variation, Induction, and Subcellular Localization of the
Liver Vitamin K-Dependent Carboxylase
  T. L. Carlisle, D. V. Shah, and J. W. Suttie 443
Effect of Pyridoxal Phosphate on the Vitamin K-Dependent Carboxylase
  *J. W. Suttie, L. O. Geweke, J. L. Finnan, S. R. Lehrman, and
  D. H. Rich* 450
Vitamin K Analogs in the Study of Vitamin K-Dependent Carboxylation
  *B. C. Johnson, D. O. Mack, R. Delaney, M. R. Wolfensberger,
  C. Esmon, J. A. Price, E. Suen, and J.-M. Girardot* 455
Stimulation of Vitamin K_1 Protein Carboxylation by Several
1,4-Naphthoquinones
  D. O. Mack, T. A. Curtis, and B. C. Johnson 467
Rat Liver Vitamin K-Dependent Carboxylase: Substrate Specificity
  *Daniel H. Rich, S. Russ Lehrman, Megumi Kawai,
  Hedda L. Goodman, and J. W. Suttie* 471
Glutamic Acid Derivatives as Substrates for the Vitamin K-Dependent
Carboxylase
  J. L. Finnan, H. L. Goodman and J. W. Suttie 480
Regulation of Vitamin K-Dependent Carboxylation
  A. Dubin, E. T. Suen, R. Delaney, and B. C. Johnson 484
Purification of the Rat Liver Vitamin K-Dependent Carboxylase
  R. Wallin, L. M. Canfield, T. A. Sinsky, and J. W. Suttie 490
Reconstitution of Vitamin K-Dependent Carboxylation Activity
  Joy A. Price and B. Connor Johnson 500
High Pressure Liquid Chromatographic Analysis of the Vitamin
K-Dependent Carboxylase System
  Louise M. Canfield, Jane Ma, and E. G. Sander 505
Carboxylation of Low-Molecular-Weight Substrates by the Rat Liver
Vitamin K-Dependent Carboxylase: Characterization of Products
  J. L. Finnan and J. W. Suttie 509
Vitamin K-Dependent Carboxylation of Peptides Containing the Glu-Glu
Sequence: Localization of γ-Carboxyglutamic Acid
  *H. Rikong-Adie, P. Decottignies-Le Maréchal, R. Azerad, and
  A. Marquet* 518

PROTHROMBIN BIOSYNTHESIS 527

Biosynthesis and Processing of Precursor Prothrombins
  C. Bruce Graves, Gary G. Grabau, and Theodore W. Munns 529
Synthesis of Factor VII in Morris Hepatoma (MH_1C_1) Cells
  H. Prydz and F. Haffner 542

Biosynthesis of Bovine Prothrombin in a Cell-Free System
    R. T. A. MacGillivray, D. W. Chung, and E. W. Davie 546
Vitamin K-Dependent Carboxylation of a Specific Prothrombin
   Precursor and Other Proteins in Rat Liver
    Allan K. Willingham 553
Some Characteristics of Purified Bovine Prothrombin Synthase
    M. de Metz, C. Vermeer, B. A. M. Soute, and H. C. Hemker 560
Mechanism of Warfarin Inhibition of Prothrombin Complex
   Glycosylation
    D. Couri and R. G. Meeks 571
Humoral Substances Regulating the Level of Coagulation Factors:
   Coagulopoietins
   Evidence for a Specific Coagulopoietin for Prothrombin
    M. Karpatkin and S. Karpatkin 576
Studies of Humoral Factor Influencing Prothrombin Levels in the Rat
    D. V. Shah, L. J. Nyari, J. C. Swanson, and J. W. Suttie 584

Index 589

Preface

This year marks the 50th anniversary of the discovery by Henrik Dam that chicks fed a lipid-free diet developed a previously unrecognized hemorrhagic condition. These studies led, a decade later, to the complete characterization and synthesis of the physiologically active quinone now known as vitamin K. Early investigations established a relationship between the dietary adequacy of vitamin K and synthesis of the plasma procoagulant prothrombin. Subsequent investigations demonstrated the essentiality of vitamin K for the biosynthesis of four plasma proteins: prothrombin (Factor II), Factor VII, Factor IX, and Factor X, and these became collectively known as the vitamin K-dependent clotting factors. It is not surprising, considering our lack of general knowledge of plasma protein biosynthesis, that little progress in elucidating the role of vitamin K in the synthesis of these clotting factors was made until the mid 1960s. Studies at that time indicated that prothrombin was formed from a liver precursor protein and that the conversion of this protein to prothrombin was the vitamin K-dependent step in prothrombin synthesis. These studies culminated in 1974 with the demonstration that prothrombin contained a number of residues of a previously unidentified amino acid, γ-carboxyglutamic acid. With this knowledge, the molecular role of vitamin K was clear. It functions as a cofactor for an enzyme that carboxylates peptide-bound glutamyl residues and converts them to γ-carboxyglutamyl residues.

This discovery set the stage for investigations in a number of related areas that were discussed in depth in this symposium. The functional role of γ-carboxyglutamic acid in proteins has been the subject of recent intense investigation, and there has been a rapid advance in the development of in vitro systems to probe the molecular actions of vitamin K in the carboxylase reaction. A successful search for other vitamin K-dependent proteins has been initiated and a physiological role for these proteins is being sought. The opening of these problem areas over the last 5 years has resulted in a stimulation of vitamin K research, and this year appears to be a particularly appropriate time to attempt to bring together workers in this field for a discussion of their results. Seldom is it possible to bring together as large a percentage of the active workers in a particular field for a meeting as it was at this symposium. This was the first meeting at which this group of researchers has been assembled, and this interaction contributed to a free exchange of information in this rapidly growing field. Because the participants at the symposium were all researchers actually engaged in vitamin K research, there were no lengthy review or general orientation presentations. Rather, an attempt was made to concentrate on what was new and ongoing in the various laboratories participating. Much of the new information was presented at poster sessions and the data presented in this form are included in these proceedings as short manuscripts.

This symposium was the eighth in a series supported by the Harry Steenbock Symposium Trust Fund, which was made available by Mr. Harry Steenbock to the Department of Biochemistry, University of Wisconsin-Madison through the Wisconsin Alumni Research Foundation. This support is gratefully appreciated. Professor Steenbock had a distinguished career as a member of the University of Wisconsin biochemistry staff from 1916 to 1956. He was a pioneer in the study of a number of the fat soluble vitamins, but is probably best known for his discovery that ultraviolet irradiation of foods induces vitamin D activity. The proceedings of this symposium are a tribute to his interest in and contribution to this area of nutritional biochemistry.

I would like to express my appreciation to all participants in the symposium, to those who aided in the organization of the symposium, and to the chairmen of sessions. I am particularly indebted to Mrs. Karen Davis, who was responsible for registration and assisted in planning all aspects of the symposium and publication of this manuscript.

J. W. Suttie

Vitamin K Metabolism and Vitamin K-Dependent Proteins

CHEMISTRY AND FUNCTIONING OF PLASMA VITAMIN K-DEPENDENT PROTEINS

STRUCTURAL PROPERTIES OF THE VITAMIN K-DEPENDENT PLASMA PROTEINS

E. W. DAVIE

University of Washington,
Seattle, WA 98195

INTRODUCTION

It is a pleasure for me to begin this conference by making a few comments on the structural properties of the vitamin K-dependent proteins of plasma. Vitamin K was discovered in 1929 by Henrik Dam who noted that chicks on diets extracted with polar solvents developed bleeding problems (1-5). This led to the discovery of a new lipid soluble vitamin which was called vitamin K. Dam and coworkers also noted that the defect in coagulation was due to a decrease in the amount of prothrombin in the plasma of the deficient chicks. Similar effects were then reported for reduced plasma levels of Factor VII, Factor IX, and Factor X in humans and cows following the administration of vitamin K antagonists such as dicumarol (6-10). More recently, two additional vitamin K-dependent plasma proteins have been added to this list, including protein C and protein S (11-13). In a preliminary report, a seventh vitamin K-dependent protein of plasma has been described (14). The characterization of this protein, called protein Z, has not been completed thus far.

A number of proposals have been suggested over the years for the mechanism of action of vitamin K. For instance, Dam and coworkers (15) proposed that the vitamin was part of the prothrombin molecule, whereas Martius and Nitz-Litzow (16) suggested that the primary role of the vitamin was in oxidative phosphorylation. In another proposal, Olson (17) suggested that the rate of prothrombin synthesis was due to an effect of the vitamin on transcription. A number of investigators then reported the presence of an inactive prothrombin molecule in humans and cows treated with vitamin K antagonists, such as dicumarol (18-23). These abnormal prothrombins had molecular weights and amino acid compositions essentially identical to normal prothrombin. The abnormal prothrombin, however, did not bind to barium sulfate and it also had a different calcium-dependent electrophoretic mobility. These data indicated that prothrombin was synthesized in humans and cows in the absence of vitamin K, but it had little biological activity. Furthermore, the lack of biological activity appeared to be due to the inability of the abnormal protein to bind calcium.

γ-CARBOXYGLUTAMIC ACID AS A STRUCTURAL FEATURE

A major advance in defining the role of vitamin K came with the discovery of γ-carboxyglutamic acid by Stenflo and coworkers in 1974 (24). This new amino acid was shown to be present in positions 7 and 8 of bovine prothrombin. In contrast, the abnormal prothrombin contained glutamic acid in positions 7 and 8. Shortly thereafter, Magnusson and coworkers (25) and Nelsestuen and coworkers (26) independently reported the presence of γ-carboxyglutamic acid in prothrombin. Furthermore, Magnusson identified the location of the 10 γ-carboxyglutamic acid residues in the aminoterminal region of prothrombin. The γ-carboxyglutamic acid content has now been determined for six of the well defined proteins from human and bovine plasma (Table I). These proteins contain 10, 11 or 12 residues of γ-carboxyglutamic acid. The location of the γ-carboxyglutamic acid residues has also been established for factor X and protein C. As shown in Figure 1, the γ-carboxyglutamic acid occurs in nearly the same position in the amino-terminal portion of all of these proteins. Furthermore, it often occurs in pairs. These data indicate that vitamin K is involved in the carboxylation of 10-12 specific glutamic acid residues that are located in the amino-terminal region of the vitamin K-dependent proteins of plasma.

TABLE I. γ-Carboxyglutamic Acid Content of the Vitamin K-dependent Plasma Proteins

	γ-Carboxyglutamic acid[a]	Molecular weight
Bovine prothrombin	10.0	71,600[b]
Human prothrombin	10.1	72,000[c]
Bovine factor VII	9.4	45,500[d]
Bovine factor IX	12.2	55,400[e]
Human factor IX	12.4	57,100[f]
Bovine factor X_1	12.3	55,100[g]
Bovine factor X_2	11.8	55,100[g]
Human factor X	11.6	58,900[f]
Bovine protein C	10.8	57,000[h]
Human protein C	10.4	57,000[i]
Bovine protein S	10.0	64,200[i]
Human protein S	10.3	69,000[i]

[a]Expressed in residues per molecule of glycoprotein. [b]From Magnusson et al. (27). [c]From Kisiel and Hanahan (28). [d]From Kisiel and Davie (29). [e]From Fujikawa et al. (30). [f]From DiScipio et al. (12). [g]From Fujikawa et al. (31). [h]From Kisiel et al. (32). [i]From DiScipio and Davie (13).

The various structural properties of the vitamin K-dependent proteins of plasma are quite similar. Present evidence suggests that they all are precursors of serine proteases (33). This is well established for prothrombin, factor VII, factor IX, factor X and protein C. Furthermore, these proteins that are present in plasma in precursor or zymogen forms are converted to serine proteases via limited proteolysis. In these activation reactions, one or two specific internal arginine-containing peptide bonds are split.

The sequence analysis of the vitamin K-dependent proteins of plasma has also proceeded rapidly during the past few years. Magnusson and co-workers (27) completed the amino acid sequence of bovine prothrombin in 1975 and have shown that it is composed of 582 amino acids, including 10 γ-carboxyglutamic acid residues and 12 disulfide bridges. The three carbohydrate chains are attached to Asn-77, Asn-101, and Asn-376.

Bovine factor X is composed of two polypeptide chains held together by a disulfide bond. The light chain (molecular weight 16,500) contains 140 amino acids, including 12 γ-carboxyglutamic acid residues (34). It does not contain carbohydrate. The heavy chain (molecular weight 55,800) is composed of 307 residues with carbohydrate bound to Asn-36 and Thr-300 (35).

```
                1                          10                         20                         30                    40
Prothrombin    A N K G F L Y Y - V R K G N L Y R Y C L Y Y P C S R Y Y A R Y A L Y S L S A T D A F W A
Factor X       A N S - F L Y Y - V K N G N L Y R Y C L Y Y A C S L Y Y A R Y V F Y D A Y Q T D Y F W S
Protein C      A N S - F L Y Y - L R P G N V Y R Y C S Y Y V C Y F Y Y A R Y I F Q N T Y D T M A F W S
Factor VII     A N - G F L Y Y L L - P G
Protein S      A N T - L L Y Y - T K K G N L
```

FIGURE 1. Amino-terminal sequences of bovine prothrombin, the light chains of factor X and protein C, factor VII, and protein S employing the one letter code. Dashes have been inserted for better homology. γ-Carboxyglutamic acid, referred to as γ, is shown in boxes to emphasize the homology between the five proteins.

Bovine factor IX is a single chain molecule containing 416 amino acids, including 12 γ-carboxyglutamic acid residues (36). The four carbohydrate chains are attached to Asn-158, Asn-168, Asn-173, and Asn-261.

The sequence of the light chain of protein C of bovine plasma has also been completed (37). This protein is composed of a heavy and a light chain, and these two chains are held together by a disulfide bond. The light chain contains 155 amino acids, including 11 γ-carboxyglutamic acid residues. A single carbohydrate chain is linked to Asn-97.

With these few brief words of introduction, I will step aside so that we can proceed with detailed reports on the various vitamin K-dependent proteins and the role of vitamin K.

REFERENCES

1. Dam, H. (1929a) Biochem. Z. 215, 468.
2. Dam, H. (1929b) Biochem. Z. 215, 475.
3. Dam, H. (1930) Biochem. Z. 220, 158.
4. Dam, H. (1935a) Nature (London) 135, 652.
5. Dam, H. (1935b) Biochem. J. 29, 1273.
6. Owen, C. A., Jr., Magath, T. B., and Bollman, J. L. (1951) Am. J. Physiol. 166, 1.
7. Koller, F., Loeliger, A., and Duckert, F. (1951) Acta Haematol. 6, 1.
8. Aggeler, P. M., White, S. G., Glendening, M. B., Page, E. W., Leake, T. B., and Bates, G. (1952) Proc. Soc. Exp. Biol. Med. 79, 692.
9. Biggs, R., Douglas, A. S., MacFarlane, R. G., Dacie, J. V., Pitney, W. R., Merskey, C., and O'Brien, J. R. (1952) Br. Med. J. 2, 1378.
10. Hougie, C., Barrow, E. M., and Graham, J. B. (1957) J. Clin. Invest. 36, 485.
11. Stenflo, J. (1976) J. Biol. Chem. 251, 355.
12. DiScipio, R. G., Hermodson, M. A., Yates, S. G., and Davie, E. W. (1977) Biochemistry 16, 698.
13. DiScipio, R. G., and Davie, E. W. (1979) Biochemistry 18, 899.
14. Prowse, C. V., and Esnouf, M. P. (1977) Biochem. Soc. Trans. 5, 255.
15. Dam, H., Schønheyder, F., and Tage-Hansen, E. (1936) Biochem. J. 30, 1075.
16. Martius, C., and Nitz-Litzow, D. (1954) Biochim. Biophys. Acta 13, 152.
17. Olson, R. E. (1964) Science 145, 926.
18. Hemker, H. C., Veltkamp, J. J., Hensen, A., and Loeliger, E. A. (1963) Nature (London) 200, 589.
19. Ganrot, P. O., and Nilehn, J. E. (1968) Scand. J. Clin. Lab. Invest. 22, 23.
20. Stenflo, J. (1970) Acta Chem. Scand. 24, 3762.
21. Nelsestuen, G. L., and Suttie, J. W. (1972) J. Biol. Chem. 247, 8176.
22. Reekers, P. M., Lindout, M. J., Kop-Klassen, B. H. M., and Hemker, H. C. (1973) Biochim. Biophys. Acta 317, 559.
23. Suttie, J. W. (1978) Handbook of Lipid Research, Vol. 2, pp. 211-277, Plenum Press, New York.
24. Stenflo, J., Fernlund, P., Egan, W., and Roepstorff, P. (1974) Proc. Natl. Acad. Sci. U.S.A. 71, 2730.
25. Magnusson, S., Sottrup-Jensen, L., Petersen, T. E., Morris, H. R., and Dell, A. (1974) FEBS Lett. 44, 189.
26. Nelsestuen, G. L., Zytkovicz, T. H., and Howard, J. B. (1974) J. Biol. Chem. 249, 6347.

27. Magnusson, S., Petersen, T. E., Sottrup-Jensen, L., and Claeys, H. (1975) Proteases and Biological Control (Reich, E., Rifkin, D. B., and Shaw, E., Eds.), Vol. 2, pp. 123-149, Cold Spring Harbor Laboratory, New York.
28. Kisiel, W., and Hanahan, D. J. (1973) Biochim. Biophys. Acta 304, 103.
29. Kisiel, W., and Davie, E. W. (1975) Biochemistry 14, 4928.
30. Fujikawa, K., Thompson, A. R., Legaz, M. E., Meyer, R. G., and Davie, E. W. (1973) Biochemistry 12, 4938.
31. Fujikawa, K., Legaz, M. E., and Davie, E. W. (1972) Biochemistry 11, 4882.
32. Kisiel, W., Ericsson, L. H., and Davie, E. W. (1976) Biochemistry 15, 4893.
33. Davie, E. W., and Fujikawa, K. (1975) Annu. Rev. Biochem. 44, 799.
34. Enfield, D. L., Ericsson, L. H., Walsh, K. A., Neurath, H., and Titani, K. (1975) Proc. Natl. Acad. Sci. U.S.A. 72, 16.
35. Titani, K., Fujikawa, K., Enfield, D. L., Ericsson, L. H., Walsh, K. A., and Neurath, H. (1975) Proc. Natl. Acad. Sci. U.S.A. 72, 3082.
36. Katayama, K., Ericsson, L. H., Enfield, D. L., Walsh, K. A., Neurath, H., Davie, E. W., and Titani, K., manuscript to be submitted to Proc. Natl. Acad. Sci. U.S.A.
37. Fernlund, P., Stenflo, J., and Tufvesson, A. (1978) Proc. Natl. Acad. Sci. 75, 5889.

CRYSTALLOGRAPHIC INVESTIGATION OF THE A-FRAGMENT (FRAGMENT-1) FROM BOVINE PROTHROMBIN

GUSTAV OLSSON[x], OLIVER LINDQVIST[x],
TORBEN E. PETERSEN, STAFFAN MAGNUSSON and
LARS SOTTRUP-JENSEN

Department of Inorganic Chemistry[x],
Chalmers University of Technology and University of Göteborg,
S-41296 Göteborg, Sweden and Department of Molecular Biology,
University of Aarhus, DK-8000 Århus C, Denmark

INTRODUCTION

Since we started to investigate the primary structures of thrombin (1-4) and prothrombin (5) in 1967, and particularly since the completion of the primary structure of prothrombin (6-9) in May 1974, we have more or less continously tried to crystallize these proteins and also the S-fragment (fragment 2; residues 157-274), neoprothrombin-S (prethrombin 1; residues 157-582) and the A-fragment (fragment 1; residues 1-156). It is obvious that both prothrombin and thrombin are native proteins with biological activity as a zymogen and its corresponding active serine protease and that therefore their crystal structures will be useful and relevant for the interpretation of their biological functions and mechanism in terms of structure. It may, however, be less obvious why the crystal structures of the A- and the S-fragments would be biologically interesting. There are three criteria that would argue in favor. The first is that if a fragment retains any binding activty or enzymatic activity also shown by the parent molecule, then it has essentially retained the conformation that it had in the native parent molecule. The second criterium is that if a fragment can be crystallized this means that a large proportion of the molecules must still have the same conformation and extensive denaturation is unlikely to have occurred. The third criterium is that if a protein contains domains of structure and function, an isolated domain is likely to have its own folding pattern independent of that of the rest of the protein and when cleaved off and isolated from the rest of the protein it is likely to still have the same structure as in the parent protein. In the case of the A-fragment all three criteria are satisfied. The first criterium is that the fragment shows essentially the same Ca^{2+} and phospholipid-binding properties as the parent prothrombin molecule (10-14) which is consistent with the fact that the A-fragment contains all the 10 γ-carboxyglutamic acid (Gla) residues of prothrombin (6, 15-17). The second criterium is that crystals have been obtained both in our own laboratories, not only of the A-fragment, but also of the S-fragment from bovine prothrombin, and of the K4-fragment (kringle structure number 4, residues 354-439) from human plasminogen (18). The third criterium comes from a detailed comparison of the primary structures of prothrombin (8, 9), plasminogen (18, 19), and the amino acid sequence of factor X_1 (20, 21), which shows that the A-fragment contains two major structural and probably functional domains, namely the vitamin K-dependent, Gla-containing domain, residues 1-42 which is derived from the same ancestral protein sequence as residues 1-41 in Factor X_1 and X_2 with their 12 Gla-residues (22) and secondly the kringle domain, residues 66-144, derived from the same ancestral protein sequence as the kringle domain, residues 171-249 in the S-fragment (7, 9) and the five kringle domains, residues 83-161, 165-242, 255-332, 357-434, and 461-540, of the heavy chain part of human plasminogen (18, 19), whereas the corresponding regions of factor

X (20) and protein C (23) apparently have a different ancestral origin. The domain character (independent folding and independent function from the rest of the protein) of a kringle region is proved by the fact that the K-4 fragment contains one of the at least two lysine-binding sites (18) of the parent plasminogen molecule and by the fact that it has been crystallized. Thus, knowledge of the tertiary structure of the A-fragment seems highly desirable.

EXPERIMENTAL

Until now we have obtained crystals of sufficient size and regularity to be useful for structural work only from the A-fragment. Crystals have been obtained in the pH range 6.5-7.5 in the presence of 100 mM Ca^{2+}. Crystallization conditions have been approached by vapor diffusion either in a Conway-type vessel containing two concentric chambers, or using the hanging-drop technique. In the early phase of this investigation (1975-1978) the crystals could not always be obtained reproducibly. However, once formed, the crystals grew rapidly and large crystals up to 0.8 x 0.8 x 1.2 mm could be obtained in a few days. Two types of crystal have been observed (Fig. 1). In both cases the space group is $P2_12_12_1$

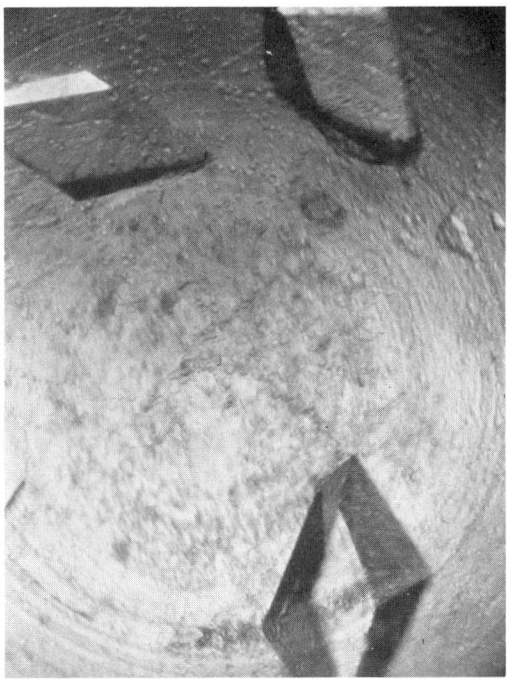

FIGURE 1. Bovine prothrombin A-fragment crystals type I obtained in the presence of 100 mM Ca^{2+}. Length along c axis appr. 0.9 mm.

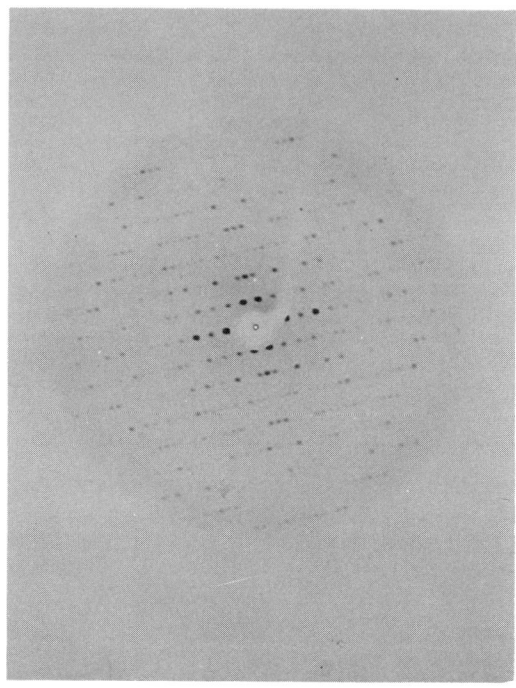

FIGURE 2. Precession photograph of a crystal of A-fragment from bovine prothrombin. Projection: h0l; $\mu = 9°$; F = 100 mm.

(Fig. 2), Z = 4, a = 39.5 Å, b = 54.0 Å. For crystals of type I c = 129.0 Å, of type II c = 133.5 Å. For type I crystals that are now being used for the structural studies V = 272,000 Å^3. With a molecular weight of 25,500 and 20% carbohydrate the water content of the crystals is estimated to be 55%. Although the crystals diffract to a resolution of 2.5 Å it is now attempted to collect data to a resolution of 4 Å using a Syntex P2$_1$ diffractometer. The crystallization procedure has been somewhat modified since about a year to include a small volume of redissolved old crystals in the crystallization mixture. Using this modification cyrstals of type I are now reproducibly obtained in all crystallization vials in 7 - 10 days. Redissolved crystals give rise to a single band with the same mobility as the original A-fragment on polyacrylamide gel electrophoresis of reduced material in sodium dodecyl sulfate containing buffer. However, peptide mapping of a tryptic digest of redissolved crystals that had been reduced and carboxymethylated, indicated that the fragment may have been "nicked" at the C-terminal end corresponding to a loss of residues 150/151-156 and possibly of some of the carbohydrate. Whether this is due to contaminating microorganisms in the redissolved old crystals now used for "seeding" crystallization mixtures has not been investigated.

Heavy metal derivatives have been obtained by soaking crystals of the native A-fragment in solutions of mercuric acetate, osmiate, or potassium-hexachloroplatinate. Patterson summation indicated that the derivatives are isomorphous, but preliminary interpretation of the results with a refinement program indicates insufficient occupancy of heavy-metal substituted sites in two of the derivatives and raise doubts about the isomorphous nature of the third derivative.

The A-fragment material used for crystallization was obtained by incubation of purified prothrombin with purified thrombin (ratio 200:1, w/w) for 2 h at room temperature. The A-fragment was then separated using a tris-chloride buffer with a linear gradient in NaCl on a 2.5 x 50 cm column of DEAE-Sephadex A-50 as described previously (7), then resalted to 50 mM NH_4HCO_3 pH 8.3 on a Sephadex G-100 column (4 x 100 cm) and finally freeze-dried.

DISCUSSION

Because the A-fragment contains the Gla residues and the first of the two kringle structures of prothrombin, a high-resolution structure of this fragment is likely to give information on the nature of Ca^{2+} and phospholipid-binding of the A-fragment itself and probably also on that of prothrombin. Furthermore, the homology of residues 1-42 with the vitamin K-dependent domains in factors X, IX and protein C and the homology of the kringle structure residues 62-144 with the single kringle of the S-fragment (fragment 2) and with the five kringle structures in plasminogen probably implies that knowledge of the tertiary structure of the A-fragment will give at least a basic idea of what the tertiary structures of the respective homologous structures look like. Crystals of fragment 1 in the absence of Ca^{2+} have been described (24). It is to be hoped that if both structures can be solved, a comparison will show the difference between the two conformations (with and without Ca^{2+}).

ACKNOWLEDGEMENTS

Supported by the U.S. National Institutes of Health (grant HL-16238), Bethesda, Md., U.S.A. (to S.M.) and by the Swedish Science Research Council (to O.L.).

REFERENCES

1. Magnusson, S. (1968) Biochem. J. 110, 25-26P.
2. Hartley, B. S. (1970) Phil. Trans. Roy. Soc. London, Ser.B 257, 77-86.
3. Magnusson, S. (1971) The Enzymes, Vol. III (P. Boyer, ed.), pp. 277-321, Academic Press, New York.
4. Magnusson, S. (1970) Methods in Enzymology, Vol. 19 (Perlmann, G. E. and Lorand, L., eds.), pp. 157-184, Academic Press, New York.
5. Magnusson, S. (1969) Biochem. J. 115, 2-3P.
6. Magnusson, S., Sottrup-Jensen, L., Petersen, T. E., Morris, H. R., and Dell, A. (1974) FEBS Letters 44, 189-193.
7. Magnusson, S., Sottrup-Jensen, L., Petersen, T. E., and Claeys, H. (1975) Prothrombin and Related Coagulation Factors (Hemker, H. C. and Veltkamp, J. J., eds.), pp. 25-46, Leiden University Press, Leiden.

8. Dayhoff, M. O. (1976) Atlas of Protein Sequence and Structure, 5. Suppl. 2, p. 95. National Biomedical Research Foundation, Washington.
9. Magnusson, S., Petersen, T. E., Sottrup-Jensen, L., and Claeys, H. (1975) Proteases and Biological Control (Reich, L., Rifkin, D., and Shaw, E., eds.), pp. 123-149, Cold Spring Harbor Laboratory, CSH, New York.
10. Gitel, S. N., Owen, W. G., Esmon, C. T., and Jackson, C. M. (1973) Proc. Natl. Acad. Sci. U.S.A. 70, 1344-1348.
11. Stenflo, J., and Ganrot, P. O. (1973) Biochem. Biophys. Res. Commun. 50, 98-104.
12. Henriksen, R. A., and Jackson, C. M. (1975) Arch. Biochem. Biophys. 170, 149-159.
13. Benarous, R., Elion, J., and Labie, D. (1976) Biochimie 58, 391-394.
14. Bajaj, S. P., Butkowski, R. J., and Mann, K. G. (1975) J. Biol. Chem. 250, 2150-2156.
15. Fernlund, P., Stenflo, J., Roepstorff, P., and Thomsen, J. (1975) J. Biol. Chem. 250, 6125-6133.
16. Howard, J. B., Fausch, M. D., and Nelsestuen, G. L. (1975) J. Biol. Chem. 250, 6178-6180.
17. Morris, H. R., Dell, A., Petersen, T. E., Sottrup-Jensen, L., and Magnusson, S. (1976) Biochem. J. 153, 663-679.
18. Sottrup-Jensen, L., Claeys, H., Zajdel, M., Petersen, T. E., and Magnusson, S. (1978) Progress in Chemical Fibrinolysis and Thrombolysis (Davidson, J. F., Rowan, R. M., Samama, M. M., and Desnoyers, P. C., eds.) 3, pp. 191-209, Raven Press, New York.
19. Dayhoff, M. O. (1978) Atlas of Protein Sequence and Structure, 5, Suppl. 3, p. 91.
20. Enfield, D. L., Ericsson, L. H., Walsh, K. A., Neurath, H., and Titani, K. (1975) Proc. Natl. Acad. Sci. U.S.A. 72, 16-19.
21. Titani, K., Enfield, D. L., Ericsson, L. H., Walsh, K. A., and Neurath, H. (1975) Proc. Natl. Acad. Sci. U.S.A. 72, 3082-3086.
22. Thøgersen, H. C., Petersen, T. E., Sottrup-Jensen, L., Magnusson, S., and Morris, H. R. (1978) Biochem. J. 175, 613-627.
23. Fernlund, P., Stenflo, J., and Tufvesson, A. (1978) Proc. Natl. Acad. Sic. U.S.A. 75, 5889-5892.
24. Aschaffenburg, R., Blake, C. C. F., Burridge, J. M., and Esnouf, M. P. (1977) J. Mol. Biol. 114, 575-579.

PROTEIN SUBSTRATES FOR γ-CARBOXYLATION: EVIDENCE FOR ALANINE HYDROXYLATION TO SERINE IN VITAMIN K-DEPENDENT ENZYMES

KARL J. MATTHES

Zentrum für Innere Medizin am Klinikum
der Justus-Liebig-Universität,
Giessen, West Germany

INTRODUCTION

γ-carboxylation of glutamic acid residues is a specific feature of vitamin-K-dependent proteins (1,2). It remains unexplained, why γ-carboxylation only occurs in specific areas of these proteins and not in other proteins of similar structure, and why all glutamic acids in the specific area of these proteins are carboxylated.

RESULTS AND DISSCUSSION

We have previously shown, that the hydroxylation of an alanine residue to serine at position 34-36 of prothrombin, which is close to the polypeptide area specific for γ-carboxylation, is an essential vitamin-K-dependent step required for γ-carboxylation of prothrombin (3). In contrast to human and bovine prothrombin (4-6) both Factor X and Protein C (7) contain an extra γ-carboxyglutamate which is positioned near the point of alanine hydroxylation in prothrombin, namely at position 36 of the polypeptide chain, alanine, however, is present at position 35 in Factor X. We present evidence now for the hydroxylation of an alanine residue to serine in positions 43 of bovine Factor X and Protein C. Position 43 contains alanine in both human and bovine prothrombin. Positions corresponding to 34-36 and 43 have not yet been sequenced in other vitamin-K-dependent proteins (Factor IX, Protein S and the bone protein). There are several other alanine residues along the amino acid sequence chain from position 28 to 47 of the prothrombins. Thus it is conceivable, that other vitamin-K-dependent proteins may have still other alanine residues which have to be hydroxylated to serine prior to γ-carboxylation of glutamic acid residues in the protein.

There is no γ-carboxylation of glutamic acid residues beyond the point of alanine hydroxylation in any of these proteins thus far sequenced. Since both alanine hydroxylation to serine and γ-carboxylation of glutamic residues occur on the surface of the vesicles of smooth endoplasmatic reticulum, it is suggested that alanine hydroxylation to serine, a step which has been shown to be Vitamin-K-dependent (3), is essential for positioning the polypeptide chains to the proper area on the surface of smooth endoplasmatic reticulum where carboxylation of all glutamic acids can proceed. Therefore, a close structural relationship between an alanine residue, which can be hydroxylated to serine, with glutamic acid residues, which can be carboxylated along a polypeptide chain, seems to be essential for γ-carboxylation to proceed. This explains, why in other regions of vitamin-K-dependent proteins and in other proteins of

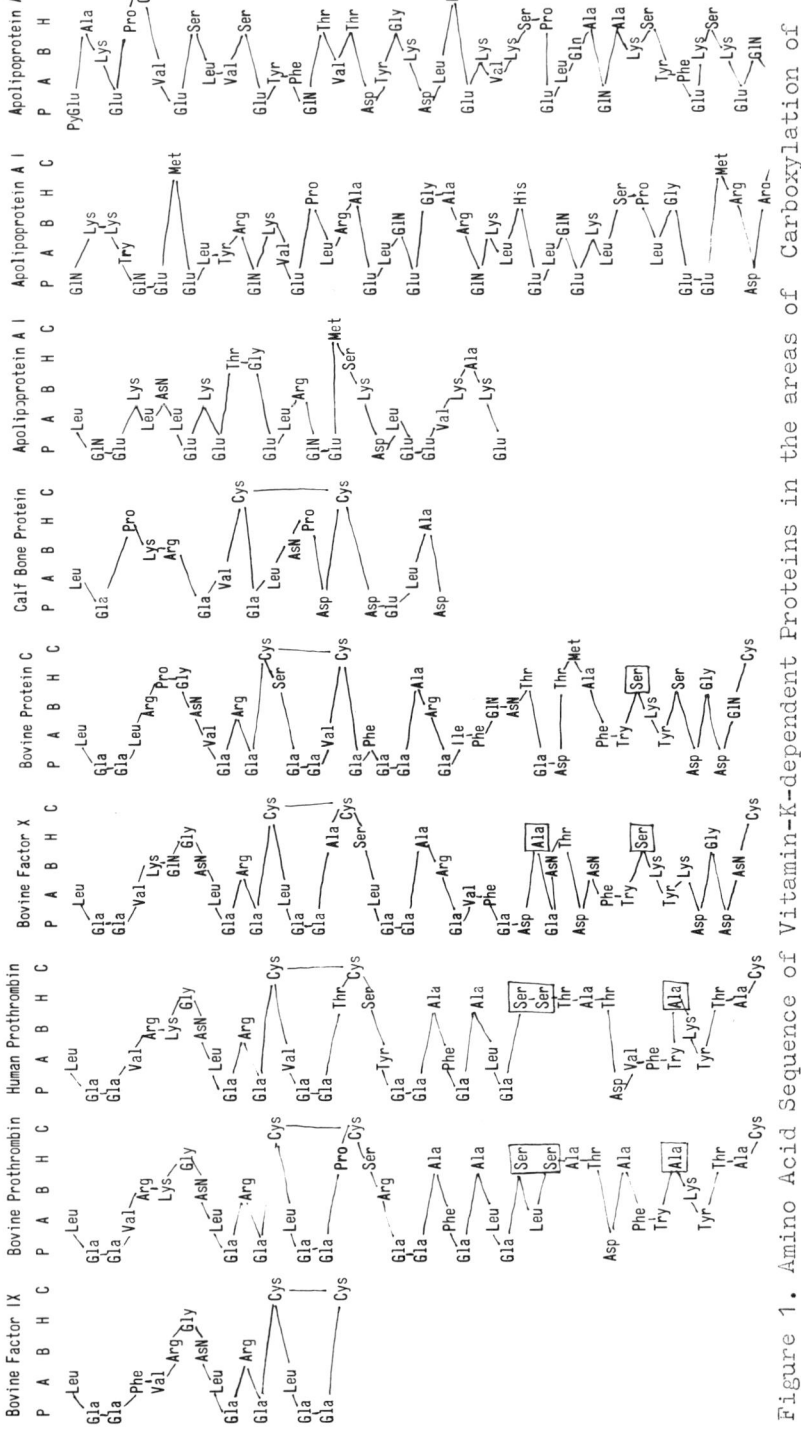

Figure 1. Amino Acid Sequence of Vitamin-K-dependent Proteins in the areas of Carboxylation of Glutamates and similar Amino Acid Sequences in Apolipoproteins, where no carboxylation occurs. Positions of alanine hydroxylation to serine are marked by ☐, in proteins where it occurs and where it does not. Gla is used as symbol for γ-carboxyglutamate. P = acidic, A = hydrophobic, B = basic, H = hydrophilic amino acids, C = sulfur-containing amino acids and S-S-bridges.

very similar structure and glutamate positions (such as phospholipase-A_2 or several apolipoproteins (see figure 1 for APO-A I and APO-A II) no carboxylation occurs. Nevertheless location of glutamic acid residues along the polypeptide chain seems to be of great importance for γ-carboxylation. This can be demonstrated with the vitamin-K-dependent bone protein (8), which although it has an entirely different structure and origin, presents a very similar, frequently mirrorlike, sequence homology to the structure of the vitamin-K-dependent serine proteinases in the area around the γ-carboxylated glutamic residues (Figure 1).

REFERENCES

1. Girardot, J. M., Delaney, R., and Johnson, B. C. (1974) Biochem. Biophys. Res. Comm. 59, 1197-1200.
2. Stenflo, J., Fernlund, P., Egan, F., and Roepstorff, P. (1974) Proc. Natl. Acad. Sci. USA 71, 2740-2744.
3. Matthes, K. J. (1975) Med. Welt (N.F.) 26, 1777-1782.
4. Walz, D. A., Reuterby, J., Meloy, L. E., and Seegers, W. H. (1975) Thrmobosis Research 7, 227-231.
5. Walz, D. A., Hewett-Emmett, D., and Seegers, W. H. (1977) Proc. Natl. Acad. Sci. USA (1977) 74, 1969-1972.
6. Suttie, J. W., and Jackson, C. M. (1977) Physiol. Reviews 57, 1-44.
7. Fernlund, P., Stenflo, J., and Tufvesson, A. (1978) Proc. Natl. Acad. Sci. USA 75, 5889-5891.
8. Price, P. A., Poser, J. W., and Rman, N. (1976) Proc. Natl. Acad. Sci. USA 73, 3374-3375.

COOPERATIVITY OF CALCIUM ION BINDING TO BOVINE PROTHROMBIN, PROTHROMBIN FRAGMENT-1 AND FACTOR X. AN ALTERNATIVE TO CONFORMATIONAL CHANGES FOR EXPLAINING SUCH BEHAVIOR

CRAIG M. JACKSON

Department of Biological Chemistry
Washington University School of Medicine
St. Louis, MO 63110

INTRODUCTION

The observation of a link between Ca^{2+} binding to the vitamin K related coagulation proteins (1,2) and the action of vitamin K led immediately to intense investigation of both the structural basis for Ca^{2+} binding by these proteins and the properties of the binding process. The structural modification, carboxylation of 10 to 12 glutamic acid residues to form γ-carboxyglutamic acid residues is now well established. In marked contrast to this situation, however, the Ca^{2+} and other divalent cation binding properties of the vitamin K related proteins remain poorly understood, in part at least as a result of what appear to be very divergent results from apparently similar binding measurements. Variability in the number of binding sites is large, e.g. from 4 (2) to 14 (3) for prothrombin, and from 20 (4,5) to 40 (6) for Factor X. Even more perplexing perhaps than the ambiguity in the estimated number of binding sites is the fact that Ca^{2+} binding exhibits positive cooperativity when examined in some laboratories but not in others. In order to illustrate this situation, divalent ion binding parameters reported in the literature for prothrombin, Prothrombin Fragment 1 and Factor X are summarized in Table 1. Observations made on some human proteins are also included as a significant difference in Ca^{2+} binding kinetics exists between bovine and human Prothrombin Fragment 1 (7). Although it is always easy to disregard observations made in laboratories other than one's own, a switch from positively cooperative Ca^{2+} binding to binding usually described as, but not necessarily reflecting multiple classes of binding sites, was observed in my laboratory when Prothrombin Fragment 1 concentration was decreased to ascertain the dependence of binding on protein concentration. This forced us to attempt to understand this complex Ca^{2+} binding process without recourse to the convenient device of disregarding a particular set or sets of data in our interpretations. In the sections which follow I will attempt to outline the considerations and observations that have been made during our attempts to understand this complex Ca^{2+} binding behavior. The specific objective of our studies has been to determine what process or processes are responsible for the cooperativity of Ca^{2+} binding which we and others (see Table 1) observe. More specific considerations related to this limited objective are detailed below. Although almost too obvious to merit noting, the underlying premises of this attempt are that all recurrent observations, even when not reproducible at will, must be acknowledged and in principle explainable by the model to be proposed and that the correct explanation obviously must be a member of the set of consistent explanations. The first premise attempts to force into the data base used in creating the set of consistent explanations, as many constraints as possible.

RESULTS AND DISCUSSION

Characteristics of Ion Binding to a Multisite System

Whenever ions bind to a macromolecule which possesses more than one binding site for the ion, the apparent affinity for each successive site to be

TABLE 1. Metal ion binding characteristics of prothrombin, Prothrombin Fragment 1 and Factor X.

Protein, Concentration Divalent Ion, pH Conc(mg/ml) Me^{2+} pH			Methodology	Type of Binding Sites	n_1	Binding Parameters $k_1(M)$	n_2	$k_2(M)$	a	Reference
Prothrombin (bovine)										
2	Ca^{2+}	7.4	Rate dialysis	Cooperative	7-8	5x10^{-4}	3-4	–	1.35	(1)
?	Ca^{2+}	7.4	Equilibrium dialysis	Cooperative	4-5	2x10^{-3}	6	3x10^{-4}	> 1	(8)
1-10	Ca^{2+}	7.0	Hummel-Dreyer column	Multiclass	6-7	6.3x10^{-4}	3-4	–	–	(3)
> 7	Ca^{2+}	7.5	Hummel-Dreyer column	Cooperative	7	1.3x10^{-3}	4	1.2x10^{-4}	> 1	(9)
0.7	Ca^{2+}	7.95	Membrane filtration	?	4	4x10^{-4}				(2)
.05	Ca^{2+}	7.5	Fluorescence quenching	Cooperative			3-4	4x10^{-4}	2.6	(10)
.05	Mg^{2+}	7.5	Fluorescence quenching	Cooperative, ?				4x10^{-4}		(11)
.05	Sr^{2+}	7.5	Fluorescence quenching	Cooperative, ?				8.5x10^{-4}		(11)
.05	Mn^{2+}	7.5	Fluorescence quenching	Cooperative, ?				< 5x10^{-5}		(11)
.08	Gd^{3+}	6.8	Rate dialysis	Multiclass	2	7.5x10^{-7}				(12)
.72	Gd^{3+}	6.8	Rate dialysis	Cooperative	9					(13)
7.5	Mn^{2+}	6.5	NMR, EPR	Cooperative and 1 class	2-3	1.3x10^{-5}	2	1.2x10^{-4}		(14)
Prothrombin (human)										
2	Ca^{2+}	7.4	Equilibrium dialysis	Cooperative	7	1.3x10^{-3}	4	1.2x10^{-4}	> 1	(15)
Fragment 1 (bovine)										
1	Ca^{2+}	7.4	Equilibrium dialysis	Cooperative			6	5x10^{-4}	> 1	(7)
1.2-2.7	Ca^{2+}	8.0	Equilibrium dialysis	Cooperative			10	6.3x10^{-4}	1.5	(4)
.05	Ca^{2+}	7.5	Fluorescence quenching	Cooperative			ca 3	4x10^{-4}	2.6	(10)
.05	Ca^{2+}	7.5	Fluorescence quenching	Cooperative			?	4.3x10^{-4}		(11)
?	Ca^{2+}	7.0	Hummel-Dreyer column	Multiclass	3-4	–	8-11	6.8x10^{-4}		(8)
< 2-4	Ca^{2+}	7.5	Hummel-Dreyer column	?			3-5	–		(9)
.10	Ca^{2+}	7.5	Hummel-Dreyer column	?				3.5x10^{-4}		(7)

Cooperativity of Calcium Ion Binding 17

TABLE 1 (Continued)

Protein, Concentration Divalent Ion, pH	Conc (mg/ml)	Me^{2+}	pH	Methodology	Type of Binding Sites	n_1	$k_1(M)$	n_2	$k_2(M)$	a	Reference
Prothrombin (bovine)											
	.10	Mg^{2+}	7.5	Fluorescence quenching	Cooperative				4.5×10^{-4}		(7)
	.05	Sr^{2+}	7.5	Fluorescence quenching	Cooperative				9×10^{-4}		(11)
	.05	Ba^{2+}	7.5	Fluorescence quenching	Cooperative				6.6×10^{-3}		(11)
	2	Mn^{2+}	6.5	NMR, ESR	Multiclass	2	2.2×10^{-5}	2	2.5×10^{-4}		(14)
	.10	Mn^{2+}	7.4	Fluorescence quenching					1.3×10^{-5}		(7)
	.10	Gd^{3+}	6.8	Rate dialysis	1 Class	2	1.6×10^{-7}				(12)
(human)											
	.10	Ca^{2+}	7.5	Fluorescence quenching	Cooperative				2.2×10^{-4}		(7)
	.10	Mg^{2+}	7.5	Fluorescence quenching	Cooperative ?				2.2×10^{-4}		(7)
	.10	Gd^{3+}	7.5	Fluorescence quenching	Cooperative ?				3.6×10^{-6}		(7)
Factor X (bovine)											
	1.2-2.0	Ca^{2+}	7.5	Equilibrium dialysis	Cooperative			20	7×10^{-4}	1.26	(4)
	0.75	Ca^{2+}	7.5	Rate dialysis	Cooperative			20	5×10^{-4}	1.5	(5)
	10	Ca^{2+}	8.0	Rate dialysis	Multiclass	1	5×10^{-5}	39	3.7×10^{-3}	–	(6)
	10	Ca^{2+}	6.8	Rate dialysis	Multiclass	2	3.1×10^{-4}	?	$> 1 \times 10^{-3}$	–	(16)
	.05	Ca^{2+}	7.5	Fluorescence quenching	Cooperative ?				2×10^{-3}		(11)
	.05	Mg^{2+}	7.5	Fluorescence quenching					1×10^{-3}		(11)
	.05	Sr^{2+}	7.5	Fluorescence quenching					4×10^{-4}		(11)
	3.3	Mn^{2+}	6.5	NMR, ESR	Cooperative	2	4×10^{-7}	6	9×10^{-5}	> 1	(17)
		Gd^{3+}	6.8	Rate dialysis		2	4×10^{-7}	4-6	2×10^{-5}	–	(16)
		Sm^{3+}	6.8			2	5×10^{-7}	4-6	6×10^{-6}	–	(16)
		Xb^{3+}	6.8			2	4×10^{-7}	4-6	5×10^{-6}	–	(16)

occupied is reduced because of electrostatic interaction between the macromolecule and the ion which is binding to it (18-21). Even if all sites possessed the same intrinsic affinity for the ion, simple behavior such as would be expected for an uncharged ligand would not be observed, e.g. a linear Scatchard plot. Rather, as shown in Figure 1, the Scatchard plot would be concave upward, reflecting the decreased affinity with in-

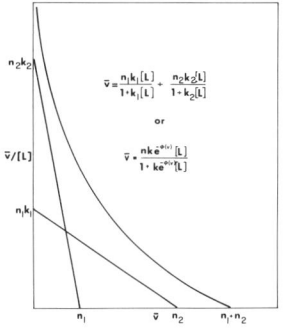

FIGURE 1 Scatchard plot observed with 2 classes of binding sites (n_1, k_1) and (n_2, k_2) where n is the number of sites and k the site association. When attenuating electrostatic interactions exist, the term $e(\exp\phi(\bar{v}))$ is a generalized interaction parameter (18).

creased site occupancy (18-21). In the absence of a large body of very good data, this situation can be difficult to distinguish from that usually interpreted as reflecting the presence of several classes of sites. In Figure 1, these are purposely not distinguished to simplify the illustration. It is virtually certain that the values for the binding constants which are used to describe the properties of the binding sites and are summarized in Table 1 are biased and are more variable than is truly the situation because of the absence of consideration of and correction for the electrostatic effects which exist within the ion-protein system. This is particularly so when attempting to compare trivalent and divalent ion binding constants.

Alteration of the electrostatic contribution to ion binding is usually obtained by changing the ionic strength of the aqueous buffer solution. The large contribution that the electrostatic attraction makes to the binding of Ca^{2+} to Prothrombin Fragment 1 is shown in Figure 2. In view of the

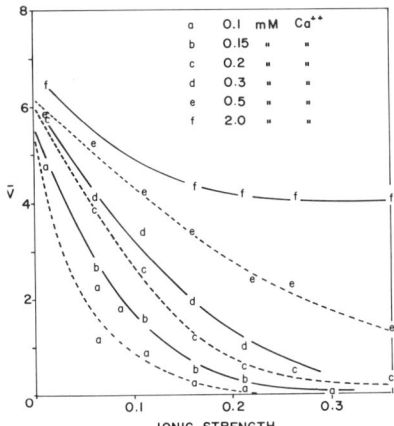

FIGURE 2 Ionic strength dependence of Ca^{2+} binding to Prothrombin Fragment 1. 0.01 M Tris-HCl, pH 7.5, Fragment 1 concentration, 25 µM. $\bar{v}$ is the number of Ca^{2+}/Fragment 1.

magnitude of this contribution, which is particularly apparent at low Ca^{2+} concentration, any analysis which attempts to distinguish sites on the basis of their relative affinities necessarily must include consideration of the electrostatic contribution. To date no such detailed examination of the electrostatic contribution to ion binding by the vitamin K related proteins has been made, undoubtedly because of the difficulty and uncertainty in doing so.

Cooperative binding is more frequently observed than "multiple class-like" binding (see Table 1). When such behavior is observed, another process in addition to binding itself must be occuring in order to produce such behavior (this is discussed below). An example of a Scatchard plot calculated as an alternative to that published (4) to describe our studies on Ca^{2+} binding to Fragment 1 is shown in Figure 3. In this particular example, a "class" of sites exhibiting positive cooperativity and a class

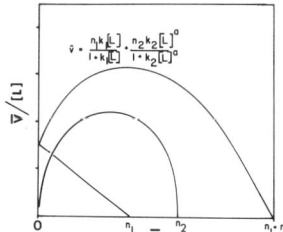

FIGURE 3 Scatchard plot calculated for two categories of sites and their sum. One class of cooperative sites and 1 class of non-interacting sites are summed to give the composite (upper) curve.

of non-interacting sites are added to produce a composite curve which "fits" the data. No specific significance exists for the parameters used for generating these curves and they are thus not given here. However, some sources of the ambiguity in the binding constants summarized in Table 1 can be identified by inspection of the curves of Figure 3. Examination of the "cooperative sites" (concave downward curves) shows that unless saturation is obtained, or nearly so, extrapolations to obtain the number of sites easily can be incorrect, tending to be high. Similarly, the practice of estimating the binding constant from the slope of a tangent to the cooperative Scatchard curve in the region in which it approaches the $\bar{v}$ axis does not yield a number which is simply interpretable as a binding constant (22) and can be seen to represent neither the binding constant for the cooperative or non-interacting sites. Until binding parameter (n,k) estimates are freed from these several types of bias and ambiguity, valid comparison between data from different laboratories will be almost impossible. In an empirical analysis of the data from cooperative systems, the Hill coefficient (a) which is greater than one for this case may frequently be interpreted as an index of the minimum number of sites participating in the cooperative process (22). When electrostatic interactions are acting in a direction opposite to the positively cooperative process, this number of sites becomes biased and yields a lower value than would be estimated for systems without such attenuating processes. Further limitations on interpretation of the Hill coefficient arise when indirect measures such as spectral perturbations are used to assess the extent of binding in a multisite system (23). Specifically, if the magnitude of the perturbation is not the same for each ion which binds, binding curves suggesting either apparent positive or negative cooperativity may arise depending upon whether successive perturbation magnitudes increase or decrease, respectively, with successive occupancy of the binding site (23, 24). In ideal situations, all parameters may be determined (23), however such is probably not the case with the vitamin K related coagulation proteins because of their multiple (see below) sites and the protein-protein association which accompanies ion binding.

Coupled Processes Potentially Capable of Accounting for Positively Cooperative Ion Binding

Several processes may be proposed which can fulfill the requirement for the coupled process in addition to cooperative ion binding. Among these are ion induced conformation changes, ion induced self-association, and ion binding dependent creation of previously non-existent sites. In perhaps an overly mechanical way the first may be envisioned as bringing groups on the macromolecule closer together so that interaction with the binding ion can occur in the concentration range of interest, the second as forming divalent ion bridges between different protein molecules, and thus create sites involving ligands from different macromolecules which interact with the metal ion and lastly, promoting dissociation of a group which can serve as a ligand to the divalent ion only in its dissociated form. None of these are mutually exclusive and all may occur in the system of interest. Criteria exist which, if fulfilled, force inclusion of these separately describable processes in the explanation for the observed behavior. However, as is well recognized, proof that any one of them does not occur is impossible, at least for the intramolecular processes. In this regard it is important to restate our objective, i.e. determination of the minimal process or processes responsible for the cooperativity of Ca^{2+} and other divalent (and trivalent (13)) ion binding. The role of the intermolecular process, i.e. protein-protein association, can be readily examined. If protein self-association is involved, Ca^{2+} binding should depend on the protein concentration. If such an intermolecular process is unrelated to the cooperativity of ion binding, then Ca^{2+} binding should be independent of protein concentration. In addition to this consideration, the question of how specific the spectral changes which are observed are for divalent ions will also be asked as such data may aid in deciding how much emphasis should be placed on interpretation of each of the types of data.

Observations Suggesting Ion Induced Conformation Changes

There can be little doubt that conformation changes occur when ions bind to the γ-carboxyglutamic acid residues of the vitamin K related coagulation proteins. The presence of 10 to 12 Gla residues, equivalent to 20-24 negative charges within a 30-40 amino acid sequence, confers a potentially very high charge density on a small portion of the surface of the molecule. When neutralization of some of these charges occurs as a result of divalent ion binding, a relaxation of the repulsion among these groups seems a forgone conclusion. Obviously to date we know too little about the real spatial distribution of the Gla residue charges to permit an estimate of the magnitude of this relaxation, although it is clear that spatial distribution is important (4,9,25). Changes in the state of ionization of some of the Gla residues may occur upon binding of divalent ions as it is not clear that all are fully deprotonated at neutral pH because of pKs reported for Gla peptides (26-28) and the relatively high local H^+ concentration which may exist in the vicinity of the Gla residues because of the high negative charge density on the Gla-containing region of the molecule. Such divalent ion-induced ionization will fall into the category of site formation (29,30). Electrostatic phenomena such as this can also promote protein-protein association (31), and thus be involved in the cooperativity of the ion binding process by an intermolecular process as well.

Changes in both the near and far ultraviolet circular dichroism spectra occur upon Ca^{2+} binding to prothrombin (32,33) and to Fragment 1 (33, 34) and suggest ion induced conformational changes (see also Carlisle, T. L., Morita, T. and Jackson, C.M., this volume). The changes in the near ultraviolet (aromatic amino acid side chain region) spectrum which implicate significant side chain contributions to the changes in the far ultraviolet (backbone) region make it difficult to unambiguously interpret the changes in the circular dichroism spectra in terms of specific conformational changes which might be related to cooperative ion binding. Tryptophan fluorescence quenching occurs upon ion binding to prothrombin, Prothrombin Fragment 1 and Factor X (7,10,11,35), and clearly demonstrates that a change in the environment of one or several of the tryptophan residues of these proteins occurs. Based on comparison of Fragment 1 with 3 tryptophanyl residues and Factor X, with one in the light (Gla-containing) chain, the preferred candidate is tryptophan number 42 in Fragment 1 and 41 in Factor X. Calcium ion-induced ultraviolet difference spectra (see Brenckle, G.M. and Jackson, C.M., this volume) support this tentative identification. The fact that monovalent ions, albeit at high concentration, also perturb the molecule and yield similar but definitely not identical difference spectra and also quench the protein fluoresence raise some doubt about the specificity of the relationship between the spectral changes and a conformation change which is linked to the cooperativity of ion binding. Hydrogen ion concentration changes also alter the fluorescence emission characteristics of Fragment 1 (35) suggesting that perhaps the aforementioned changes in the degree of ionization of Gla residues or other groups in the vicinity of the reporting aromatic residue may be responsible for the spectral changes. Analysis of the divalent ion induced difference spectra (see Brenckle, G.M. and Jackson, C.M., this volume) suggests that these are most likely charge-induced (36) difference spectra. Difference spectra determined Ca^{2+} titration curves at the lowest protein concentration at which we have been able to make measurements (ca. 2 μM) remain sigmoid in shape and suggests: 1) that a cooperative binding process exists which is almost certainly the result of a conformation change which may be related to the Ca^{2+} binding process, or 2) the magnitude of the spectral perturbation for each of the ions that binds is quite different in a way that mimics cooperativity (23,24). Until the issue raised in item 2 is resolved, the interpretation of the titration curve shape must remain open or in favor of a binding-linked conformation change. If individual ion binding site related perturbation magnitudes are varying in a way which mimics cooperativity, then explicit determination of the individual site constants and absorptivity changes may be practically impossible because of the large number of microscopic equilibria which exist for such multisite proteins (37). It has been demonstrated that the Ca^{2+} concentration required to give one-half maximal difference spectral response depends on the Fragment 1 concentration (Brenckle, G.M. and Jackson, C.M., this volume) and thus indicates that interpretation of the spectral changes must also include consideration of intermolecular interactions as well as complex multiequilibria. Comparison of equilibrium Ca^{2+} binding data with the difference spectral data also indicates that the extent to which the Ca^{2+} binding sites are occupied is not the same as the extent to which the spectral change has occurred at different protein concentrations in a way that indicates that Ca^{2+} binding at higher protein concentrations interfers with the Ca^{2+} ion dependent spectral changes. These observations must also be considered and included into the difference spectral titration curve shape analysis. Taken altogether, these observations and the earlier comments about the analysis of such data suggest that the relationship between cooperativity of divalent ion binding and the environment (or conformation) changes observed by spectral techniques is not necessarily a causal one and is a particularly complex one in these multisite systems.

The distinctions which can be made by antibodies between prothrombin in the presence and absence of Ca^{2+} (38) almost certainly indicate detailed conformational differences. However, how to test the relationship between these changes and cooperativity of Ca^{2+} binding escapes the author!

Divalent Ion Induced Self Association and Protein Concentration Dependent Calcium Ion Binding

Divalent ion induced self association (which is almost undoubtedly dimerization) of Prothrombin Fragment 1 has been demonstrated to occur independently in two laboratories (7,25). Evidence has also been presented for a Ca^{2+} mediated association of prothrombin (25) as well as the previously demonstrated dimerization in the absence of Ca^{2+} (39,40). Formation of a complex between prothrombin and Fragment 1 in the presence of Ca^{2+} but not in its absence has also been reported (25). Data on Ca^{2+} mediated Fragment 1 dimerization are in good agreement, when the total Ca^{2+} concentration reported in the one study (7) is converted to free Ca^{2+} concentration (25). The free Ca^{2+} concentration for half maximal dimerization, 0.5 ± 0.1 mM, is essentially the same as the half saturation concentration (Table 1) for Ca^{2+} binding. These data clearly suggest a linkage between Ca^{2+} binding and Ca^{2+} induced self association. Direct examination of Ca^{2+} binding to Fragment 1 as a function of Fragment 1 concentration has been made using the Hummel-Dreyer column technique (41,42). Results for 0.25 mM Ca^{2+} (roughly the concentration giving the maximum in the Scatchard plot from Ca^{2+} binding to Fragment 1 (4)) and 5 mM are shown in Figures 4 and 5, respectively. A protein concentration dependence consistent with protein association and binding being linked is evident in the data of Figure

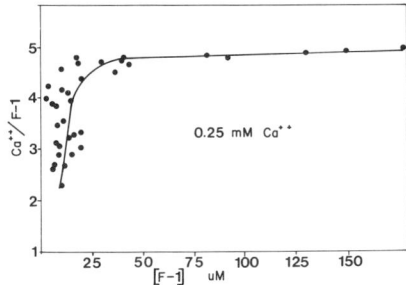
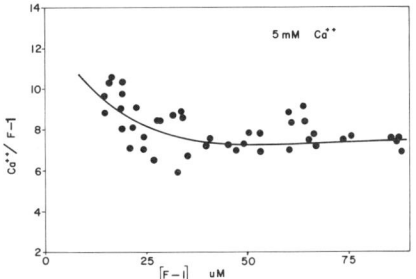

FIGURE 4 Calcium ion binding to Prothrombin Fragment 1 as a function of Fragment 1 concentration at 0.25 mM Ca^{2+}. $\bar{v}$ is the number of Ca^{2+} ions/Fragment 1 molecule. Buffer, 0.01 M Tris-HCl, 0.10 M NaCl, pH 7.5.

FIGURE 5 Calcium ion binding to Prothrombin Fragment 1 as a function of Fragment 1 concentration at 5.0 mM Ca^{2+}. $\bar{v}$ is the number of Ca^{2+} ions/Fragment 1 molecule. Buffer, 0.01 M Tris-HCl, 0.10 M NaCl, pH 7.5.

4, where the number of Ca^{2+} ions bound increases from 2.4 at the lowest protein concentration (10 µM) to 4.6 at the highest concentration (i.e. greater than 40 µM). Similar data are observed between 0.1 and 0.5 mM Ca^{2+} (Brenckle, G.M., Kohm, D.G. and Jackson, C.M., unpublished observations). A clearly different situation is observed at 5 mM Ca^{2+}. At this concentration the number of binding sites increases with decreasing protein concentration with an apparent extrapolated value of ca. 14 sites per protein molecule. Similar behavior is observed at 2 and 10 mM Ca^{2+} as well. At 10 mM Ca^{2+}, 10 sites are observed at 40 µM Fragment 1, consistent with previously reported values from this laboratory (4). The increase in number of sites at low protein concentration (5 mM Ca^{2+}) yields a number, i.e. 14, remarkably similar to the total number of sites observed by one group who did not observe cooperative Ca^{2+} binding (3) and suggests that the number of sites may vary depending upon whether they involve ligands from one or two protein molecules (see below). At very low Ca^{2+} concentrations, i.e. 0.01-0.1 mM, the binding curves appear similar to those observed at high Ca^{2+}, i.e. the number of sites appears to increase with decreasing protein concentration. Such behavior leads to Scatchard plots which appear to change from "multiclass type" to cooperative as protein concentration is increased. What is very clear from all these binding data and the Ca^{2+} mediated dimerization is that Ca^{2+} dependent association and cooperativity of Ca^{2+} binding must be considered together and the protein dimerization process included into any models used for interpreting the cooperativity of Ca^{2+} binding. Protein concentration dependence in Gd^{3+} binding to prothrombin has also been reported (13) with cooperative binding being observed at higher protein concentration and multiclass site behavior at lower concentration, consistent with the Ca^{2+} binding related observations described above. It perhaps should be noted that none of these data provide any evidence against concomitantly occuring conformation changes which may be involved in the binding and association processes, in fact conformation changes in the monomeric protein species are expected to occur as a result of the interaction between monomers in the dimer.

Models for Ligand Induced Self Association Potentially Capable of Explaining the Divalent Ion Binding Characteristics of the Vitam K Dependent Coagulation Proteins

Mechanisms describing the behavior of systems exhibiting ligand induced association have been reported and described in detail by Nichol and Winzor (43) and by Cann (44,45) and Cann and Hinman (42). In Figure 6a and 6b are

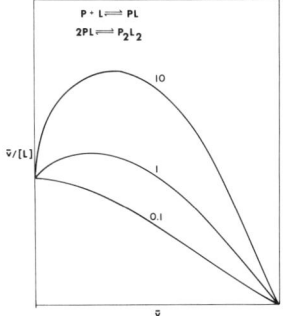

FIGURE 6a Scatchard plot for ligand induced dimerization of two liganded monomers. The numbers adjacent to each curve represent the relative magnitude of the dimerization constants (from reference 43).

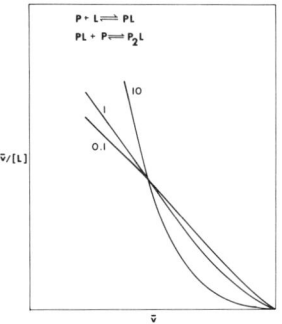

FIGURE 6b Scatchard plot for ligand induced dimerization of one liganded and one unliganded monomer. The numbers adjacent to each curve represent the relative magnitude of the equilibrium constant for the dimerization reaction (from reference 43).

shown two types of Scatchard plots predicted from the simplest example of such types of mechanisms. In Figure 6a it can be seen that ligand binding to a protein molecule which subsequently dimerizes leads to concave downward Scatchard plots, i.e. positive cooperativity. The mechanism of Figure 6b, in which one liganded protein molecule associates with an unliganded protein molecule leads to behavior which, with the coupled electrostatic effects discussed above, can look very much like "multiclass site" binding. It must be noted that these models are for a protein molecule with a single site, whereas the vitamin K related proteins possess many sites. It seems entirely possible that a situation in which both partially liganded protein molecules dimerize and monomers in which sites which might participate in dimerization are already liganded inhibit dimerization, can explain the binding behavior of the vitamin K related proteins. Scatchard plots from models which involve sites participating in dimerization and sites unrelated to dimerization have also been reported (45), which although involve fewer sites look very much like the Scatchard plots reported for prothrombin, Fragment 1 and Factor X. Such a "model", which is a combination of the two simple models of Figure 6a and 6b permits inclusion of virtually all the published data if allowance is made for some heterogeneity in the individual preparation of proteins which would alter the protein concentration dependence of binding. Batches of protein with tightly bound ions (7,8) and which may be altered during storage (10) have been reported. If some maximum number of potential sites exist on a monomer protein molecule, e.g. 20 from the 20 carboxylates of 10 Gla residues, then a monomer may bind as many as 20 Ca^{2+} ions, albeit very weakly. If dimer formation occurs between two protein molecules, then carboxylate ligands from each may interact with individual Ca^{2+} ions leading to "Ca^{2+} bridges" between the two proteins. Such a mechanism would be consistent with the stoichiometry of Ca^{2+} binding which is calculated per monomeric protein and would permit protein-protein association variability to alter the apparent number of sites on a monomer. A schematic representation of such a model for Ca^{2+} liganded dimers is shown in Figure 7, which is consistent with a large body of data, including that from investigations of

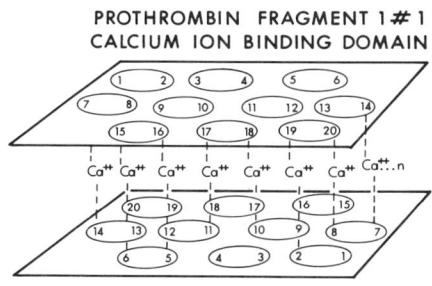

FIGURE 7 A schematic representation of Ca^{2+} induced dimer formation between two Gla containing regions of Fragment 1 molecules. Adapted from reference 25.

Fragment 1 binding to phospholipid vesicle surfaces (46) which has been interpreted to involve as many as 20 Ca^{2+} bridges. Such a model requires particular binding site symmetry (47) which can be shown to be possible from molecular models, but which must await completion of the crystallographic studies on Fragment 1 (48) and (Magnusson et al., this volume) for an unambiguous test.

The advantages of a ligand (divalent cation) mediated self association model for explaining the cooperativity of divalent ion binding to the vitamin K dependent coagulation proteins are several. First, such a process must be considered because of the demonstrated divalent cation dependent dimerization (7,25). The fact that Ca^{2+} and Gd^{3+} (13) binding are protein concentration dependent clearly links the two processes. The possibility of explaining the observations of many laboratories by such a hybrid model must also be considered an advantage, as bases for disregarding the apparently divergent results are difficult to justify. When inclusion of the electrostatic effects, along with the binding and association into a single model has been achieved, the details will undoubtedly appear complex, but the processes involved are well documented and the unification of observations which can be expected should overshadow the complexity of the details. In view of all the observations discussed above, it is the author's opinion that a model involving ion induced self association is preferable to an explanation involving an intramolecular conformational change for explaining the cooperativity of Ca^{2+} and other divalent ion binding to these Gla containing proteins. Conformational changes which undoubtedly occur may be related or even be more important than the intermolecular interaction among protein molecules, however until both more data can be obtained and very rigorous analysis of such data made, this will remain uncertain.

ACKNOWLEDGMENTS

This work was supported by grants HL 12820 and HL 14147 from the National Heart, Lung and Blood Institute. CMJ was an Established Investigator of the American Heart Association during the performance of this work.

REFERENCES

1. Stenflo, J. and Ganrot, P.O. (1973) Biochem. Biophys. Res. Comm. 50, 98-104.
2. Nelsestuen, G.L. and Suttie, J.W. (1972) Biochemistry 11, 4961-4964.
3. Benson, B.J. and Hanahan, D.J. (1975) Biochemistry 14, 3265-3277.
4. Henriksen, R.A. and Jackson, C.M. (1975) Arch. Biochem. Biophys. 170, 149-159.
5. Lindhout, M.J. and Hemker, H.C. (1978) Biochim. Biophys. Acta 533, 318-326.
6. Yue, R.H. and Gertler, M.M. (1978) Thrombos. Haemostas. (Stuttg.) 40, 350-357.
7. Prendergast, F.G. and Mann, K.G. (1977) J. Biol. Chem. 252, 840-850.
8. Bajaj, S.P., Butkowski, R.J. and Mann, K.G. (1975) J. Biol. Chem. 250, 2150-2156.
9. Nelsestuen, G.L., Broderius, M., Zytkovicz, T.M. and Howard, J.B. (1975) Biochem. Biophys. Res. Comm. 65, 233-240.
10. Nelsestuen, G.L. (1976) J. Biol. Chem. 251, 5648-5656.
11. Nelsestuen, G.L., Broderius, M. and Martin, G. (1976) J. Biol. Chem. 251, 6886-6892.
12. Furie, B.C., Mann, K.G. and Furie, B. (1976) J. Biol. Chem. 251, 3235-3241.
13. Nemerson, Y. and Furie, B. (1979) Critical Rev. Biochem. 6, in press.
14. Bajaj, S.P., Nowak, T. and Castellino, F.J. (1976) J. Biol. Chem. 251, 6294-6299.
15. Benarous, R., Elion, J. and Labie, D. (1976) Biochemie 58, 391-394.
16. Furie, B.C. and Furie, B. (1975) J. Biol. Chem. 250, 601-608.
17. Bajaj, S.P., Byrne, R., Nowak, T. and Castellino, F.J. (1977) J. Biol. Chem. 252, 4758-4761.
18. Tanford, C. (1961) Physical Chemistry of Macromolecules. John Wiley and Sons, New York, pp. 457-586.
19. Edsall, J.T. and Wyman, J. (1958) Biophysical Chemistry, Academic Press, New York, pp. 645-651.
20. Scatchard, G. (1949) Ann. N.Y. Acad. Sci. 51, 660-672.
21. Klotz, I.M. (1953) In Neurath, H. and Bailey, K., eds., The Proteins, Vol. I, Part B, Academic Press, pp. 727-806.

22. Dahlquist, F.W. (1978) Meth. Enzymol. 48, Academic Press, New York, pp. 270-299.
23. Greenfield, N. (1975) Critical Rev. Biochem. 3, 71-110.
24. Deranleau, D.A. (1969) J. Am. Chem. Soc. 91, 4050-4054.
25. Jackson, C.M., Peng, C.W., Brenckle, G.M., Jonas, A. and Stenflo, J. (1979) J. Biol. Chem. 254, in press.
26. Maike, W., Oppliger, M. and Schwyzer, R. (1977) Helv. Chim. Acta 60, 807-815.
27. Robertson, Jr., P., Hiskey, R.G. and Koehler, K.A. (1978) J. Biol. Chem. 253, 5880-5883.
28. Sperling, R.A., Furie, B.C., Blumenstein, M., Keyt, B. and Furie, B. (1978) J. Biol. Chem. 253, 3898-3906.
29. Parsons, D.L. and Vallner, J.J. (1978) Math. Biosciences 41, 189-215.
30. Parsons, D.L. and Vallner, J.J. (1978) Math. Biosciences 41, 217-230.
31. Timasheff, S.N. (1966) Biopolymers 4, 107-120.
32. Bjork, I. and Stenflo, J. (1973) FEBS Lett. 32, 343-346.
33. Bloom, J.W. and Mann, K.G. (1978) Biochemistry 17, 4430-4438.
34. Gabriel, D.A., Schaefer, D.J., Roberts, H.R., Aronson, D.L. and Koehler, K.A. (1975) Thromb. Res. 7, 839-846.
35. Scott, M.E., Koehler, K.A. and Hiskey, R.G. (1979) Biochem. J. 177, 879-886.
36. Andrews, G.T. and Forster, L.S. (1972) Biochemistry 11, 1875-1879.
37. Klotz, I.M. and Hunston, D.L. (1975) J. Biol. Chem. 250, 3001-3009.
38. Furie, B., Provost, K.L., Blanchard, R.A. and Furie, B.C. (1978) J. Biol. Chem. 253, 8980-8987.
39. Cox, A.C. and Hanahan, D.J. (1970) Biochim. Biophys. Acta 207, 49-64.
40. Agarwal, G.P., Gallagher, J.G., Aune, K.C. and Armeniades, C.D. (1977) Biochemistry 16, 1865-1870.
41. Hummel, J.P. and Dreyer, W.J. (1962) Biochim. Biophys. Acta 63, 530-532.
42. Cann, J.R. and Hinman, N.D. (1976) Biochemistry 15, 4614-4622.
43. Nichol, L.W. and Winzor, D.J. (1976) Biochemistry 15, 3015-3019.
44. Cann, J.R. (1970) Interacting Macromolecules, Academic Press, New York.
45. Cann, J.R. (1978) Methods in Enzymology 48, Academic Press, New York, pp. 299-307.
46. Dombrose, F.A., Gitel, S.N., Zawalick, K. and Jackson, C.M. (1979) J. Biol. Chem. 254, in press.
47. Morgan, R.S., Miller, S.L. and McAdon, J.M. (1979) J. Mol. Biol. 127, 31-39.
48. Aschaffenburg, R., Blake, C.C.F., Burridge, J.M. and Esnouf, M.P. (1977) J. Mol. Biol. 114, 575-579.

PROTHROMBIN FRAGMENT 1 MODIFICATIONS: EFFECTS ON PROTEIN-MEMBRANE INTERACTION

G. L. NELSESTUEN, R. M. RESNICK, C. S. KIM and
C. PLETCHER

Dept. of Biochemistry, University of Minnesota
St. Paul, MN 55108

INTRODUCTION

The vitamin K-dependent proteins of the plasma display calcium-dependent interactions with phospholipid membranes (see ref. 1 and references therein). While the γ-carboxyglutamic acid residues are essential for calcium binding and protein-membrane interactions (2-4), it is clear that other portions of these proteins are also essential. A peptide corresponding to residues 12-44 of prothrombin (containing 8 γ-carboxyglutamic acid residues) has shown decreased calcium binding and does not bind to membranes in the manner of the parent molecule (5). Furthermore, a peptide corresponding to residues 4-45 of factor X (5,6) (containing all of the γ-carboxyglutamic acid residues of this protein (7,8)) also has low calcium-binding affinity and fails to bind to the membranes.
In another study, Henrickson and Jackson observed that disulfide bond reduction of prothrombin fragment 1 results in a loss of tight calcium binding (9). Derivatization of the carboxyl groups results in complete loss of the activities attributed to γ-carboxyglutamic acid (10). These rather drastic protein modifications reveal that functionality of γ-carboxyglutamic acid is dependent on protein structure beyond a simple primary amino acid sequence containing these residues. Nelsestuen (11) has demonstrated that a calcium-dependent protein transition is essential for prothrombin-membrane interaction. This transition can be monitored by intrinsic protein fluorescence (11,12), u.v. (9) or CD measurements of prothrombin fragment 1 (13,14). Further studies have revealed that a metal ion-phospholipid interaction must also precede protein-membrane binding (15,16). The manner of expressing these interactions has been presented as (16):

$$\left.\begin{array}{c} P + iCa \rightleftarrows P_{iCa} \rightleftarrows P'_{iCa} \\ + \\ PL + jCa \rightleftarrows PL_{jCa} \end{array}\right\} + mCa \rightleftarrows P' \cdot PL_{i+j+mCa} \quad (1)$$

where P is protein, P' is the protein after the cation-dependent transition and PL is the phospholipid membrane. These equilibria appear to apply to all vitamin K-dependent plasma proteins (1). The transition helps to illustrate the fact that considerable portions of the protein are essential for the protein-membrane interaction.
 A naturally occurring protein modification is the activation of the vitamin K-dependent proteins by partial proteolysis. Recent studies have indicated that activation has relatively little effect on the membrane-binding properties of these proteins (1,15,16).
 Prothrombin fragment 1 contains two complex carbohydrate chains (17,18). Nelsestuen and Suttie (19) have reported the removal of a majority of the sugar residues of prothrombin without effect on its usefulness as a substrate for thrombin formation in the two-stage

prothrombin assay. This indicates that the carbohydrate is one portion of the molecule which is not essential to protein-membrane interaction.
Further protein modifications are considered here.

MATERIALS AND METHODS

The protein preparations used as well as the techniques have all been described in the literature and are cited in the figure legends or in the text.

RESULTS AND DISCUSSION

Naturally occurring protein modifications

The vitamin K-dependent proteins of the plasma are a closely-related group of proteins. This is very evident from sequence homology in the amino-terminal, γ-carboxyglutamic acid-containing region (1,20-24). These proteins undoubtedly descend from a common ancestral gene so that the amino acid substitutions occurring in different proteins constitute modifications brought about by evolutionary means. Comparisons of protein-membrane binding for the different proteins can indicate the effects of the observed amino acid substitutions. Such comparisons have provided an evolutionary scheme for the appearance of these proteins (1). More detailed comparisons of the γ-carboxyglutamic acid-containing regions of these proteins is presented in figure 1. The proteins are listed in order of their membrane-binding affinity. They break down into three or four classes: the highest affinity is displayed by factor X; prothrombin and protein S form a second category; factor IX binds much less tightly; and protein C and factor VII bind with such low affinity that their binding cannot be detected by some techniques. Prothrombin and factor X were postulated to be the parental molecules in evolution with protein C and factor VII developing later (1). Evolution actually seems to have developed a poorer phospholipid binding site.
   When analyzed by the method of Chou and Fasman (25), it was found that the γ-carboxyglutamic acid residues reside in regions which have high potential for helix formation (Fig. 1). There appears to be no tendency to form a β-sheet in this region of the protein and such analysis is not included in figure 1. Comparisons of protein C and factor X, the two extremes of binding affinity, reveal little difference except in positions 10-14. In this region there occurs a strong inverse correlation between helix breaking potential and tight membrane binding. For example, factor X has only two helix breaking residues and has the tightest membrane binding. Prothrombin, protein S and factor IX each have three helix-breaking residues but only factor IX contains these in a continuous sequence. Four helix breaking residues in a continuous sequence abolish a helix entirely (25). Factor IX theoretically can form a continuous helix through this region but only with the greatest of difficulty. In agreement with this, factor IX shows the poorest membrane binding of these three proteins. Factor VII and protein C contain a proline residue which entirely eliminates the possibility of a continuous helix through this region of the protein (25). These latter two proteins have by far the poorest membrane-binding.
   This analysis is of course subject to the potential error of the Chou and Fasman method (25) as well as the assumption that γ-carboxyglutamic acid would be a helix-forming amino acid. The differences which account for varying membrane-binding affinities could reside in

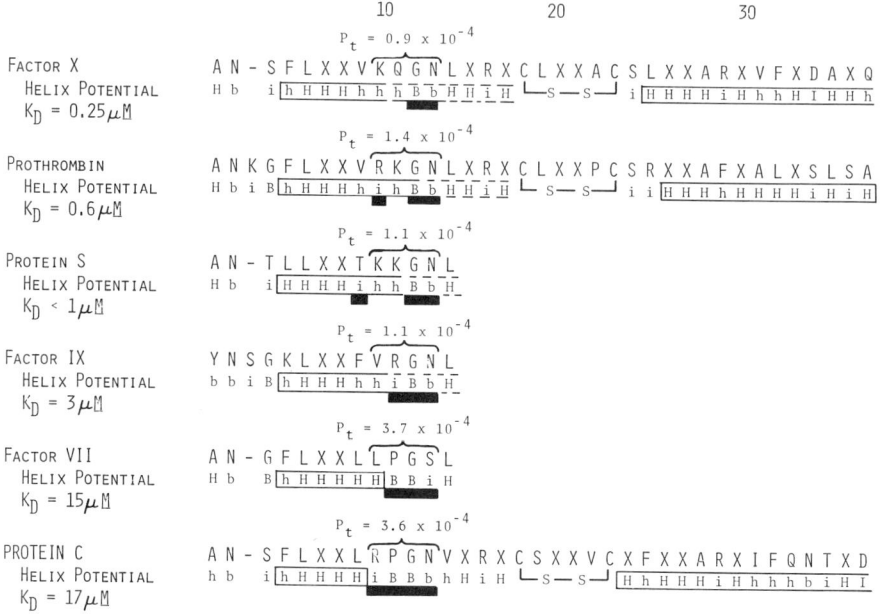

FIGURE 1 Amino acid sequence and membrane-binding potential of the vitamin K-dependent proteins of bovine plasma. The proteins are ranked in order of their affinity for a given phospholipid at 2 mM calcium (K_D values from Nelsestuen et al. and are more accurately described as K_4Ca^* (1)). The helix forming potential is according to Chou and Fasman (25) where H and h are strong and weak helix forming amino acids, I and i are indifferent and slight helix-breaking residues and b and B are weak and strong helix breaking residues. An assumption in this analysis is the classification of γ-carboxyglutamic acid in the H category with glutamic acid. Possible α-helix regions are enclosed in the solid line with a dotted line indicating areas where a helix might be extended. P_t is $f_i \times f_{i+1} \times f_{i+2} \times f_{i+3}$ (25) and indicates the tendency to form a β-turn; a value of greater than 0.75×10^{-4} is consistent with β-turn formation. The helix-breaking residues between 9 and 13 are underlined to draw attention to the correlation of helix breaking in this region with loss of membrane-binding ability. The factor X sequence is from Enfield et al. (7), prothrombin from Magnusson et al. (17), Protein S from DiScipio and Davie (21), factor IX from Fujikawa et al. (22), factor VII from Kisiel and Davie (23) and Protein C is from Fernlund et al. (24). Some of the γ-carboxyglutamic acid residues are assigned by extrapolations from other studies. The single letter code is used for the amino acids and X indicates γ-carboxyglutamic acid.

other regions of the molecule. Nevertheless, the correlation of membrane binding and the ability to form a continuous helix through residues 5-14 is very striking and seems worthy of further consideration. Breaking a helix in this region of the protein will clearly change the relationship of the γ-carboxyglutamic acids at positions 7 and 8 with the remainder of the molecule. Bloom and Mann (13) have estimated that the calcium-dependent prothrombin protein transition involves an increase in helix conformation. Perhaps some of this increase involves residues 5-14. It is also possible that helix formation occurs only at the protein-membrane interface.

Another feature of these proteins is the tendency to form a β-turn at residues 10-13. There is a general inverse relationship between β-turn potential and tight membrane-binding (Fig. 1). The only exception is factor IX which has no greater potential for β-turn formation than prothrombin or protein S but still binds with lower affinity. Consequently, the best correlation with membrane binding affinity is the ability to form a continuous helix.

Tryptophan

Other, more sutble protein modifications have been performed in order to help pinpoint essential and non-essential portions of the protein. A large change in intrinsic tryptophan fluorescence occurs during the protein transition (11). This suggests that the environments of the indole side chains undergo considerable change. The study of tryptophan was therefore initiated. The results from iodide quenching are shown in figure 2. An intercept of 1.0 on the ordinate of this plot indicates that complete quenching of fluorescence is possible at infinite iodide ion concentration and that the tryptophan residues are all accessible to the solvent. In the presence and absence of calcium, essentially all of the tryptophan fluorescence was accessible to quenching by iodide ion (Fig. 2). The slopes of the quenching curves, however, indicate that higher iodide ion concentrations are required in the presence of calcium and that the tryptophan moieties are less accessible. The amount which

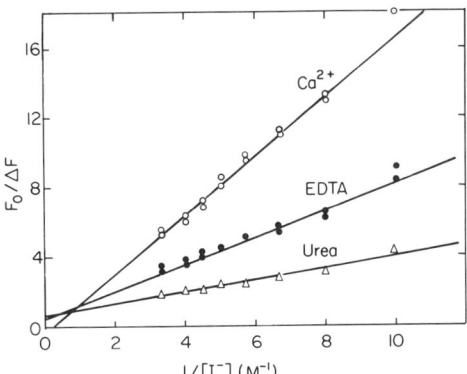

FIGURE 2 Modified Stern-Volmer plot of fragment 1 fluorescence quenching by iodide ion. Fragment 1 (0.09 mg/ml) fluorescence in 0.05 $\underline{M}$ tris buffer (pH 7.5) was analyzed at varying potassium iodide concentrations. The salt concentration was maintained at a constant level by additions of KCl. All solutions contained 0.1 mM $Na_2S_2O_3$. The analysis is that described by Lehrer (26). F_o is the integrated fluorescence emission spectrum (300-400 nm) in the absence of added iodide ion and ΔF is the change in the integrated fluorescence emission spectrum in the presence of iodide ion (F_o-F). Excitation was at 280 nm. An intercept of 1.0 on the ordinate indicates that all of the fluorescence is accessible to iodide ion quenching. The values of less than 1.0 would imply the same. Quenching curves in the presence of 3 mM calcium (-o-), 5 mM EDTA (-●-) and 8 $\underline{M}$ urea (-△-) are shown. The calcium concentration is adequate to bring about the full protein fluorescence change at this ionic strength.

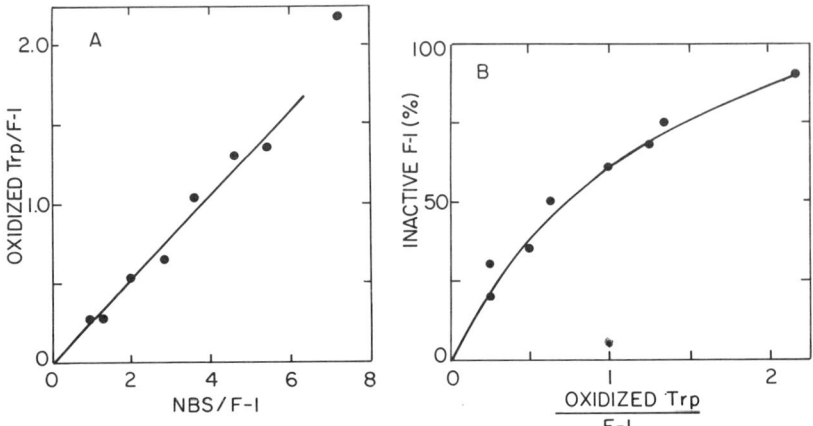

FIGURE 3 Oxidation of tryptophan by N-bromosuccinimide. Freshly prepared, recrystallized N-bromosuccinimide (NBS) was added to a solution of prothrombin fragment 1 (1.7 mg/ml) in .05 M acetate buffer (pH 5.0). The absorbance at 280 nm was monitored and the number of oxidized tryptophan residues calculated by the method described by Patchornick et al. (27). This calculation assumes a molar extinction coefficient for tryptophan (5500) and that no other components interfere at 280 nm. The molar ratio of NBS per oxidized tryptophan obtained from figure 3A is 3.5 which is within the typical range of 2 to 4 (28). Figure 3B shows the relationship of tryptophan oxidation and inactive protein. Inactive F-1 is protein that does not bind to the membrane and the method of calculation is given in the text.

calcium-dependent protein dimerization (12) contributes to this accessibility is not known.

Oxidation of tryptophan with N-bromosuccinimide was also conducted. The conditions used (Figure 3) are reported to minimize side reactions (28). The estimated relationship of inactive protein to oxidized tryptophan is presented in figure 3B. The amount of inactive fragment 1 ($F-1_i$) was estimated by solving equations 2 and 3 simultaneously:

$$K_D = \frac{[F-1][PL]}{[F-1 \cdot PL]} \quad (2) \qquad K' = \frac{[F-1+F-1_i][PL]}{[F-1 \cdot PL]} \quad (3)$$

where F-1 is fragment 1, PL is the molar concentration of protein binding sites, F-1·PL is the protein-phospholipid complex, K_D is the dissociation constant for native fragment 1-membrane interaction under the conditions used and K' is the value obtained for partially oxidized fragment 1 under the same conditions. The K_D and K' values were determined by the relative light scattering technique described by Nelsestuen and Lim (15) assuming $\frac{\partial n}{\partial c}$ values of 0.172 and 0.192 for phospholipid and protein, respectively (15). A molecular weight of 23,500 for fragment 1 and an $E^{1\%}_{280}$ of 10.1 (29) for native fragment 1 were used in these calculations.

SDS-gel electrophoresis (30) showed no detectable change in the molecular weight of the oxidized fragment 1 indicating that major fragmentation of the peptide chain had not occurred. The results shown in figure 3 therefore indicate that oxidation of tryptophan has an adverse affect on protein-membrane interaction.

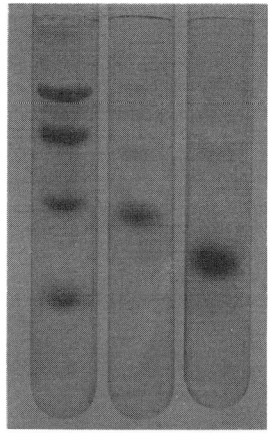

FIGURE 4 SDS gel electrophoresis of normal and aglycofragment 1. Gel 1 shows the standards (bovine serum albumin (66,000 daltons), ovalbumin (40,000 daltons), carbonic anhydrase (29,000 daltons) and myoglobin (17,000 daltons)). Gel 2 is normal fragment 1 (estimated molecular weight = 26,500) while gel 3 shows the aglycofragment 1 (estimated molecular weight = 20,500) derived from anhydrous HF treatment of fragment 1.

This conclusion must still be viewed with some caution however. Kalayama and Titani have reported that the peptide linkages of γ-carboxyglutamic acid residues can be cleaved by N-bromosuccinimide (31). Cleavages at positions 7 or 8 would result in small molecular weight changes which probably would not be detected by the electrophoresis method used. The destruction of membrane-binding could therefore be due to tryptophan oxidation or loss of the amino terminal hepta- or octapeptide.

Carbohydrate Removal

Mort and Lamport (32) have shown that fluorolysis in anhydrous HF removes O-glycoside-linked carbohydrate moieties of glycoproteins without hydrolysis of the peptide chain. This technique was applied to prothrombin fragment 1. The resulting aglycofragment 1 was purified by ion exchange chromatography. Neutral sugar assay (33) indicates no neutral carbohydrate (≤10% of the initial carbohydrate content) on the HF-treated protein. Gel electrophoresis (Figure 4) also indicated a loss of molecular weight which corresponds approximately to the loss of two complex carbohydrate chains (NANA$_2$ Gal$_2$ Man$_3$ GlcNAc$_4$ = 2200 daltons each (18)).

Several characteristics indicate that the membrane-binding site of the aglycofragment 1 is still intact. Figure 5 gives the calcium titration of protein fluorescence which is indicative of the calcium-dependent protein transition. Comparison to normal fragment 1 reveals approximately the same total fluorescence change, similar cooperativity and a similar slow rate and activation energy (11) for the transition (rate studies not shown). The only difference observed is in the calcium concentration requirement; the midpoint of the aglycofragment 1 titration occurs at a higher calcium concentration (Fig. 5). This difference is not great but is experimentally significant.

Comparisons of the CD spectra of the aglyco and normal fragment 1 in the presence and absence of calcium also show no substantial differences (Fig. 6). This is in agreement with other studies which have detected no changes in the peptide backbone when carbohydrate is removed from glycoproteins (e.g. ref. 34,35). Calcium does cause a significant change in the CD spectra of both proteins (compare Figs. 6A and B). This change agrees with the studies of Bloom and Mann (13).

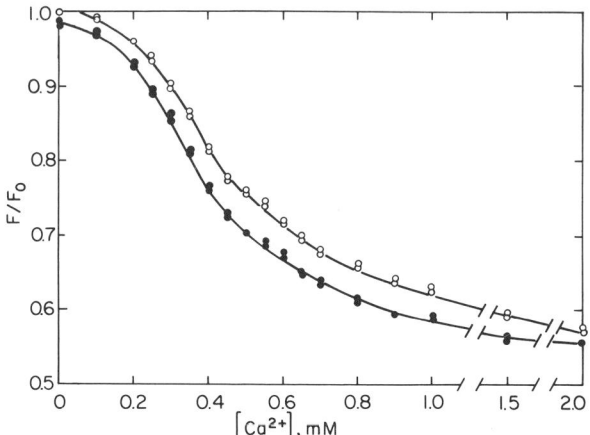

FIGURE 5   Calcium titration of fragment 1 (-●-) and aglycofragment 1 (-o-) fluorescence. The protein concentration was 100 μg/ml. Each point represents one determination. F is the fluorescence observed in the presence of calcium and F_o is the fluorescence after addition of excess EDTA. This technique has been described in full previously (11).

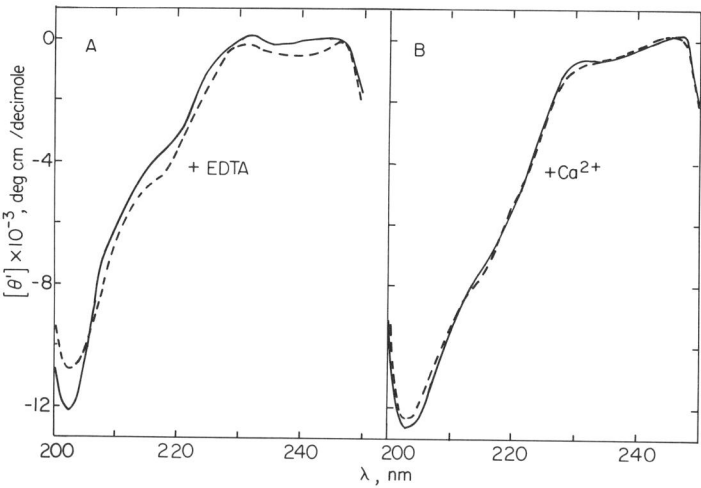

FIGURE 6   CD spectra of normal (---) and aglycofragment 1 (——) in the presence of 2 mM EDTA (6A) and the presence of 2 mM calcium (6B). The spectra were taken on a Jasco 41C spectropolarimeter with a digital processor. The path length was 0.1 cm, the protein solutions used had an A_{280} = 0.11 and were in 0.05 M tris buffer (pH 7.5)-0.1 M NaCl. The sample chamber was flushed with N_2 gas at ambient temperature. Four scans were obtained for each spectrum. [Θ'] is the mean residue ellipticity at the wavelengths indicated.

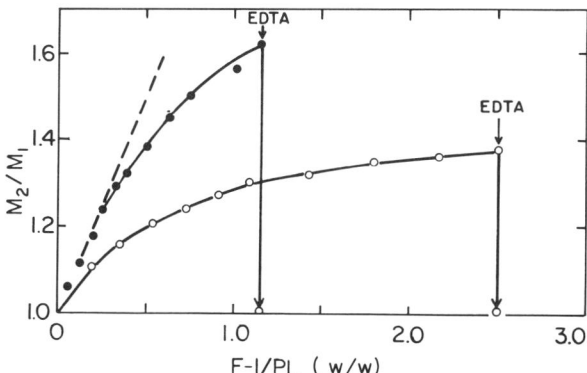

FIGURE 7 Binding of normal (-o-) and aglycofragment 1 (-●-) to acidic phospholipids. Phospholipid vesicles containing 20% phosphatidyl serine were prepared and quantitated as described previously (15). M_2 is the average molecular weight of the fragment 1-phospholipid vesicle complex and M_1 is the molecular weight of the vesicles alone. This ratio was estimated by the relative light scattering method described by Nelsestuen and Lim (16) using their conditions at 2 m$\underline{M}$ calcium and a phospholipid concentration of 0.1 mg/ml. The dotted line shows the theoretical curve if all of the added protein were bound to the phospholipid vesicles. EDTA indicates the addition of an excess of this chelating agent to dissolve the complex.

The membrane-binding characteristics of aglycofragment 1 have undergone changes as evidenced by the results shown in figure 7. Normal fragment 1 binds to the membrane in an equilibrium manner (some bound and free protein) with a maximum corresponding to approximately a monolayer of protein on the surface of the vesicle (based on previous calculations for prothrombin (16) a monolayer of spherical hexagonally packed fragment 1 molecules on the vesicle would give an M_2/M_1 ratio of 1.5). The aglycofragment 1 however binds much tighter (essentially all of the protein is bound up to a protein:phospholipid ratio of about 0.3) and clearly exceeds a monolayer on the vesicle surface (Fig. 7). The fact that this binding is entirely reversed with EDTA (Fig. 7) indicates that calcium-dependent processes are responsible for the protein-membrane contact and that the γ-carboxyglutamic acid residues are functioning normally. We feel that this enhancement of binding is due to protein-protein interactions which allow for multiple layering of protein on the vesicle surface and provide for tighter binding. The carbohydrate may mask hydrophobic sites which are involved in these interactions. Fundamentally however, the carbohydrate appears to have no direct function in protein-membrane interaction.

Peptide cleavages

Partial proteolysis with plasmin was studied in an attempt to isolate smaller peptides which retain their membrane-binding ability. Excess proteolytic digestion will cause inactivation of fragment 1 as shown in figure 8. This study examined both the protein fluorescence change in the presence of calcium and the amount of functional or membrane-binding protein. The slope of the line drawn in figure 8 is nearly 1.0 (actual value = 0.85). This indicates that either method can be used to approximate the amount of inactive protein. For very accurate analysis, the

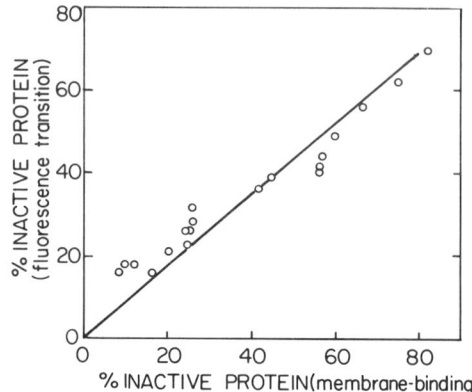

FIGURE 8 Inactivation of fragment 1 by protease digestion. Fragment 1 (2.5 mg/ml) in 0.05 M tris buffer (pH 7.5)-0.1 M NaCl was treated with 0.025 mg/ml of plasmin (purchased from the Sigma Chemical Co.; 0.45 units/mg, suppliers units) at 25°. At various time intervals (0-2 hr), samples were chilled to 0°, 20 mM lysine plus 2 mM calcium were added to inhibit plasmin digestion. The maximum calcium-dependent fluorescence change was determined and used to estimate the amount of inactive fragment 1 (defined as protein which shows no calcium-dependent fluorescence change). Fully active fragment 1 gives a 45% decrease in protein fluorescence in the presence of 2 mM Ca^{2+}. The K_D for fragment 1-phospholipid binding was determined by the relative light-scattering technique described for figure 7. The percentage of inactive fragment 1 (that which does not bind to the membrane) was determined from equations 2 and 3 as described in the text. These values are plotted on the abscissa.

membrane-binding assay would appear to be superior. The maximum intrinsic protein fluorescence change observed is 45 percent and a few preparations have shown changes up to 48 percent in the presence of calcium. Earlier reports of a maximum change of 35 percent (11,12) were undoubtedly made with protein containing some non-functional molecules. Quantitative measurements with prothrombin fragment 1 therefore require caution to ascertain that fully functional protein is used. This caution has also been indicated previously (5).

Calcium was found to inhibit the proteolysis very considerably (data not shown). The calcium-dependent conformational change and perhaps dimer formation (12) appear to make the protein less accessible to proteases.

A proteolytically modified fragment 1 molecule which retained its membrane-binding properties was isolated. Mild digestion with plasmin was followed by cochromatography of the protein with phospholipid vesicles (containing 30% phosphatidyl serine) on an agarose A 0.5m gel filtration column. The eluting buffer (0.05 M tris (pH 7.5)-0.1 M NaCl) contained 2 mM $CaCl_2$ plus 20 mM lysine. Membrane-bound (and therefore functional) protein elutes at the exclusion volume of the column and is clearly separated from unbound protein (e.g. see ref. 11). The membrane-bound fractions were pooled and mixed with EDTA. The released protein was then separated from the phospholipid by rechromatography on the same column which was now eluted with buffer containing 2 mM EDTA. The eluted protein was desalted, lyophylized and the amino terminal sequence analyzed. The amino terminal sequence consisted primarily of Gly-Phe-Leu (residues 4-6 of fragment 1, Fig. 1) with only a residual level of Ala-Asn-Lys and no other detected sequences. Based on both calcium-dependent fluorescence change and membrane-binding characteristics, this protein appeared to fully retain its function. These results indicate that the amino terminal tripeptide is not essential for fragment 1-membrane binding.

No evidence for other proteolytically cleaved but active fragment 1 molecules was obtained. The high degree of disulfide-crosslinking in fragment 1 (17) together with the essential γ-carboxyglutamic acid residues at positions 7 and 8 (see above) indicate that isolation of smaller but active fragment 1 molecules is unlikely. Fragment 1 (156 residues) appears to approximate the smallest functional peptide which can be isolated.

ACKNOWLEDGEMENTS

This work was supported in part by grant HL 15728 from the NIH. The authors are indebted to Dr. Finn Wold and Dr. Christopher Chin for the amino acid sequence analysis and Dr. John Gander and Dr. Sheri Tonn for performing the anhydrous HF treatments.

REFERENCES

1. Nelsestuen, G. L., Kisiel, W. and DiScipio, R. G. (1978) Biochemistry 17, 2134-2138.
2. Nelsestuen, G. L. and Suttie, J. W. (1972) Biochemistry 11, 4961-4964.
3. Stenflo, J. and Ganrot, P.-O. (1973) Biochem. Biophys. Res. Commun. 50, 98-104.
4. Esmon, C. T., Suttie, J. W. and Jackson, C. M. (1975) J. Biol. Chem. 250, 4095-4099.
5. Nelsestuen, G. L., Broderius, M., Zytkovicz, T. H. and Howard, J. B. (1975) Biochem. Biophys. Res. Commun. 65, 233-240.
6. Howard, J. B. and Nelsestuen, G. L. (1975) Proc. Natl. Acad. Sci. USA 72, 1281-1285.
7. Enfield, C. L., Ericsson, L. H., Walsh, K. A., Neurath, H. and Titani, K. (1975) Proc. Natl. Acad. Sci. USA 72, 16-19.
8. Thøgersen, H. C., Petersen, T. E., Sottrup-Jensen, L., Magnusson, S. and Morris, H. R. (1978) Biochem. J. 175, 613.
9. Henrickson, R. A. and Jackson, C. M. (1975) Arch. Biochem. Biophys. 170, 149-159.
10. Howard, J. B. and Nelsestuen, G. L. (1974) Biochem. Biophys. Res. Commun. 59, 757-763.
11. Nelsestuen, G. L. (1976) J. Biol. Chem. 251, 5648-5656.
12. Prendergast, F. and Mann, K. G. (1977) J. Biol. Chem. 252, 840-850.
13. Bloom, J. W. and Mann, K. G. (1978) Biochemistry 17, 4430-4438.
14. Gabriel, D. A., Schaefer, D. J., Roberts, H. R., Aronson, D. L. and Koehler, K. A. (1975) Thrombosis Res. 839-846.
15. Nelsestuen, G. L., Broderius, M. and Martin, G. (1976) J. Biol. Chem. 251, 6886-6893.
16. Nelsestuen, G. L. and Lim, T. K. (1977) Biochemistry 16, 4164-4171.
17. Magnusson, S., Petersen, T. E., Sottrup-Jensen, L. and Claeys, H. (1975) in Proteases and Biological Control, Reich, E., Rifkin, D. B. and Shaw, E. Cold Spring Harbor Laboratory, p. 123-150.
18. Nelsestuen, G. L. and Suttie, J. W. (1972) J. Biol. Chem. 247, 6096-6102.
19. Nelsestuen, G. L. and Suttie, J. W. (1971) Biochem. Biophys. Res. Commun. 45, 198-203.
20. Fujikawa, K., Coan, M. H., Enfield, D. L., Titani, K., Ericsson, L. H. and Davie, E. W. (1974) Proc. Natl. Acad. Sci. USA 71, 427-430.
21. DiScipio, R. G. and Davie, E. W. (1979) Biochemistry 18, 899-904.

22. Fujikawa, K., Thompson, A. R., Legaz, M. E., Meyer, R. G. and Davie, E. W. (1973) Biochemistry 12, 4938.
23. Kisiel, W. and Davie, E. W. (1975) Biochemistry 14, 4928-4934.
24. Fernlund, P., Stenflo, J. and Tufvesson, A. (1978) Proc. Natl. Acad. Sci. USA 75, 5889-5892.
25. Chou, P. Y. and Fasman, G. D. (1978) Ann. Rev. Biochem. 47, 251-276.
26. Lehrer, S. S. (1971) Biochemistry 10, 3254-3263.
27. Patchornik, A., Lawson, W. B. and Witkop, B. (1958) J. Am. Chem. Soc. 80, 4747-4749.
28. Spande, T. F., Witkop, B. (1967) Meth. Enz. 11, 498-522.
29. Heldebrant, C. M. and Mann, K. G. (1973) J. Biol. Chem. 248, 3642-3652.
30. Weber, K. and Osborn, M. (1969) J. Biol. Chem. 244, 4406-4412.
31. Katayama, K. and Titani, K. (1978) FEBS Lett. 95, 157-160.
32. Mort, A. J. and Lamport, D. T. A. (1977) Anal. Biochem. 82, 289-309.
33. Dubois, M., Gilleo, K. A., Hamilton, J. K., Rebers, P. A. and Smith, F. (1956) Anal. Chem. 28, 350.
34. Wang, F.-F. C. and Hirs, C. H. W. (1977) J. Biol. Chem. 252, 8358-8364.
35. Chu, F. K., Trimble, R. B. and Maley, F. (1978) J. Biol. Chem. 253, 8691-8693.

CORRELATION OF METAL ION-INDUCED FLUORESCENCE TRANSITIONS WITH CONFORMATIONAL CHANGES IN PROTHROMBIN FRAGMENT 1

F. G. PRENDERGAST, J. BLOOM, M. R. DOWNING and
K. G. MANN

Mayo Foundation,
Rochester, MN 55901

INTRODUCTION

Data first published by Nelsestuen et al. (1) and later confirmed by work in our laboratory (2) have shown that a variety of metal ions upon interaction with prothrombin fragment 1 lead to quenching of intrinsic fluorescence. The data suggest, moreover, that these changes in fluorescence herald alterations in the structure of the prothrombin fragment 1 molecules which are essential for the eventual expression of lipid binding properties of this component of the prothrombin molecule and hence for promotion of the activation of prothrombin to thrombin. Other data further indicate that the metal ion binding sites on the prothrombin fragment 1 component of prothrombin are formed by γ-carboxyglutamic acid residues in the 1 to 42 aminoacid segment of the aminoterminus of prothrombin fragment 1, a fact which is underscored by the finding that warfarin treatment results in the formation of a defective prothrombin fragment 1 which is devoid of γ-carboxyglutamic acid residues (3) Apparently there is a connection between the interaction of metal ions at these binding sites and some intramolecular event that results in a fluorescence change and subsequent expression of functional activity. The most obvious interpretation of these phenomena is that metal ions induce a conformational transition in the protein molecule but this conclusion cannot be drawn solely on the basis of changes in intrinsic fluorescence, and the issue therefore remains as to how we may make the correlation between the transitions observed in intrinsic fluorescence and the putative configurational change in the prothrombin fragment 1 molecule.

The data presented in this paper are meant to provide a review of our data concerning the metal ion-prothrombin fragment 1 interaction, and the nature of various alterations induced by metal ion binding to this protein. Our final interpretation of the data is that metal ion induced fluorescence transitions indeed reflect configurational changes in prothrombin fragment 1 and that dimerization occurs subsequent to these transitions.

MATERIALS AND METHODS

For all titrations with calcium, a volumetric 1 M $CaCl_2$ stock solution obtained from British Drug House, Poole, England, was used. All other metal salts used in this study were obtained from Ventron Corporation and were the purest available. Proteins were purified by the methods outlined by Heldebrant et al. (4), and protein concentrations were determined as described by Prendergast and Mann (2). Measurements of fluorescence intensity and emission spectra were made on an SLM spectrofluorometer. Experiments were performed in a buffer comprising 0.15 M KCl, 0.01 M PIPES, pH 6.8 at 25°. For experiments involving tryptophan fluorescence an excitation wavelength of 295 nm was employed to minimize the contribution of tyrosine to the fluorescence emission observed at 340 nm. For spectra and fluorescence intensity measurements the excitation monochromator slits were 8 nm, the excitation beam was isolated using a Corning 7-54 filter, and 2 nm slit widths were employed on the emission monochromators. Fluorescence intensity was recorded as a voltage from a digital voltmeter. An SLM series 800 subnanosecond lifetime instrument, which employs the differential phase and modulation technique, was used for the measurement of fluorescent lifetimes. The excitation signal (λ excitation = 295 nm) was isolated from the emission detector by use of a Corning 0-52 filter. The 0-52 filter is itself fluorescent when excited by UV radiation scattered from the sample; to avoid interference from this fluorescence a filter filled with 1 M sodium nitrite was placed in front of the 0-52 glass preventing excitation by the scattered UV radiation. Measurements of sedimentation velocity and sedimentation equilibrium were made on a Beckman Model E analytical ultracentrifuge and data were analyzed using standard formulation (5). A Durrum stopped flow rapid mix apparatus was employed for studies of the rapid phase of fluorescence quenching observed when prothrombin fragment 1 interacts with metal ions. Circular dichroic spectra were recorded on a Jasco spectropolarimeter. Metal ion binding studies were carried out using conventional or flow equilibrium dialysis.

RESULTS AND DISCUSSION

The concentration-effect curves for the quenching of intrinsic fluorescence of prothrombin fragment 1 by metal ions are shown in Figure 1.

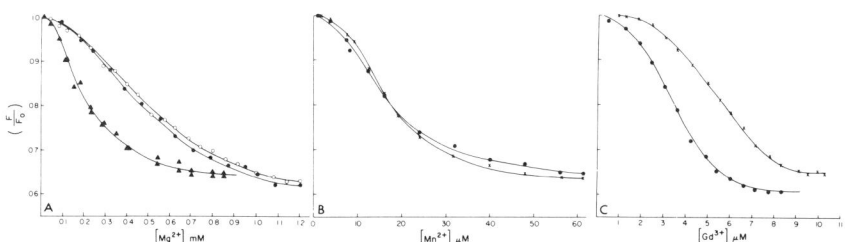

Figure 1. Fluorescence quenching of human and bovine prothrombin fragment 1 by Mg^{++}, Mn^{++} and Gd^{+++}. Fractional fluorescence (F/F_o) is plotted versus the concentration of the respective ion. A, fluorescence quenching of human (▲——▲) and bovine (CIRCLES) prothrombin fragment 1 by Mg^{++}. Bovine prothrombin fragment 1 was employed at two concentrations, 0.10 mg/ml (●——●) and 0.44 mg/ml (O——O). B, fluorescence quenching of human (●——●) and bovine (X——X) prothrombin fragment 1 by Mn^{++}. C, fluorescence quenching of human (●——●) and bovine (X——X) prothrombin fragment 1 by Gd^{+++}. Concentration-effect curves for Ca^{++} binding are given in Figure 5.

The curves are grossly sigmoidal but are skewed. It is clear that a host of divalent cations (within and outside of the group IIA cation series), and also lanthanide ions, are capable of effecting this fluorescence transition and these data are amply corroborated by those of Nelsestuen and co-workers (1,6,7). Calcium and magnesium are approximately equivalent in their ability to effect this fluorescence transition, but manganese is more efficient than either and lanthanides more effective yet.

In part, the increased quenching of manganese may be attributable to its paramagnetic character, but in large measure, the increased effectiveness of manganese as a quenching agent over calcium or magnesium appears to be attributable to its tighter binding to the protein. Bajaj et al. (8) used ESR spectroscopy to determine the binding parameters for manganese to prothrombin fragment 1 and showed that there are apparently two binding sites for this ion per molecule of prothrombin fragment 1 with an affinity of about 10^{-5}M Kd. The tervalent lanthanides might be expected to bind more tightly than divalent cations; it is also known that they may act as isomorphic replacements for calcium (9,10). It is therefore not surprising to find that, in general, the lanthanides are effective at micromolar concentrations. In addition, the data of Furie et al. (11) clearly demonstrate that prothrombin fragment 1 has two high affinity sites for lanthanides. The significance of the binding of magnesium, manganese and lanthanides to prothrombin fragment 1 is underscored by the finding that these ions can partially support the activation of prothrombin to thrombin. Prendergast and Mann (2) showed, for example, that whereas 1 mM magnesium by itself would not support the activation of prothrombin to thrombin, that concentration of magnesium in the presence of 0.3 mM of calcium added several minutes subsequent to the addition of magnesium would fully promote the activation of bovine prothrombin to thrombin. These data, taken together, suggest rather strongly that there must be two classes of binding sites for metal ions to prothrombin fragment 1, especially with respect to the binding of calcium. By inference, we may deduce that the first class of sites comprises a minimum of two binding sites which are fairly degenerate in the sense that they can bind a variety of divalent and tervalent cations. We infer that metal ion binding to these sites results in quenching of intrinsic fluorescence. The metal ion binding data for prothrombin fragment 1 are summarized in Table 1.

TABLE 1. Bovine Prothrombin Fragment 1 Metal Ion Binding.

Metal Ion	# Sites	K_d (M)
Calcium[a]	5-6	6.3×10^{-4}
Calcium[b]	10-12	6.3×10^{-4}
Magnesium[c]	---	2×10^{-4}
Manganese[d]	2	2.2×10^{-5}
Gadolinium[e]	2	1.6×10^{-7}

The superscripts a through e relate to references 2 & 17, 16, 2, 8, and 11, respectively.

Nelsestuen also showed that in bovine prothrombin fragment 1 the fluorescence quenching process was not instantaneous upon the addition of metal ion but showed a fast phase amounting to about 20% of the total fluorescence followed by a slow decrease in fluorescence intensity which was highly temperature dependent (1). These data are corroborated by those of Prendergast et al. (10) (Fig. 2) who have also evaluated this temperature dependence; the activation enthalpy for this temperature dependent quenching process was 19 kcal/mole, very similar to the values obtained by Nelsestuen et al. (1). In order to fully describe the quenching process, at least phenomenologically, however, it is clear that we need to be able to describe the entire quenching profile, which includes the rapid initial phase. The reaction is, however, far too rapid

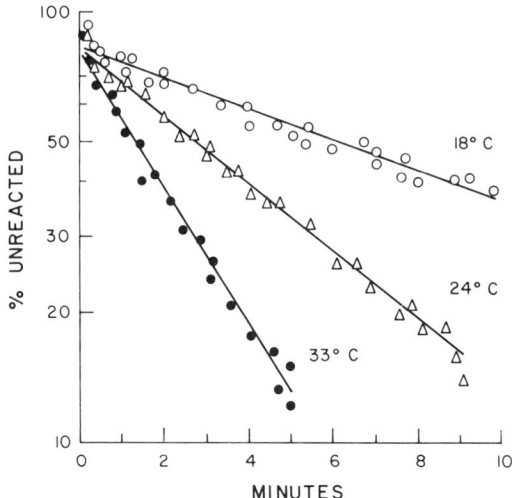

Figure 2. Temperature dependence of the rate of fluorescence quenching of bovine prothrombin fragment 1 by Ca^{++}. Protein concentration was 5×10^{-6} M and the concentration of Ca^{++} was 2 mM.

to be followed by a conventional fluorometer and for that reason the experiments have been done in a stop-flow rapid mix apparatus which allowed us to probe the quenching of fluorescence in a millisecond time frame. The reduced data from stop-flow rapid mix experiments with prothrombin fragment 1 and calcium are given in Figure 3. It is clear from

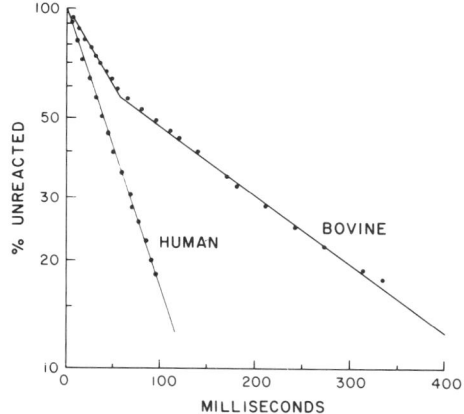

Figure 3. Kinetics of Ca^{++}-induced fluorescence quenching of human and bovine prothrombin fragment 1. The Y axis is given as the percentage quenching and the X axis is time in milliseconds. Percentage quenching was determined at $(F_t - F_\infty / F_o - F_\infty)$ where F_o is the fluorescence intensity in the absence of metal ions, F_∞ the minimum fluorescence intensity observed for the rapid phase of the fluorescence quenching, and F_t the fluorescence intensity at chosen points in time during the rapid phase of fluorescence quenching.

the data presented in Figures 2 and 3 that the kinetics of rapid fluorescence quenching in the bovine and human system are quite different. In the bovine system the initial phase accounts for approximately 20 to 25% of the total quenching observed in prothrombin fragment 1 upon the addition of metal ion; the slow phase clearly predominates. In human prothrombin fragment 1 the rapid phase accounts for 80% of the total quenching observed. The subsequent slow phase accounts for the remaining 20% of the transition and has a rate constant of approximately 2.5 min^{-1}. The initial phase of the quenching in the bovine system is clearly biphasic whereas that in the human system is apparently a single phase.

While fluorescence signal changes provide a useful measure of a phenomenological event occurring in a peptide or protein, by themselves they are insufficient to allow a conclusion to be drawn regarding configurational changes in the molecule. This is especially true of steady-state fluorescence measurements such as the measurement of fluorescence intensity, but considerably more insight into the mechanisms involved in fluorescence quenching may be obtained from measurements of fluorescence lifetimes. We have made such measurements on prothrombin fragment 1 in presence and absence of metal ions and the data are given in Table 2.

TABLE 2. Intrinsic Fluorescence Lifetimes (in n sec) of Human Prothrombin, Prothrombin Fragment 1, and Bovine Prothrombin Fragment 1 and N-acetyl Tryptophanamide (25°C, λex = 295 nm, 30 MHz modulation frequency).

Protein	Additions	τ_ϕ	τ_m
Prothrombin	None	1.54	2.9
	Ca^{++}	1.44	2.8
	6 M GuHCl	2.1	2.5
Prothrombin fragment 1 (human)	None	0.90	1.1
	Ca^{++}	0.67	0.9
	6 M GuHCl	2.1	2.53
Prothrombin fragment 1 (bovine)	None	1.13	2.24
	Ca^{++}	0.76	1.67
	6 M GuHCl	2.34	2.88
N-Acetyl tryptophanamide	6 M GuHCl	2.81	2.84

The data show that in prothrombin fragment 1 the intrinsic fluorescence lifetime is short in both the bovine and human systems and all emitting tryptophan residues are affected. The splitting of the values for fluorescence lifetime observed by phase and modulation (especially in prothrombin) is probably indicative of the heterogeneity of the environments of the multiple tryptophans. Addition of guanidinium chloride tends to equalize the fluorescence lifetimes, but the fact that the values are still split indicates that microdomains of structure in the region of the tryptophan residues are probably retained even when the proteins are placed in guanidinium chloride, probably due to the retention of disulfide bonds. The fact that the fluorescence lifetime of N-acetyltryptophan amide is the same in guanidinium chloride as it is in water validates this latter conclusion.

The fluorescence lifetimes of the tryptophyl moieties in prothrombin fragment 1 are significantly shorter than that of N-acetyltryptophan amide which suggests further that the tryptophan residues in prothrombin fragment 1 even in the absence of any metal ion are already being quenched. There are two ways in which fluorescence of tryptophan residues, and in fact of all fluorophores, may be quenched. First, if there are substances which form ground state complexes with the tryptophan moieties, then the quantum yield (fluorescence intensity) will inevitably decrease since the ground state complex is non-fluorescent. Second, if the quenching molecule must diffuse to the site of the fluorophore and collide with the fluorophore during the fluorescence lifetime of that residue, then the quenching is dynamic and the fluorescence lifetime will be shortened by the quenching process. Since fluorescence lifetimes of the tryptophan residue in prothrombin fragment 1 are considerably less than those observed for tryptophan and analogues in an aqueous environment, it is clear that this low intrinsic fluorescence lifetime of prothrombin fragment 1 in the absence of metal ion must be attributable to dynamic, intramolecular events; it is known from the work of Weinryb and Steiner (11) that carboxyl groups, histidine, disulfide bond and amino moieties can all effectively quench the fluorescence of tryptophan. It seems plausible therefore that one or more of such groups may be sufficiently near the main tryptophan residue responsible for the intrinsic fluorescence of prothrombin fragment 1 and that intramolecular fluctuations rapidly approximate this quenching moiety and the tryptophan side chain and causes an apparent dynamic quenching of the tryptophan fluorescence. Certainly, the low quantity yield (and therefore lifetime) in this particular protein cannot be due to solvent effects on tryptophan fluorescence. Somehow the addition of metal ions and binding of these to two sites on prothrombin fragment 1 triggers an enhanced ability for intramolecular residues to quench intrinsic fluorescence; this could arise either from an increased <u>rate</u> of intramolecular motions or a configurational change in prothrombin fragment 1 that brings the fluorophore and the intrinsic quenching agent closer together. The latter explanation seems more likely. It would appear from the sequence of prothrombin fragment 1 that tryptophan 41 may be the particular residue affected but there are no data to support this at present.

Further evidence that there are two classes of sites involved in the binding of metal ions to prothrombin fragment 1 may be adduced from the studies of hydrodynamic properties of that protein that are caused by metal ion binding. In Figure 4, for example, data are shown on the

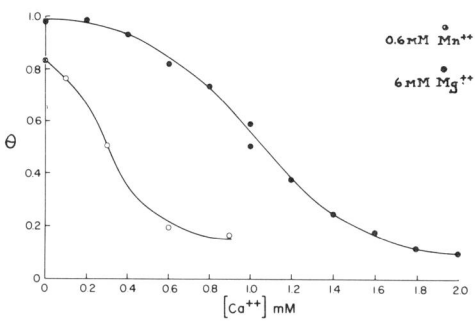

Figure 4. Titration of prothrombin fragment 1 (bovine) sedimentation behavior with Ca^{++} alone, and Ca^{++} in the presence of 1 mM Mg^{++} (●). The fraction of prothrombin fragment 1 (○) is plotted versus absolute Ca^{++} concentration. The values inserted on the right hand side of the graph are the calculated fraction monomer in the presence of 0.6 mM Mn^{++} and 6 mM Mg^{++}.

sedimentation velocity behavior of prothrombin fragment 1 when exposed to metal ions. The sedimentation data indicate that calcium induces a dimerization of prothrombin fragment 1 (2) and these data have been corroborated by the work of Agarwal et al. (12) working with prothrombin. In Figure 4 the Y axis denotes and gives values for the fraction monomer while the X axis gives the concentration of added calcium. The graphs are again sigmoidal and show that upon the addition of calcium to a solution of prothrombin fragment 1 (at 6 mg/ml of protein) there is a progressive dimerization transition of the protein which is essentially complete at 2 mM Ca^{++}, interestingly, the concentration of Ca^{++} found in plasma. Although not shown in the figure, 6 mM magnesium causes no significant dimerization. However, if 1 mM of magnesium is added and the sedimentation velocity determined as before while the calcium ion concentration is varied, the concentration-effects curve is shifted markedly to the left; apparently magnesium is playing a permissive role in allowing calcium ions to mediate the dimerization process. This differentiation of the fluorescence transition in the dimerization process is even more strikingly shown by manganese, for which the fluorescence transition is essentially complete at 60 µM metal ion. Ten times this concentration or 600 µM manganese shifts the sedimentation coefficient by only 4%.

All these data taken together strongly support the notion of two classes of sites, the first class of sites being largely responsible for the fluorescence transition while the second class of sites are responsible for dimerization or, as Prendergast and Mann have shown (2), for the lipid binding process which determines the ability of prothrombin to be activated to thrombin. It seems reasonable to suppose that the initial binding of metal ions to prothrombin fragment 1 triggers a change in conformation of the molecule to allow the second phenomenon. The fact that the fluorescence change is observed at very low protein concentrations (ca 10^{-6} M) and that the midpoint of the transition occurs at low ion concentrations, while the dimerization process occurs only at high protein concentration, and maximally at 2 mM Ca^{++} indicates that the fluorescence transitions cannot be attributed to this dimerization process. Neither the fluorescence data nor the information gleaned from sedimentation velocity experiments is sufficient to sustain a conclusion that metal ions induce conformational transition in prothrombin fragment 1. More direct evidence is provided by measurements of circular dichroic

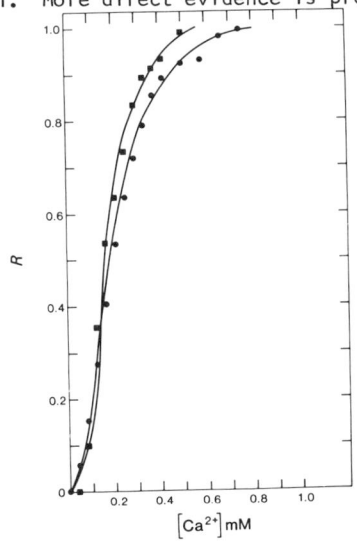

Figure 5. Ca^{++} titration by CD at 231 nm and fluorescence quenching (15) of bovine prothrombin fragment 1 (0.11 mg/ml) in a 1 cm cuvette. For the CD experiment, R is the mean residue ellipticity at a given Ca^{++} concentration divided by the value obtained when no further change in the spectrum occurs upon Ca^{++} addition. For the fluorescence quenching experiment, R is defined as $(F-F_o)/(F_\infty-F_o)$ where F is the observed fluorescence, F_o is the untitrated value, and F_∞ is the value obtained when no further quenching occurs upon Ca^{++} addition.

spectra. Such data are given in Figure 5. These show that the binding
of calcium ions to prothrombin fragment 1 induces a shift in the CD
spectra of that protein to the right, the changes in molar ellipticity
being consistent with the interpretation of an apparent increase in helical content in prothrombin fragment 1 as a consequence of metal ion binding. The involvement of the γ-carboxyglutamic acid residues and of metal
binding thereto in the change in the CD spectrum is, however, indicated
by the fact that prothrombin fragment 1, when decarboxylated by heat
treatment, ment, shows a CD spectrum essentially identical to that of
prothrombin fragment 1 when no metal ions are bound and this CD spectrum
of decarboxylated prothrombin fragment 1 is unchanged by the subsequent
addition of calcium ions (Tuhy and Mann, manuscript submitted for
publication).

TABLE 3. T_m Values for Metal Ions Which Induce Circular Dichroism
Transitions in Human and Bovine Prothrombin Fragment 1.

Metal Ion	T_m (CD)	T_m (Fluorescence)	
Ca^{++}	0.25 mM (H)[a]	0.22 mM (H)[b]	
	0.20 mM (B)[a]	0.35 mM (B)[b]	0.40 mM (B)[c]
	0.17 mM (B)[d]	0.19 mM (B)[d]	
Mg^{++}	0.23 mM (H)	0.22 mM (H)[b]	
	0.21 mM (B)	0.25 mM (B)[b]	
Mn^{++}	22.8 μM (H)	12.6 μM (H)	

The letters H and B in parentheses refer to human and bovine prothrombin
fragment 1, respectively. [a] The circular dichroism T_m values are from
ref. 15. [b] These refer to T_m values determined from fluorescence data
in ref. 2. [c] These refer to T_m values from ref. 1. These are T_m values
obtained by Bloom and Mann (15) on a freshly purified sample of bovine
prothrombin fragment 1; as Bloom and Mann (15) point out, the "age" of
the prothrombin fragment 1 influences the concentration-effect curve
for metal ion induced fluorescence transitions. This may explain the
disparity in T_m values given above (and see Fig. 1).

   An examination of the T_m values for the CD change (Table 3) indicate
that the midpoint of the sigmoidal transition observed with various metal
ions are close to or identical with those obtained from fluorescence
measurements. This indicates that the change in conformation observed in
the CD spectra is associated with metal ion filling of the first two sites
on prothrombin fragment 1 and that thereafter the liganding of calcium
to the protein causes no further change in gross configuration. In most
instances at equivalent protein concentrations, transition midpoints
observed for CD and fluorescence data are exactly equivalent except for
the data obtained with manganese. The fluorescence transition midpoint
for manganese appears to be at a somewhat lower concentration of this
metal ion but this divergence can be interpreted in terms of paramagnetic
quenching by bound manganese. In contrast, the CD transition, which is
not influenced by paramagnetic factors, occurs with a transition midpoint equivalent to the dissociation constant obtained by Bajaj et al.
(8) from spin resonance data. The stoichiometry observed by Bajaj et al.
on the filling of these sites with manganese is 2 moles Mn^{++} per mole
of prothrombin fragment 1. This same stoichiometry was obtained by
Furie et al. (11) for the binding of gadolinium to prothrombin fragment 1
at low concentrations of protein and metal ion.

   These data led us to suggest the following model for the binding of
metal ions to prothrombin fragment 1 and subsequent expression of func-

tion in this particular domain of prothrombin (15). We propose that there are eight potential sites on prothrombin fragment 1 that are capable of binding metal ions (Fig. 6). The first two are non-selective in that they will bind a host of different metal ions and that upon interaction with metal ligands a change in the conformation of the protein is induced which approximates the residue or residues capable of quenching tryptophan fluorescence (for example, histidine, carboxylate, disulfide groups or cationic amino groups). The metal ion binding sites exposed

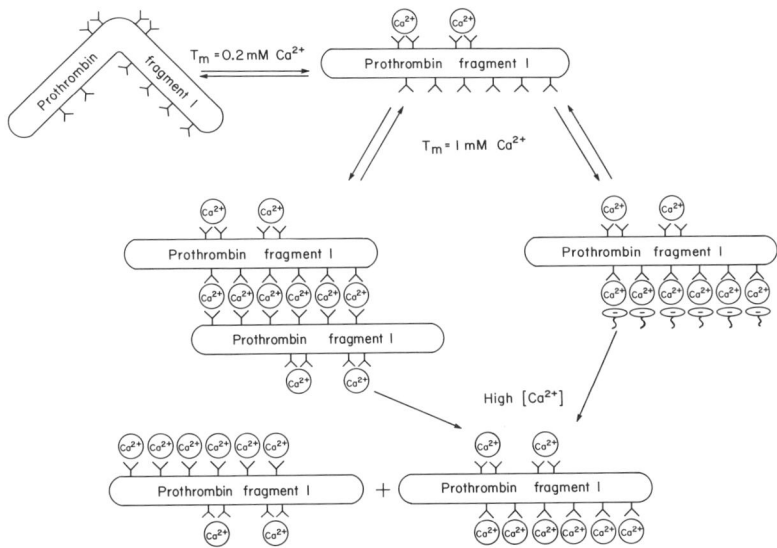

Figure 6. Models of Ca^{++} binding to prothrombin fragment 1. The stoichiometries for the interaction of prothrombin fragment 1 with Ca^{++} are calculated to be 5 moles Ca^{++} per mole protein where complete dimerization occurs and 8 moles Ca^{++} per mole of protein in the presence of lipid or at high concentrations of Ca^{++}.

by this initial reaction bind calcium relatively specifically. The protein may dimerize through calcium bridging but the data indicate that that such an event will occur only at high concentrations of protein and calcium, well outside the concentration limits observed for the metal ion effects on either fluorescence or circular dichroic spectra. If there is an appropriate lipid surface available, interaction of prothrombin fragment 1 will occur preferentially with that surface, again minimizing the tendency for dimer formation. Finally, at concentrations of calcium much higher than the concentration of protein, it is likely that once again the monomeric species will prevail but with all the sites filled with calcium ions as shown in Figure 6. There is some divergence in the literature with regard to equilibrium dialysis derived calcium binding data, both with respect to curve shape and the potential number of binding sites on prothrombin fragment 1. Since conventional equilibrium dialysis experiments with prothrombin fragment 1 must be conducted at relatively high protein concentrations under which all transitions would be observed to a greater or lesser degree, it is likely that some divergence in data may be resolved with appropriate consideration of the various transitions in prothrombin fragment 1.

ACKNOWLEDGEMENTS

This work was supported by Grants HL 17430-D and HL 07069 from the National Heart Lung and Blood Institute (to K.G.M.), and the Mayo Foundation. We especially thank Mrs. E. Webster for her help in preparation of this manuscript.

REFERENCES

1. Nelsestuen, G. L. (1976) J. Biol. Chem. 251, 5648-5656.
2. Prendergast, F. G. and Mann, K. G. (1977) J. Biol. Chem. 252, 840-850.
3. Suttie, J. W. and Jackson, C. M. (1977) Physiol. Rev. 57, 1-70.
4. Heldebrant, C. M., Butkowski, R. J., Bajaj, S. P. and Mann, K. G. (1973) J. Biol. Chem. 248, 7149-7163.
5. Chervenka, C. H. (1970) A Manual of Methods for the Analytical Ultracentrifuge, Beckman Instruments, Inc., Palo Alto, California.
6. Nelsestuen, G. L., Broderius, M. and Martin, G. (1976) J. Biol. Chem. 251, 6886-6893.
7. Lim, T. K., Bloomfield, V. A. and Nelsestuen, G. L. (1977) Biochemistry 16, 4177-4181.
8. Bajaj, S. P., Nowak, T. and Castellino, F. J. (1976) J. Biol. Chem. 251, 6294-6299.
9. Barry, C. D., North, A. C. T., Glasel, J. A., Williams, R. J. P. and Xavier, A. V. (1971) Nature 232, 236-245.
10. Dwek, R. A., Morallee, K. G., Nieboer, E., Richard, R. E., Williams, R. J. P. and Xavier, A. V. (1971) Eur. J. Biochem. 21, 204-209.
11. Furie, B. C., Mann, K. G. and Furie, B. (1976) J. Biol. Chem. 251, 3235-3241.
12. Prendergast, F. G., Downing, M. R., Morris, R. G. and Mann, K. G. Submitted for publication: Biochemistry.
13. Weinryb, I. and Steiner, R. F. (1971) Excited States of Proteins and Nucleic Acids (Weinryb, I. & Steiner, R. F., eds.) pp. 277-316, Plenum Press, New York.
14. Agarwal, G. P., Gallagher, J. G., Aune, K. C. and Armeniades, C. D. (1977) Biochemistry 16, 1865-1870.
15. Bloom, J. W. and Mann, K. G. (1978) 17, 4430-4438.
16. Henriksen, R. A. and Jackson, C. M. (1975) Arch. Biochem. Biophys. 170, 149-159.

CALCIUM INDUCED CONFORMATIONAL CHANGE IN HUMAN PROTHROMBIN

RICHARD BENAROUS, GÉRARD GACON, MARIE-JOSÈPHE RABIET and DOMINIQUE LABIE

Institut de Pathologie Moléculaire INSERM,
CHU Cochin Port-Royal 24,
rue du faubourg Saint-Jacques,
75014 Paris, France

INTRODUCTION

Prothrombin and the other vitamin K dependent coagulation factors contain γ-carboxyglutamic acid residues (1-3) which are apparently essential for their Ca^{++} binding ability (4,5). The binding of Ca^{++} to prothrombin as well as to isolated prothrombin fragment 1 (F 1) is a highly cooperative process (5-7), which implies presumably a protein conformation change. Such conformational transition has been reported essentially with isolated F 1 by changes in circular dichroism and Trp fluorescence quenching (8-11). Changes in the UV absorption spectra due to binding of Ca^{++} to bovine prothrombin fragment 1 have been mentioned by Henrikson and Jackson (12). But, up to now, no extensive studies have been reported about this phenomenon, and there are no available data concerning the whole prothrombin molecule. In the present study the UV spectral changes induced by Ca^{++} binding to human prothrombin and F 1 are described. Tentative correlations with structural modifications occurring within the protein structure upon Ca^{++} binding are proposed.

MATERIAL AND METHODS

Human prothrombin fragment 1 and fragment 2 were prepared according to Mann (13). UV absorption spectra were recorded on a Cary 118 C spectrometer. All experiments were performed at 25° in 0.025 M Tris HCl, 0.1 M NaCl, pH 7.4. Solvent perturbation studies were performed according to the method of Herkovitz and Laskowski (14). Fluorescence experiments were performed in an Aminco spectrofluorometer according to Prendergast and Mann (10).

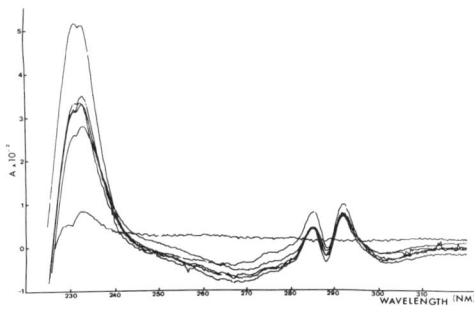

Figure 1. Ultra-violet absorption difference spectrum induced by Ca^{++} binding to prothrombin fragment 1 (0.4 mg/ml) in 0.025 M Tris HCl, pH 7.4, NaCl 0.1 M and Ca^{++} (0-2 mM). Analogous spectra were obtained with human prothrombin (not shown).

RESULTS

Absorption Difference Spectroscopy

The binding of Ca^{++} ions to human prothrombin or to F 1 is associated with a UV absorption difference spectrum characterized in the aromatic region by two maxima at 292 nm and 284-285 nm, and a large maximum at about 233 nm (Fig. 1). The magnitude of the difference spectrum is maximum for 2 mM Ca^{++}. Such spectrum is characteristic of a red shift Trp difference spectrum (15), although a small contribution of tyrosine residues perturbation cannot be excluded. An identical spectrum is obtained with Mg^{++} instead of Ca^{++}. No spectral changes could be detected with F 2 where the weak affinity Ca^{++} binding sites are located (6). The difference spectra induced by Ca^{++} in both isolated F 1 and intact prothrombin are qualitatively identical, and the magnitude of the differences at 292 nm (table I) are roughly similar. The titration curve of

Table I. Comparison between the magnitude of the Ca^{++} induced spectral changes in human prothrombin and prothrombin fragment 1, with respect to their molar concentration.

Table I

	HUMAN PROTHROMBIN	PROTHROMBIN FRAGMENT 1
Concentration	1.16 mg/ml = $1.6 \cdot 10^{-5}$ M	0.41 mg/ml = $1.8 \cdot 10^{-5}$ M
A_{280}	1.70 (E 1 % = 14.7)	0.487 (E 1 % = 1.19)
ΔA_{292}	$12 \cdot 10^{-3}$	$11.5 \cdot 10^{-3}$
$\dfrac{\Delta A_{292}}{\text{molar concentration}}$	$7.5 \cdot 10^2$	$6.4 \cdot 10^2$

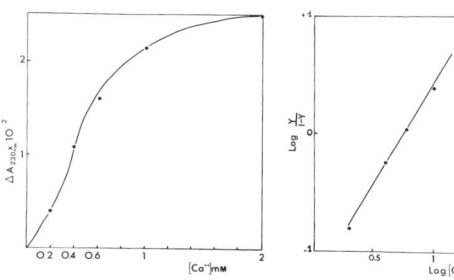

Figure 2. Titration curve for UV spectral changes in fragment 1 (0.4 mg/ml). Difference spectra showing maxium difference at 240 nm. ΔA_{230} was plotted vs. Ca^{++} concentration. Similar curve with smaller difference was also obtained at ΔA_{292}.

the calcium induced spectral change of F 1 is sigmoidal (Fig. 2). The midpoint of transition occurs at 0.4 mM and the n value can be estimated at 1.8. The UV difference spectroscopy experiments were performed in apolar solvent (20 % glycerol) instead of aqueous solution. The major feature observed (Fig. 3) was the persistance of a red shift Trp difference spectrum of similar magnitude when compared to the one obtained in aqueous solution. Thus the spectral modifications are insensitive to changes in the solvent polarity. The main source of the difference spectrum seems therefore to be a local vicinity charge effect of Ca^{++} ions on a Trp residue.

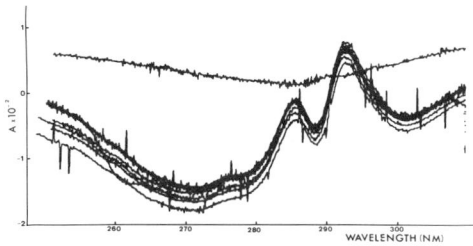

Figure 3. UV absorption difference spectra induced by Ca^{++} binding to prothrombin in the presence of 20 % glycerol. Prothrombin (1 mg/ml) in buffer with 20 % glycerol and Ca^{++} (0.5-2 mM) was compared to prothrombin in the same conditions, but without Ca^{++}.

Solvent Perturbation Studies

However, more substantial conformational changes in the overall protein structure cannot be excluded. We looked for such modifications by using solvent perturbation methods. With no Ca^{++} present (Fig. 4A) the spectrum obtained is due to a perturbation by glycerol of solvent exposed Trp and Tyr residue (16). In the presence of Ca^{++} (Fig. 4B) the magnitude of the glycerol induced spectral changes is markedly reduced. Thus the number of aromatic residues accessible to the solvent must be smaller in prothrombin having bound Ca^{++} as compared to prothrombin without Ca^{++}. Therefore, the binding of Ca^{++} to prothrombin appears also to be associated with an alteration of chromophores environment from an exposed to a buried region in the protein.

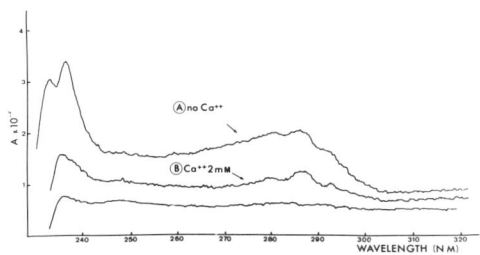

Figure 4. Solvent perturbation studies of prothrombin. <u>A</u>. Prothrombin (1 mg/ml) in Tris buffer was added to one compartment and glycerol 40 % to the second compartment. After establishing a base-line, the sample cuvette was inverted and mixed, and the spectrum recorded. <u>B</u>. Same conditions as in A except that prothrombin and glycerol compartments contained 2 mM Ca^{++}.

DISCUSSION

UV difference spectra of roughly similar magnitude could be recorded either with intact human prothrombin or with isolated F 1. From these results, it can be assumed that the conformational state of the F 1 region, as well as the changes induced by Ca^{++} binding are identical, regardless whether the F 1 is isolated or within the intact prothrombin molecule. This confirms also the idea that the F 1 region within the prothrombin molecule would be a structural domain relatively independent from the two other domains, namely : F 2 and prethrombin 2. Human F 1 contains 3 Trp residues (17) and further investigations are obviously necessary to localize the residue(s) involved in the Ca^{++} induced spectral perturbations. However, comparisons with the results reported by Lindhout and Hemker (18) on Ca^{++} binding to factor X lead us to postulate that the Trp residue 41 in prothrombin might be involved in the observed spectral changes. This assumption is based on the following points: (i) Ca^{++} induced difference spectra on both factor X and prothrombin are strikingly similar; (ii) F 1 and the light chain of factor X present a high degree of structural homology (19); (iii) among the 3 Trp residues of human F 1, Trp 41 is exactly homologous to the unique Trp residue of factor X. The nearly pure red shift Trp difference spectra obtained in aqueous solution with both isolated F 1 and intact prothrombin suggest strongly a minor local change due to a vicinity charge effect around a Trp residue located close to the Ca^{++} binding sites. This is substantiated by the persistance of a clear red shift difference spectrum even in the presence of apolar solvent (glycerol 20 %). Put together these data lead to the conclusion that Trp 41 is located in the close vicinity of some of the Ca^{++} binding sites.

Besides the local effect, a conformational transition in the overall structure of the protein can be demonstrated by the solvent perturbation studies. Why the experiments performed in the aqueous solution failed to demonstrate this overall structural change is still uncertain. But taking into account the difference in molecular diameter between H_2O and glycerol, it appears likely that, a crevice or crevices in which some of the chromophores are located decrease(s) sufficiently in size during the conformational change, to exclude glycerol but not H_2O.

ACKNOWLEDGEMENTS

This research was supported by grants from the "Délégation Générale á la Recherche Scientifique et Technique" (grant n° 77-0235) and the "Institut National de la Santé et de la Recherche Médicale (ASR 5).

REFERENCES

1. Stenflo, J., Fernlund, P., Egan, W. and Roepstorff, P. (1974) Proc. Natl. Acad. Sci. US 71, 2730-2733
2. Nelsestuen, G., Zytkovicz, T.H. and Howard, J.B. (1974) J. Biol. Chem. 249, 6347-6350
3. Magnusson, S., Sottrup-Jensen, L., Petersen, T.E., Morris, H.R. and Dell, A. (1974) FEBS Lett. 44, 189-193
4. Stenflo, J. and Ganrot, P.O. (1973) Biochem. Biophys. Res. Commun. 50, 98-104
5. Suttie, J.W. and Jackson, C.M. (1977) Physiol. Rev. 57, 1-70
6. Bajaj, S.P., Butkowski, R.J. and Mann, K.G. (1975) J. Biol. Chem. 250, 2150-2156
7. Benarous, R., Elion, J.E. and Labie, D. (1976) Biochimie 58, 391-394
8. Bjork, I. and Stenflo, J. (1973) FEBS Lett. 32, 343-346

9. Nelsestuen, G.L. (1976) J. Biol. Chem. 251, 5648-5656
10. Prendergast, F.G. and Mann, K.G. (1977) J. Biol. Chem. 252, 840-850
11. Bloom, J.W. and Mann, K.G. (1978) Biochemistry 17, 4430-4438
12. Henrikson, R.A. and Jackson, C.M. (1975) Arch. Biochem. Biophys. 170, 149-159
13. Mann, K.G. (1976) Meth. Enzymol. XLV, 123-156
14. Herkovitz, T.T. and Laskowski, M.J. (1962) J. Biol. Chem. 237, 2481-2492
15. Donovan, J.W. (1973) Meth. Enzymol. XXVII, 497-525
16. Herkovitz, T.T. Meth. Enzymol. XI, 748-775
17. Mann, K.G. and Elion, J.E. (1977) Prothrombin in CRC Handbook Series in Clinical Lab. Science, Section I : Hematology (Schmidt, R.M. ed.) CRC Press, Cleveland, Ohio (in press)
18. Lindhout, M.J. and Hemker, M.C. (1978) Biochim. Biophys. Acta 584, 66-75
19. Enfield, D.L., Ericsson, L.H., Walsh, K.A., Neurat, H.H. and Titani, K. (1975) Proc. Natl. Acad. Sci. USA 72, 16-19

CALCIUM BINDING TO PROTHROMBIN FRAGMENT-1 BY ULTRAVIOLET DIFFERENCE SPECTROSCOPY

G. M. BRENCKLE, C. W. PENG, and C. M. JACKSON

Department of Biological Chemistry
Washington University School of Medicine
St. Louis, MO 63110

INTRODUCTION

The spectral properties of prothrombin and Prothrombin Fragment 1 are altered upon calcium binding as demonstrated by both fluorescence and ultraviolet difference spectroscopy (1,2). The reporting chromophore is tryptophan, although there is a small contribution (6-8%) from tyrosine (3). Bovine Factor X, which has only one tryptophan in its light chain, has a calcium induced difference spectrum almost identical with Fragment 1. Although there are three tryptophan residues in Fragment 1, by comparison with Factor X one may assume that the spectral perturbation is due mainly to the common tryptophan residue (trp 41 in Factor X, trp 42 in Fragment 1). However, contributions from the other two tryptophans cannot be ruled out.

Fluorescence quenching titration data have shown that divalent metal ions bind with apparent positive cooperativity and have been interpreted as indicating a protein conformation change which occurs after the bind-binding of two to five calcium ions (4,5). Recently it has been reported that divalent metal ions induce dimerization of Fragment 1 (2,5). As ligand induced self association can be responsible for cooperative ligand binding (6,7), an investigation of the possibility that self association might account for the cooperativity observed in the spectral and divalent metal ion binding properties of Fragment 1 has been undertaken. The following experiments were performed in an attempt to investigate the nature of the shift in the electronic transitions of the reporting tryptophan and to assess the possible contribution of self association to the spectral perturbation.

RESULTS

Ion Induced Ultraviolet Difference Spectra

Divalent and monovalent metal ion induced difference spectra are shown in Figure 1. From comparison with model compounds, it can be concluded that these spectra satisfy the criteria for charge induced perturbations of the tryptophan electronic transitions (8,9). The monovalent ion induced spectra also appear to be charge induced and, while not the same, are similar to the divalent ion spectra. As fluorescence and absorption are essentially reciprocal processes, the ion induced perturbations can also be monitored by fluorescence quenching. At 1.25 M NaCl the fluorescence is decreased 5-10%, while at 4.5 M LiCl the signal is decreased by 20-30% from its initial value. Calcium at 10 mM quenches the fluorescence by about 40%. These observations are consistent with the interpretation that the spectral perturbation is due to alteration of the electrostatic environment of the reporting tryptophan either by specific divalent ion binding or by a different, weaker process at high ionic strength.

Ultraviolet Difference Spectral Titration of Divalent Ion Binding

Calcium induced difference spectral titration curves are sigmoid, Figure 2, in agreement with fluorescence titration data reported previously (3).

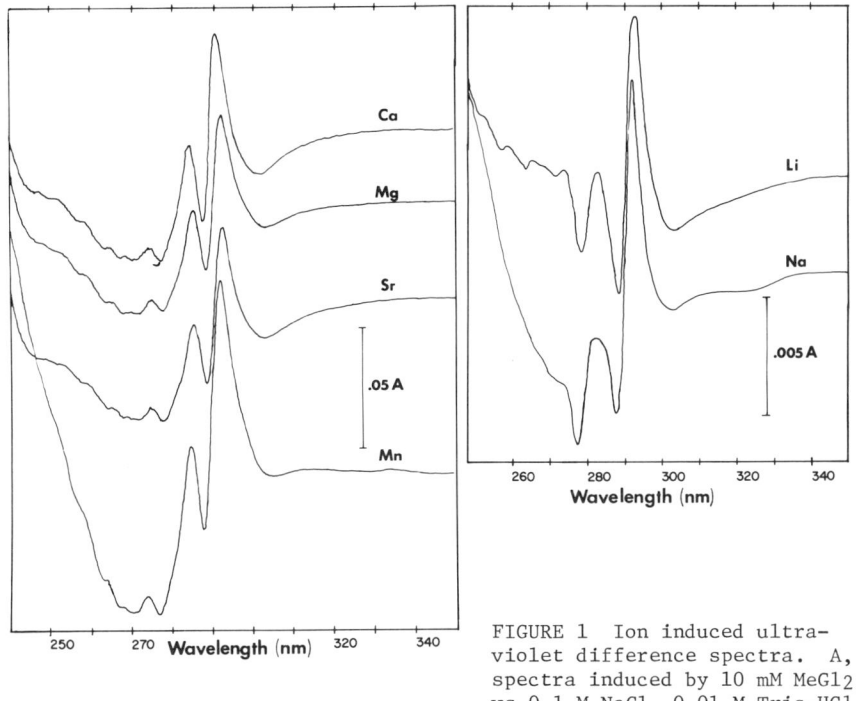

FIGURE 1 Ion induced ultraviolet difference spectra. A, spectra induced by 10 mM MeGl$_2$ vs 0.1 M NaCl, 0.01 M Tris-HCl, pH 7.5 reference buffer. B, Spectra induced by 1.2 M NaCl, or 4.8 M LiCl vs 0.01 M Tris-HCl, pH 7.5 reference buffer.

If the binding and spectral behavior of Fragment 1 are affected only by an intramolecular process, such as a protein conformation change, the calcium titration data should be independent of the concentration of Fragment 1. However, if divalent ion induced dimerization, an intermolecular process, is altering the binding behavior, it should be possible to observe protein concentration dependence. The maximum spectral shift, $\Delta\varepsilon_{max}$, is independent of the concentration of Fragment 1, Figure 3, indicating that the same final state can be reached at all protein concentrations. However, the calcium concentration at which the half maximal spectral shift is obtained is dependent upon the concentration of Fragment 1, Figure 4. The protein concentration dependence on calcium binding was observed directly by equilibrium binding studies using the Hummel-Dreyer column technique. Using this data, it is possible to relate the spectral shift directly to the average number of sites occupied. At low Fragment 1 concentrations, 2 μM, $\Delta\varepsilon_{max}$ is reached when an average of 3 gram atoms of calcium are bound. At higher protein concentrations, 40 to 80 μM, an average of 7 or 8 sites are occupied. The observation that the spectral change is not a linear function of site occupancy is an indication that certain sites contribute more to the total spectral change than others. If the same binding sites which are necessary to obtain the maximum spectral perturbation at low protein concentration are responsible for the perturbation at high concentration, it is apparent that, as the protein concentration is raised, up to four extra binding sites are filled before the maximum perturbation is obtained. This indicates that the order in which the calcium binding sites are filled is dependent on the protein concentration. These observations demonstrate that the ion binding behavior of Fragment 1 cannot be interpreted by spectral titration data without related equilibrium binding measurements.

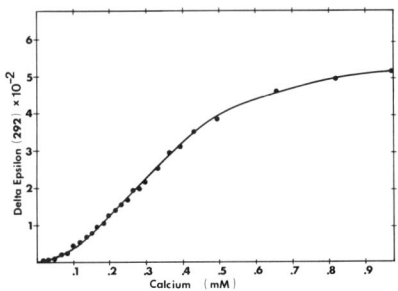

FIGURE 2 Calcium induced difference spectral titration curve. The spectral perturbation is presented as the relative change in the extinction coefficient at 292 nm in reference to 350 nm.

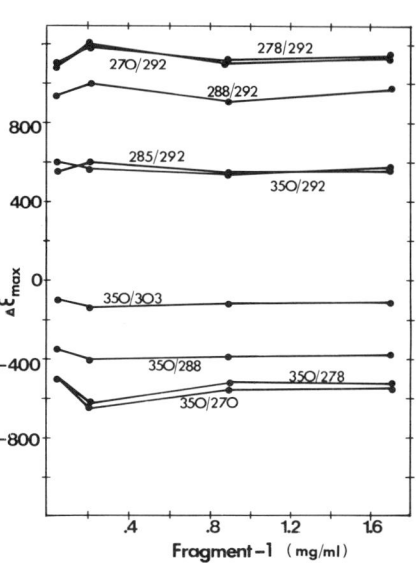

FIGURE 3 The effect of protein concentration on the maximum spectral perturbation at different wavelengths.

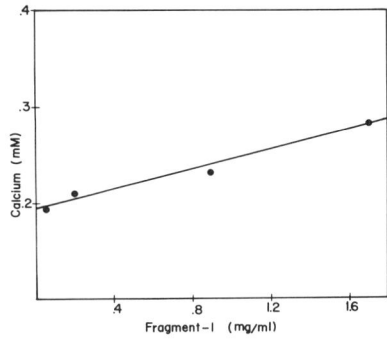

FIGURE 4 The effect of protein concentration on the calcium concentration at which half the maximal spectral perturbation has been obtained.

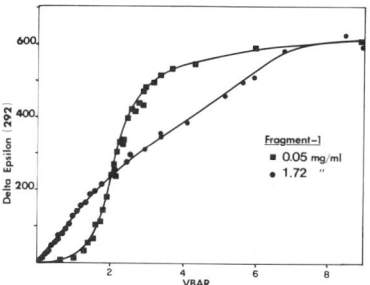

FIGURE 5 The change in the extinction coefficient at 292 nm as a function of the average site occupancy.

DISCUSSION

The ion induced spectral behavior of Fragment 1 may be explained by charge induced perturbation of the electronic transitions of the tryptophan residues, most probably trp 42. Such an explanation would require that the occupation of certain divalent ion binding sites alter the charge environment around tryptophan, either by charge neutralization or by altering the dissociation of another ionizable group. Binding to these sites would introduce shifts in the two electronic transitions of the tryptophan indole, depending on the relative orientation of the transitions and the altered charge. Ion binding to other sites would be less able to perturb the electrostatic environment and therefore make a smaller contribution to the spectral change. High concentrations of monovalent ions would most likely introduce similar, much weaker perturbations of the environment by screening effects and altering hydrogen ion activity. The difference spectral titration curves would exhibit apparent cooperativity and complex protein concentration dependence due to the different relative contributions of various sites to the total spectral change and to the effects of ion induced self association on binding.

This simple model, while consistent with the data, is most certainly one of many such models. The presence of protein concentration dependence in the interaction of Fragment 1 with calcium indicates that a protein conformation change is not sufficient to explain the data, and that the effects of ligand induced self association must be included. While a protein conformation change may affect the calcium binding, a skeptical analysis shows that the data do not force such a conclusion.

ACKNOWLEDGMENTS

This work was supported by grant HL 14147 from the National Heart, Lung and Blood Institute. One of us, CMJ held an Established Investigatorship from the American Heart Association during the time that these studies were performed.

REFERENCES

1. Nelsestuen, G.L. (1976) J. Biol. Chem. 251, 5648-5656.
2. Jackson, C.M., Peng, C.W., Brenckle, G.M., Jonas, A. and Stenflo, J. (1979) J. Biol. Chem., in press.
3. Jonas, A. and Jackson, C.M., unpublished observations.
4. Nelsestuen, G.L., Broderius, M. and Martin, G. (1976) J. Biol. Chem. 251, 6886-6893.
5. Prendergast, F.G. and Mann, K.G. (1977) J. Biol. Chem. 252, 840-850.
6. Nichol, L.W. and Winzor, D.T. (1976) Biochemistry 15, 3015-3019.
7. Cann, J.R. and Hinman, N.D. (1976) Biochemistry 15, 4614-4622.
8. Strickland, E.H., Billups, C. and Kay, E. (1972) Biochemistry 11, 3657-3662.
9. Andrews, G.T. and Forster, L.S. (1972) Biochemistry 11, 1875-1879.

GLA-REGION SECONDARY STRUCTURE IN PROTHROMBIN AND FACTOR X

T. L. CARLISLE, T. MORITA and C. M. JACKSON

Department of Biological Chemistry
Washington University School of Medicine
St. Louis, MO 63110

INTRODUCTION

The gamma-carboxy glutamic acid (Gla)-containing region of prothrombin functions in the calcium-mediated binding of prothrombin to phospholipid. Prothrombin Fragment 1 (F1) binds calcium cooperatively. A conformational change of F1 has been suggested to explain this cooperativity. We are thus interested in the structure of F1 and in any structural change which may occur during calcium binding. Several studies of the circular dichroism (CD) spectra of prothrombin and F1 have previously appeared (1,2). Recently (3) it was shown that CD spectral changes similar to those which occur when F1 binds Ca^{2+} occur also when Mg^{2+} or Mn^{2+} are bound, and that these spectral changes correlate well with the quenching of intrinsic F1 fluorescence by the metal ions.

The goals of the present study include: 1. Obtaining preliminary and qualified estimates of the secondary structure of F1, 2. Refining these estimates by separate measurements on the Gla-region and the "kringle" domain, and 3. Further characterizing any structural change which may occur during calcium binding. In addition to the peptide backbone, aromatic amino acids, cystine, and carbohydrate can also contribute to UV CD thereby complicating its interpretation in terms of secondary structure. Several possible contributions of this kind to the CD of F1 or of its Gla-containing domain are excluded.

RESULTS AND DISCUSSION

The far UV CD spectrum of bovine F1 (in 0.1 M NaCl, 0.01 M Tris-HCl, pH 7.5), shown in Figure 1, is in good agreement with previous results. In addition, a maximum of 2,000 $\pm$ 1,000 deg-cm^2/dmol at about 188 nm was detected using 0.100 M NaF as the supporting electrolyte. Using the reference spectra of Chen, Yang, and Chau (4) to estimate a secondary structure consistent with the spectrum yields values for helix, beta sheet, and nonrepetitive structure of 12, 44, and 98 residues, respectively. The near UV CD spectrum had a strong signal attributable to tryptophan and a negative signal above 300 nm as notable features. The addition of 10 mM $CaCl_2$ results in an increased negative CD signal between 205 and 235 nm and increased positive signal below 200 nm. The change is consistent with 3-5 residues more helix and about 8 residues more beta sheet. Similar but smaller changes occur when the NaCl concentration is increased to 1.0 M, or when the pH is lowered to 5. In addition, a strong positive peak appears near 245 nm, and the 280-290 region signal decreases about 20%. These results confirm previous observations of the CD spectrum of F1 and suggest a preliminary estimate of about 5-15% helix, 25-35% beta sheet, and 50-60% nonrepeating structure.

The similarity of the sequence of the F1 Gla-domain to that of the corresponding region of Factor X light chain suggested that, as for Factor X (T. Morita and C.M. Jackson, this volume), chymotrypsin cleavage might separate intact the Gla-domain and the remainder of F1. The time course by SDS-polyacrylamide gel electrophoresis, and the isolation and structural characterization of the Gla-domain peptide and of F1 less the Gla-domain (F1(-GD)) showed that α-chymotrypsin can cleave both the

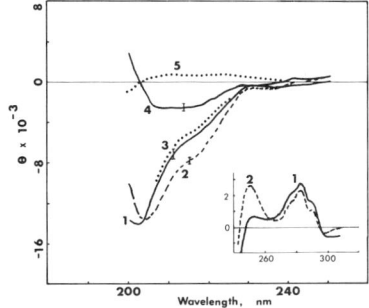

FIGURE 1 CD spectrum of F1: effect of Ca^{2+} or chymotrypsin. F1 without (1) or with (2) 10 mM $CaCl_2$, and after proteolysis with chymotrypsin (3). Computed CD difference spectra resulting from the addition of Ca^{2+} (4) or chymotrypsin (5) are also shown; the inset shows curves 1 and 2 in the near UV. Units are mean residue ellipticity x 10^{-3} (or molar ellipticity x 10^{-4} in the inset) in degree-cm^2/decimole.

tyrosyl-serine peptide bond (45-46) and the tryptophanyl-alanine bond (42-43). F1(-GD) was very resistant to α-chymotrypsin. SDS and alkaline polyacrylamide gel electrophoresis patterns of reaction mixtures of F1 with several other proteases (elastase, subtilisin, plasmin, and trypsin) suggested that these enzymes also rapidly cleaved the same region (40-45) of F1.

In order to assess the effect of these cleavages on its structure, the CD of F1 was monitored during incubation with chymotrypsin. Little change occurred. The signal increased by a maximum of 700 ± 500 deg-cm^2/dmol between 210 and 225 nm, and decreased 20% in the near $\overline{UV}$. The Gla- and kringle domains appear to retain much the same secondary structure present in F1.

The spectra of the isolated Gla-region (1-42) and of F1(-GD) tend to support this conclusion (Fig. 2). About 80% of the near UV CD intensity (280 nm) of F1 is present in the kringle region. An intense peak at 231 nm suggests that the similar feature of the F1 spectrum is contributed by the kringle region. Estimated secondary structure is largely nonrepetitive (66 residues), with 39 residues beta sheet, and 6 of helix. Neither $CaCl_2$ nor $MgCl_2$ (10 mM) produce a significant change in the far UV spectrum of the kringle domain. In contrast, the Gla-domain far UV CD signal changes markedly in 40 mM $MgCl_2$, decreasing by about 5,000 deg-cm^2/dmol at 220 nm (Fig. 2). The estimated values for helix, beta sheet, and non-repetitive are 3, 6, and 33 residues without, and 7, 5, and 30 residues with $MgCl_2$. The Gla-region in isolation appears to have largely nonrepetitive secondary structure, with little helix or beta sheet. Addition of $MgCl_2$ gives rise to changes similar, but not identical, to those seen when F1 binds calcium. As previously reported, $CaCl_2$ precipitates this peptide, and thus could not be tested (5). The different behavior of this peptide with Ca^{2+} and Mg^{2+} ions underscores that the Mg^{2+}-induced changes cannot be interpreted as exactly analogous to those caused by Ca^{2+}.

In a second approach to estimating the structure of the Gla-containing region of F1, the CD difference spectrum for F1 minus the kringle region was calculated (on a molar basis) and divided by the number of residues in the Gla domain, 45 (Fig. 3). The resulting spectrum is similar to that of the isolated peptide. The estimated secondary structure is about 6 residues helix and 9 of beta sheet, marginally higher than for the Gla region in isolation.

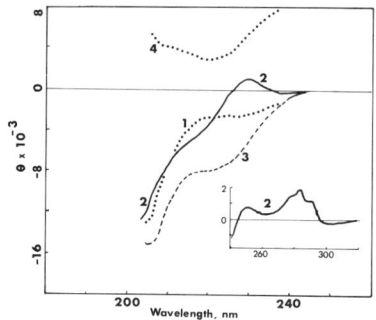

FIGURE 2 CD spectra of F1 residues 1-42 (1) and 46-156 (2), and the effect on residues 1-42 of 40 mM $MgCl_2$ (3). Curve (4), the computed CD difference spectrum for addition of Mg^{2+} to F1 residues 1-42, is displaced upward 8,000 deg-cm^2/dmol. The inset shows the near UV CD spectrum of F1 residues 46-156.

The peptide F1 (1-40) which lacks the tryptophan and one of three phenylalanines gives spectra (with or without Mg^{2+}) similar to those of residues 1-42, demonstrating that Trp 42 and Phe 41 cannot account for the observed change. Reduction and carboxamidomethylation of the Gla-domain was likewise without major effect. An attempt to decarboxylate the Gla residues by the method of Poser and Price (6) gave a derivative with a far UV CD spectrum similar to the intact Gla domain. The spectrum of this putative Glu-containing Gla peptide did not change on the addition of Mg^{2+}.

The far UV CD spectrum of glycopeptides derived from F1 by pronase digestion was found to contribute a negative signal equivalent to a mean residue ellipticity of 260 deg-cm^2/dmol (calculated per dmol of F1) at 211 nm, and did not change on the addition of 10 mM Ca^{2+}.

Residues 1-44 of Factor X yielded spectra similar to those of the F1 Gla domain, and gave similar estimates of secondary structure: 2 residues

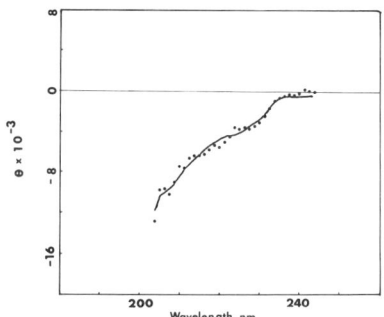

FIGURE 3 Computed CD difference spectrum between F1 and F1 residues 46-156 expressed as mean residue ellipticity for the 45 residue Gla domain of F1 (filled circles). Also shown (solid line) is the calculated lease squares best fit of this spectrum to the reference spectra for helix, beta sheet, and aperiodic structure of Chen et al. (4).

of helix, 4 of beta sheet, and 35 residues nonrepetitive. The change with addition of Mg^{2+} (40 mM) was somewhat larger, giving 9 residues helix, 11 residues beta sheet, and 24 nonrepetitive. Residues 1-41 of Factor X (like Prothrombin F1 (1-42)) lack an intense near UV CD signal. Factor X residues (1-44) also lack intense near UV CD, but develop a signal peaking at 245 nm with a broad negative band at higher wavelengths when 40 mM $MgCl_2$ is added. The magnitude of this signal is about half that generated by addition of Ca^{2+} to F1. This demonstrates that residues 1-44 of Factor X alone are sufficient to give rise to a signal such as that seen for F1 with Ca^{2+}, and supports the suggestion that the Ca^{2+}-induced difference CD peak of F1 at 245 nm originates in the Gla region, probably in the disulfide which links residues 18-23 of that region.

Prothrombin F1 has been separated into kringle and Gla domains by limited proteolysis with chymotrypsin. CD spectra suggest that only minor secondary structural rearrangements accompany the cleavage process. Guarded estimates of the secondary structure were made by fitting the CD spectra of F1 and the two domains with empirically derived reference spectra. The estimates suggested that the secondary structure of F1 is largely nonrepetitive (98 residues) with a substantial component (44 residues) of beta sheet and a small amount of helix (12 residues). The isolated kringle region was also estimated as primarily nonrepetitive (66 residues), and accounted for most (39/44 residues) of the beta sheet of F1. The isolated Gla domain was also estimated to be largely aperiodic with about 3 residues of helix and 6 of beta sheet. A second estimate of the structure of residues 1-45, obtained by fitting the difference spectrum of F1 minus F1 residues 46-156, suggested a marginally higher content of ordered structure in this portion of F1. These estimates must be viewed with caution, in that interpretation of far UV CD spectra is complicated by the contributions of non-peptide chromophores and several other factors.

The CD spectrum of F1 has been reported to change on addition of calcium in a way consistent with small increases in helix and beta sheet structure. The present study demonstrated that spectrum of the isolated kringle region does not change on the addition of Ca^{2+} or Mg^{2+} ions, but that of the Gla region shows a spectral change similar to that of F1 on addition of Mg^{2+}. This change was shown to occur in the absence of the Phe-Trp sequence (residues 41-42), and in reduced-carboxamidomethylated Gla-region peptide, but to be abolished by treatment known to decarboxylate Gla residues. The possibility that some of the CD spectral change during divalent ion binding to F1 might originate in its carbohydrate was eliminated.

ACKNOWLEDGMENTS

This work was supported by grant HL 14147 from the National Heart, Lung and Blood Institute. One of us, CMJ, held an Established Investigatorship from the American Heart Association during the time that these studies were performed.

REFERENCES

1. Bjork, I. and Stenflo, J. (1973) FEBS Lett. 32, 343-346.
2. Gabriel, D.A., Schaefer, D.J., Roberts, H.R., Aronson, D.L. and Koehler, K.A. (1975) Thromb. Res. 7, 839-846.
3. Bloom, J.W. and Mann, K.G. (1978) Biochemistry 17, 4430-4438.
4. Chen, Y.H., Yang, J.T. and Chau, K.H. (1974) Biochemistry 13, 3350-3359.
5. Jackson, C.M., Peng, O.W., Brenckle, G.M., Jonas, A. and Stenflo, J. (1979) J. Biol. Chem. 254, in press.
6. Poser, J.W. and Price, P.A. (1979) J. Biol. Chem. 254, 431-436.

EFFECT OF γ-CARBOXYGLUTAMIC ACIDS ON PROPERTIES OF PROTHROMBINS AND THEIR FRAGMENTS

O. P. MALHOTRA

Veterans Administration Medical Center
Cleveland, OH 44106

INTRODUCTION

Since prothrombin holds a singular position in the blood clotting mechanism, purification, characterization, kinetics of activation, and its biosynthesis continue to be studied intensively. In early 1971, we reported the isolation of atypical prothrombin (1); a year later, different forms of these atypical molecules, induced by dicoumarol (2,3), an antagonist of Vitamin K, were isolated. Vitamin K has now been found essential for the carboxylation of the γ-carbon atoms in the first ten glutamyl residues of normal prothrombin to form γ-carboxyglutamic acids (gla) (4-6). Of our atypical proteins, one form adsorbs and elutes from barium citrate in much the same way as does normal prothrombin, but contains 7 gla's instead of the 10 present in the normal molecule. A second variant which adsorbs onto barium oxalate but not onto barium citrate contains 5 gla's; while the third atypical material which adsorbs onto alumina gel and not onto the insoluble barium salts contains 2 gla's (7).

For the physiological generation of thrombin, prothrombin is cleaved by factor X_a at the Arg^{274}-Thr peptide bond to generate Prothrombin fragment 1·2 and Prethrombin 2 (P_2). The single chain P_2 is then transformed into a biologically active molecule, thrombin, after another cleavage by factor X_a at the Arg^{323}-Ile bond (8). Since Ca^{2+} increases the rate and amount of thrombin formation and since the extra carboxyl group present in gla is the calcium-binding site of prothrombin (4-6), the gla's, therefore, should affect the activation of prothrombin. We have been differentiating the normal and various atypical prothrombins according to Ca^{2+}-binding capacities, electrophoretic mobilities, immunological criteria, structural circular dichroism, and fluorescence studies, pI, and physiological and nonphysiological activation. These studies have further taken into account both the parent prothrombin molecule, as a whole, as well as its fragments, viz., the gla-containing portion, Prothrombin fragment 1 (F_1) and the thrombin-containing portion, Prethrombin 1(P_1). The F_1 and P_1 are generated from prothrombin by undergoing cleavage at the Arg^{156}-Ser peptide bond with thrombin (9). We have found that thrombin also cleaves the Arg^{52}-Asn bond of F_1, and the rates of the two cleavages (at Arg^{156}-Ser and at Arg^{52}-Asn) are related to the number of gla's (10). Furthermore, gla's affect the immunoprecipitation reaction between the F_1's and the antibodies produced against normal prothrombin. The differences amongst the normal and each of the atypical proteins can be related solely to the extent of carboxylation of the 10 glutamyl residues directly or indirectly through their Ca^{2+}-binding ability. In this paper, we shall describe some properties of the normal and atypical prothrombins with particular reference to their activation characteristics and shall compare these properties with those of the P_1's derived from each of the proteins. Our results document that the partially acarboxylated (atypical) prothrombins do have some bioactivity and the amount as well as the time required for the generation of thrombin correlate directly with their gla contents.

MATERIALS AND METHODS

Isolation and purification of bovine normal (10-gla) (11), Ba citrate atypical (7-gla), Ba oxalate (5-gla), and pH 4.6 alumina atypical (2-gla) prothrombins have been described previously (7). The P_1's from each of the prothrombins were generated by digesting the proteins with thrombin and subjecting the digest to DEAE-cellulose chromatography followed by gel filtration on Sephadex G-100 (Pharmacia).

Analytical polyacrylamide (disc-)gel (12) and sodium-dodecyl sulfate (SDS-)gel (13) electrophoresis were performed as described previously (7). For pI determination, column and gel electrofocusing were performed according to the manufacturer's instructions (LKB). Physiological activity was determined by the two stage procedure of Ware and Seegers (14) with some modifications. Bovine serum, without prior absorption, obtained from clotted blood kept for approximately 30 h at room temperature was used as a source of factors V, VII and X. Activation was carried out in polystyrene or nitrocellulose tubes.

RESULTS AND DISCUSSION

By SDS-gel electrophoresis, normal and each of the atypical prothrombins showed a single component, consisting of one polypeptide chain with a molecular mass of about 70,000 daltons. Also by disc-gel (and agar gel) electrophoresis, each material showed a single component; however, the 10-gla (normal) prothrombin moved fastest, the 7-gla protein was the second fastest, followed by the 5-gla variant, and lastly the 2-gla prothrombin (Fig. 1). Understandably then, a mixture of the 10- and 2-gla prothrombins showed two distinct bands. These differences are related to the negative charges contributed by the extra carboxyl groups present in gla's, which are also responsible for the lowering of their pI's. For example, the pI's of normal (10-gla) and 2-gla prothrombins were 4.55 and 4.82, respectively. The gla effect, in differentiating the F_1's, becomes even more profound because the pI of 10-gla F_1 was 3.58 <u>vs</u> the pI of 4.29 for 2-gla F_1.

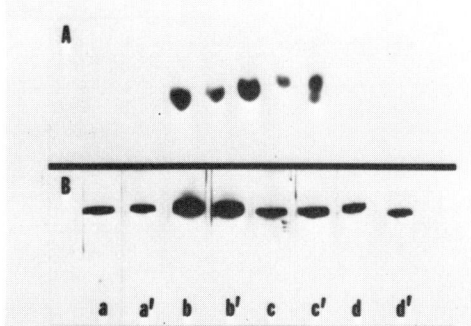

FIGURE 1. Polyacrylamide (disc-) (A) and sodium dodecyl sulfate (SDS-) (B) gel electrophoresis of normal and dicoumarol-induced prothrombins. Separatory gel lengths approximated 12 cm (A). A: Gels from left to right represent normal (10-gla), 7-, 5-, 2-, and 10- plus 2-gla prothrombins. The mobility decreased with the reduction of gla-content. Therefore, the admixture of 10- and 2-gla prothrombins showed two components. B: SDS-gels of 10-gla (a, a'), 7-gla (b,b'), 5-gla (c,c'), and 2-gla (d,d'). Samples a,b,c, and d were reduced with mercaptoethanol.

Normal bovine prothrombin generates thrombin (shortest clotting time) in 6 to 8 min. When glass tubes instead of plastic ones are used, the shortest clotting time begins to rise rapidly (Table 1) because of the adsorption of thrombin onto glass. To avoid this loss, which otherwise would affect the assay of prothrombin (particularly for our atypical prothrombins which have long activation times), we used plastic tubes. The 7-gla prothrombin took about 1.5 h to generate thrombin which, although long in comparison with normal protein (6 to 8 min), was significantly shorter than the approximately 3 to 5 and 7 to 9 h taken, respectively, by the 5- and 2-gla prothrombins. These results show that the time requirement for the formation of thrombin relates to the number of gla's. This conclusion is further strengthened by the fact that the P_1's from each of the prothrombins take approximately 5 h to activate.

The specific biological activity of normal (10-gla) prothrombin was about 3,000 U per mg prothrombin. The activity correlated with the number of gla's because the physiological activities of 7-, 5-, and 2-gla prothrombins approximated 52, 35, and 18 to 25% of normal. These values were, however, higher than the reported value of approximately 3% (15-16). Since we found that the bioactivity of the P_1's, calculated on a molar basis, was 40% that of 10-gla prothrombin, it becomes apparent that the partially acarboxylated prothrombins will, to a certain extent, convert to thrombin. Furthermore, the recent corrective studies of prothrombin time of plasma from dicoumarol-treated steers with the newly discovered plasma protein M support our conclusions (17).

TABLE 1. Physiological activation of normal and atypical prothrombins. Normal prothrombin activated in 6 to 8 min. In glass tubes, the shortest clotting time begins to rise rapidly; while in nitrocellulose tubes, it remains constant for several minutes. For this reason, the atypical prothrombins were activated in nitrocellulose tubes. The shortest clotting times of 7-, 5-, and 2-gla prothrombins approximated 1.5, 3 to 5, and 7 to 9 h.

Prothrombin	6	8	14	30	60	90	120	180	220	345	560
			Activation Time in Minutes								
			Clotting Time in Seconds								
Normal (10-gla)	[a]15.0	15.8	19.4								
		15.2	15.0	15.2							
7-gla		>30.0	21.4	19.2	16.8	15.0	18.0				
5-gla		>30.0		24.8			16.8	15.2	15.2	14.8	
2-gla						>30.0				21.0	14.0

[a]Activation in glass tubes

Despite the above results, we feel that in 'living plasma (or blood)' the bioactivities of atypical prothrombin may not be important, primarily because of their long activation times and presence of inhibitors like antithrombin III, which inactivates several clotting factors including thrombin and factor X_a (18). As a result, atypical prothrombin preparations containing some antithrombin III activity failed to generate thrombin activity (7). Moreover, antithrombin III can affect the assay of normal prothrombin in dicoumarol-induced plasma. For example, plasma containing approximately 8% of normal activity may show 4% when thrombin used for defibrinogenation is decreased (unpublished data).

We have found that gla's induce some conformational changes in the prothrombin molecule so as to affect availability of the Arg^{156}-Ser and Arg^{52}-Asn peptide bonds to thrombin. Whether or not gla's also directly affect the rate of the two cleavages, at Arg^{274}-Thr and Arg^{323}-Ile, which are catalyzed by factor X_a to generate thrombin from prothrombin, remains to be investigated.

ACKNOWLEDGEMENTS

This work was supported by the Veterans Administration. The author gratefully appreciates the interest and council of Dr. J.R. Carter and the technical assistance of Mrs. Peggy Mendelson.

REFERENCES

1. Malhotra, O.P., and Carter, J.R. (1971) J. Biol. Chem. 246, 2665-2671.
2. Malhotra, O.P. (1972) Life Sciences 11 (Part II),901-907.
3. Malhotra, O.P. (1972) Nature New Biol. 239, 59-60.
4. Magnusson, S., Sottrup-Jensen, L., Peterson, T.E., Morris, H.R., and Dell, A. (1974) FEBS Letters 44, 189-193.
5. Fernlund, P., Stenflo, J., Roepstorff, P., and Thomson, J. (1975) J. Biol. Chem. 250, 6125-6133.
6. Nelsestuen, G.L., and Zytkovicz, T.H. (1974) J. Biol. Chem. 249, 6347-6350.
7. Malhotra, O.P. (1979) Thromb. Res. In press.
8. Esmon, C.T., and Jackson, C.M. (1974) J. Biol. Chem. 249, 7782-7790.
9. Stenn, K.S., and Blout, E.R. (1972) Biochemistry 11, 4502-4515.
10. Malhotra, O.P. (1979) Fed. Proceedings 38, 3047.
11. Malhotra, O.P., and Carter, J.R. (1968) Thromb. Diathes. Haemorrh. 19, 178-185.
12. Davis, B.J. (1964) Ann. N.Y. Acad. Sci. 121, 404-427.
13. Weber, K., and Osborn, M. (1969) J. Biol. Chem. 244, 4406-4412.
14. Ware, A.G., and Seegers, W.H. (1949) Amer. J. Clin. Pathol. 19, 471-482.
15. Nelsestuen, G.L., and Suttie, J.W. (1972) J. Biol. Chem. 247, 8176-8182.
16. Stenflo, J., and Ganrot, P.O. (1972) J. Biol. Chem. 247, 8160-8166.
17. Seegers, W.H., and Ghosh, A. Personal communication.
18. Rosenberg, R.D. (1977) Semin. Hematol. 14, 427-440.

CONFORMATION-SPECIFIC ANTIBODIES TO ABNORMAL PROTHROMBIN AND PROTHROMBIN

R. A. BLANCHARD, B. FURIE, and B. C. FURIE

Tufts-New England Medical Center and
Tufts University School of Medicine,
Boston, MA 02111

INTRODUCTION

Prothrombin is a vitamin K-dependent blood coagulation zymogen whose conversion to thrombin by activated factor X requires calcium, phospholipid and factor V. Abnormal prothrombin is a form of prothrombin which circulates in the plasma of mammals deficient in vitamin K or treated with vitamin K antagonists. Abnormal prothrombin is assumed to have an identical primary amino acid sequence to prothrombin except in the NH_2-terminal region where some or all of the glutamic acid residues remain uncarboxylated (1,2). The presence of γ-carboxyglutamic acid is critical to the calcium binding properties and hence the biologic activity of prothrombin (3). Indeed, we have shown that γ-carboxyglutamic acid has unique metal binding properties which allow its participation in intramolecular and intermolecular bridging (4). Studies of prothrombin with lanthanide ions are consistent with the presence of two high affinity and multiple lower affinity metal binding sites (5). If as proposed, two γ-carboxyglutamic acid residues bind a single metal ion in forming a high affinity metal binding site, binding of metal ions to the high affinity site will alter the three dimensional structure of that region. In fact, fluorescence (6,7) and circular dichroism (8) studies suggest a metal-induced conformational change in prothrombin upon metal binding. Whether this change is a general one or localized to the immediate area of metal binding is unknown. Lacking γ-carboxyglutamic acid, abnormal prothrombin does not bind calcium and would not be expected to undergo this metal-induced conformational change.

To investigate this and other structure-function relationships of prothrombin and abnormal prothrombin, we have used conformationally specific antibodies as probes of protein structure. In this article we summarize our studies on the interaction of three conformationally specific antibody subpopulations with prothrombin, abnormal prothrombin, and fragments of prothrombin. Two of these antibody subpopulations are isolated from antiprothrombin antisera and their binding is either enhanced by or dependent on the presence of calcium. One is isolated from anti-abnormal prothrombin antisera and is specific for abnormal prothrombin.

MATERIALS AND METHODS

Abnormal prothrombin was purified from warfarinized bovine plasma (gift of Dr. K.G. Mann, Mayo Clinic) by DEAE Sephacel chromatography, affinity chromatography using anti-prethrombin 1 covalently bound to agarose, and Sephacryl S 200 gel filtration (9). Abnormal prothrombin was active in the E. carinatus assay system but not in the standard prothrombin assay, and did not contain detectable γ-carboxyglutamic acid.

Des-γ-carboxy fragment 1 was prepared by decarboxylation of prothrombin fragment 1 followed by gel filtration on Sephacryl S 200 to remove high molecular weight protein aggregates (9).

Rabbits were immunized by the subcutaneous injection of 1 mg of prothrombin or abnormal prothrombin emulsified in complete Freund's adjuvant bimonthly for two months. Antibody titres as measured by quantitative precipitin analysis were maintained by monthly injection of protein in incomplete Freund's adjuvant.

RESULTS

Purification and Characterization of Metal-dependent Anti-prothrombin Antibody Subpopulations

Antibodies that were calcium-dependent or directed against a γ-carboxyglutamic acid-rich region of prothrombin (residues 12-44) were fractionated by affinity chromatography using columns of Sepharose to which prothrombin or prothrombin fragments were covalently coupled. A calcium dependent antiprothrombin antibody subpopulation was purified from the antiprothrombin antibodies by affinity chromatography in the presence of $CaCl_2$ using prothrombin covalently bound to Sepharose and elution with 3 mM EDTA (10). These antibodies represented about 10% of the total antibody population directed against prothrombin and were totally dependent upon calcium for their interaction with prothrombin (Fig. 1A). A direct binding assay employed ^{125}I-labeled prothrombin, calcium-dependent antiprothrombin antibodies and a double antibody precipitation method in the presence of 1 mM calcium chloride or 3 mM EDTA. Prothrombin fragment 1 exhibited identical interaction with the calcium-dependent antiprothrombin antibodies. In contrast, radiolabeled abnormal prothrombin bound minimally to the calcium dependent anti-prothrombin antibody subpopulation (Fig. 1B).

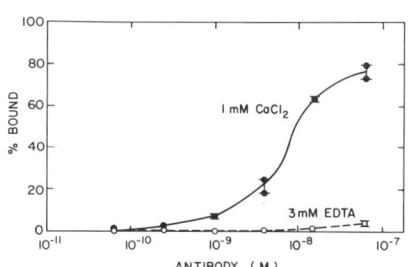
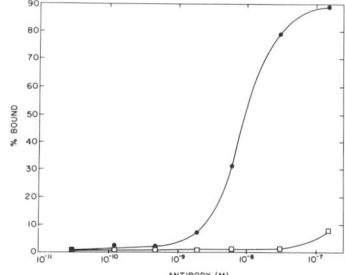

Fig. 1A. Interaction of the calcium dependent anti-prothrombin with ^{125}I-labeled prothrombin in the presence of 1 mM $CaCl_2$ (●) or 3 mM EDTA (o) (reference 10)

Fig. 1B. Interaction of calcium-dependent anti-prothrombin antibodies in the presence of Ca(II) with abnormal prothrombin (□) and prothrombin (●) (reference 10)

Another antibody subpopulation, one whose binding was enhanced by but not dependent on the presence of calcium, was isolated from antiprothrombin antisera. These antibodies were directed against a region in prothrombin from amino acid residue 12 to residue 44 which contains eight of the ten γ-carboxyglutamic acid residues of prothrombin. The anti-$(12-44)_N$ subpopulation was purified by sequential immunoabsorption using columns in which prothrombin, fragment 1, prethrombin 1, and prothrombin fragment

(12-44) were covalently bound to Sepharose (11). The final anti-(12-44)$_N$ antibody subpopulation represented about 5% of the total antibody population directed against prothrombin.

In a competitive radioimmunoassay anti-(12-44)N antibodies exhibited interaction with prothrombin and fragment 1. Unlabeled prothrombin fragment 1 competed with equal effectiveness to unlabeled prothrombin for anti-(12-44)N (Fig. 2A), but almost a 100-fold greater concentration of abnormal prothrombin than prothrombin was required to effect a 50% displacement of ^{125}I-labeled prothrombin from anti-(12-44)N antibodies (Fig. 2B). The interaction of other vitamin K dependent coagulation proteins with anti-(12-44)N was also examined. Approximately a 25-fold molar excess of factor X, a 100-fold molar excess of factor IX and a 200-fold molar excess of human prothrombin over prothrombin was required to effect 50% inhibition of binding of the ^{125}I-labeled prothrombin to anti-(12-44)N (12).

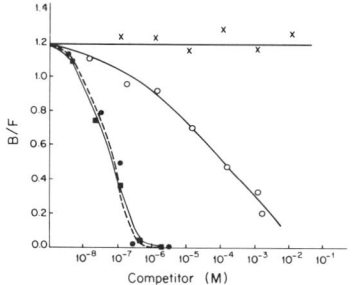

Fig. 2A. Interaction of anti-(12-44)N with prothrombin and prothrombin fragments. Prothrombin (■), fragment 1 (●), fragment 12-44, (o), and γ-carboxyglutamic acid (X) was measured by the displacement of ^{125}I-labeled prothrombin from anti-(12-44)N (reference 11).

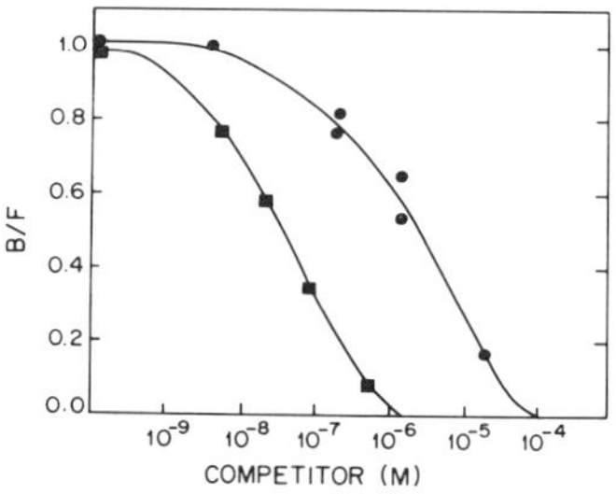

Fig. 2B. Interaction of anti-(12-44)N with prothrombin and abnormal prothrombin. The binding of anti-(12-44)N to prothrombin (■) and abnormal prothrombin (●) was measured by the displacement of ^{125}I-labeled prothrombin from anti-(12-44)$_N$ (reference 11).

Purification and Characterization of Anti-abnormal Prothrombin-Specific Antibody Subpopulation

Antibodies specific for abnormal prothrombin were isolated from anti-abnormal prothrombin antisera by sequential immunoabsorption using affinity chromatography (9). Antisera was absorbed on des-γ-carboxy fragment 1 coupled to Sepharose followed by elution with 4M guanidine HCl. Approximately one third of the anti-abnormal prothrombin antibodies bound to the des-γ-carboxy fragment 1-Sepharose column, despite the fact that crude anti-abnormal prothrombin antisera showed minimal crossreactivity with prothrombin fragment 1. The portion of the antisera which bound to the des-γ-carboxy fragment 1-Sepharose column was applied to a Sepharose-prothrombin column to remove antibodies which crossreacted with both prothrombin and abnormal prothrombin. The final antibody subpopulation, anti-abnormal prothrombin-specific antibodies, represented about 3% of the original antibodies directed against abnormal prothrombin.

Anti-abnormal prothrombin-specific antibodies bound radiolabeled abnormal prothrombin but not radiolabeled prothrombin as seen in the direct binding assay (Fig. 3A). The interaction of either radiolabeled antigen was unaltered by the presence of 1 mM $CaCl_2$ or 1 mM EDTA. In a competition assay similar results were observed. (Fig. 3B). Unlabeled abnormal prothrombin was able to displace the antibody from radiolabeled abnormal prothrombin, but unlabeled prothrombin in 1600-fold excess of abnormal prothrombin effected no displacement.

Using a competitive radioimmunoassay the interaction of anti-abnormal prothrombin-specific antibodies with normal and warfarinized plasmas was studied (Fig. 4). Bovine plasma from a calf treated with sodium warfarin displaced labeled antigen from antibody, but normal bovine plasma and normal human plasma showed no displacement. Human plasma from a patient treated with sodium warfarin also effected no displacement. These results would indicate that abnormal prothrombin is not a significant component of normal bovine plasma.

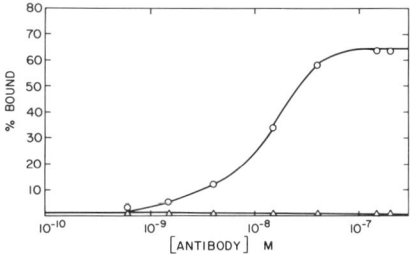

Fig. 3A. Interaction of anti-abnormal prothrombin-specific antibody with abnormal prothrombin and prothrombin. ^{125}I-labeled abnormal prothrombin in the presence of 1 mM $CaCl_2$ or 1 mM EDTA (o) or ^{125}I-labeled prothrombin in presence of 1 mM $CaCl_2$ or 1 mM EDTA (Δ) and anti-abnormal prothrombin-specific antibody (reference 9)

Fig. 3B. The interaction of antibody with abnormal prothrombin and prothrombin was studied using a competition assay. Anti-abnormal prothrombin-specific antibody, ^{125}I-labeled abnormal prothrombin, and unlabeled abnormal prothrombin (o) or prothrombin (•) as indicated (reference 9)

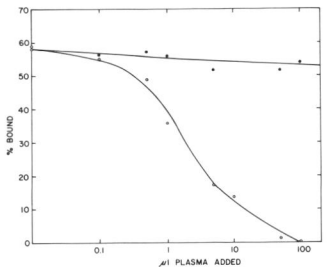
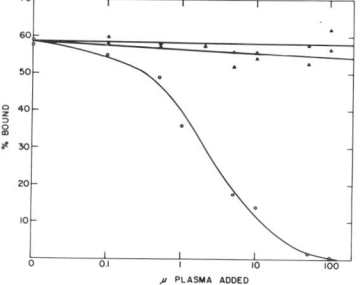

Fig. 4A. Interaction of anti-abnormal prothrombin-specific antibody with plasma proteins. The displacement of antibody-^{125}I-labeled bovine abnormal prothrombin binding by bovine plasma (•) or plasma from a calf treated with warfarin (o) (9)

Fig. 4B. Interaction of human plasma proteins with anti-abnormal prothrombin-specific antibodies. Human plasma (Δ) or plasma obtained from a patient treated with warfarin (▲). A control from a calf treated with warfarin is presented (o) (ref. 9)

DISCUSSION

Conformationally specific antibodies have been used successfully to investigate the tertiary structural differences of proteins and their fragments (13), proteins whose primary structure differs minimally (14), and the effects of ligands on the stabilization of conformational motility (15). The existence of calcium dependent antibody subpopulations in anti-prothrombin antisera argues strongly in favor of a conformationally induced change in prothrombin on metal binding. This change appears to be limited to the fragment 1 region since both calcium dependent antibodies interacted fully with fragment 1. Isolation of a population of antibodies specific for anti-$(12-44)_N$ implies that this region was immunogenic and hence at least partially exposed on the surface of the protein. Furthermore it may be assumed that the region of prothrombin from 12 to 44 was immunogenic in its native conformation since anti-$(12-44)_N$ antibodies showed minimally crossreactivity with fragment 12-44. The exposure of prothrombin region 12-44 on the protein surface is in accord with the idea that the γ-carboxyglutamic acid residues must be accessible to interact with the platelet membrane. In addition to localizing areas of conformational change in prothrombin, these calcium dependent antibody subpopulations have been used to study in detail the interaction of prothrombin with various metal ions and to confirm previous studies (6-8) of metal-induced conformational change at concentrations where protein-protein interaction should be minimal (12).

Bovine prothrombin shares considerable sequence homology in the fragment 1 region with regions in factor IX and factor X. Considerable crossreactivity of these factors with the metal-dependent antibody subpopulations might be expected. However, studies with anti-$(12-44)_N$ demonstrated little interaction with bovine factor IX or factor X. Similarly, bovine and human prothrombin have substantial primary sequence homology and so should their respective abnormal prothrombins. However, neither anti-$(12-44)_N$ antibodies nor anti-abnormal prothrombin-specific antibodies showed significant crossreactivity with human prothrombin or human abnormal prothrombin.

It has been assumed that abnormal prothrombin has a similar primary amino acid sequence to prothrombin with the exception of the substitution of glutamic acid for γ-carboxyglutamic acid residues in the fragment 1 region. This lack of γ-carboxyglutamic acid accounts for the failure of abnormal prothrombin to bind calcium and, presumably, to undergo the putative tertiary structural change seen in prothrombin upon metal binding. Our observations on the interaction of abnormal prothrombin with two subpopulations of metal-dependent anti-prothrombin antibodies would seem to substantiate this. Conversely, we have isolated an antibody subpopulation from anti-abnormal prothrombin antisera which binds to abnormal prothrombin but not to prothrombin. As expected the binding of this antibody subpopulation was not influenced by the presence or absence of calcium. Specifically, the absence of calcium did not enhance the binding of prothrombin, i.e. make it more like abnormal prothrombin, to the abnormal prothrombin-specific antibody. This suggests that there are major antigenic differences in the tertiary structure of the fragment 1 regions of prothrombin and abnormal prothrombin.

The calcium dependent anti-prothrombin antibody subpopulations and the anti-abnormal prothrombin-specific antibody subpopulation are highly specific for the carboxylated and decarboxylated forms of prothrombin respectively. These antibody subpopulations, one specific for prothrombin and one for abnormal prothrombin, should be useful reagents in investigating and distinguishing the levels of decarboxylated, partially carboxylated and fully carboxylated forms of prothrombin which may occur naturally both in the plasma and during prothrombin biosynthesis in the liver.

ACKNOWLEDGEMENTS

This work was supported by Grants HL-21543 and HL-18834 from the National Institutes of Health. Dr. Blanchard is the recipient of the Samuel A. Levine Fellowship of the American Heart Association, Massachusetts Affiliate and of a postdoctoral fellowship of the National Institutes of Health (1 F32 HL 05630). Dr. Bruce Furie is an Established Investigator of the American Heart Association and its Massachusetts affiliate. Dr. Barbara C. Furie is the recipient of a Research Career Development Award (HL-00235) from the National Institutes of Health. The authors are indebted to M. Tai for generously providing experimental data contained in manuscripts in preparation. We are grateful to Ms. Nancy Kane for her assistance in the preparation of the manuscript.

REFERENCES

1. Stenflo, J., Fernlund, P., Egan, W., and Roepstorff, P. (1974) Proc. Nat. Acad. Sci. USA 71, 2730-2733.
2. Nelsestuen, G.L., Zytkovicz, T.H., and Howard, J.B. (1974) J. Biol. Chem. 249, 6347-6350.
3. Nelsestuen, G.L., and Suttie, J.W. (1972) Biochemistry 11, 4961-4964.
4. Sperling, R., Furie, B.C., Blumenstein, M., Keyt, B., and Furie, B. (1978) J. Biol. Chem. 253, 3898-3906.
5. Furie, B.C., Mann, K.G., and Furie, B. (1976) J. Biol. Chem. 251, 3235-3241.
6. Nelsestuen, G.L. (1976) J. Biol. Chem. 251, 5648-5656.
7. Prendergast, F.G., and Mann, K.G. (1977) J. Biol. Chem. 252, 840-850.
8. Bloom, J.W., and Mann, K.G. (1978) Biochemistry 17, 4430-4438.
9. Blanchard, R.A., Furie, B.C., and Furie, B. (1979) submitted.
10. Tai, M., Furie, B.C., and Furie, B. (1979) Fed. Proc. 38, 792.
11. Furie, B., Provost, K.L., Blanchard, R.A., and Furie, B.C. (1978) J. Biol. Chem. 253, 8980-8987.
12. Furie, B., and Furie, B.C. J. Biol. Chem. in press.
13. Furie, B., Schechter, A.N., Sachs, D.H., and Anfinsen, C.B. (1974) Biochemistry 13, 1561-1566.
14. Curd, J.G., Young, N.S., and Schechter, A.N. (1976) J. Biol. Chem. 251, 1290-1295.
15. Furie, B., Schechter, A.N., Sachs, D.H., and Anfinsen, C.B. (1975) J. Mol. Biol. 92, 497-506.

FUNCTIONS FOR PROTEIN C

C. T. ESMON, P. C. COMP, and F. J. WALKER

The University of Oklahoma Health Sciences Center
Oklahoma City, OK 73104

INTRODUCTION

For years it was generally accepted that the sole effect of either vitamin K deficiency or the vitamin K antagonists on the coagulation sysem was to produce deficiencies in prothrombin and coagulation Factors VII, IX and X. The first suggestion that there might exist an additional vitamin K dependent factor or factors came from the observations of Seegers' group (1). They found that partially purified prothrombin complex, when treated with thrombin, elicited anticoagulant activity. This activity was not appreciated as a new factor at that time, but rather was believed to be derived from prothrombin (1). No direct evidence was provided that this protein was dependent on vitamin K for normal biosynthesis. In retrospect, its absorption onto Ba^{++} salts suggested its structural relationship with the other vitamin K dependent proteins. In 1976 Stenflo isolated a protein, Protein C, from bovine plasma that was distinct from the other vitamin K dependent clotting factors (2). It contained γ-carboxyglutamic acid residues, and its biosynthesis was inhibited by dicoumarol. Immunological and structural comparisons revealed that this protein was similar or identical to the inhibitor studied by Seegers' group (3). The existence of a similar activity in human plasma was shown by Marciniak (4) and the human protein has recently been purified by Kisiel (5).

The mechanism by which activated Protein C inhibits coagulation remains controversial. Early reports (6,7) indicated that activated Protein C was a competitive inhibitor of prothrombin activation, and that the inhibitory effect could be reversed by increasing concentrations of Factor V. The concept of activated Protein C functioning as competitive inhibitor is supported by the sequence homology between Factor Xa (8) and activated Protein C (9), but is difficult to reconcile with observations indicating that activated Protein C is a protease. Diisopropylfluorophosphate was shown to inactivate the anticoagulant activity of activated Protein C, indicating that proteolytic activity is necessary for anticoagulation (10). This view is supported by the observation (11) that activated Protein C inhibited the activity of partially purified Factor V. The inhibitory capacity was blocked when activated Protein C was inhibited with diisopropylfluorophosphate, and it was concluded that activated Protein C inhibited blood clotting by proteolytic inactivation of Factor V.

Recently, Factor Va has been demonstrated to be bound either in or on platelets (12,13). This platelet associated Factor V activity can be inhibited by anti-Factor V antibodies (12,13). The platelet-Factor V activity can be expressed by freeze-thawing platelet suspensions (12) or by thrombin treatment of platelets (13). Expression of platelet-Factor V activity during platelet activation (12,13) or aggregation (14) appears to correlate with the surface (13,15). Since activated Protein C has a narrow substrate specificity, it is an ideal reagent for investigating the role of platelet derived Factor V in prothrombin activation.

In addition to the inhibition of coagulation, activated Protein C has been observed to facilitate clot lysis (16,17). This appears to be an indirect effect since the activated Protein C does not activate plasminogen directly (16). One of the major problems in studying the role of activated Protein C in clot lysis has been to establish a reproducible system in which lysis is always observed. Unlike the coagulation system, the study of fibrinolysis has been difficult, primarily because no adequate in vitro system has been available to study the process. Whereas coagulation occurs rapidly upon removal of blood, lysis of the human or bovine whole blood clots in vitro occurs very slowly, if at all. Contributing to the complexities and problems of studying fibrinolysis is the observation that a potent plasminogen activator is contained within the vascular endothelium (18). Factors controlling the release and function of this activator may be essential to fibrinolysis and to achieving a model system in which in vitro fibrinolysis can be studied.

Since whole blood clots do not lyse, other model systems have been developed. They rely on dilution and/or selective precipitation of inhibitors. In such systems, clot lysis can be observed. In one of these, the dilute whole blood clot lysis system, the involvement of the platelet in fibrinolysis has been implicated (19,20). Protein C and activated Protein C, which are known to bind phospholipids (21,22) and trigger aggregation of platelets under certain conditions (3), may provide a link between the platelet and fibrinolysis.

Our initial studies sought to combine the findings from these earlier studies into a system in which the participation of activated Protein C, platelets, the vascular plasminogen activator and other regulators of fibrinolysis might be studied. We have found that activated Protein C mediated lysis can be routinely observed in systems containing platelet-rich plasma, vein segments, activated Protein C and Ca^{++}.

MATERIALS AND METHODS

Preparation of Proteins: Activated Factor X (Xa) was prepared from purified Factor X (23) by activation of the Factor X with the Factor X activator from Russell's viper venom as described earlier (24). Prothrombin and thrombin were prepared as described earlier (23). Factor V was purified and converted to Factor Va by incubation with thrombin (25). Factor Va was separated from activation products and thrombin by chromatography on QAE Sephadex Q50 (25).

Protein C was isolated by a modification (26) of the method of Stenflo (2). The modification involved chromatography on heparin agarose and elution with a linear gradient (0 to 0.6 M NaCl) in 0.05 M imidazole HCl, 0.01 M $CaCl_2$ 1 mM benzamidine HCl pH 6.0. The resulting protein appreared homogeneous following sodium dodecyl gel electrophorsis or alkaline gel electrophoresis.

Activation of Protein C: Protein C (6 mg, 0.5 mg/ml) in 0.1 M NaCl, 0.02 M Tris-HCl, 0.01 M $CaCl_2$, pH 7.5, was activated at 37° with the Factor X activator from Russell's viper venom (12.5 μg/ml final concentration). The extent of activation was monitored by the hydrolysis of N-α-p-tosyl-L-arginine methyl ester, and activation was allowed to proceed until no further increase in hydrolytic activity occurred.

Following complete activation of Protein C, the Factor X activator was quantitatively separated from activated Protein C by chromatography on a column (0.6 x 10 cm) of QAE Sephadex. Prior to chromatography the reaction mixture was made 2.0×10^{-3} M benzamidine HCl. The column was washed with 20 ml of 0.2 M NaCl, 0.02 M Tris-HCl, 2×10^{-3} M benzamidine, pH 7.5 to remove the venom protein. Activated Protein C was eluted from the column with 0.6 M NaCl, 0.02 M Tris-HCl, 2×10^{-3} M benzamidine, pH 7.5.

Clotting Factor Assays: Factor V (27) and activated Factor X (28) were assayed by standard methods employing deficient plasmas. Thrombin was assayed by its ability to clot fibrinogen.

Phospholipid Preparation: Phospholipid was prepared from acetone dried bovine brain by the method of Bligh and Dyer (29). Phospholipid vesicles were prepared by mixing the phospholipid in chloroform and then drying under nitrogen onto the walls of a glass tube. The lipid was dispersed into buffer (0.1 M NaCl, 0.02 M Tris-HCl, pH 7.5) by sonicating the tube with a Bronson bath sonicator for four hours at room temperature.

Platelet collection and gel filtration: Nine parts bovine blood was collected by jugular venipuncture into 1 part 3.8% sodium citrate, pH 5.5. Platelet rich plasma was obtained by centrifuging the blood for 5 min at 895 X g at 25° C. The platelet rich plasma was drawn off and 8 ml layered on a 3 X 25 cm column of Bio-Gel A-15 m equilibrated with a modified Tangen-HEPES buffer (30) containing 5 mg/ml bovine albumin and gel filtered in the same buffer. The collection and isolation of platelets was in plastic.

Iodination of Factor X: The method of Hunter (31) was used to iodinate Factor X. The iodination was performed at room temperature with 1 mCi Na^{125}I added to 300 µg Factor X in 1.2 ml of buffer. Final chloramine T concentration was 0.71 mM and sodium meta-bisulfite 1.26 mM. Chloramine T was added 3.5 sec prior to the sodium meta-bisulfite. Immediately following iodination, the Factor X was chromatographed on a 0.9 x 20 cm Sephadex G 25 column equilibrated with 0.1 M NaCl, 20 mM Tris-HCl and 1 mM benzamidine, pH 7.4, to remove the unbound ^{125}Iodine. The ^{125}I-Factor X was then activated with the Factor X activator from Russell's viper venom. The Factor Xa activity which resulted was identical to that generated from non-iodinated control Factor X. Activation of the ^{125}I-Factor X was also complete as judged by disc gel electrophoretic analysis with reduced samples on sodium dodecyl sulfate containing gels. The resulting specific radioactivity was 600-700 cpm per ng.

Binding assays: The binding of Factor Xa to platelets was determined by centrifugation of the platelets through oil to separate the platelets from unbound Factor Xa. The method described by Miletich et al (13) was employed. Platelets were activated directly with thrombin. Prothrombin was not present during the binding studies.

Characterization of the assay for platelet prothrombin converting activity. The ability of thrombin treated platelets to enhance the conversion of prothrombin to thrombin was measured as follows: gel filtered platelets were diluted to 1.0×10^8 per ml in 0.15 M NaCl, 20 mM Tris HCl buffer, pH 7.4, containing 1 mg/ml bovine albumin and to 100 µl of the diluted platelets, 0.1 u thrombin (10 µl) was added. Then following incubation at 37°C for 45 sec, 100 µl 25 mM CaCl$_2$ was added and 15 sec later 100 µl Factor Xa at 2 µg/ml was added. The mixture was incubated for 1 min and then 100 µl of prothrombin at 200 µg/ml was added. After 60 sec incubation, 100 µl fibrinogen at 6 mg/ml was added and the clotting time determined. Thrombin units generated were determined by reference to a thrombin curve. Under these conditions, 5.4-5.8 units of thrombin were generated per min per 10^8 platelets. This platelet cofactor activity will be referred to as platelet prothrombin converting activity. In this assay thrombin formation was directly proportional to the length of incubation with prothrombin. To assure rapid saturation of the platelet sites, Factor Xa at 400 ng/ml was used for PPCA determination with one min incubation of the Factor Xa with the platelets and calcium prior to prothrombin addition.

Euglobulin fractions were prepared from citrated platelet poor plasma by 20 fold dilution into 10 mM Na acetate, pH 5.5, at 4°. After incubation at 4° for 30 min, the euglobulin precipitate was centrifuged and then resuspended in 0.15 M NaCl, 0.02 M Tris-HCl, pH 7.5, to the original volume of the plasma. Clots were formed by the addition of thrombin (1 u/ml) and $CaCl_2$ (6 mM). All samples were run in duplicate and individuals judging the visual lysis times did not know the contents of the tubes.

Sapheneous vein of human origin was obtained fresh and diced and homogenized before inclusion in the clot lysis system.

RESULTS

Plasma clotting initiated by Factor Xa is inhibited by activated Protein C (Figure 1). The ability of activated Protein C to inhibit clotting is minimized by either of two independent manipulations. When the plasma is supplemented with low levels of Factor Va, the plasma becomes resistant to inhibition by activated Protein C. Alternatively, if the plasma Factor V is converted to activated Factor V by incubation with the Factor V activating enzyme from Russell's viper venom, the plasma becomes similarly resistant to anticoagulation by activated Protein C. These results suggest that either Factor V levels or the form of Factor V play a key role in the expression of anticoagulant activity. In agreement with previous investigators (10,11), we find that diisopropylphosphoryl-activated Protein C is not active as an anticoagulant. This suggests that the active site is required for anticoagulant activity and suggests that some form of Factor V is a substrate for the activated Protein C.

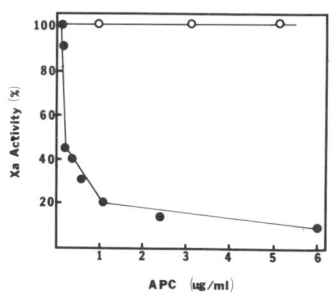

Figure 1: Effect of activated Protein C on Factor Xa initiated clotting of plasma. 0.05 ml of Factor Xa (0.2 µg/ml), 0.1 ml phospholipid (500 µg/ml), 0.1 ml $CaCl_2$ (0.025 M), APC (final concentration indicated on the figure) and buffer (0.1 M NaCl, 0.02 M Tris-HCl, pH 7.5, and 1 mg/ml bovine serum albumin) were mixed to give a final volume of 0.3 ml. Clotting was initiated by the addition of 0.1 ml of Factor X deficient plasma. Percent activity was derived from a standard curve made with the Factor Xa used in the assay. (●—●) Activity determined in Factor X deficient plasma, (○—○) Activity determined in Factor X deficient plasma treated with the Factor V activator from Russell's viper venom (6 ug/ml). This activator did not change the clotting time of the control Factor X deficient plasma. APC is used as an abbreviation for Activated Protein C.

The effect of activated Protein C on Factor V activity was investigated directly by incubating purified Factor V with activated Protein C (Figure 2). Activated Protein C had little effect on Factor V activity. The Factor V retained its ability to "activate" when treated with thrombin, but unlike Factor V activated in the absence of activated Protein C, Factor V activated in the presence of activated Protein C was rapidly inactivated (Figure 2). These results indicate that Factor Va is the preferred substrate for activated Protein C. Similar rates of inhibition of Factor Va are observed when purified Factor Va is inactivated with activated Protein C in the absence of thrombin (data not shown).

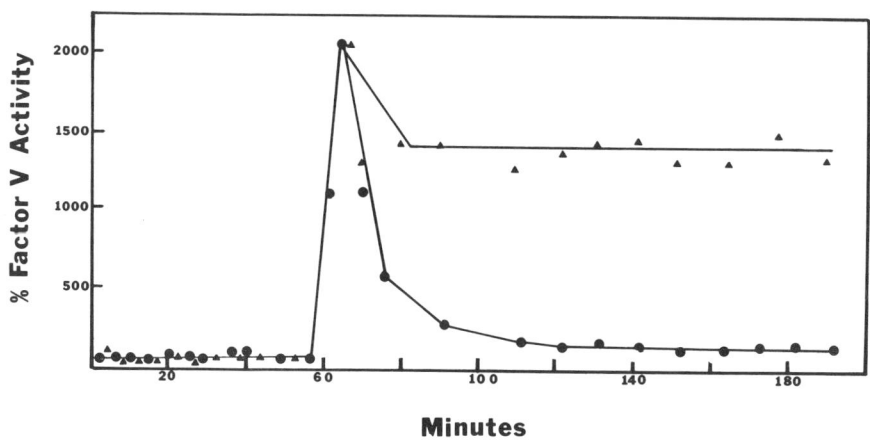

Figure 2: The effect of Activated Protein C on the extent of Factor V activation by thrombin. Factor V (60 units/ml in 10 mM $CaCl_2$) was equilibrated at 37° for 5 minutes. At that time activated Protein C (30 µg/ml) (●—●) and no addition (▲—▲) were incubated for 60 min with Factor V. At that time thrombin (2.3 µg/ml) was added. At the time indicated Factor V was assayed by the one-stage assay described in "Methods." % Factor V activity was calculated by dividing the activity of the sample after thrombin treatment to that before thrombin treatment.

All of the known vitamin K dependent clotting factors bind to, and their activity is enhanced by, phospholipid. The inactivation of Factor Va by activated Protein C is also accelerated by phospholipid. This effect is very large at low concentrations of Factor Va but much less at higher concentrations (Figure 3). These results are consistent with the idea that a primary role of the phospholipid is to concentrate enzyme and substrate on the membrane surface. The rate of Factor Va inactivation was saturated at approximately 60 mM Factor Va. (Figure 4)

Inhibition of Factor Va by activated Protein C is a complex process which is subject to regulation by the level of Factor Xa present during inactivation. The rate of inhibition of Factor Va is decreased by the presence of Factor Xa and the extent of the protection increases with increasing concentrations of Factor Xa (Figure 5). This protection is specific since Factor X does not afford protection. In the absence of phospholipid, Factor Xa has little effect on the rate of inactivation of Factor Va.

Functions for Protein C   77

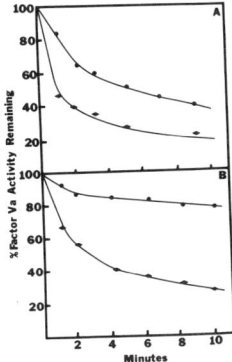

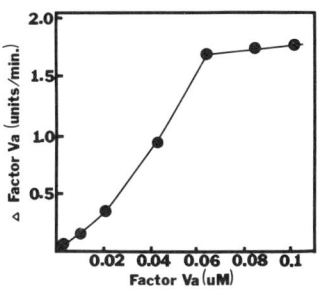

Figure 3: The effect of phospholipid on the inactivation of Factor Va at two Factor Va concentrations. Activated Protein C (0.5 ug/ml) was incubated with CaCl$_2$ (5 mM) with (•—•) or without (◆—◆) phospholipid (0.08 mg/ml) in 0.1 M NaCl, 0.02 M Tris-HCl, pH 7.5 and bovine serum albumin (1 mg/ml) at 37°. The reactions were initiated by the addition of Factor Va, A. (35 ug/ml) or B. (16.2 ug/ml).

Figure 4: The effect of Factor Va concentration on the rate of Factor Va inactivation by activated Protein C. Factor Va at the indicated concentration was incubated with CaCl$_2$ (5 mM), phospholipid (0.08 mg/ml) and activated Protein C (0.005 mg/ml) in 0.1 M NaCl, 0.02 M Tris-HCl, pH 7.5 and bovine serum albumin (1 mg/ml) at 37°. The inactivation of Factor Va was initiated by the addition of activated Protein C. One and two minutes after the reaction was started samples were removed and the Factor Va activity remaining was measured. The results are expressed as the average change in Factor Va activity per minute.

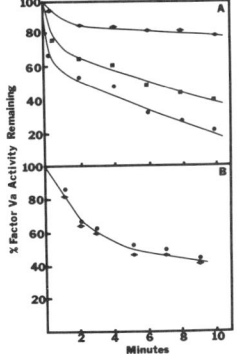

Figure 5: The effect of Factor Xa and phospholipid on the inactivation of Factor Va by activated Protein C. A. Factor Va (16.2 ug/ml) was incubated at 37° with CaCl$_2$ (5 mM), phospholipid (0.08 mg/ml) and activated Protein C (0.5 ug/ml) in NaCl (0.1 M) Tris-HCl (0.02 M), pH 7.5 and bovine serum albumin (1 mg/ml) with no addition (•—•), with Factor Xa (1.2 ug/ml) (■—■) or Factor Xa (2.4 ug/ml) (◆—◆). The reaction was initiated by the addition of Factor Va. At the indicated times samples were removed and Va activity was determined as described in "Methods" B. Factor Va (35 ug/ml) was incubated as above except that phospholipid was ommited with no addition (•—•) or with Factor Xa (6.5 ug/ml) (◆—◆).

Recent studies have now shown that Factor V is located in (13) platelets and that activation of platelets leads to expression of the Factor V activity. The platelet surface appears to have a low number of high affinity sites for Factor Va (14), and when Factor Va is bound to these sites in the presence of Factor Xa, rapid prothrombin activation occurs. Thus, if activated Protein C is to serve as an anticoagulant, it must be able to inactivate the platelet procoagulant activity. As seen above in the purified system, activated Protein C rapidly inactivates the platelet procoagulant activity (Figure 6). Factor Xa also protects the procoagulant activity from inactivation. Thus, although the Factor Va is probably bound to a surface receptor, it is nonetheless susceptible to inactivation by activated Protein C.

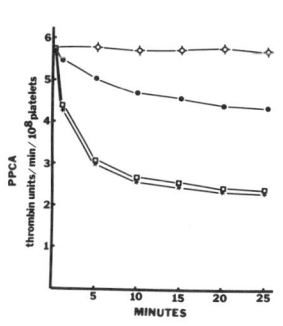

Figure 6: Time dependent inactivation of platelet prothrombin converting activity (PPCA) by activated Protein C. Activated Protein C (1 ug/ml) was added to platelets which had been activated by thrombin (0.2 U/ml) at 37° for the times indicated prior to the addition of Factor Xa (400 ng/ml) for 1 min and sequential addition of prothrombin and fibrinogen (★). In a parallel experiment Factor Xa (20 ng/ml) was added to the platelets for 20 min prior to the addition of the activated Protein C (●). Factor X (200 ng/ml) also added to the activated platelets prior to activated Protein C (■). Platelets not treated with activated Protein C were also examined (◆).

Factor Va appears to provide a portion of the platelet Factor Xa receptor activity (13). If activated Protein C destroys the platelet activity, then it would be anticipated that it would destroy the platelet Factor Xa receptor activity. The inhibition of platelet procoagulant activity of suboptimal levels of activated Protein C appear essentially biphasic. After a rapid initial loss of activity, the activity remains more stable. The cause of this biphasic inhibition remains unknown, but it provides a convenient means to examine the relationship between loss of receptor and loss of procoagulant activity. Following activation with thrombin, platelets were incubated with selected levels of activated Protein C for 30 minutes after which time both procoagulant and Factor Xa receptor activity were determined (Figure 7). These results suggest that the inactivation of the procoagulant activity results from the loss of the ability of the platelet receptor to bind Factor Xa.

In addition to being an anticoagulant, Seegers (16) has suggested that activated Protein C facilitates clot lysis. Under normal conditions, whole blood clots do not lyse. Even when diced or homogenized vein is added as a source of plasminogen activator, clot lysis is very slow. Our initial interest in the lytic capacity of activated Protein C arose when we observed on one occasion that nonanticoagulated bovine blood lysed spontaneously only if activated Protein C was present. This observation, although reproducible on that day, failed to be reproducible on reexamination of new blood samples. This observation lead us to investigate more

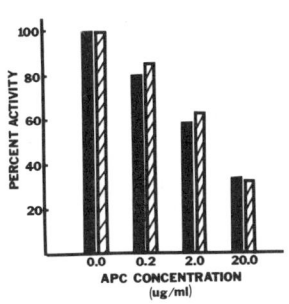

Figure 7: Effect of activated Protein C on platelet prothrombin converting activity and specific binding of Factor Xa. Activated Platelets were incubated with 0 ng APC/ml, 0.2 ng/ml, 2 ng/ml, and 20 ng/ml, for 30 minutes at 25° and then 20 ng ^{125}I-Factor Xa was added and the incubation continued at 25° for 30 min. Platelet prothrombin converting activity (dark bars) and specific binding of Factor Xa (crosshatched bars) were then measured and are expressed as percentage of the activity of the platelets which were not incubated with activated Protein C.

complex systems in order to establish an in vitro lytic system which would respond to activated Protein C. As mentioned previously, vascular endothelium contains a plasminogen activator which can be released by certain trauma. We reasoned that perhaps the activator had been released due to unknown causes into the blood clots that lysed in response to activated Protein C and had not been released in those samples that failed to lyse. A system which could be used to test this possibility required the presence of a source of plasminogen activator: vein segments or ground vein were chosen. In this system, clot lysis was stimulated by activated Protein C. A description of the requirements for clot lysis are indicated in Table 1.

REQUIREMENTS FOR ACTIVATED PROTEIN C STIMULATED CLOT LYSIS

APC	VEIN	PLATELET RICH PLASMA	PLATELET POOR PLASMA	Ca^{2+}	LYSIS TIME
+	+	+	-	+	4-12 hrs.
-	+	+	-	+	>4 days
+	-	+	-	+	>4 days
-	-	+	-	+	>4 days
+	+	+	-	-	>4 days
+	+	-	+	+	>4 days

The Concentrations of Components are Listed Below.

1) 0.1 ml fresh bovine platelet rich plasma in citrate.

2) 0.1 ml of APC in 0.1 M NaCl 0.02 M Tris HCl (10 ug/ml)

3) 0.1 ml of diced or homogenized vein (100 mg wet weight /ml in the above buffer).

4) 0.1 ml of 0.025 M $CaCl_2$.

5) Incubation is at 37° in glass tubes.

Rapid clot lysis required activated Protein C, vein, platelets, plasma and Ca^{++}. Reproducible responses to activated Protein C in this system requires that the donor, either bovine or human, be exercized prior to plasma preparation. The factor of factors present in the exercised plasma are unknown. Such complex systems are difficult to manipulate and too complex to allow characterization of the interaction between components. To simplify this system, we chose to examine the effect of activated Protein C on euglobulin lysis to determine if this acceleration of lysis has an absolute requirement for cells. The euglobulin lysis system is relatively inhibitor-free. We find that activated Protein C does decrease the euglobulin lysis time, but that it does so reproducibly only when the euglobulin fraction is formed from plasma from exercised donors (Table 2). Factor Va speeds the lysis time, but this effect is not strictly dependent on the addition of activated Protein C. These results indicate that whatever the nature of the exercise factor, it is carried into the euglobulin lysis system and can facilitate lysis in a cell-free system.

EFFECT OF ACTIVATED PROTEIN C ON EUGLOBULIN LYSIS

	Resting Donor Plasma Euglobulin Fraction				Exercised Donor Plasma Euglobulin Fraction			
APC	−	+	+	−	−	+	+	−
Va	−	−	+	+	−	−	+	+
Lysis Time (min)	200	170	160	156	98	52	43	72

Legend - Activated Protein C (1 ug/ml) and/or Factor Va (1 u/ml) was added to whole blood for 1 min prior to euglobulin fractionation.

It is well established that exercise enhances the fibrinolytic activity of plasma (32). Furthermore, it is often assumed that this increase in lytic activity is due to release of the activator from the vascular endothelium. Radcliffe and Heinze (33) have recently established an affinity chromatographic system using lysine-agarose which allows rapid and essentially quantitative recovery of a highly purified plasma plasminogen activator. Chromatographic and functional properties suggest that this activator is similar to the vascular activator. Whether this activator is directly involved in expression of activated Protein C dependent clot lysis is currently under investigation in both the euglobulin and plasma systems.

DISCUSSION

The dual functions of activated Protein C as an inhibitor of coagulation and as a stimulator of fibrinolysis make this protein a possible candidate for a key role in the regulation of blood clotting and fibrinolysis. Unfortunately, unlike the case with the clotting factors, no congenital deficiency has been observed. Thus, it is not possible to infer the role of Protein C in normal haemostasis. An additional problem related to establishing Protein C as an integral part of the regulation of coagulation or fibrinolysis is to establish the extent and timing of the activation of Protein C. Although thrombin can activate Protein C <u>in vitro</u>, only small amounts of Protein C are activated during intrinsic coagulation (34). In the platelet vein-system there is no evidence for the activation of endogenous Protein C. This is supported by the observation that levels of activated Protein C below those of the endogenous zymogen will stimulate clot lysis. If only a small percentage of Protein C is activated, then the functions ascribed to the activated Protein C may not be of physiological significance. Thus, the question of the physiological activation of Protein C remains open.

Assuming that Protein C is activated under certain conditions, then it clearly becomes an effective anticoagulant. Its anticoagulant activity is expressed, in part by its ability to inactivate Factor Va, whether the Factor Va is of plasma or platelet origin. The inactivation is complex, being modulated by the availability of phospholipid and the level of Factor Xa. The extent of Factor X activation may also be controlled by activated Protein C as suggested by Marciniak (4). Activated Protein C may block Factor X activation sufficiently to prevent significant protection of Factor V. The specificity of activated Protein C for the activated form of Factor V may prevent total depletion of Factor V levels and prevent the onset of secondary bleeding problems.

Inactivation of platelet Factor Va appears similar to that of plasma Factor Va. The rate of inactivation is increased by increasing levels of activated Protein C and decreased by increasing levels of Factor Xa. The protection does not appear to be competitive since the protection effect is saturable with Factor Xa and at this level inactivation is not totally blocked.

The effect of activated Protein C on coagulation appears to be due to the inactivation of activated Factor V of either plasma or platelet origin. The function of APC in the stimulation of fibrinolysis has proven to more intractable. We have defined a whole blood system which includes veinous tissue, and plasminogen activator, as well as exercise as requirements for the APC effect upon lysis. Our data indicates activated Protein C involvement in two apparently distinct processes: one platelet dependent and the other platelet independent. The euglobulin lysis time is shortened by addition of activated Protein C, provided that the euglobulin fraction is prepared with plasma from exercised donors. Since this system is essentially inhibitor free, the effect of activated Protein C is probably to enhance plasminogen activation. The enyzmatic pathway remains unknown. The platelet dependent system requires the presence of vascular tissue and Ca^{2+} ions for reproducible response. To our knowledge the influence of Factor V on the euglobulin lysis time shown here represents the first evidence that Factor V may participate in clot lysis. This involvement is supported by the ability of purified Factor Va to shorten the euglobulin lysis time. Factor Va sometimes shortens the euglobulin lysis time even without added activated Protein C. Whether this stimulation requires endogenous Protein C activation remains to be determined.

Several experiments suggest that the effect of activated Protein C on the euglobulin lysis system is less dramatic than on the complex system containing vein or endothelial cells. Thus it appears that the vein may contain some factor which responds to activated Protein C. A distinct possiblity is that activated Protein C triggers release of the activator from vein. This possibility is currently under investigation. In addition, the ability of activated Protein C to block anti-plasmin inhibitors (16) may contribute to this effect.

If Protein C proves to be important in the physiological regulation of coagulation and fibrinolysis as the in vitro data imply, then this may be an important consideration in selecting between coumarin and heparin as anticoagulants, since activated Protein C is not inhibited by heparin and antithrombin III.

ACKNOWLEDGEMENTS

This work was supported by a grant-in-aid from the American Heart Association with funds contributed in part by the Oklahoma Heart Association and National Heart, Lung and Blood Institute Grants HL 17812 and HL 07207. This work was done during the tenure of the John L. Dickson Memorial of the American Heart Association. Frederick J. Walker was supported by a postdoctoral fellowship from the Oklahoma Affiliate of the American Heart Association.

ABBREVIATIONS

Activated Protein C : APC
Platelet Prothrombin Converting Activity; PPCA

REFERENCES

1. Mammen, E.F., Thomas, W.R., and Seegers, W.H., (1960) Thromb. Diath. Haemorrh. 5, 218-250.

2. Stenflo, J., (1976) J. Biol. Chem. 251, 355-363.

3. Seegers, W.H., Novoa, E., Henry, R.L., and Hassouna, H.I., (1976) Thromb. Res. 8, 543-552.

4. Marciniak, E., (1972) J. Lab. Clin. Med. 79, 924-934.

5. Kisiel, W., (1978) Circulation 58, 822 Abst.

6. Murano, G., Seegers, W.H., and Zolton, R.P., (1974) Thromb. Diath. Haemorrh. 57, 305-313.

7. Seegers, W.H., Marlar, R.A., and Walz, D.A., (1978) Thromb. Res. 13, 233-243.

8. Titani, K., Fujikawa, K., Enfield, D.L., Ericsson, L.H., Walsh, K.A., and Neurath, H., (1975) Proc. Nat. Acad. Sci. USA 72, 3082-3086.

9. Fernlund, P., and Stenflo, J., This symposium.

10. Seegers, W.H., Marciniak, E., and McCoy, L., (1969) Thromb. Diath. Haemorrh. 22, 32-34

11. Kisiel, W., Canfield, W.M., Ericsson, L.H., and Davie, E.W., (1977) Biochemistry 16, 5824-5839.

12. Osterud, B., Rapaport, S.I., and Lavine, K.K., (1977) Blood 49, 819-834.

13. Miletich, J.P., Jackson, C.M., and Majerus, P.W., (1978) J. Biol. Chem. 253, 6908-6919.

14. Cox, A.C., Ingyangetor, P., Esmon, C.T., and White, B.J., (1979) Blood in press.

15. Dahlback, B., and Stenflo, J., (1978) Biochemistry 17, 4938-4946.

16. Zolton, R.P., and Seegers, W.H., (1973) Thromb. Res. 3, 23-33.

17. Comp, P.C., and Esmon, C.T., (1978) Circulation 58, 819 Abst.
18. Luskutoff, D.J., and Edgington, T.S., (1977) Proc. Nat. Acad. Sci. USA 74, 3903-3907.
19. Taylor, F.B., and Müller-Eberhard, H.J., (1970) J. Clin. Inv. 49, 2068-2085.
20. Lockhardt, M.L., Comp, P.C., and Taylor, F.B., (1979) J. Lab. Clin. Med. (in press)
21. Esmon, C.T., Stenflo, J., Suttie, J.W., and Jackson, C.M., (1976) J. Biol. Chem. 251, 355-363.
22. Nelsestuen, G.L., Kisiel, W., and Di Scipio (1978) Biochemistry 17, 2134-2138.
23. Owen, W.G., Esmon, C.T., and Jackson, C.M., (1974) J. Biol. Chem. 249, 594-605.
24. Esmon, C.T., (1973) Ph.D. Thesis, Washington University, St. Louis.
25. Esmon, C.T., (1979) J. Biol. Chem. 254, 964-973.
26. Walker, F.J., Sexton, P.W., and Esmon, C.T., Biochem. Biophys. Acta. submitted.
27. Kappeler, R., (1955) Z. Klin. Med. 153, 103-113.
28. Bachmann, F., Ruckert, F., and Koller, F., (1958) Thromb. Diath. Haemorrh. 2, 24-38.
29. Bligh, E.G., and Dyer, W.J., (1959) Canad. J. Biochem. Biophys. 37, 911-917.
30. Tangen, O., Berman, H.J., and Marfey, P., (1971) Thromb. Diath. Haemorrh. 25, 268-278.
31. Hunter, W., (1969) The preparation of radioactive proteins of high activity, their reaction with antibody in vitro. Handbook of Experimental Immunology. Blackwell, London.
32. Iatridis, S.G., and Ferguson, J.H., (1963) J. Appl. Physiol. 18, 337-351.
33. Radcliffe, R., and Heinze, T., (1978) Arch. Biochem. Biophys. 189, 185-194.
34. Kisiel, W., and Davie, E.W., (1976) Biochemistry 15, 4893-4900.

AMINO ACID SEQUENCE OF BOVINE PROTEIN C

PER FERNLUND and JOHAN STENFLO

Department of Clinical Chemistry,
University of Lund, General Hospital,
S-214 01 Malmö, Sweden

INTRODUCTION

Protein C is a vitamin K-dependent glycoprotein from bovine plasma (1). The activated form of protein C seems to be identical to autoprothrombin II-A described by Seegers et al. (2). Protein C can be activated to a serine amidase by thrombin and by the factor X activator from Russels viper venom (3). Activated protein C prolongs the kaolin-cephalin clotting time of bovine plasma and inactivates purified bovine factor V in the presence of calcium ions and phospholipid (4). Protein C may thus have a regulatory effect on the rate of prothrombin activation.
Protein C has two polypeptide chains linked by one or more disulfide bridges. The amino acid sequence of the light chain is homologous to that of factor X (5). To be able to compare protein C with other serine proteases and in particular with the closely related vitamin K-dependent proteins in bovine plasma we have determined the complete amino acid sequence of protein C.

MATERIAL AND METHODS

Protein C was isolated from bovine plasma as previously described (1). After reduction and alkylation of protein C with iodo (^{14}C) acetic acid in 6 M guanidine-HCl the light and heavy chains were separated by chromatography on a AcA 44 column in 0.1 M NH_4HCO_3 (1). The procedures used for the degradation of the light chain of protein C have already been described as well as the methods used to isolate the fragments (5). The intact heavy chain was subjected to cyanogen bromide degradation, partial acid hydrolysis and to tryptic digestion after temporary blocking of NH_2-groups by citraconylation. Complete separation of the cyanogen bromide fragments was obtained by chromatography on a column (1.6cmx100cm) packed with Sephacryl S-200 in 50 mM Tris-HCl, 2 mM EDTA, 6 M guanidine hydrochloride pH 8.0. The tryptic peptides were separated by chromatography on a column (1.5cmx194cm) of Sephadex G-50 superfine in 0.1 M NH_4HCO_3. In some instances further purification of the tryptic peptides by high voltage paper electrophoresis at pH 6.5 was required.
Cyanogen bromide fragments 1, 2 and 5 were subdigested with trypsin either with or without previous citraconylation, with chymotrypsin and with the protease from Staphylococcus aureus which has a high specificity for glutamyl bonds. The resulting peptides were isolated by chromatography on Sephadex G 50 as described above for whole chain tryptic peptides. Amino acid analyses were performed with standard methods. Half-cystine was determined as S-carboxymethylcysteine. γ-Carboxyglutamic acid was determined after alkaline hydrolysis as already described (6). Sequence analyses were performed with a Beckman Sequencer (model 890 C) using a modi-

```
                    10                                      20                                      30
Ala-Asn-Ser-Phe-Leu-Gla-Gla-Leu-Arg-Pro-Gly-Asn-Val-Gla-Arg-Gla-Cys-Ser-Gla-Gla-Val-Cys-Gla-Phe-Gla-Gla-Ala-Arg-Gla-Ile-
                    40                                      50                                      60
Phe-Gln-Asn-Thr-Gla-Asp-Thr-Met-Ala-Phe-Trp-Ser-Lys-Tyr-Ser-Asp-Gly-Asp-Gln-Cys-Glu-Asp-Arg-Pro-Ser-Gly-Ser-Pro-Cys-Asp-
                    70                                      80                                      90
Leu-Pro-Cys-Cys-Gly-Arg-Gly-Lys-Cys-Ile-His-Gly-Leu-Gly-Gly-Phe-Arg-Cys-Asp-Cys-Ala-Glu-Gly-Trp-Glu-Gly-Arg-Phe-Cys-Leu-
                    100                                     110                                     120
His-Glu-Val-Arg-Phe-Ser-Asn-Cys-Ser-Ala-Glu-Asx-Gly-Gly-Cys-Ala-His-Tyr-Cys-Met-Glu-Glu-Glu-Gly-Arg-Arg-His-Cys-Ser-Cys-
                    130                                     140                                     150
Ala-Pro-Gly-Tyr-Arg-Leu-Glu-Asp-Asp-His-Gln-Leu-Cys-Val-Ser-Lys-Val-Thr-Phe-Pro-Cys-Gly-Arg-Leu-Gly-Lys-Arg-Met-Glu-Lys-

Lys-Arg-Lys-Thr-Leu


                    10                                      20                                      30
Asp-Thr-Asn-Gln-Val-Asp-Gln-Lys-Asp-Gln-Leu-Asp-Pro-Arg-Ile-Val-Asp-Gly-Gln-Glu-Ala-Gly-Trp-Gly-Glu-Ser-Pro-Trp-Gln-Ala-
                    40                                      50                                      60
Val-Leu-Leu-Asp-Ser-Lys-Lys-Lys-Leu-Val-Cys-Gly-Ala-Val-Leu-Ile-His-Val-Ser-Trp-Val-Leu-Thr-Val-Ala-His-Cys- X -Arg-Lys-
                    70                                      80                                      90
Lys-Leu-Ile-Val-Arg-Leu-Gly-Glu-Tyr-Asp-Met-Arg-Arg-Trp-Glu-Ser-Trp-Glu-Val-Asp-Leu-Asp-Ile-Lys-Glu-Val-Ile-Ile-His-Pro-
                    100                                     110                                     120
Asn*-Tyr-Thr-Lys-Ser-Tyr-Ser-Asp-Asn-Asp-Ile-Ala-Leu-Leu-Arg-Leu-Ala-Lys-Pro-Ala-Thr-Leu-Ser-Gln-Thr-Ile-Val-Pro-Ile-Cys-
                    130                                     140                                     150
Leu-Pro-Asp-Ser-Gly-Leu-Ser-Glu-Arg-Lys-Leu-Thr-Gln-Val-Gly-Gln-Glu-Thr-Val-Val-Thr-Gly-Trp-Gly-Tyr-Arg-Asp-Glu-Thr-Lys-
                    160                                     170                                     180
Arg-Asn*-Arg-Thr-Phe-Val-Leu-Ser-Phe-Ile-Lys-Val-Pro-Val-Val-Pro-Tyr- X -Ala-Cys-Val-His-Ala-Met-Glu-Asn-Lys-Ile-Ser-Glu-
                    190                                     200                                     210
Asn-Met-Leu-Cys-Ala-Gly-Ile-Leu-Gly-Asp-Pro-Arg-Asp-Ala-Cys-Glu-Gly-Asp-Ser-Gly-Gly-Pro-Met-Val-Thr-Phe-Phe-Arg-Gly-Thr-
                    220                                     230                                     240
His-Phe-Leu-Val-Gly-Leu-Val-Ser-Trp-Gly-Glu-Gly-Cys-Gly-Arg-Leu-Tyr-Asn-Tyr-Gly-Val-Tyr-Thr-Lys-Val-Ser-Arg-Tyr-Leu-Asp-
                    250
Trp-Ile-Tyr-Gly-His-Ile-Lys-Ala-Gln-Glu-Ala-Pro-Leu-Glu-Ser-Gln(Val,Pro)
```

FIGURE 1. Amino acid sequence of the light chain (top) and the heavy chain (bottom) of protein C.

fied Beckman 1 M Quadrol program (7) for intact chains and large cyanogen bromide fragments. Smaller peptides were sequenced with Polybrene (Aldrich) as a carrier in the sequenator cup using the standard Beckman 1 M Quadrol program (Beckman 122974). The phenylthiohydantoin (PTH) amino acid derivatives were identified by high pressure liquid chromatography and thin-layer chromatography as described (5). PTH carboxymethylcysteine was also identified by measurements of radioactivity.

RESULTS AND DISCUSSION

The amino acid sequence of the light and heavy chains of bovine protein C are shown in Figure 1. The 155 amino acid residues long light chain sequence was derived from data obtained by sequenator analysis of the intact chain and of fragments isolated after cyanogen bromide cleavage, tryptic digestion of citraconylated light chain and BNPS-skatole treated light chain (Fig. 2). Further data about how the structure of the light chain was determined will not be given here since it has already been published (5).

Five unique cyanogen bromide fragments were isolated from the heavy chain (Fig. 2). They could be aligned essentially with the aid of peptides from the tryptic digest of the intact heavy chain. Partial acid hydrolysis resulted in a cleavage between Asp 12 and Pro 13 and between Asp 190 and Pro 191. Isolation of the resulting COOH-terminal fragment

TABLE I
Amino Acid Composition of Protein C

Amino Acid	Light chain		Heavy chain	
	Composition after acid hydrolysis[1]	Found in sequence[1]	Composition after acid hydrolysis	found in sequence
Lysine	6.3	7	11.5	15
Histidine	3.5	5	3.6	6
Arginine	12.4	14	11.9	14
Half-cystine	17.9	17	9.6	7
Aspartic acid	14.3	13	25.4	23
Threonine	4.2	4	12.6	14
Serine	10.5	10	14.6	15
Glutamic acid	23.5	24	28.3	26
Proline	6.3	6	13.9	12
Glycine	17.2	16	22.7	21
Alanine	7.9	7	16.0	13
Valine	4.7	5	22.7	26
Methionine	3.3	3	5.1	4
Isoleucine	2.0	2	14.1	14
Leucine	8.0	9	22.6	24
Tyrosine	2.9	3	7.3	9
Phenylalanine	8.0	8	7.8	5
Tryptophan	2.5	2	6.1	8

1 From Fernlund, P., Stenflo, J., and Tufvesson, A. (5).

made possible the proper alignment of CB 4 and CB 5. CB 5 was the only cyanogen bromide fragment lacking homoserine and thus constituted the COOH-terminal part of the heavy chain. The tryptic peptide (TR 4) containing residues 66 to 72 did not give a satisfactory overlap between CB 1 and CB 2. Due to incomplete cyanogen bromide cleavage between CB 1 and CB 2, a large fragment was isolated which had the same NH_2-terminal sequence as CB 1 and an amino acid composition that was identical with the sum of the compositions of CB 1 and CB 2.

To determine the complete sequences of CB 1, CB 2 and CB 5 subdigestion with proteolytic enzymes was necessary (Fig. 2). In CB 1 the residue in position 58 could not be identified, presumably because it was washed out from the sequenator cup. Since CB 1 was resistant to digestion with the Glu-specific protease from S. aureus we have not yet been able to establish an overlap between CH 1 (residues 51-58) and TR 3 (residues 60-65) in CB 1. The overlap between residues 153 and 154 in CB 2 is also tentative. All peptides isolated from digests of the intact heavy chain as well as from digests of the individual cyanogen bromide fragments have been accounted for in the sequence.

The two Asn residues (no 91 and 152) marked with asterisks (Fig. 2) are assumed to have carbohydrate side chains attached to them. The corresponding sequenator cycles were blank and the assignments have been made on the basis of 1. the presence of Thr residues in positions 93 and 154 i.e. necessary conditions for the attachment of carbohydrate side chains were fulfilled, 2. the corresponding peptides tarred on acid hydrolysis and glukosamine was found on amino acid analysis. We have not yet been

Amino Acid Sequence of Protein C

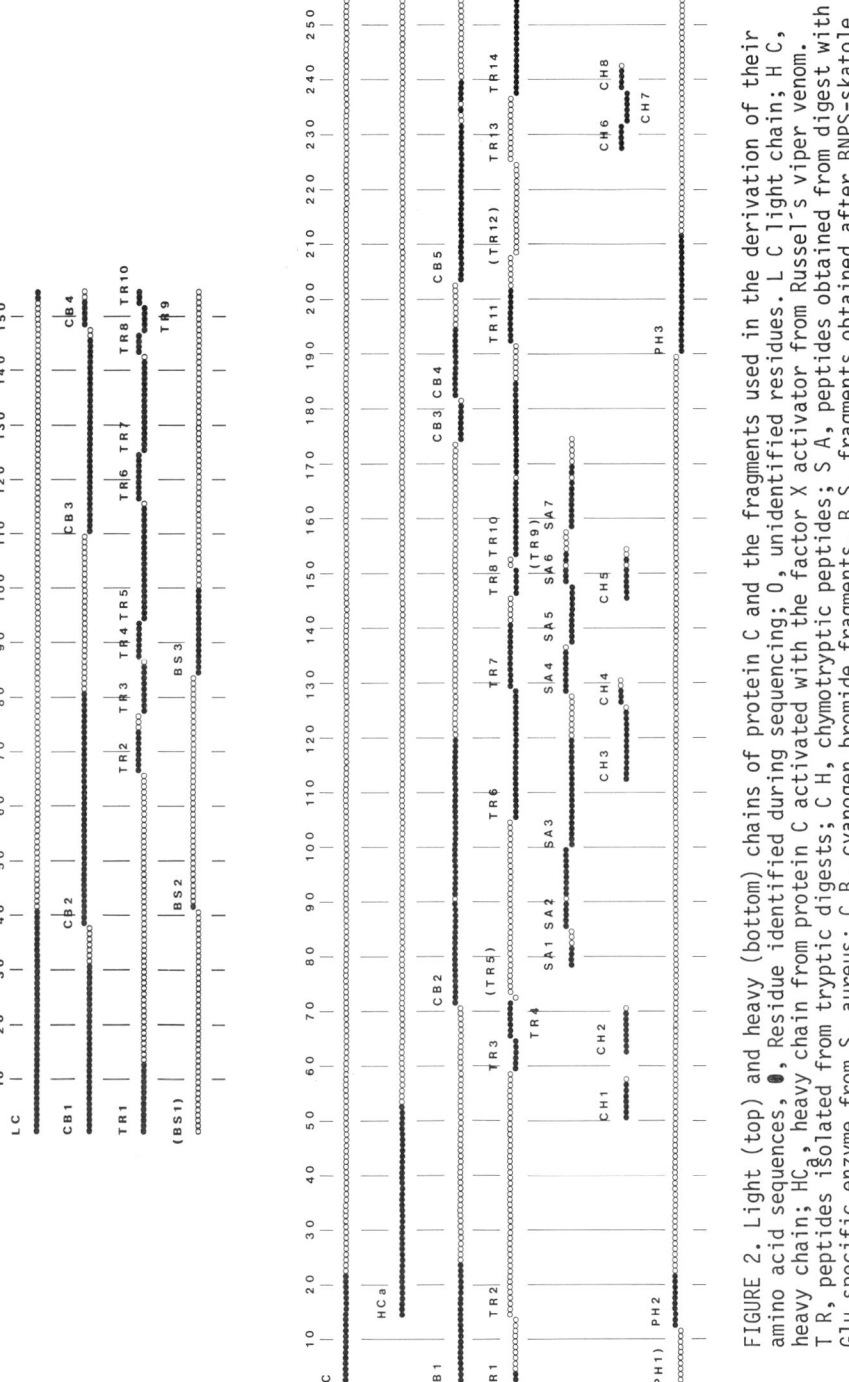

FIGURE 2. Light (top) and heavy (bottom) chains of protein C and the fragments used in the derivation of their amino acid sequences, ●, Residue identified during sequencing; O, unidentified residues. L C light chain; H C, heavy chain; HC$_a$, heavy chain from protein C activated with the factor X activator from Russel's viper venom. T R, peptides isolated from tryptic digests; C H, chymotryptic peptides; S A, peptides obtained from digest with Glu specific enzyme from S. aureus; C B, cyanogen bromide fragments, B S, fragments obtained after BNPS-skatole cleavage; P H, fragments obtained by partial acid hydrolysis.

able to make a positive identification in position 168. Carboxypeptidase Y digestion of the intact heavy chain did not release any amino acids and the order of the two carboxyterminal residues of the chain is unknown.

The amino acid compositions predicted from the sequences of the light and heavy chains of protein C are given in Table I. They are in accordance with those obtained after acid hydrolysis. The γ-carboxyglutamic acid content in three different preparations of the light chain was 10.3, 11.4 and 9.6 moles per mol of light chain, respectively. Eleven residues were found by sequencing.

The NH_2 terminal region of the light chain of protein C, which has the vitamin K-dependent γ-carboxyglutamic acid residues shows a pronounced homology with the corresponding part of prothrombin and factor X. The rest of the sequence of the light chain, i.e. approximately from residue 45 shows more homology with factor X than with prothrombin (5). On activation of protein C by thrombin or by the factor X activator from Russel´s viper venom the peptide bond between residues 14 and 15 is cleaved (3). The sequence of the heavy chain of protein C is homologous to those of other plasma and pancreatic serine proteases (8). The components of the "charge-relay" system of pancreatic serine proteases are all found in the heavy chain of protein C, i.e. His 56, Asp 100, and Ser 199. These results suggest that the conformation of active protein C is similar to that of the other serine proteases.

ACKNOWLEDGEMENTS

The expert technical assistance of Mrs Monica Jönsson and Mr Roland Nilsson is gratefully acknowledged. The authors are also indebted to Mr Arne Tufvesson who purified protein C. This investigation was supported by grants from the Swedish Medical Research Council (projects no B79-13X-4487-5C and B79-13X-00581-15B) and by grants from Magnus Bergvalls Stiftelse and from Thorsten and Elsa Segerfalks Stiftelse. The sequenator was procured by a grant from the Wallenberg Foundation.

REFERENCES

1. Stenflo, J. (1976) J. Biol. Chem. 251, 355-363.
2. Seegers, W.H., Novoa, E., Henry, R.L., and Hassouna, H.J. (1976) Thromb. Res. 8, 543-552.
3. Kisiel, W., Ericsson, L.H., and Davie, E.W. (1976) Biochemistry 15, 4893-4900.
4. Kisiel, W., Caufield, W.M., Ericsson, L.H., and Davie, E.W. (1977) Biochemistry 16, 5824-5831.
5. Fernlund, P., Stenflo, J., and Tufvesson, A. (1978) Proc. Natl. Acad. Sci. USA 75, 5889-5892.
6. Fernlund, P., Stenflo, J., Roepstorff, P., and Thomsen, J. (1975) J. Biol. Chem. 250, 6125-6133.
7. Thomsen, J., Bucher, D., Brunfeldt, K., Nexof, E., and Olesen, H. (1976) Eur. J. Biochem. 69, 87-96.
8. Woodbury, R.G., Katunuma, N., Kobayashi, K., Titani, K., and Neurath, H. (1978) Biochemistry 17, 811-819.

INTERACTION BETWEEN PROTHROMBIN AND THE PLATELET RECEPTOR FOR FACTOR X_A INHIBITORY EFFECT OF PROTEIN C

JOHAN STENFLO and BJÖRN DAHLBÄCK

Department of Clinical Chemistry,
University of Lund, General Hospital,
S-214 01 Malmö, Sweden

INTRODUCTION

Activation of prothrombin to thrombin by limited proteolysis is the last zymogen activation in the clotting cascade. It has been carefully studied in vitro with purified components and involves the cleavage of two peptide bonds in prothrombin by activated factor X (factor X_a) (Fig. 1) (1-3). The activation rate of prothrombin is greatly increased when factor X_a is part of a macromolecular complex, the prothrombinase complex, in which the following interactions have been demonstrated: factor X_a - Ca^{2+} ions - phospholipid; factor X_a - factor V; factor V - phospholipid (3,4). Prothrombin fragment 1 interacts with phospholipid, and fragment 2 with factor V in the prothrombinase complex. Although platelets have been shown to substitute for phospholipid in clotting assays detailed knowledge about the interaction of the vitamin K-dependent proteins with platelets was lacking, until Miletich et al. (5,6) demonstrated binding of human factor X_a to a platelet receptor. The receptor was exposed after the release reaction had been induced and had properties in common with plasma factor V. Factor X_a bound to platelets activated prothrombin more effectively than when bound to phospholipid and factor V. The importance of the factor X_a binding to platelets was further documented when Miletich et al. (7) demonstrated low or absent factor X_a binding to platelets from factor V deficient patients.
 The recently discovered vitamin K-dependent protein C (8) is, after activation by thrombin, a potent inhibitor of factor V-activity (9). Presumably activated protein C (protein C_a) is identical with autoprothrombin II-A described by Seegers et al. (10). The inactivation of factor V requires the presence of phospholipid and calcium ions. Whether protein C has a regulating effect on prothrombin activation in vivo has not yet been established.
 The purpose of the present study was to investigate the interaction between platelets and the vitamin K-dependent proteins, prothrombin, factor X, and protein C. Bovine coagulation factors and platelets were used.

BINDING OF FACTOR X_a TO PLATELETS

A previously described experimental model (5,11), utilizing highly purified bovine coagulation factors and washed bovine platelets, was used to study the effect of platelets on prothrombin activation. Measurements were made of ^{14}C serotonin release, binding of ^{125}I factor X_a to platelets, and of thrombin generation. Following the addition of factor X_a ^{14}C serotonin was rapidly released by a very small amount of thrombin probably formed on the surface of disintegrated platelets. Subsequent to the

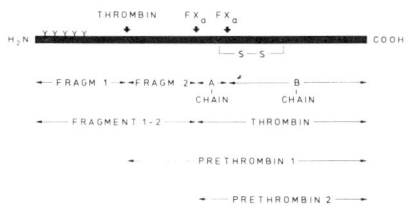

FIGURE 1. Schematic structural model of the prothrombin molecule. Activation of prothrombin by factor X_a involves two peptide bond cleavages. The first one gives rise to fragment 1-2 and prethrombin 2. Prethrombin 2 is activated to thrombin by the second cleavage. Thrombin can cleave fragment 1-2 yielding fragment 1 and fragment 2. If thrombin acts on intact prothrombin the NH_2-terminal fragment 1 and prethrombin 1 are formed. The symbol (Y) denotes γ-carboxyglutamic acid residues.

release reaction, factor X_a bound to the platelet surface and thrombin was generated. To avoid possible interference from high concentrations of prothrombin activation fragments and thrombin, formed during the prothrombin activation, the ^{125}I factor X_a binding was initially characterized in the absence of prothrombin. The binding of factor X_a to platelets, in which the release reaction had been induced with a low concentration of thrombin, had the properties of a true receptor interaction. It was saturable, reversible, and correlated with the biological response i.e. the thrombin formation rate. At low factor X_a concentrations the rates of prothrombin activation measured in the presence of platelets were higher than those obtained with optimum concentrations of phospholipid and factor V. No factor X_a binding was found if the platelet release reaction had not been induced. Furthermore the zymogen factor X was not bound whether platelet release had been induced or not.

The specific binding of factor X_a was saturable at levels of 2-3 ng bound per 1×10^8 platelets corresponding to 290-420 binding sites per platelet. The association constant, estimated from Scatchard plots, was approximately $5 \times 10^9 M^{-1}$ (2.8×10^9 to $1.0 \times 10^{10} M^{-1}$). Platelet bound ^{125}I factor X_a was rapidly displaced by the addition of an excess of unlabeled factor X_a or diisopropylphosphofluoridate inactivated factor X_a (DIP-factor X_a). Direct binding of ^{125}I DIP-factor X_a was also demonstrated. Prothrombin activation was effectively inhibited by the displacement of factor X_a from the platelet receptor by DIP-factor X_a. It would thus appear that an intact active site is not a prerequisite for binding of factor X_a to the platelet surface. The difference in binding between zymogen and active enzyme can instead presumably be attributed to the conformational change that takes place upon activation of the zymogen.

STRUCTURAL REQUIREMENTS ON PROTHROMBIN FOR ACTIVATION IN THE PRESENCE OF PLATELETS

Both the fragment 1 and fragment 2 parts are important for the interaction of prothrombin with the prothrombinase complex (3). Detailed knowledge about the activation of prothrombin by factor X_a in the presence of platelets has, however, been lacking. Efforts to demonstrate direct binding of prothrombin to platelets, with the methods used for measurements of factor X_a binding, have been unsuccessful probably due to a much lower binding constant with a rapid dissociation of prothrombin from a platelet receptor (11,12). The platelet prothrombin interaction was therefore studied by indirect means i.e. by determining the structural requirements on prothrombin for its activation by platelet bound factor X_a. Activation of prothrombin by factor X_a in the presence of platelets gave rise to the same activation fragments and products as previously identified in the phospholipid-factor V system. To elucidate the roles of prothrombin fragment 1 and fragment 2 for activation of prothrombin by platelet bound factor X_a the thrombin formation rates in incubations with equimolar concentrations of prothrombin, prethrombin 1 and prethrombin 2 were compared (Fig. 2). The thrombin formation rate in an incubation with

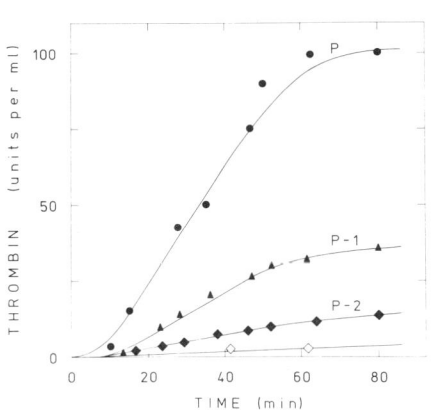

FIGURE 2. Structural requirements on prothrombin for activation by factor X_a in the presence of platelets. Release was induced with the calcium ionophore A 23 187 (1 μM final concentration) in parallel incubations at 22°C with platelets (1x10^8 per ml) in 50 mM Tris-HCl, 0.15 M NaCl, 2.5 mM CaCl, pH 7.5 containing albumin (5 mg per ml) and glucose (1 mg per ml). The incubations contained equimolar concentrations of prothrombin (0.22 mg per ml, 3 μM), prethrombin 1 (0.15 mg per ml, 3 μM) or prethrombin 2 (0.11 mg per ml, 3 μM). Reactions were initiated by addition of factor X_a (200 ng per ml) and thrombin formation was followed. (●), Normal prothrombin; (▲), prethrombin 1; (◆), prethrombin 2; (◇), a parallel incubation with prethrombin 2 without platelets. If platelets were omitted from the incubations with prothrombin and prethrombin 1 no thrombin was formed.

prethrombin 2 and fragment 2 was approximately the same as in the incubation with prethrombin 1. The reason for this is that fragment 2 and prethrombin 2 associate noncovalently (13). We conclude that both the phospholipid binding fragment 1 and the factor V binding fragment 2 are required for rapid prothrombin activation in the presence of platelets.

After administration of vitamin K antagonists prothrombin as well as the other vitamin K-dependent coagulation factors are synthesized in abnormal forms (14-16) lacking γ-carboxyglutamic acid residues. The fragment 1 part of acarboxyprothrombin (dicoumarol induced abnormal prothrombin) does not bind to phospholipid (17), and the rate of activation of acarboxyprothrombin to thrombin by factor X_a is accordingly uninfluenced by the addition of phospholipid. The factor V binding fragment 2 parts are identical in acarboxy and normal prothrombin. To elucidate the functional significance of the γ-carboxyglutamic acid residues an incubation with a-carboxyprothrombin instead of normal prothrombin was performed. No thrombin activity of ^{14}C serotonin release was detected during 40 to 50 min of incubation. When the incubation was extended further, thrombin was slowly generated after a submaximal serotonin release. If the release reaction was induced with the calcium ionophore A 23 187 (Lilly) the slow thrombin generation started immediately. This was presumably due to interaction between the fragment 2 part of acarboxyprothrombin and the now exposed platelet factor X_a receptor.

The rate of activation in incubations with prothrombin was a function of the amount of factor X_a bound to platelet factor X_a receptors. This was the case also when platelets and factor X_a mixtures were incubated with prethrombin 1 or acarboxyprothrombin illustrating that these substrates have an affinity for the factor X_a receptor and that they are activated to thrombin on the platelet surface (Fig. 3). Compared with pro-

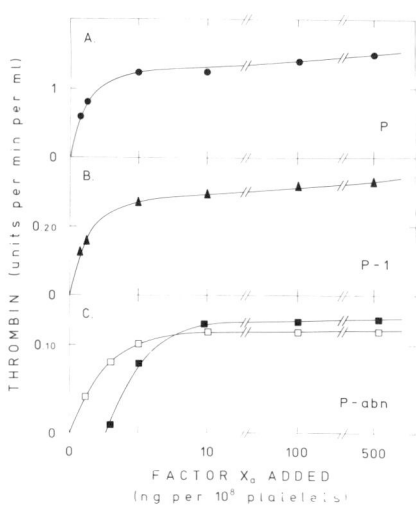

FIGURE 3. Comparison between thrombin formation rates in platelet incubations with normal prothrombin, prethrombin 1 or a-carboxyprothrombin, and increasing factor X_a concentrations. The thrombin formation rates were calculated from the maximum slopes of the thrombin formation curves, determined in parallel incubations, at 22°C in the standard buffer, with platelets (1×10^8 per ml), different factor X_a concentrations, and A, (●) normal prothrombin (0.15 mg per ml, 2 μM); B, (▲) prethrombin 1 (0.10 mg per ml, 2 μM); C, (□) acarboxyprothrombin (0.15 mg per ml, 2 μM). (■) A-carboxyprothrombin with the release reaction induced with the calcium ionophore A 23 187.

thrombin the maximum rate of activation was however tenfold lower with acarboxyprothrombin and fourfold lower with prethrombin 1, at the particular substrate concentration used. K_M and k_{cat} for prothrombin, prethrombin 1, and acarboxyprothrombin in the factor X_a - platelet system were determined. Maximal thrombin formation rates were estimated in parallel incubations with varied substrate concentrations. The K_M for prothrombin was found to be approximately 0.6 μM. The k_{cat}, calculated by using the amount of factor X_a bound (6×10^{-14} moles per 1×10^8 platelets (11)) as E_T, was found to be $10^a sec^{-1}$. The K_M for acarboxyprothrombin and prethrombin 1 were equal and found to be 3.6 μM or approximately 6 times higher than the K_M determined for prothrombin. The k_{cat} for acarboxyprothrombin was 1.3 sec^{-1} and 3.0 sec^{-1} for prethrombin 1. The coefficient for proteolytic efficiency k_{cat}/K_M (18) was thus approximately 50 times higher for normal prothrombin than for acarboxyprothrombin. This illustrates the importance of the carboxylated glutamic acid residues for normal phospholipid binding and for rapid activation of prothrombin by platelet bound factor X_a.

The data obtained by Miletich et al. (5-7) and by ourselves (11) thus indicate that a receptor is exposed on the surface on platelets as a result of the release reaction. The receptor binds factor X_a with high affinity and prothrombin with low affinity effectively exposing susceptible bonds in prothrombin for factor X_a. The receptor consists of a negatively charged phospholipid and of a protein, closely related to plasma factor V, both exposed upon the release reaction. The γ-carboxyglutamic acid residues in factor X_a and prothrombin are required for the Ca^{2+}-ion-dependent interaction with the phospholipid. High affinity binding of factor X_a and rapid activation of prothrombin also require the factor V related part of the receptor.

PROTEIN C_a. AN IN VITRO INHIBITOR FOR PROTHROMBIN ACTIVATION

Protein C is a zymogen of a serine amidase (19,20). It can be activated both by the factor X-activator from Russel's viper venom and by thrombin (9). On activation an Arg-Ile bond in the aminoterminal part of the heavy chain is cleaved, and an activation peptide 14 amino acid residues long is released. Bovine activated protein C, but not the zymogen, markedly prolongs the kaolin-cephalin clotting time of bovine plasma but not of human plasma as shown by Kisiel et al. (9). Plasma factor V, which enhances the rate of prothrombin activation about 200-fold, is readily inactivated by protein C_a in the presence of calcium ions and phospholipid (9). Since the platelet factor X_a - prothrombin receptor has many properties in common with plasma factor V, the inhibitory effect of protein C_a on the rate of prothrombin activation in this system was investigated. Such an inhibition actually occurred although to a slight extent at a protein C_a concentration of 1 μg per ml. At higher concentrations the effect was more pronounced. To explore the possibility that proteolysis of the platelet factor X_a-prothrombin receptor by protein C_a caused the inhibition of prothrombin activation the following experiments were performed. Protein C_a was incubated at 37°C with platelets in which the release reaction had been induced with thrombin. After various preincubation periods ^{125}I factor X_a and prothrombin were added to aliquots of the suspension. Thrombin generation and factor X_a binding were then measured (Fig. 4).

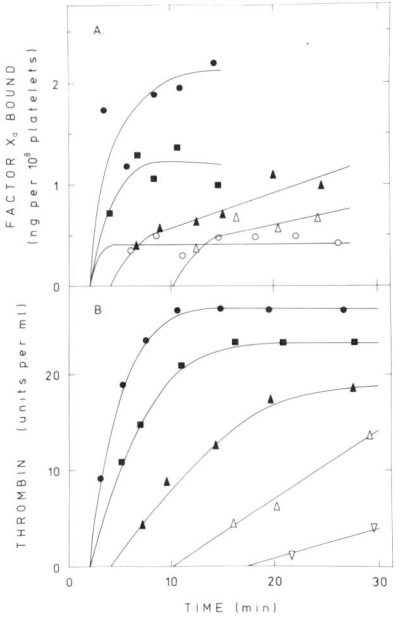

FIGURE 4. Platelet factor X_a receptor sites are destroyed by protein C_a. Platelets (1×10^8 per ml) were treated with thrombin (1 unit per ml) to induce the release reaction and then incubated with protein C_a (1 μg per ml). ^{125}I-factor X_a (20 ng per ml) and prothrombin (0.1 mg per ml) were added to aliquots of the reaction mixture at different times and factor X_a binding (A) and thrombin formation (B) were followed. (●), An incubation without protein C_a; (■), protein C_a, ^{125}I factor X_a, and prothrombin added simultaneously; (▲), two minutes preincubation with protein C_a; (△) eight minutes preincubation; (▽), fifteen minutes preincubation.(0) nonspecific binding of factor X_a.

Protein C_a was found to destroy the factor X_a receptor after a short incubation with a concomitant decrease in thrombin generation rate. If ^{125}I factor X_a, prothrombin, and protein C_a were added simultaneously, the amount of factor X_a bound was constant during the first ten minutes and approximately 50 % of that in a parallel incubation without protein C_a. The effect on the thrombin formation rate was small and similar to that obtained with unreleased platelets. The factor X_a binding sites on the receptors thus seemed to be protected from proteolysis by protein C_a when occupied by factor X_a. To investigate if the binding sites for prothrombin on the receptor were destroyed by protein C_a, ^{125}I-factor X_a and protein C_a were added simultaneously to a platelet suspension after the release reaction had been induced. Prothrombin was added to aliquots of the platelet suspension after various intervals. No difference in the amount of factor X_a bound was found in these aliquots. There was, however, a gradual decrease in thrombin formation rates as shown in Figure 5. Apparently pro-

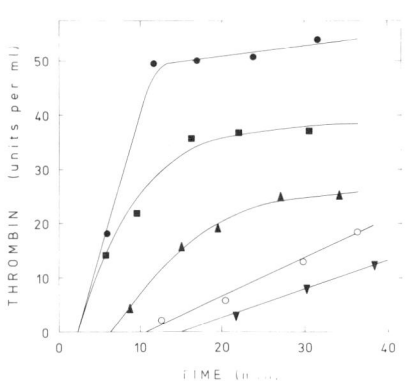

FIGURE 5. Protein C_a destroys the site interacting with prothrombin on the platelet surface. ^{125}I factor X_a (20 ng per ml) and protein C_a (1 µg per ml) were added simultaneously to a platelet incubation (1x10^8 per ml) pretreated with thrombin (1 unit per ml) to induce release. The incubation was performed at 37°C in the standard buffer. Prothrombin (0.1 mg per ml) was added after various intervals and thrombin formation was measured. (●), incubation without protein C_a; (■), ^{125}I factor X_a, protein C_a and prothrombin added simultaneously; (▲) prothrombin added after 3 min; (O), prothrombin added after 7 min; (▼), prothrombin added after 12 min.

tein C_a not only destroys the receptor site for factor X_a but also inhibits the interaction between the platelet receptor and prothrombin. No measurable effect on factor X_a binding and thrombin generation was found if protein C_a had previously been incubated with diisopropyl phosphorofluoridate. Furthermore protein C_a binding to platelets was undetectable with the technique used to measure factor X_a binding. The conclusion that protein C_a destroys the factor X_a-prothrombin receptor by proteolysis was supported by the time course of the reactions.

Thrombin, which readily activates protein C at an enzyme-to-substrate ratio of 1:50 (9) may be the physiological activator of protein C. Kisiel et al. (20) have, however, reported that protein C isolated from serum was indistinguishable from that isolated from plasma. Furthermore fluoresceinisothiocyanate labeled protein C did not appear to be activated during clotting of plasma in the presence of brain thromboplastin or a kaolin-phospholipid mixture. These experiments do not preclude that protein C may be activated during blood coagulation in vivo. Possible activation of protein C during prothrombin activation in the presence of platelets was studied by including ^{125}I labeled protein C in a standard platelet-prothrombin-factor X_a incubation. Aliquots were drawn during the incubation and subjected to SDS-slab-gel electrophoresis. After 20 min incubation approximately 20 % of the added ^{125}I protein C, corresponding to 1 µg per ml, was activated, and after 60 min the activated form accounted for approximately 40 %. Although the experiment does not simulate in vivo hemostasis it suggests that protein C may be activated during blood clotting in vivo and may have a physiological effect as one of the regulators of the rate of prothrombin activation.

ACKNOWLEDGEMENT

The expert technical assistance of Mrs Bergisa Hildebrand is gratefully acknowledged. This investigation was supported by a grant from the Swedish Medical Research Council (project no. B79-13X-4487-5C).

REFERENCES

1. Davie, E.W., and Fujikawa, K. (1975) Ann. Rev. Biochem. 44, 799-829.
2. Mann, K.G. (1976) Methods Enzymol. 45, 123-156.
3. Suttie, J.W., and Jackson, C.M. (1977) Physiol. Rev. 55, 1-70.
4. Freeman, J.P., Guillin, M.C., Begeand, A., and Jackson, C.M. (1977) Fed. Proc. 36, 675.
5. Miletich, J.P., Jackson, C.M., and Majerus, P.W. (1977) Proc. Natl. Acad. Sci. USA 74, 4033-4036.
6. Miletich, J.P., Jackson, C.M., and Majerus, P.W. (1978) J. Biol. Chem. 253, 6908-6916.
7. Miletich, J.P., Majerus, D.W., and Majerus, P.W. (1978) J. Clin. Invest. 62, 824-831.
8. Stenflo, J. (1976) J. Biol. Chem. 251, 355-363.
9. Kisiel, W., Canfield, W.M., Ericsson, L.H., and Davie, E.W. (1977) Biochemistry 16, 5824-5831.
10. Seegers, W.H., Novoa, E., Henry, R.L., and Hassouna, H.J. (1976) Thromb. Res. 8, 543-552.
11. Dahlbäck, B., and Stenflo, J. (1978) Biochemistry 17, 4938-4945.
12. Tollefsen, D.M., Jackson, C.M., and Majerus, P.W. (1975) J. Clin. Invest, 56, 241-245.
13. Jackson, C.M., Esmon, C.T., and Owen, W.G. (1975) in Proteases and Biological Control (E. Reich, D.B. Rifkin and E. Shaw, eds.), pp 95-109, Cold Spring Harbor Laboratory, New York.
14. Reekers, P.P.M., Lindhout, M.J., Kop-Klaassen, B.H.M., and Hemker, H.C. (1973) Biochim. Biophys. Acta 317, 559-562.
15. Stenflo, J., and Suttie, J.W. (1977) Ann. Rev. Biochem. 46, 157-172.
16. Stenflo, J. (1978) Adv. Enzymol. 46, 1-31.
17. Esmon, C.T., Suttie, J.W., and Jackson, C.M. (1975) J. Biol. Chem. 250, 4095-4099.
18. Fruton, J. (1975) in Proteases and Biological Control (E. Reich, D.B. Rifkin and E. Shaw, eds.), pp 33-50, Cold Spring Harbor Laboratory, New York.
19. Esmon, C.T., Stenflo, J., Suttie, J.W., and Jackson, C.M. (1976) J. Biol. Chem. 251, 3052-3056.
20. Kisiel, W., Ericsson, L.H., and Davie, E.W. (1976) Biochemistry 15, 4893-4900.

FUNCTION OF PREVIOUSLY UNRECOGNIZED PLASMA PROTEIN M IN THROMBIN GENERATION

WALTER H. SEEGERS, ABHA GHOSH, and VAN-YU WU

Wayne State University School of Medicine
Detroit, MI 48201

INTRODUCTION

By 1939 methods had been developed for quantitative analysis of prothrombin and thrombin, and valuable preparations of bovine prothrombin complex and thrombin were obtained. Prothrombin lost all of its activity when thrombin was added to it (1). The reasons for this loss is now partly understood. Among the reactions that took place, Protein C was converted to the inhibitor called autoprothrombin II-A. This retarded the reagents used for the two-stage assay of prothrombin. Additionally, thrombin divided the prothrombin molecule into prothrombin fragment 1 and prethrombin 1. In the bovine species the former consists of 156 amino acid residues including ten γ-carboxyglutamic acid residues important for the transformation of prothrombin to thrombin. This loss of prothrombin fragment 1, due to the addition of thrombin to prothrombin, left the thrombin precursor refractory to the two-stage reagents. When prethrombin 1 was isolated for the first time (2), it did not convert to thrombin when the two-stage analytical reagents were used. It was, however, converted to thrombin slowly, after a prominent lag phase, with only purified Factor Xa (2,3). The activity of Factor Xa was enhanced by the addition of purified Ac-globulin (Factor V), phospholipid and calcium ions (3,4). Thus, a five-component system consisting of substrate (prethrombin 1), activating enzyme (Factor Xa) and accessories (phospholipid, Ac-globulin and calcium ions) generated thrombin rapidly. For a given amount of substrate the enzyme and accessories were used at "optimum" concentrations in a manner which would reduce the thrombin yield in association with reduction in concentration of either Factor Xa, Ac-globulin, phospholipid or calcium ions. One could then summarize the five-component system as follows:

$$\text{Prethrombin 1} \xrightarrow{\begin{array}{c}Ca^{2+}\\ \text{Ac-globulin}\\ \text{Phospholipid}\\ \text{Factor Xa}\end{array}} \text{Thrombin + Fragment 2}$$

The thrombin generating characteristics of the above five-component system were altered appreciably when prothrombin complex or prothrombin preparations were substituted for prethrombin 1 (5,6). With prothrombin complex or purified prothrombin, activation was more rapid than with prethrombin 1 and ten times less Factor Xa was sufficient. The yield of thrombin from these substrates was also higher than from prethrombin 1 (5,6). For accelerating thrombin generation from prothrombin complex or prothrombin, best results were obtained with the simultaneous presence of optimal concentrations of calcium ions, Ac-globulin and lipids such as phosphatidyl serine or phosphatidyl inositol (5). Reducing any one of the three accessories to zero concentration reduced the rate and yield of thrombin generation.

One might suppose that the difference in activation characteristics of prethrombin 1 and either the prothrombin preparation or prothrombin complex could be due to the binding of phospholipid to prothrombin via calcium ions, and failure to do so with prethrombin 1. This could not occur with prethrombin 1 because there are no γ-carboxyglutamic acid residues in the molecule. They are in prothrombin fragment 1. But even with prothrombin certain bile salts can be substituted for phospholipid (5), and unlike lipids, the bile salts do not bind to prothrombin even in the presence of calcium ions (7). Thus, the formation of a complex consisting of prothrombin, phospholipids and calcium ions does not completely account for the main events in the transformation of prothrombin to thrombin.

OBJECTIVES

Using the five-component system we compared the activation characteristics of our prethrombin 1 preparation of 1967 (2) with our so-called DEAE-prothrombin preparation of 1972 (8) and with our isolated prothrombin of 1976 (9). The latter can be regarded as clean on the basis of numerous criteria, and has a higher specific activity than any other bovine product. Using the five-component system we have found that the highly purified prothrombin activates more nearly like prethrombin 1 than DEAE-prothrombin or prothrombin complex. This implies that the latter contains a factor of importance for thrombin generation, and we succeeded in isolating small amounts of a protein with procoagulant properties. Until a better term is found we can call this material Protein M. The five-component system becomes modified as follows:

$$\text{Prothrombin} \xrightarrow{\begin{array}{c} Ca^{2+} \\ Ac\text{-globulin} \\ \text{Phospholipid} \\ \text{Protein M} \\ \text{Factor Xa} \end{array}} \text{Thrombin + Fragments}$$

Prothrombin Complex Fractionation

The prothrombin complex preparations were obtained and fractionated as previously described (8,9). However, step-wise elution was used in place of a gradient. The results of this approach are outlined by means of Table 1. Protein C and F-VII were eluted with 0.15 M sodium chloride. The eventual yield of purified Factor VII was about 0.8 mg/liter plasma, and is more than obtained in the extensive work of Nemerson and associates (10-12). Kisiel and Davie (13) obtained only a milligram from 25 liters of plasma. By the methods outlined (Table 1), the following were obtained as purified single components: Protein C, Factor VII, prothrombin, Protein M-2, Factor IX, Protein M, Factor X, and Factor X similar inert protein. Protein M was obtained in the 0.30 M sodium chloride eluate and then purified using a Sephadex G-100 column. For reasons still to be determined, the protein was not always obtained. One possibility is that it occurs in plasma in precursor form.

TABLE 1. Fractionation of bovine prothrombin complex on DEAE-Sephadex A-50 column (2.5 x 15 cm).

Molar NaCl	Eluted Material*	Remarks
0.15	Protein C + F-VII + Unknown Component	Resolved on Sephadex G-100 Column (2.5 x 180 cm) to Obtain Clean Protein C and Factor VII
0.20	Multiple Components	No Activity Identified
0.25	Prothrombin + Protein M-2 + F-IX + Trace Protein M + Unknown Component	Resolved on Heparin-Sepharose Column (1.5 x 18 cm) to Obtain Pure Prothrombin and F-IX, and Nearly Pure Protein M-2**
0.30	Protein M + Unknown Components	Resolved on Sephadex G-100 Column (2.5 x 180 cm) Clean Protein M
0.50	F-X + Inactive Material	Resolved on Sephadex G-100 Column (2.5 x 180 cm)***

*In all cases a single symmetrical elution curve.
**Some protein is removed from this Protein M-2 fraction on Sephadex G-100 column (2.5 x 180 cm). Protein M-2 modifies the initial velocity of thrombin generation from purified prothrombin when Ac-globulin is left out of the five-component system.
***F-X is obtained as a single component. The inactive material is also pure, with amino acid composition and with some other properties similar to Factor X.

Five-Component System

The concentration of purified prothrombin, DEAE-prothrombin, or prothrombin complex was set near 1,200 U/ml on the basis of our two-stage prethrombin assay (2). That assay generates as much thrombin as possible by any known means and thus the results obtained by that method served as a standard base for comparison. For the five-component system, other assay procedures and methods, including concentrations of procoagulants, were also the same as in previous work from this laboratory (4-6). Figure 1 is intended as an illustration to represent confirmation and duplication of previous work. All of the prothrombin in the prothrombin complex was converted to thrombin. By contrast, the yield of thrombin from purified prothrombin, under the same conditions, was incomplete unless a small amount of Protein M was added (Fig. 2). With purified prethrombin 1 the yield of thrombin was also less than with purified prothrombin complex. Nevertheless, the addition of Protein M resulted in complete conversion of prethrombin 1 to thrombin even though less effectively than with prothrombin (Fig. 3). Protein M thus functions as a procoagulant irrespective of whether the thrombin precursor contains γ-carboxyglutamic acid residues or not. The same function could not be demonstrated with purified Factor VII.

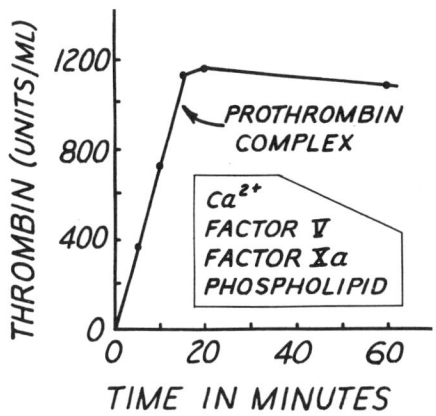

FIGURE 1. Prothrombin concentration in the prothrombin complex preparation was 1200 U/ml in the final reaction mixture. At the same time the Factor Xa concentration 12 U/ml (Bovine plasma = 34 U/ml Factor X). The Factor V concentration was 50 U/ml, the lipid concentration 0.3 mg/ml, and the calcium ion concentration 0.01 M. Results confirm previous work (5,6).

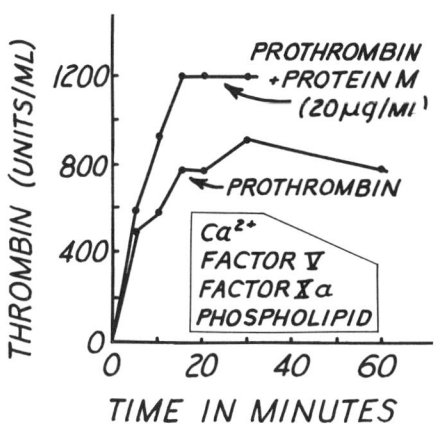

FIGURE 2. Five-component system with purified prothrombin instead of prothrombin complex as in Figure 1. Note incomplete yield of thrombin, except when Protein M was supplied. Factors Xa, V, lipid and calcium ion concentrations the same as for data of Figure 1.

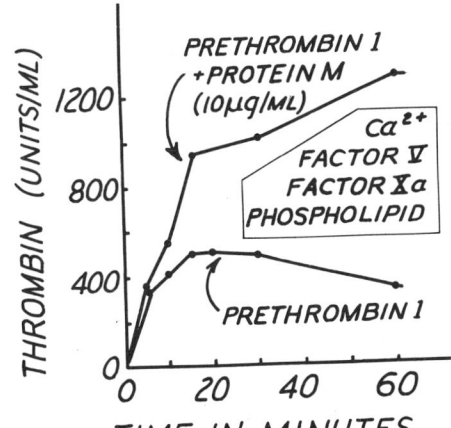

FIGURE 3. Five-component system with purified prethrombin 1. Compare with Figure 2. Thrombin yield from prethrombin 1 was less than with prothrombin. The thrombin yield was brought to 100% with the addition of Protein M. With 20 µg of Protein M instead of ten, thrombin generation was more rapid. Lower curve comparable to data presented in 1967 by Baker and Seegers (4).

Prothrombin Time

The prothrombin time of plasma from a steer treated with dicumarol was 204 sec. About 50 μg of Protein M brought this to 26.8 sec. or close to the control value for normal steer plasma (Table 2). One hundred μg brought the time down to 22.4 sec. The same could not be accomplished with either purified prothrombin, Factor X, prethrombin 1, or Factor VII. All of these proteins did, however, have an effect.

TABLE 2. Prothrombin time of plasma from dicumarol treated steer.

Steer Plasma (Control).	26.0 sec.
Plasma from Dicumarol Treated Steer	204 sec.
+ Purified Protein M	
50 μg/ml.	26.8 sec.
100 μg/ml.	22.4 sec.
+ Purified Prothrombin*	
10 U/ml	147 sec.
200 U/ml	105 sec.
600 U/ml	92 sec.
1000 U/ml	88 sec.
+ Purified Factor X*	
50 U/ml	77 sec.
100 U/ml	72 sec.
200 U/ml	66 sec.
+ Purified Prethrombin 1*	
10 U/ml	118 sec.
50 U/ml	157 sec.
600 U/ml	144 sec.
1000 U/ml	136 sec.
+ Purified Factor VII*	
75 μg/ml.	92 sec.
110 μg/ml.	80 sec.
550 μg/ml.	48 sec.
1100 μg/ml.	36 sec.
+ Purified Factor X + Prothrombin	
25 U/ml 250 U/ml	57 sec.
50 U/ml 500 U/ml	40 sec.

*The concentrations given are for the solution that constituted one fourth of the one-stage prothrombin time reaction mixture.

DISCUSSION

Protein M was found to be a single chain protein with an apparent molecular weight near 50,000 as determined by SDS polyacrylamide gel electrophoresis. Under the same conditions the result for Factor VII was 54,000 and thus close to carefully determined values previously published (11, 12). A mixture of purified Factor VII and Protein M separated into two distinct bands by gel electrophoresis.

From our work it is evident that prothrombin complex preparations may contain a previously unrecognized procoagulant. It has been isolated but not consistently from one attempt to another. It functions in the conversion of prothrombin to thrombin as demonstrated with purified factors in the system consisting of prothrombin precursor, Ac-globulin, Factor Xa, phospholipid and calcium ions. Until further experiments are completed, we can assume that the shortening of the prothrombin time of plasma taken from steers treated with dicumarol was due to an effect on thrombin generation from normal as well as atypical prothrombin molecules. A combination of highly purified factors, especially prothrombin, and quantitative analytical work made the discovery of Protein M possible. Most likely Protein M is a vitamin K-dependent protein, but further evidence is required for deciding the question, and for further differentiation from other factors.

ACKNOWLEDGEMENTS

This work was supported by grant HL-03424-22 from the National Heart, Lung and Blood Institute, National Institutes of Health, U.S. Public Health Service, the McGregor Fund and the Skillman Foundation. Om Malhotra, Veterans Administration Hospital, Cleveland, Ohio supplied generous quantities of plasma taken from steers given dicumarol. Emily Poulik's technical assistance is much appreciated.

REFERENCES

1. Mertz, E. T., Seegers, W. H. and Smith, H. P. (1939) Proc. Soc. Exp. Biol. Med. 41, 657-661.
2. Seegers, W. H., Marciniak, E., Kipfer, R. K. and Yasunaga, K. (1967) Arch. Biochem. Biophys. 121, 372-383.
3. Seegers, W. H. and Marciniak, E. (1965) Life Sci. 4, 1721-1726.
4. Baker, W. J. and Seegers, W. H. (1967) Thromb. Diath. Haemorrh. 17, 205-213.
5. Barthels, M. and Seegers, W. H. (1969) Thromb. Diath. Haemorrh. 22, 13-27.
6. Seegers, W. H., Sakuragawa, N., McCoy, L. E., Sedensky, J. A. and Dombrose, F. A. (1972) Thromb. Res. 1, 293-310.
7. Bajwa, S. S. and Hanahan, D. J. (1976) Biochim. Biophys. Acta 444, 118-130.
8. McCoy, L. E. and Seegers, W. H. (1972) Thromb. Res. 1, 461-472.
9. Novoa, E., Seegers, W. H. and Hassouna, H. I. (1976) Prep. Biochem. 6, 307-338.
10. Radcliffe, R. and Nemerson, Y. (1976) Methods in Enzymology: Proteolytic Enzymes, Part B, pp. 49-56, Academic Press, New York.
11. Jesty, J. and Nemerson, Y. (1974) J. Biol. Chem. 249, 509-515.
12. Radcliffe, R. and Nemerson, Y. (1975) J. Biol. Chem. 250, 388-395.
13. Kisiel, W. and Davie, E. W. (1975) Biochemistry 14, 4928-4934.

PURIFICATION OF PROTEIN S FROM BOVINE PLASMA

JOHAN STENFLO

Department of Clinical Chemistry,
University of Lund, General Hospital,
S-214 01 Malmö, Sweden

INTRODUCTION

Prothrombin, factor VII, factor IX, and factor X are the four vitamin K-dependent proteins active in blood coagulation (1). A fifth vitamin K-dependent plasma protein called protein C was isolated and characterized only recently (2-5). Activated protein C is presumably identical with autoprothrombin IIA described by Seegers et al. (6). Kisiel et al. (7) have presented evidence indicating that protein C has a regulatory function in blood coagulation. All the vitamin K-dependent proteins contain γ-carboxyglutamic acid residues (8). In the course of large scale purification of protein C from bovine plasma we have found a previously unknown vitamin K-dependent protein. Its amino-terminal sequence was similar to that of human protein S (9) a new vitamin K-dependent protein. A recent paper by DiScipio and Davie (10) describing the purification and characterization of bovine protein S has clarified that we have independently purified bovine protein S. This communication describes our purification procedure for bovine protein S and some of the properties of the purified protein.

MATERIALS AND METHODS

The initial steps in the purification of protein S from slaughterhouse blood (barium citrate adsorption, ammonium sulphate fractionation, and DEAE-Sephadex A 50 chromatography) were performed as described previously (2) except that the ammonium sulphate fractionation was between 20 and 67 % saturation instead of 40 and 67 %. The pooled fractions from the DEAE-Sephadex chromatography (Fig. 1) were dialyzed against 50 mM Tris HCl, 0.1 M NaCl pH 7.4 and applied to a column (2.5x40 cm) of Blue Dextran Sepharose. Protein S was not retained on the column in contrast to prothrombin. Traces of factor IX were removed by chromatography on heparin Sepharose as described by Fujikawa et al. (11). The purified protein S was either stored at -20°C or dialyzed against distilled water and lyophilized. Standard electrophoretic (12,13) and immunochemical techniques (14-16) were used. The antisera against bovine factor IX, factor X, prothrombin, and protein C were the same as used previously (2) whereas the antiserum against bovine factor VII was a gift from dr Earl W. Davie. The amino acid composition of protein S was determined in acid hydrolysates (24,48 and 72 hours in 6 M HCl at 110°C in vacuo) with standard procedures (17) using a single column program. γ-Carboxyglutamic acid was determined in base hydrolysates as described previously (18) with synthetic γ-carboxyglutamic acid as a standard. The amino terminal sequence of protein S was determined in a Beckman model 890 C sequencer using the technique of Edman and Begg (19). Two programs were used, a modified Beckman 1 M Quadrol

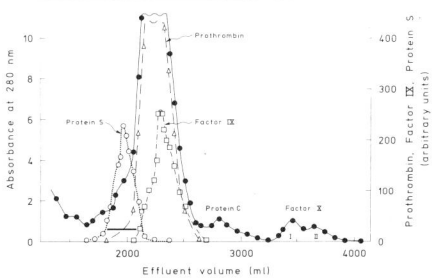

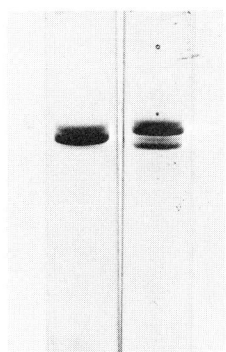

FIGURE 1. DEAE-Sephadex A 50 chromatography of ammonium sulphate-fractionated material on a column (5x52 cm) in 0.1 M phosphate buffer 1 mM benzamidine-HCl pH 6.0. Elution was accomplished with a linear gradient of NaCl (0.15 to 0.55 M) 2000 ml in each chamber. The flow rate was 90ml per hour. The column effluent was monitored immunochemically with antisera against protein S, prothrombin and factor IX. The positions of the peaks containing protein C and factors X_1 and X_2 were known from previous experiments.

FIGURE 2. SDS polyacrylamide gel electrophoresis of purified bovine protein S. Unreduced sample to the left and reduced to the right. Approximately 7 µg of protein was loaded on the gels. The anode was at the bottom.

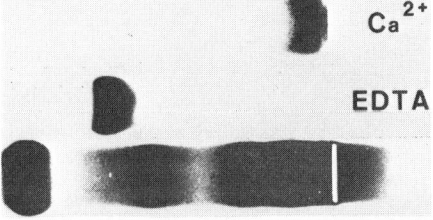

program which allowed simple identification of γ-carboxyglutamic acid (20) and a standard program for protein sequencing (21). The phenylthiohydantoin residues were identified by high pressure liquid chromatography and thin-layer chromatography as previously described (5).

FIGURE 3. Electrophoresis of purified bovine protein S on agarose gel in 0.075 M barbital buffer pH 8.6 with 2 mM Ca^{2+} or 2 mM EDTA. The electrophoretic pattern of bovine plasma is shown as a reference. The anode was to the left.

RESULTS AND DISCUSSION

During purification of protein C a previously unrecognized protein, later identified as protein S, was found at the front of the prothrombin peak during DEAE-Sephadex chromatography (Fig. 1). Protein S was further purified by Blue Dextran Sepharose chromatography and by heparin agarose chromatography (10). A typical preparation from 100 liters of bovine blood gave 140 mg of protein S. A monospecific antiserum against protein S was used for quantitation of the protein by electroimmunoassay. The method did not allow precise measurements of protein S in plasma due to the low concentration of the protein. Barium citrate adsorption of the plasma however appeared to remove the protein quantitatively. The recovery of protein S, measured from the barium citrate eluate, was 35 %.
    Purified protein S die not react with antisera against any of the previously characterized K-dependent plasma proteins i.e. prothrombin, factor VII, factor IX, factor X, and protein C. Despite this the purified protein S, both reduced and unreduced, appeared as a doublet on SDS poly-

TABLE I
Amino Acid Composition of Acid Hydrolysate of Bovine Protein S[1]

Amino Acid	Residues/molecule
Lysine	35.0
Histidine	7.2
Arginine	17.2
Half-cystine	26.0
Aspartic acid	58.1
Threonine[2]	27.5
Serine[2]	41.7
Glutamic acid	64.0
Proline	24.9
Glycine	37.9
Alanine	30
Valine[3]	39.0
Methionine[3]	9.4
Isoleucine[3]	25.9
Leucine	41.7
Tyrosine	15.8
Phenylalanine	20.6
Tryptophan[4]	5.3
TOTAL	527.2

1. Calculated relative to thirty residues of alanine which gives a molecular weight of 57 100 for the apoprotein.
2. Extrapolated zero time hydrolysis.
3. Seventy-two hours' hydrolysis value.
4. Determined spectrophotometrically.

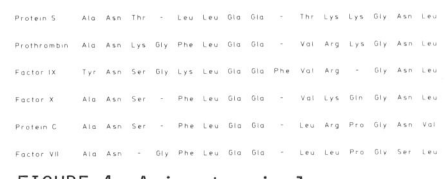

FIGURE 4. Amino terminal sequences of bovine vitamin K-dependent plasma proteins.

acrylamide gel electrophoresis (Fig. 2). The anodal electrophoretic mobility of protein S in agarose gel was lower in buffer containing Ca^{2+} ions than in EDTA containing buffer indicating that it binds Ca^{2+} ions (Fig. 3). The protein appeared homogenous in both buffers. The reason for the heterogeneity of the purified protein on SDS acrylamide gels is not known.

Protein S consists of a single polypeptide chain as judged by SDS acrylamide gel electrophoresis. The apparent molecular weight of the major component was 65 000. Its amino acid composition (Table I) arbitrarily calculated relative to 30 residues of alanine, gives a molecular weight of the apoprotein of 57 000. The hexoseamine content of protein S was not quantitated. The γ-carboxyglutamic acid content of protein S was 9.3 moles per mole of protein when calculated relative to aspartic acid in a base hydrolysate. The amino-terminal sequence of bovine protein S was Ala-Asn-Thr-Leu-Gla-Gla-Thr-Lys-Lys-Gly-Asn-Leu where Gla stands for γ-carboxyglutamic acid. Only thirteen residues could be identified using either the modified program which allowed unambigous identification of γ-carboxyglutamic acid in positions 6 and 7 or a standard program for sequenator degradation of proteins. The reason for the drop in yield after residue 13 is not known. The sequence of bovine protein S shows a striking homology to the sequences of the other vitamin K-dependent plasma proteins (Fig. 4). The results presented in this communication are in good agreement with those obtained by DiScipio and Davie (10).

ACKNOWLEDGEMENTS

The expert technical assistance of Mrs Monica Jönsson is gratefully acknowledged. I want to thank Dr Rickard, DiScipio and Dr Earl W Davie for making their manuscript on protein S available prior to publication and for testing our antiserum against their protein S preparations. This investigation was supported by a grant from the Swedish Medical Research Council (B79-13X-04487-05C).

REFERENCES

1. Davie, E.W., and Fujikawa, K. (1975) Ann. Rev. Biochem. 44, 799-829.
2. Stenflo, J. (1976) J. Biol. Chem. 251, 355-363.
3. Kisiel, W., Ericsson, L.H., and Davie, E.W. (1976) Biochemistry 15, 4893-4900.
4. Esmon, C.T., Stenflo, J., Suttie, J.W., and Jackson, C.M. (1976) J. Biol. Chem. 251, 3052-3056.
5. Fernlund, P., Stenflo, J., and Tufvesson, A. (1978) Proc. Natl. Acad. Sci. USA 75, 5889-5892.
6. Seegers, W.H., Novoa, E., Henry, R.L., and Hassouna, H.I. (1976) Thromb. Res. 8, 543-552.
7. Kisiel, W., Canfield, W.M., Ericsson, L.H., and Davie, E.W. (1977) Biochemistry 16, 5824-5831.
8. Stenflo, J., and Suttie, J.W. (1977) Ann. Rev. Biochem. 46, 157-172.
9. DiScipio, R.G., Hermodson, M.A., Yates, S.G., and Davie, E.W. (1977) Biochemistry 16, 698-706.
10. DiScipio, R.G., and Davie, E.W. (1979) Biochemistry 18, 899-904.
11. Fujikawa, K., Thompsen, A.R., Legaz, M.E., Meyer, R.G., and Davie, E.W. (1973) Biochemistry 12, 4938-4945.
12. Laemmli, V.K. (1970) Nature 227, 680-685.
13. Johansson, B.G. (1972) Scand. J. Clin. Lab. Invest. 29 (Suppl. 124), 7-19.
14. Ganrot, P.O. (1972) Scand. J. Clin. Lab. Invest. 29 (Suppl. 124), 39-47.
15. Ouchterlony, Ö. (1958) Progr, Allergy 5, 1-78.
16. Laurell, C.-B. (1966) Anal. Biochem. 15, 45-52.
17. Spackman, D.H., Stein, W.H., and Moore, S. (1958) Anal. Chem. 30, 1190-1206.
18. Fernlund, P., Stenflo, J., Roepstorff, P., and Thomsen, J. (1975) J. Biol. Chem. 250, 6125-6133.
19. Edman, P., and Begg, G. (1967) Eur, J. Biochem. 1, 80-91.
20. Fernlund, P., and Stenflo, J. (1979) in Biosynthesis and Function of Vitamin K-Dependent Proteins (J.W. Suttie, ed.).
21. Thomsen, J., Bucher, D., Brunfeldt, K., Nexö, E., and Olesen, H. (1976) Eur. J. Biochem. 69, 87-96.

ACTIVATION OF HUMAN PROTHROMBIN: KINETICS AND REGULATION

CAROLYN L. ORTHNER, SAM MORRIS, FRANK A. ROBEY and DAVID P. KOSOW

Plasma Fractions Laboratory,
American Red Cross Blood Services
Bethesda, MD 20014

INTRODUCTION

It has been established that the presence of γ-carboxyglutamic acid residues is necessary for both high affinity calcium and phospholipid binding to the vitamin K-dependent blood coagulation proteins (1-3). The rate of conversion of prothrombin to thrombin catalyzed by Factor X_a is markedly enhanced by calcium and phospholipid. Since both prothrombin and Factor X_a contain γ-carboxyglutamic acid residues and can, therefore, bind calcium and phospholipid, the mechanism by which these ligands enhance the reaction rate is not easily discernible. The enhancement of the rate of the reaction may be due to ligand binding to either the enzyme, the substrate, or both. The effect of the ligands may be on the catalytic rate constant or on the equilibrium constants for the interaction of the enzyme with the substrates and products of the reaction. Enyzme kinetics, the experimental tool most frequently used for studying enzyme mechanisms, has only recently been employed to study the coagulation cascade. This is due to the fact that steady-state kinetic measurements cannot be performed using the clotting assay. With the availability of chromogenic and isotopically labelled substrates, several laboratories have begun kinetic investigations of the coagulation pathway (4-7). We have utilized the techniques of steady-state kinetics to investigate the kinetic mechanism of thrombin formation from prothrombin catalyzed by Factor X_a in the presence of calcium and phospholipid.

KINETIC ANALYSIS

Kinetic mechanisms are divided into two major groups (8). Those in which all substrates and effectors must combine with the enzyme before product formation takes place and the products are released are called sequential. When one or more products are released before all the reactants have combined with the enzyme, the mechanism is called ping-pong. It is difficult to conceive of thrombin formation occurring by a ping-pong mechanism as the reaction has only one substrate (phospholipid and calcium are effectors of the reaction). Furthermore, initial rate studies give data which is compatible with a sequential mechanism and not with a ping-pong mechanism (9).

Sequential enzyme mechanisms may be ordered or random with respect to the binding of reactants and release of products. Since the rate equations for ordered and random reaction mechanisms differ, it is possible to differentiate between these two types of mechanisms. However, in considering the kinetic mechanism of thrombin formation, there are several complications. The calcium and phospholipid may need to bind to both the enzyme, Factor X_a, and the prothrombin substrate before reaction can occur. Also, if calcium and phospholipid need to bind to Factor X_a for the reaction to occur, they may or may not have to dissociate from the enzyme prior to either release of the products or the binding of another molecule of prothrombin. Thus, the kinetic mechanism for thrombin formation could be a very simple single substrate reaction, such as that shown in reaction mechanism 1, where calcium and phospholipid combine with Factor X_a. The complex then binds prothrombin (free or bound to phospholipid and/or calcium), thrombin and Fragment 1·2 are formed and released without dissociation of the calcium and phospholipid. It does not matter whether free prothrombin or a complex of prothrombin, calcium and phospholipid is the substrate since the rate equation would be the

(1) Prothrombin $\xrightarrow{\text{Factor } X_a \cdot \text{Ca} \cdot \text{Phospholipid}}$ Thrombin + Fragment 1·2

same unless both forms have different and measurable activities. On the other hand, the mechanism may include the dissociation of the calcium and phospholipid with one of the products of the reaction (presumably Fragment 1·2, the N-terminal portion of prothrombin which contains the γ-carboxyglutamic acid residues and which is cleaved from prothrombin during thrombin formation). Thus, the reaction may be a terreactant system as shown in reaction mechanism 2 where Pro is prothrombin, PL is

(2) $X_a + Ca \longrightarrow X_a \cdot Ca \xrightarrow{PL} X_a \cdot Ca \cdot PL \xrightarrow{Pro} X_a \cdot Ca \cdot Pro \cdot PL \longrightarrow$
$I \longrightarrow F1 \cdot 2 + \text{Thrombin} + Ca + PL + X_a$

phospholipid and F1·2 is Fragment 1·2 and I indicates the intermediates involved in product formation. As in the previous example, prothrombin may or may not be complexed with calcium and phospholipid. The above mechanism is for an ordered reaction, with calcium being the first and prothrombin the last reactant to bind to the enzyme. This order was chosen because calcium can bind to the vitamin K-dependent coagulation factors in the absence of other ligands, but phospholipid binding requires calcium (10,11).

In order to derive rate equations for the various reaction mechanisms, the steady-state assumption was made and, of course, all velocity measurements were made within the limits of this assumption. For mechanism 1, the rate equation is:

$$v = \frac{V}{1 + \frac{K_A}{A}}$$

while for mechanism 2, the rate equation is:

$$v = \frac{V}{1 + \frac{K_A}{A} + \frac{K_B}{B} + \frac{K_C}{C} + \frac{K_A K_B}{AB} + \frac{K_B K_C}{BC} + \frac{K_A K_B K_C}{ABC}}$$

where A, B and C are, respectively, the first, second and third ligands to bind to the enzyme, v is the observed velocity and V is the maximum velocity. This equation has an ABC term, but unlike a random mechanism lacks an AC term. This means that if $(v)^{-1}$ is graphed versus $(C)^{-1}$ at several constant A concentrations, the slopes of the lines will differ at low concentrations of B where the ABC term is significant, but the lines will be parallel when the concentration of B is much greater than K_B and K_B/B approaches zero. Figure 1 shows the results of an experiment designed to test whether equation 2 describes the reaction mechanism. Note that in Fig. 1A where the phospholipid concentration is 7.5 μM, a converging pattern is observed, while in Fig. 1B where the phospholipid concentration is 25 μM (about four times its K_m), the lines are nearly parallel. Since 25 μM is only four times the K for phospholipid and the change of slope with calcium concentration is about ten times greater at 7.5 μM phospholipid than it is at 25 μM phospholipid, it is obvious that at infinite phospholipid the change of slope with respect to calcium concentration would approach zero (i.e., the lines of double reciprocal plots such as those in Fig. 1 would be parallel). Thus, the experimental data fits the rate equation derived for the mechanism where there is an ordered addition of reactants to Factor X_a, and phospholipid is the second reactant to bind. These data do not indicate whether calcium or prothrombin is the first substrate to bind. Also, the data does not differentiate between the alternate mechanisms where either prothrombin or a prothrombin·calcium·phospholipid complex is the substrate. However, if both are substrates with different activities, the double reciprocal plots (Fig. 1) would not be linear. It is important to note that this mechanism requires that the calcium and phospholipid must dissociate from the Factor X_a with each turnover of the enzyme.

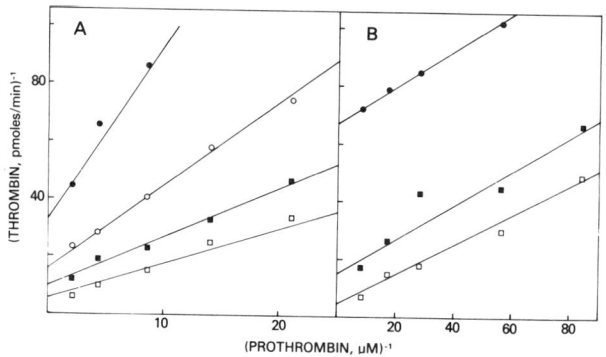

FIGURE 1. Initial velocity pattern with the phospholipid concentration constant at 7.5 μM (A) or 25 μM (B). The calcium concentration was 1.0 mM (●), 1.5 mM (○), 2.0 mM (■) or 3.0 mM (□).

In order to determine whether or not phospholipid exerts its effect by increasing the turnover of Factor X_a (V) or by altering the equilibrium constants (K) for the interaction of the various components of the system, the experiment illustrated in Fig. 2 was performed. The calcium concentration was kept constant at 5 mM and the prothrombin concentration was varied between 0.05 and 0.3 μM at four concentrations of phospholipid. It is apparent from the figure that the V increased from 0.11 to 0.31 pmoles thrombin produced per min when the phospholipid was increased from 1.5 to 6 μM. The K for prothrombin did not vary significantly, averaging 45 μM with a standard deviation of 3.6 μM.

Our results indicate that the addition of calcium, phospholipid and prothrombin to Factor X_a is an ordered reaction. The function of phospholipid is to increase the turnover number of the enzyme Factor X_a. These studies demonstrate that the coagulation cascade is amenable to study by steady-state kinetic techniques and that the coagulation enzymes are regulated by ligand-enzyme interactions in a similar fashion as enzymes of other physiological processes.

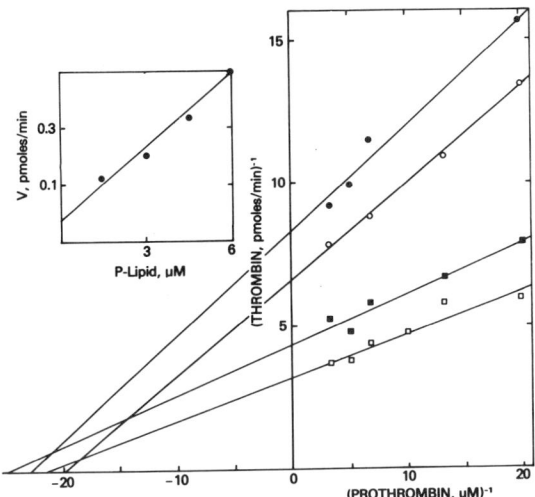

FIGURE 2. Initial velocity pattern with prothrombin the variable reactant and phospholipid held constant at 1.5 μM (●), 3.0 μM (O), 4.5 μM (■) or 6.0 μM (□). The inset is a replot of the maximum velocity vs the phospholipid concentration.

ACKNOWLEDGMENTS

This work was supported, in part, by Research Grant HL 19282 and Biomedical Research Support Grant 5 S07 RR05737 from the National Institutes of Health. Contribution No. 451 from the American Red Cross Blood Services Laboratories.

REFERENCES

1. Stenflo, J., and Ganrot, P. O. (1973) Biochem. Biophys. Res. Comm. 50, 98-104.
2. Reekers, P. P. M., Lindhout, M. J., Kop-Klaassen, B. H. M., and Hemker, H. C. (1973) Biochim. Biophys. Acta 317, 559-562.
3. Esmon, C. T., Suttie, J. W., and Jackson, C. M. (1975) J. Biol. Chem. 250, 4095-4099.
4. Kosow, D. P. (1976) Thromb. Res. 9, 565-573.
5. Morris, S., Robey, F. A., and Kosow, D. P. (1978) J. Biol. Chem. 253, 4604-4608.
6. Silverberg, S. A., Nemerson, Y., and Zur, M. (1977) J. Biol. Chem. 252, 8481-8488.
7. Lindhout, M. J., Kop-Klaassen, B. H. M., and Hemker, H. C. (1978) Biochem. Biophys. Acta 533, 327-341.
8. Cleland, W. W. (1970) in The Enzymes (Boyer, P. D. ed.), Vol. II, pp. 1-65, Academic Press, New York.
9. Kosow, D. P., and Orthner, C. L. (1979), submitted for publication.
10. Suttie, J. W., and Jackson, C. M. (1977) Physiol. Rev. 57, 1-70.
11. Davie, E. W., and Fujikawa, K. (1975) Ann. Rev. Biochem. 44, 799-829.

THE INFLUENCE OF BOVINE COAGULATION FACTORS V AND Va ON THE FUNCTION OF "PROTHROMBINASE"

MICHAEL E. NESHEIM, JAMES W. BLOOM, PAULA TRACY, and KENNETH G. MANN

Hematology Research Section,
Mayo Foundation,
Rochester, MN 55901

INTRODUCTION

Factor V, an integral component of "prothrombinase", functions as a cofactor in conjunction with Ca^{++} and phospholipid to greatly augment the Factor Xa catalyzed activation of prothrombin (1). As isolated from bovine plasma, Factor V is a high molecular weight (M_r = 330,000) single chain protein with only minimal cofactor activity (2). Upon brief exposure to catalytic amounts of thrombin, Factor V is cleaved at several points and displays a many-fold increase in cofactor activity (2-4). Consequently, prothrombin activations initiated in the presence of unactivated Factor V display characteristics of positive feedback that can be attributed to the conversion of Factor V to Factor Va by thrombin during the course of the reaction. In vivo, "prothrombinase" activity is thought to be intimately associated with the platelet, which presumably provides phospholipid and possibly Factor V. The platelet also tenaciously binds Factor Xa (5,6) through a presumed interaction with platelet-bound Factor Va (5). In previous studies, models used to elucidate presumed in vivo functions have been assembled in vitro from homogeneous Factor Xa and prothrombin, Ca^{++}, partially purified plasma Factor Va, and phospholipid from various sources (7,8).

The limitations encountered in attempts to model prothrombinase in vitro have been related to 1) a lack of procedures for isolating homogeneous Factor V, and 2) a lack of methods for precisely monitoring prothrombinase activity with sufficient detail to permit correspondingly detailed conclusions to be drawn. These limitations have been largely overcome with the isolation of homogeneous bovine Factor V (2,3) and the development of dansylarginine-N-(3-ethyl-1,5-pentanediyl) amide (DAPA) as a continuous fluorimetric marker for prothrombinase activity (9). In the studies to be described here, homogeneous Factor V and DAPA were used to assemble and study a model for prothrombinase in vitro. Results from these studies, as well as studies of the phospholipid and platelet binding properties of Factor V and Factor Va, are used to draw conclusions about aspects of the structure and function of the model prothrombinase. Comparisons of the model with a prothrombinase assembled from Factor Xa, Ca^{++}, and activated bovine platelets are also made.

Phospholipid Binding Properties

The binding interactions of Factor V and Factor Va with phospholipid were measured by right-angle light scattering (10) with data analyzed as described by Nelsestuen and Lim (11) in studies with prothrombin and Factor X. The phospholipid used was in the form of homogeneously-sized unilamellar vesicles of phosphatidyl-choline (PC) and phosphatidyl-serine (PS) prepared according to Barenholz, et al. (12). The results of these studies indicated that both Factor V and Factor Va bind the vesicles with ~10 times the avidity of either prothrombin or Factor X. The binding, in contrast to that of prothrombin or Factor X, is Ca^{++} independent. Binding to vesicles prepared exclusively from PC could not be demonstrated. With vesicles prepared from mixtures of PC-PS, the binding capacity increased with increasing PS content until a plateau was obtained between 20-40 mole percent PS.

Platelet Binding Properties

The binding of radioiodinated Factor V and Factor Va to bovine platelets was studied (13) by rapidly centrifuging platelet suspensions through oil to determine bound and free cofactor in a manner similar to that described by Miletich, et al. (14) in studies of the binding of Factor Xa to platelets. With Factor Va, Scatchard analyses of binding data were clearly bi-phasic. Scatchard plots were interpreted as indicating 800 high affinity sites per platelet with $K_d = 4.0 \times 10^{-10}M$ and 3500 lower affinity sites with $K_d = 4.0 \times 10^{-9}M$. The number of high affinity sites was similar to the number of Factor V molecules associated with well-washed platelets as measured by both bioassay (670 Factor V molecules/platelet) and radioimmunoassay (590 Factor V molecules/platelet). The binding of unactivated Factor V to platelets was also studied with results similar but not identical to those obtained with activated Factor V (Va). About 800-900 sites per platelet with $K_d = 3.2 \times 10^{-9}M$ were observed. Iodinated Factor V bound to such sites could be completely displaced by unlabelled Factor Va. In contrast, unlabelled Factor V could not completely displace bound Factor Va. The amount of Factor Va which could not be displaced by unlabelled Factor V corresponded to the number of high affinity sites for Factor Va. All bound Factor Va, however, could be displaced by unlabelled Factor Va. Thus, although both Factor V and Factor Va bind platelets similarly, the data indicate the existence of a set of high affinity sites specific for the activated cofactor that cannot be shared by the unactivated cofactor. In these studies the same results were obtained with unactivated or thrombin-activated platelets.

Effect On Kinetics Of Prothrombin Activation

The functional aspects of the model prothrombinase have been determined from measurements of the kinetics of prothrombin activation (15). Concentrations of prothrombin were typically $1.39 \times 10^{-6}M$ (0.1 mg/ml) and concentrations of Factor Xa were about $5.0 \times 10^{-9}M$ (0.28 μg/ml). Reactions were monitored by including DAPA ($3.0 \times 10^{-6}M$) which specifically and reversibly binds thrombin ($K_d = 4.3 \times 10^{-8}M$) (9), and thereby inhibits the enzyme. The binding of the probe to thrombin is characterized by a three-fold increase in fluorescence intensity that provides a convenient signal to monitor the process of prothrombin activation. The dependence of the rate of activation on concentrations of each of the components [Factor Xa, Factor Va, Ca^{++}, and PCPS vesicles (20% PS)] was studied. Activation rates reached plateaus at about 2.0 mM Ca^{++} and 15 μM PCPS. When various concentrations of Factor Xa were used, a plateau was approached as the concentration of Factor Xa approached that of Factor Va. Conversely, when the concentration of Factor Va was varied, a plateau was approached when the Factor Va concentration approached that of Factor Xa. The saturation curves obtained with Factor Xa or Factor Va, when analyzed by double reciprocal analysis, yielded an apparent 1:1 stoichiometry between the two proteins with a dissociation constant of $7.3 \times 10^{-10}M$, a value similar to that reported for the binding of radioiodinated Factor Xa to bovine platelets ($1.9 \times 10^{-10}M$) (6). Similar titrations were carried out with unactivated Factor V at fixed levels of Factor Xa. Although the observed velocities were only about 0.25 percent of those obtained under similar conditions with the activated cofactor, saturation was again observed with respect to Factor Xa at a 1:1 stoichiometry with $K_d = 2.5 \times 10^{-9}M$. These results suggest that both Factor V and Factor Va interact stoichiometrically and with high affinity with Factor Xa. In the presence of Ca^{++} and phospholipid, the interaction of Factor Va with Factor Xa is marked by a great increase in the rate of prothrombin activation. The effects of Factor Va and the other components on the rate of the process were determined by omitting the components one at a time from activation reactions which were otherwise saturated with respect to the remaining components. The relative rates observed with various combinations of the prothrombinase components (in addition to Factor Xa) were as follows: none, 1.0; PCPS, 1.0; Ca^{++}, 2.3; Ca^{++} and PCPS, 22.0; Ca^{++}, PCPS and Factor Va, 278,000. These relative rates demonstrate the pronounced influence of Factor Va on prothrombinase activity. Although PCPS, when added to Factor Xa plus Ca^{++} only, caused only a 10-fold increase in rate, its deletion from the combination of Factor Xa, Ca^{++}, and Factor Va was accompanied by an 800-fold decrease in rate. The 10-fold change in rate may reflect the influence of substrate binding to phospholipid, while the 800-fold change may reflect the combined effects of phospholipid binding interactions with both the substrate and cofactor.

In addition to studies carried out at various concentrations of the enzymatic components, experiments were performed to examine the influence of concentrations of prothrombin on rates of activation. The rate of activation varied with substrate in conformity with the Michaelis-Menton equation and yielded the apparent parameters, $K_m = 1.03 \times 10^{-6}M$ prothrombin and V_{max} = 2100 moles thrombin min^{-1} mole^{-1} Factor Xa (22° C, 0.02 M TRIS·HCl, 0.15 M NaCl, 2.0 mM $CaCl_2$, pH 7.4 with saturating concentrations of PCPS and Factor Va). The apparent V_{max} was 15-20 times greater than values previously obtained with similar model systems (5,7). The V_{max} was, however, similar to values observed by other investigators studying platelet-derived prothrombinase activity (5). Consequently, studies were undertaken to directly compare the activity of the model prothrombinase to the combination of Factor Xa, Ca^{++}, and well-washed, thrombin-activated bovine platelets (300,000/mm^3) as a source of both phospholipid and Factor V. Conditions were arranged such that in either instance (platelets or model) the concentration of Factor Va was both rate-limiting and equal (2.5 x 10^{-10}M). The Factor V level of the platelet suspension was determined both by bioassay and with a radioimmunoassay developed in this laboratory for plasma Factor V (13). Under these conditions the V_{max} values obtained, respectively, with the model system and with platelets were 1800 and 1600 moles thrombin per minute per mole Factor Va (specific activities were calculated on the basis of Factor Va rather than Factor Xa since the latter was present in molar excess). These values, in addition to being similar to each other, are quite similar to those observed with platelets in another laboratory (5). In those investigations specific-activity values were calculated on the basis of platelet-bound Factor Xa, rather than Factor Va. These observations are consistent with two conclusions: 1) in terms of maximum rates of catalysis, the prothrombinase complex consisting of Factor Xa, Ca^{++}, plasma Factor Va and phospholipid vesicles is equivalent under the present conditions to the complex utilizing platelets in place of the latter two components, and 2) since similar specific activities are observed with platelets on the basis of either Factor Va or bound Factor Xa, Factor Va is implicated as the binding site for Factor Xa on platelets. This conclusion follows since total Factor Va (when Factor Xa is present in great excess) and bound Factor Xa (under any circumstances) are equivalent to concentrations of Factor Va·Xa complex if Factor Va constitutes the binding site for Factor Xa.

Studies using DAPA were also conducted in which the activation of prothrombin was initiated with Factor Va in solutions containing activated bovine protein C (Ca) in addition to Factor Xa, Ca^{++}, and PCPS. Protein Ca has been shown to obliterate, through proteolysis, the cofactor activity of activated Factor Va (16). With protein Ca present in ongoing prethrombin-1 activations, a continuous diminution of the rate constant of the process occurred indicating a continuous loss of cofactor activity. It has not been established whether Factor Va inactivated by Ca binds Factor Xa; if it does, inactivated Factor Va could be expected to diminish rates of prothrombin activation by competing for Factor Xa.

Aspects Of The Structure And Function Of Prothrombinase

The above observations suggest several conclusions about the structure and function of the prothrombinase complex and each of its components. The titration with Ca^{++} (as measured by kinetics) displayed saturation at about 2.0 mM reminiscent of concentrations required to saturate the Ca^{++} binding sites of prothrombin (8). Thus, in part, the Ca^{++} saturation may reflect maximal binding of prothrombin to Ca^{++} and, consequently, to phospholipid (11). The titration with PCPS displayed saturation at about 15 µM phospholipid (12 µg/ml). Based on the data of Nelsestuen and Lim (11) in which prothrombin was shown to bind an equal weight of phospholipid with a µM dissociation constant with respect to concentrations of protein, the conclusion can be drawn that the plateau obtained with PCPS in activation studies with prothrombin at 0.1 mg/ml (1.39 x 10^{-6}M) does not represent saturation of the vesicle with protein or <u>vice versa</u>. Since the dissociation constant for Factor Va binding to phospholipid is about 0.1 that for prothrombin binding, the saturation profile obtained with PCPS reflects the binding of Factor Va rather than prothrombin to the vesicle surface. The binding parameters for the interactions of Factor Va and prothrombin with PCPS permit the calculation of the distribution of both the substrate and cofactor between both solution and PCPS vesicles at the onset of the activation of prothrombin. Under the initial conditions in which concentrations of prothrombin, Factor Xa, Factor Va, Ca^{++}, and PCPS are respectively, 1.39 x 10^{-6}M, 5.0 x 10^{-9}M, 1.0 x 10^{-8}M, 2.0 mM, and 15 µM, the following distributions can be calculated with prothrombin: 97 percent is in solution, 3 percent is on the vesicle surface. Even though only a small percentage is bound, it is sufficient to approximately half-saturate the available binding sites. Unlike prothrombin, Factor Va is quantitatively (>95%) bound, although the absolute amount bound contributes very little to the fractional saturation of vesicles as Factor Va is present in only relatively trace quantities. Since Factor Va is quantitatively bound, and a high affinity interaction exists between it and Factor Xa, the latter is also presumably quantitatively associated with the vesicle surface.

The results of these calculations as well as a summary of most of the results presented in this article are summarized schematically in Figure 1. The large sphere in the center of the drawing represents a PCPS vesicle. Imbedded in its surface is a molecule of activated Factor V (suggested by a "schism") in 1:1 stoichiometry with Factor Xa. Interactions of the peptides of Factor Va are promoted, as indicated, by Ca^{++} (3). Shown both in solution, on the vesicle surface, and associated with the lipid-bound complex of Factor Va and Factor Xa are molecules of prothrombin with the prothrombin fragment-1, prothrombin fragment-2 and

prethrombin-2 domains as indicated. An interaction with Factor Va
through the prothrombin fragment-2 domain is suggested in accordance
with data inferred from previously published studies of the kinetics of
prothrombin activation (8,17). The interaction of prothrombin with the
vesicle is suggested through Ca^{++} bridging mediated by the γ-carboxyglutamate residues of the fragment-1 domain. In solution a prothrombin
dimer (18) is indicated with the interaction of the two molecules most
likely promoted again by Ca^{++} bridging as proposed by Bloom and Mann (19).
The drawing in Figure 1 and the data which support it suggest that the
model prothrombinase consists of a phospholipid-bound complex of Factor
Va and Factor Xa with Ca^{++} most likely participating in at least some of
the interactions involved in the assembly of the catalyst. In this model
Factor Va constitutes a "binding site" for Factor Xa in a manner analogous to that thought to occur with prothrombinase assembled in vivo from
Factor Xa, Ca^{++} and platelets (5,6).

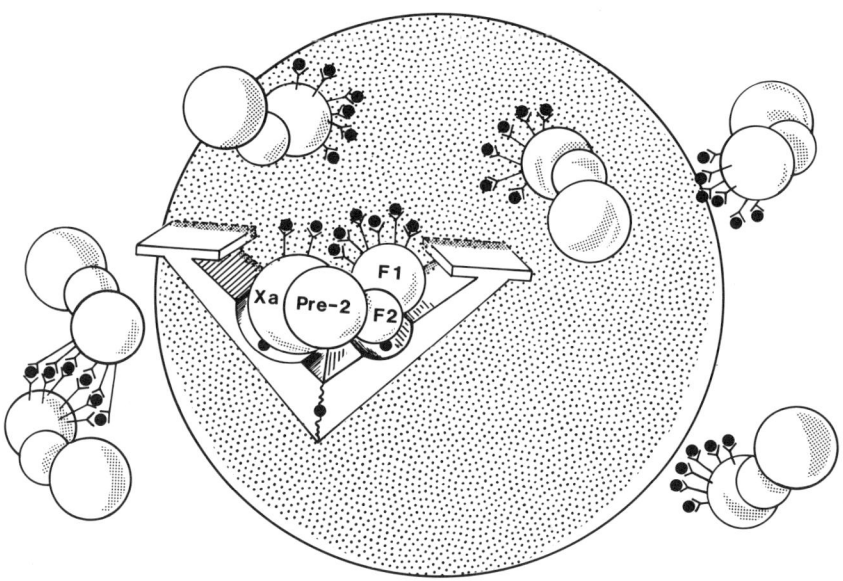

Figure 1. Schematic representation of the activation of prothrombin as
catalyzed by the prothrombinase complex.

ACKNOWLEDGEMENTS

This work was supported by NIH Grant HL-17430 D and by Blood Banking
and Hemostasis Training Grant HL-07069.

REFERENCES

1. Davie, E. W., and Fujikawa, K. (1975) Annu. Rev. Biochem. 44, 799-829.
2. Nesheim, M. E., Myrmel, K. H., Hibbard, L., and Mann, K. G. (1979) J. Biol. Chem. 254, 508-517.
3. Esmon, C. T. (1979) J. Biol. Chem. 254, 964-973.

4. Nesheim, M. E., and Mann, K. G. (1979) J. Biol. Chem. 254, 1326-1334.
5. Miletich, J. P., Jackson, C. M., and Majerus, P. W. (1978) J. Biol. Chem. 253, 6908-6916.
6. Dahlback, B., and Stenflo, J. (1978) Biochemistry 17, 4938-4945.
7. Esmon, C. T., Owen, W. G., and Jackson, C. M. (1974) J. Biol. Chem. 249, 8045-8047.
8. Bajaj, S. P., Butkowski, R. J., and Mann, K. G. (1975) J. Biol. Chem. 250, 2150-2156.
9. Nesheim, M. E., Prendergast, F. G., and Mann, K. G. (1979) Biochemistry 18, 996-1003.
10. Bloom, J. W., Nesheim, M. E., and Mann, K. G. (1979) VIIth International Congress on Thrombosis and Hemostasis (abstract), Thrombosis and Hemostasis (in press).
11. Nelsestuen, G. L., and Lim, T. K. (1977) Biochemistry 16, 4164-4171.
12. Bavenholz, Y., Gibbs, D., Litman, B. J., Goll, J., Thompson, E., and Carlson, F. D. (1977) Biochemistry 16, 2806-2810.
13. Tracy, P. B., Peterson, J. M., Nesheim, M. E., McDuffie, F. C., and Mann, K. G. (1979) VIIth International Congress on Thrombosis and Hemostasis (abstract), Thrombosis and Hemostasis (in press).
14. Miletich, J. P., Jackson, C. M., and Majerus, P. W. (1977) Proc. Natl. Acad. Sci. USA 74, 4033-4036.
15. Nesheim, M. E., Bloom, J. W., Tracy, P. B., and Mann, K. G. (1979) VIIth International Congress on Thrombosis and Hemostasis (abstract), Thrombosis and Hemostasis (in press).
16. Canfield, W., Nesheim, M., Kisiel, W., and Mann, K. G. (1978) Am. Heart Assn. 51st Scientific Sessions, Dallas, TX. Circulation, Part II, 58, 4.
17. Esmon, C. T., and Jackson, C. M. (1974) J. Biol. Chem. 249, 7791-7797.
18. Prendergast, F. G., and Mann, K. G. (1977) J. Biol. Chem. 252, 840-850.
19. Bloom, J. W., and Mann, K. G. (1978) Biochemistry 17, 4430-4438.

HUMAN PROTHROMBIN ACTIVATION: RADIOIMMUNOASSAY OF FRAGMENT 3

DANIEL A. WALZ and THOMAS R. BROWN

Wayne State University School of Medicine
Detroit, MI 48201

INTRODUCTION

The generation of thrombin from human prothrombin and its pattern of in vitro activation have been characterized. In the human prothrombin molecule there are two factor Xa susceptible peptide bonds and two thrombin susceptible bonds (1,2). Factor Xa will hydrolyze an arginyl-threonyl bond, thus forming prethrombin 2 and prothrombin fragment 1·2; factor Xa also hydrolyzes an arginyl-isoleucyl bond in prethrombin 2 giving rise to the active enzyme thrombin. Human thrombin hydrolyzes the arginyl-seryl bond between fragment 1·2, thus forming prothrombin fragments 1 and 2. Human thrombin also will autocatalytically hydrolyze an arginyl-threonyl bond near the amino-terminus of the thrombin A chain generating a third activation fragment, human prothrombin fragment 3.

The chemistry of the human prothrombin molecule is also known. Prothrombin fragment 1 is a 155 residue polypeptide which contains the 10 γ-carboxyglutamic acids (3,4); prothrombin fragment 2 is a 118 residue component (4). The amino acid sequence of the human thrombin A chain (5) gave the first indication that there was a shortened A chain and this was subsequently confirmed by additional reports on the partial sequence of thrombin (6), the primary structure of prethrombin 2 (7), and the isolated fragment 3 (8).

Immunochemical evaluations of the prothrombin molecule have not been extensively reported. A radioimmunoassay for human thrombin (9) has been developed; the assay was specific for thrombin in as much as it did not cross-react with the thrombin-antithrombin III complex and was three orders of magnitude more reactive to thrombin than prothrombin. More recently, a radioimmunoassay for human prothrombin has been reported and the quantity of prothrombin in normal plasma was 86 µg/mL (10). An alternate approach for probing prothrombin activation, using crossed immunoelectrophoresis of urine samples (11), has demonstrated the presence of prothrombin fragment 1. Finally, the question of the in vivo pathway of prothrombin activation has been explored (12) and the evidence is that during whole blood clotting prothrombin degradation proceeds only by the formation of fragment 1·2. The question we have addressed then was the nature of "physiological" thrombin; is fragment 3 generated during whole blood clotting as a free fragment or does it remain a component of thrombin?

MATERIALS AND METHODS

Human prothrombin fragment 3 was commercially synthesized by special order (Bachem Fine Chemicals, Torrence, CA) using the literature reported amino acid sequence (7,8). The peptide was coupled either to serum albumin (bovine and pig) or thyroglobulin (chicken and bovine) using the carbodiimide method (morpho CDI, Aldrich Chemical Co., Milwaukee, WI). The hapten-conjugated fragment was emmulsified with Freund's complete adjuvant and injected in 20-40 intradermal sites on the back of each white New Zealand female rabbit. After an initial incubation of 8 weeks, the animals were boosted with a second series of injections and antisera harvested 7 days later by negative pressure collection. The synthetic fragment 3 was iodinated using a standard chloramine T protocol as follows: 25 µL of 0.5 M $K-PO_4$, pH 7.2; 2.5 µg protein in 10 µL buffer; 7 µL 125-I (Amersham, 15 mCi/µg, 100 µCi/µL); 10 µL chloramine T (8 mg/10 mL); 30 seconds reaction time; 500 µL sodium metabisulfite (4 mg/10 mL); filtration on G-10 (8 x 210 mm). On some occasions the iodinated fragment 3 was additionally purified by ion-exchange chromatography.

Validation studies for the radioimmunoassay were performed on prothrombin activation components purified in our laboratory (ie. prothrombin, prethrombin 1, fragments 1,2, and 3). Human α-thrombin was a gift from Dr. J.W. Fenton.

Human sera was collected from fasting, healthy donors. Immunoprecipitation of human serum prior to gel filtration on Sephacryl 300 (Pharmacia Fine Chemicals) was made with antisera to: antithrombin III (provided by Dr. L. Williams), α_2-macroglobulin (Miles Laboratories), albumin and whole human serum. Controls were run combining similar aliquots of human sera with non-immune rabbit serum. Plasma samples were collected into an anticoagulant consisting of citrate, benzamidine and theophylline.

RESULTS AND DISCUSSION

Validation studies were conducted to ascertain the specificity and sensitivity of the assay. Using purified components, the assay was three orders of magnitude more reactive to fragment 3 than to purified prothrombin or prethrombin 1; purified thrombin did not cross-react in this assay (data not shown). The logit curve was generated with fragment 3 standards ranging from 3.9-100 ng/mL.

The concentration of human prothrombin in plasma was calculated to be approximately 100 µg/mL (10), based on a biological specific activity of 3 units/µg protein. Since the molecular weight of prothrombin is 74,000 daltons (1,2) and the molecular weight of fragment 3 is 1400, it was estimated that 1.9% of the prothrombin molecule consists of fragment 3. When normal plasma was screened with this assay at volumes up to 400 µL (equivalent of 760 ng fragment 3) no detectable label displacement occurred. However, when solutions of purified prothrombin (10 µg/100 µL) were screened, an average of 4.7 ng of fragment 3-like protein was quantitated, an observation in good agreement with the specificity (cross-reactivity less than 0.001) but not in agreement with the similar theoretical information for plasma. When similar assays were performed using purified prothrombin in a 5% albumin solution, 3.9 ng of fragment 3-like protein was quantitated, indicating that something other than bulk protein concentrations were responsible for the lack of immunoreactive material in plasma. The possibilities are that prothrombin in plasma circulates in association with some other protein(s) or that during the process of isolation, subtle yet noticeable alterations in the solute form of prothrombin are introduced which makes the fragment 3 immuno-accessible.

When the assay was used to quantitate the amount of fragment 3 in serum, the range of fragment 3 was found to be 40-100 ng/mL. The theoretical amount which should be present in serum, based on the assumption that prothrombin is completely converted to thrombin and that all of the prothrombin activation products are quantitatively present in serum, would be 1900 ng/mL. Our yields of serum fragment 3 were, therefore, only 2-6% of theoretical quantities. The possible combination of reasons for this low recovery are numerous and include: a) erroneous theoretical assumptions in the quantity of fragment 3 generated; b) failure of the prothrombin fragments to be quantitatively released into serum (i.e., entrapment in the clot, either on the platelet or fibrin); c) retention of the fragment as a component of thrombin, rendering it less immunoreactive than the free fragment.

In order to determine the nature of the serum fragment 3, an aliquot of human serum was filtered on a calibrated S-300 column. Fractions from this column were pooled, concentrated, and quantitated by the radioimmunoassay. Synthetic fragment 3 was found to filter in the total volume of the column. Serum filtration gave four distinct protein fractions. Fragment 3 was found to filter in the ascending portion of second protein fraction, corresponding to a molecular weight of 150,000 daltons. Therefore, the immediate conclusion from this observation was that "physiological" thrombin retains the fragment 3 and has an A chain of 49 amino acids. Since this thrombin is incapable of autocatalysis, we next attempted to identify the nature of the thrombin inhibition. Aronson et al (12) had been able to assay only 10 units of thrombin per mL of blood during whole blood clotting. Shapiro (13) found that approximately 70% of thrombin in plasma was inhibited by antithrombin III, the remainder being bound to α_2-macroglobulin. Accordingly, we pre-incubated an aliquot of human serum with specific antibodies to antithrombin III, α_2-macroglobulin, albumin, and whole human serum prior to S-300 chromatography (see Figure 1). The recovery from normal serum filtration averaged 96% of the fragment 3 applied. Pre-precipitation of the serum with anti-α_2-macroglobulin resulted in recoveries of approximately 80% of the pretreated serum fragment 3. Antithrombin III precipitated serum recoveries were about 57% of their pretreated values (see Figure 1). Albumin recoveries were the same as untreated serum; however, precipitation with anti whole human serum resulted in only a 23% recovery of the fragment 3.

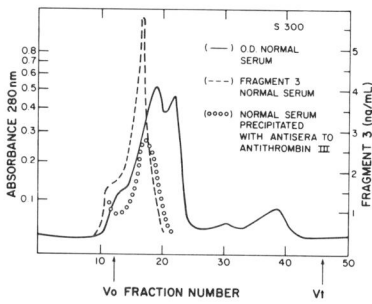

FIGURE 1 Gel filtration of 1 mL of human serum. The eluate (solid lines) represents the optical density profile; the normal quantity of fragment 3 eluted at 150,000 daltons and was reduced in quantity to 57% when the serum was pre-precipitated with antithrombin III.

The amount of precipitate formed with the antisera to antithrombin III and α_2-macroglobulin was very slight, whereas the precipitate using anti whole human serum was very substantial. The most favorable interpretation of the above data is that physical trapping of the fragment 3 has occurred during whole serum precipitation. The discrepency between our quantitation and those of Shapiro (13) probably reflect the difference in experimental design rather than any inherent disagreement in absolute values. Shapiro (13) cautions on the application of antisera to antithrombin III for quantitation purposes since the more complex high molecular forms of thrombin-antithrombin III probably are not as immunoreactive as the 1:1 complex.

In conclusion, we have identified the nature of "physiological" thrombin as one retaining the fragment 3 component when the thrombin is formed during whole blood clotting. The thrombin thus formed can be measured by the described radioimmunoassay for fragment 3 even when the thrombin is bound to the plasma inhibitors.

ACKNOWLEDGEMENTS

This work was supported by a NIH grant (05384-17) and the Michigan Heart Association. The expert assistance of Ms. June Snow and Ms. Debra McKinley are gratefully acknowledged.

REFERENCES

1. Walz, D.A., Reuterby, J., Hewett-Emmett, D., and Seegers, W.H. (1975) Fed. Proc. 34, 290.
2. Downing, M.R., Butkowski, R.J., Clark, M.M., and Mann, K.G. (1975) J. Biol. Chem. 250, 8897-8906.
3. Walz, D.A., Hewett-Emmett, D., and Seegers, W.H. (1977) Life Sci. 20, 79-84.
4. Walz, D.A., Hewett-Emmett, D., and Seegers, W.H. (1977) Proc. Natl. Acad. Sci. U.S.A. 74, 1969-1972.
5. Walz, D.A. and Seegers, W.H. (1974) Biochem. Biophys. Res. Commun. 60, 717-722.
6. Thompson, A.R., Enfield, D.L., Ericsson, L.H., Legaz, M.E., and Fenton, J.W. (1977) Arch. Biochem. Biophys. 178, 356-367.
7. Butkowski, R.J., Elion, J., Downing, M.R., and Mann, K.G. (1977) J. Biol. Chem. 252, 4942-4957.
8. Walz, D.A., Hewett-Emmett, D., Reuterby, J., and Seegers, W.H. (1976) Thromb. Res. 9, 289-292.
9. Shuman, M.A. and Majerus, P.W. (1976) J. Clin. Invest. 58, 1249-1258.
10. Lox, C.D., Strohm, G.H., and Corrigan, J.J. (1978) Am. J. Hematol. 4, 261-267.
11. Bezeaud, A., Aronson, D.L., Ménaché, D., and Guillin, M.C. (1978) Thromb. Res. 13, 551-556.
12. Aronson, D.L., Stevan, L., Ball, A.P., and Franza, B.R. (1977) J. Clin. Invest. 60, 1410-1418.
13. Shapiro, S.S. and Anderson, D.B. (1977) Chemistry and Biology of Thrombin, pp. 361-374, Ann Arbor Science, Ann Arbor, Michigan.

BOVINE FACTOR X_1 AND X_2: ACTIVATION PEPTIDE BASED CHROMATOGRAPHIC DIFFERENCES

TAKASHI MORITA and CRAIG M. JACKSON

Department of Biological Chemistry
Washington University School of Medicine
St. Louis, MO 63110

INTRODUCTION

Bovine Factor X is eluted from anion exchange chromatographic columns (1-4) in two forms (X_1 and X_2). These two variants have indistinguishable amino acid compositions, molecular weights and coagulant specific activities. Although small differences in the content of carbohydrate (3) and γ-carboxyglutamic acid (5) between Factors X_1 and X_2 have been reported, both these results have been disputed on the basis of data from other laboratories (2,4-7). The amino acid sequences of the regions which contain the γ-carboxyglutamic residues have been shown to be identical in X_1 and X_2 (8). During the process of isolating a derivative of Factor X and Xa from which the γ-carboxyglutamic acid containing region (residues 1-44 of the light chain) was proteolytically cleaved, abbreviated X(-GD) and Xa(-GD) we found that X(-GD) and the activation peptide(s) eluted as two distinguishable forms. These results led us to investigate the structural basis for these two forms of bovine Factor X. In this paper we demonstrate that the difference between X_1 and X_2 resides in the structures of the activation peptides (AP) and particularly in the structure of tyrosine at position 18.

RESULTS AND DISCUSSION

Two Forms of Factor X(-GD)

Figure 1 shows an elution profile from anion exchange chromatography of the reaction products after incubation of bovine Factor X_1 and X_2 with α-chymotrypsin. The products from a mixture of X_1 and X_2 are shown in Figure 1A, from X_1 alone in Figure 1B, and X_2 alone in Figure 1C. It is clearly evident that even after removing the Gla-domain (residues 1-44 of the light chain) from the molecule, Factor X(-GD) still exists in two forms.

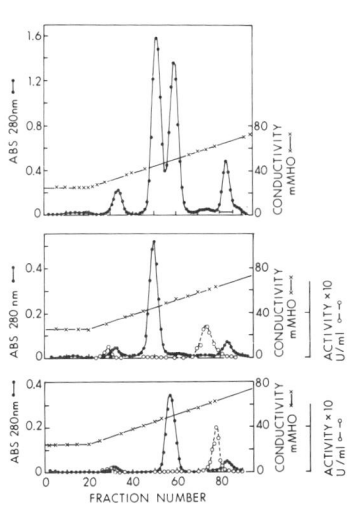

FIGURE 1 Analysis of the products from Factor X after limited proteolysis by α-chymotrypsin by QAE Sephadex column chromatography.

120

Two Forms of the Factor X Activation Peptide

Figure 2 shows an elution profile from anion exchange column chromatography of the mixture obtained after activating Factor X(-GD) with the Vipera russelli activator (X-CP). The first, large, asymmetric peak in Figure 2A contains 4 components, Factor Xa(-GD) (both α and β forms), Factor X Fragment 4 (Fr-4, heavy chain residues 291-307), and X-CP. These products were identified after separation on a column of Sephadex G-100. The second and third small peaks contained the two activation peptides, AP_1 and AP_2. These were shown to be independently derived from Factor X_1 and X_2 by activation of isolated X_1(-GD) which yielded only AP_1 (Fig. 2B) and isolated X_2(-GD) which yielded only AP_2 (Fig. 2C).

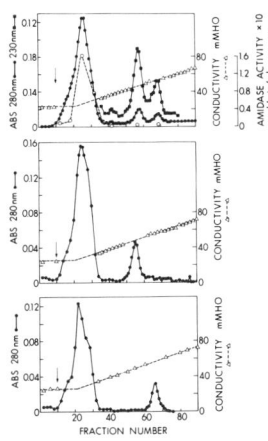

FIGURE 2 Chromatography of the Products of X(-GD) Activation on QAE Sephadex.

Direct Isolation of the Activation Peptide(s) from Factor X

The activation peptide(s) of Factor X ($X_1 + X_2$) can be separated from Factor Xa by gel filtration on Sephadex G-100 under non-denaturing conditions (Fig. 3A). The activation peptides from the mixture of X_1 and X_2 are readily separated into two forms by anion exchange chromatography (Fig. 3B).

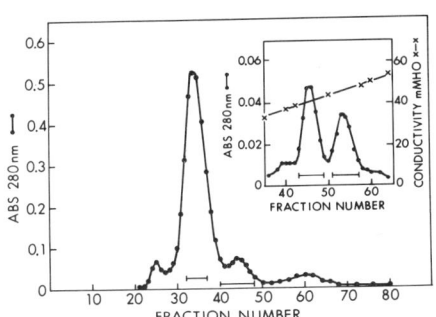

FIGURE 3 Isolation of AP_1 and AP_2 from normal Factor X.

Relative Elution Positions of the Activation Peptides and Factor Xa on Anion-Exchange Chromatographic Columns

Anion exchange column chromatography is often used to isolate Factor Xa after activation of Factor X. Because the activation peptide(s) stain poorly with Coomassie brilliant blue on acrylamide gel electrophoresis and the absorbance of AP_1 and AP_2 is only 6% and 3% of that of Factor X, respectively, the relative elution position of Xa and activation peptides have not been determined previously. The chromatographic pattern obtained from an activation mixture of tritiated bovine Factor X or a mixture of tritiated AP_1, tritiated AP_2 and Xa has been determined. AP_1 and AP_2 separately eluted before Factor Xa from the anion exchange column but the AP_2 peak overlaps the Factor Xa and cannot be easily separated completely from it under the usual chromatographic conditions.

Chromatographic Behavior of Factor X Fr-4 (Residues 291-307) on Anion Exchange Column Chromatography

Factor X Fragment 4 was isolated from an activation mixture of Factor X or of X(-GD) by gel filtration on Sephadex G-100. This peptide was also separated into two forms by anion-exchange chromatography. The ratio of the 1st peak (Fr 4') to the 2nd peak (Fr-4") from such columns is approximately 1 to 2 on the basis of absorbance at either 280 or 230 nm, whereas the ratio of Factor X_1 to X_2 and AP_1 to AP_2 is 2 to 1. Only two species of Fr-4 are isolated from the activation mixture prepared from X_1 and X_2, and the activation mixture obtained from X_1 alone. When coupled with the difference in relative amounts of X_1 and X_2, and AP_1 and AP_2, it is clear that the two forms of F-4 bear no relationship to the chromatographic properties of X_1 and X_2 or AP_1 and AP_2. Amino acid compositions of Fr-4' and Fr-4" were the same as the values which were calculated from the amino acid sequence of the heavy chain (8). However, Fr-4' and Fr-4" contained different amounts of sialic acid, 0.7 ± 0.10, and 1.6 ± 0.44 residues per mole, respectively, implying that the chromatographic difference between Fr-4' and Fr-4" is most likely the result of a sialic acid based difference in net charge.

Structural Properties of the Activation Peptides

The above mentioned results show that the difference between X_1 and X_2 which is responsible for their chromatographic behavior must reside in the structure of the activation peptides. AP_1 and AP_2 were indistinguishable in amino acid composition, number of sialic acid residues, and number of free carboxyl groups. Moreover, mixtures of asialo X_1 and asialo X_2 and asialo AP_1 and asialo AP_2 were also separable into two forms by anion-exchange chromatography. The glycopeptides obtained after pronase digestion of AP_1 and AP_2 which had been ^3H labeled in their sialic acid residues were separated by anion exchange chromatography (Fig. 4). The elution profiles showed six glycopeptide components in AP_1 and AP_2, which were indistinguishable in their elution positions and relative amounts. On the basis of their amino acid compositions, peaks 2 and 3 must be Asn linked and peaks 4, 5 and 6 Ser linked oligosaccharides. These data indicate that at least one (Ser linked) oligosaccharide chain must be present in the Factor X activation peptides in addition to the Asn linked chain previously reported (9), but that the distinction between X_1 and X_2 cannot be due to oligosaccharide chain sialic acid differences.

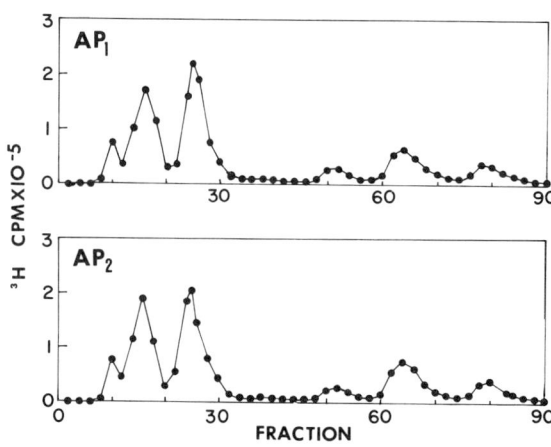

FIGURE 4 Analysis of the glycopeptides from pronase digested samples of AP_1 and AP_2 by QAE Sephadex A25 column chromatography. ^3H AP_1 and AP_2 (about 1 mg) were digested by pronase for 4 days in 0.2 M Tris-HCl, pH 8.0, respectively.

Ultraviolet Absorption Spectral Differences between AP_1 and AP_2

The ultraviolet absorption spectra of AP_1 and AP_2 can be seen from Figure 5 to be distinctly different. The amino terminal dipeptides, Trp-Ala,

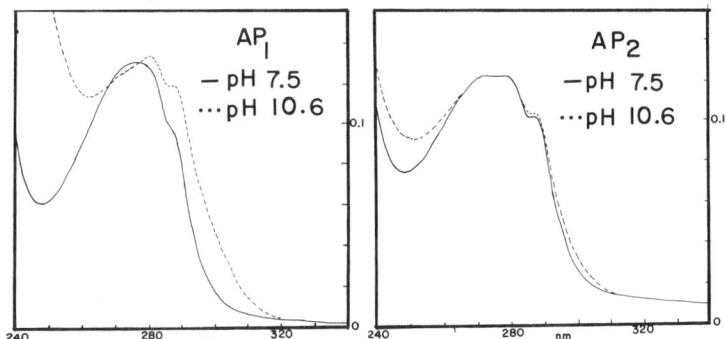

FIGURE 5 Ultraviolet adsorption spectra of AP_1 and AP_2.

were isolated from AP_1 and AP_2 and found to be indistinguishable by ultraviolet absorption. Titration of AP_1 and AP_2 demonstrated distinct differences in tyrosine ionization in these peptides. In AP_1 the pK of tyrosine (residue 18) was 10.4 and $\Delta\varepsilon_{295}$ and $\Delta\varepsilon_{245}$ were 2640 cm M^{-1} and 10,300 cm M^{-1}, consistent with the expected behavior for a single tyrosyl residue. Tyrosine ionization in AP_2 could not be unambiguously demonstrated; the small change observed being explainable by 10% contamination of the AP_2 with AP_1. This difference in tyrosine ionization can be explained by a substitution of the tyrosyl hydroxyl with a group such as sulfate, thus leading to tyrosine O-sulfate in AP_2 which could account for the chromatographic behavior. Other possibilities also exist, but in the absence of evidence for them, a substituted tyrosyl residue in AP_2 is proposed.

ACKNOWLEDGMENTS

This work was supported by a grant HL 12820 from the National Heart, Lung and Blood Institute. CMJ was an Established Investigator of the American Heart Association during the performance of this work.

REFERENCES

1. Jackson, C.M. and Hanahan, D.J. (1968) Biochemistry 7, 4506-4517.
2. Fujikawa, K., Legaz, M.E. and Davie, E.W. (1972) Biochemistry 11, 4882-4891.
3. Jackson, C.M. (1972) Biochemistry 11, 4873-4882.
4. Esnouf, M.P., Lloyd, P.H. and Jesty, J. (1973) Biochem. J. 131, 781-789.
5. Neal, G.G., Prowse, C.V. and Esnouf, M.P. (1976) FEBS Letters 66, 257-260.
6. Lindhout, M.J., Kop-Kaassen, B.H.M., Kop, J.M.M. and Hemker, H.C. (1978) Biochim. Biophys. Acta 533, 302-317.
7. DiScipio, R.G. and Davie, E.W. (1979) Biochemistry 18, 899-904.
8. Thøgersen, H.C., Peterson, T.E., Sottrup-Jensen, L., Magnusson, S. and Morris, H.R. (1978) Biochem. J. 175, 613-627.
9. Titani, K., Fujikawa, K., Enfield, D.L., Ericsson, L.H., Walsh, K.A. and Neurath, H. (1975) Proc. Nat. Acad. Sci. USA 72, 3082-3086.

STRUCTURAL AND FUNCTIONAL CHARACTERISTICS OF A PROTEOLYTICALLY MODIFIED, "GLA DOMAIN-LESS" BOVINE FACTOR X AND XA (DES LIGHT CHAIN RESIDUES 1-44)

TAKASHI MORITA and CRAIG M. JACKSON

Department of Biological Chemistry
Washington University School of Medicine
St. Louis, MO 63110

INTRODUCTION

Factor Xa can interact both with phospholipid in the presence of Ca^{2+} ions and with Factor Va. The ability of Factor Xa to activate prothrombin is increased dramatically by these cofactors (1). The sites on prothrombin responsible for interaction between prothrombin and Va, and prothrombin, phospholipid, and Ca^{2+} are well known (1). Because Fragment 1, Fragment 2 and α-thrombin are not disulfide linked to each other, these domains can be easily isolated and Fragment 1, Fragment 2 and α-thrombin shown to have the Ca^{2+} and phospholipid binding sites, Va interaction site and catalytic site, respectively (1). Although the sequence of bovine Factor X (2) and the isolation and the characterization of acarboxy-Factor X (3,4) make it virtually certain that the Gla domain region of X and Xa contains the Ca^{2+} binding sites, the polypeptide region responsible for interaction between Xa and Va is unknown. The precise location of the 20 Ca^{2+} binding sites on Factor X (5) is not clear, as the number of binding sites exceeds the number of Gla residues by 8.

Aronson (6) reported that Factor Xa may exist in two forms, normal Xa and a partially active degradation product. The activity of this latter form of Xa cannot be amplified by Ca^{2+}, phospholipid and V, but it has proteolytic and esterase activity. Milstone (7) reported that α-chymotrypsin converts Factor Xa to a Factor Xa derivative which has very similar properties to this partially active Xa. These observations suggested to us that Factor Xa may have a common peptide bond susceptible both to α-chymotrypsin (7) and an unknown protease (6) and that these derivatives of Factor Xa may be Gla-domain less Factor Xa and thus presumably have no phospholipid interaction site.

Using alpha-chymotrypsin we have developed an easy method for isolating specific Gla domain less derivatives of Factor X and Xa (des light chain residues 1-44) and two Gla domain peptides, residues 1-44 and 1-41, which can be used to deduce the location of the Va interaction site on Xa and to assess the dependence of Ca^{2+} binding and prothrombin activation on the Gla domain of Factor Xa.

RESULTS

Limited Proteolysis of Bovine Factor X by α-Chymotrypsin

Alpha-chymotrypsin rapidly inactivates Factor X as assessed by one stage clotting activity. Concomitantly, the molecular weight of light chain is decreased to about 11,000 with no decrease in molecular weight of the heavy chain (Fig. 1).

Separation and Structural Properties of X(-GD) and the Gla Domain Peptide (Gla-Peptide)

Modified Factor X and the small fragment which were released from the light chain were separated by anion exchange chromatography (see Fig. 1 in Morita, T. and Jackson, C.M., "Bovine Factor X_1 and X_2: Activation Peptide Based Chromatographic Differences"). Amino acid analysis, amino

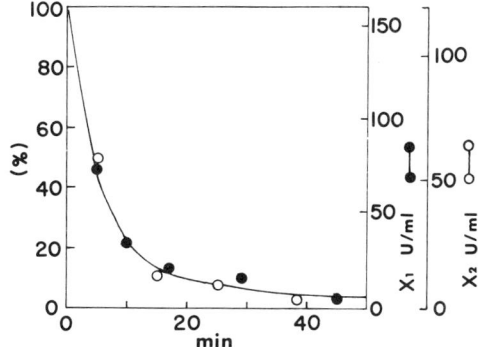

FIGURE 1 Destruction of Factor X One-Stage Clotting Activity by α-Chymotrypsin. Bovine Factor X_1 (1.66 mg/ml) ●, Factor X_2 (1.25 mg/ml) O, were incubated with α-chymotrypsin at room temperature (Enzyme to substrate ratio: 1 to 650).

terminal analysis and isolation of the tripeptide Ser-Lys-Tyr (light chain residues 42-44) demonstrated that the first cleavage site was the Tyrosyl (44)-Lysine (45) peptide bond. Alpha-chymotrypsin also cleaved the Tryptophanyl (41)-Serine (42) bond, however the rate of this latter cleavage is about 1% of the rate of the first cleavage. Whereas bovine Factor X had a specific activity of 80-120 units/mg in a one-stage clotting assay, Factor X(-GD) was virtually inactive with a specific activity of less than 0.01 unit/mg.

Activation of Factor X(-GD) by the Vipera russelli Activator (RVV-X-CP)

Factor X(-GD) could be activated by RVV-X-CP in the presence of Ca^{2+}, but not in the absence of Ca^{2+} (Fig. 2). The activation rate was very slow compared to the rate of normal Factor X activation. After full activation, the Boc-L-Val-L-Leu-Gly-L-Arg-pNA hydrolase specific activity of Factor Xa(-GD) and normal Xa differed by less than 10%. [^{3}H]DFP incorporation into Xa and Xa(-GD) was also the same. Clotting specific activity of Xa(-GD) however was less than the 0.01% of normal Factor Xa.

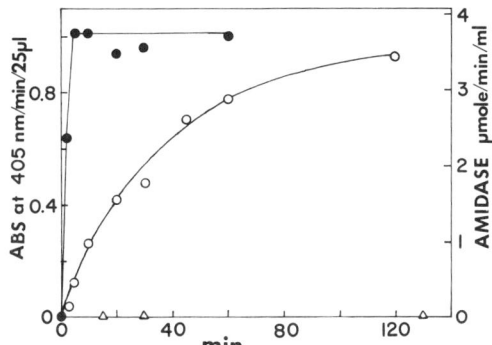

FIGURE 2 Activation of Normal Factor X and Factor X(-GD) by RVV-X-CP. Normal Factor X (●) or Factor X(-GD) (O) were activated with RVV-X-CP (Enzyme to substrate, 1 to 225) in the presence of 5 mM $CaCl_2$. Factor X(-GD) (Δ) was also treated in the presence of 0.5 mM EDTA.

Separation and Structural Properties of Xa(-GD)

After activation of Factor X(-GD) by RVV-X-CP, the α and β Xa(-GD), the activation peptides (2 species) and Fragment 4 (residues 290-307 of the heavy chain) were separated by anion-exchange chromatography and gel filtration on Sephadex G-100. The isolation of the activation peptide (heavy chain residues 1-51) and Fragment 4 showed that X(-GD) has a complete heavy chain structure (residues 1-307). Amino acid analysis of the light chain (-GD) and heavy chain of Xa(-GD) showed that the light chain (-GD) consisted of residues 45-140.

Functional Properties of Factor Xa(-GD)

Normal Factor Xa interacts both with phospholipid (in the presence of Ca^{2+}) and Va. From the data of Figure 3 it can be seen that Factor Xa(-GD) has lost the ability to interact with phospholipid, but retains fully its ability to interact with Factor Va.

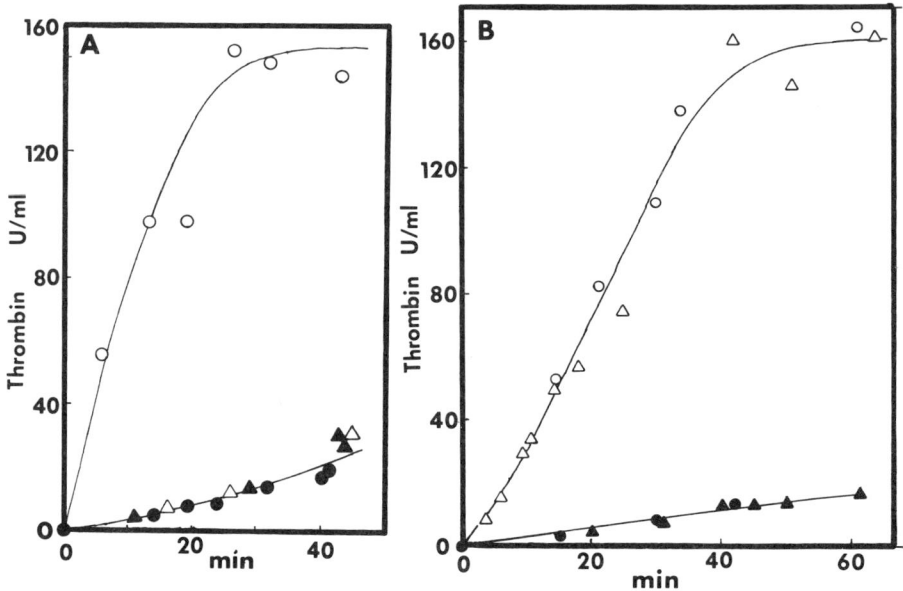

FIGURE 3 Prothrombin Activation by normal Xa and Xa(-GD) in the presence of phospholipid (A) and in the presence of Va (B). A. Non-acceleration of the activation of prothrombin by phospholipid in the case of Xa(-GD). Prothrombin (0.356 mg/ml) was activated by Xa (0.007 mg/ml) or Xa(-GD) (0.008 mg/ml) in the presence of phospholipid (0.234 mg/ml) and 10 mM $CaCl_2$. Activation by Xa+PL, O;   Xa, ●;   Xa(-GD)+PL, Δ;   Xa(-GD), ▲.
B. Acceleration of the prothrombin activation by Va. Prothrombin (0.356 mg/ml) was activated by Xa (0.0035 mg/ml) or Xa(-GD) (0.004 mg/ml) in the presence of Va (0.011 mg/ml) and 10 mM $CaCl_2$. Activation of Xa+Va, O;   Xa, ●;   Xa(-GD)+Va, Δ;   Xa(-GD), ▲.

Ca^{2+} Inhibition of the Proteolysis of Factor Xa by α-Chymotrypsin

Ca^{2+} ions inhibit chymotrypsin proteolysis of Factor X (Fig. 4). Factor X, Xa and Prothrombin Fragment 1 (8) can be "spontaneously" degraded during storage, presumably by proteases from airborne bacteria or molds. The degradation product has been identified as a Gla-domain less derivative in each case. Addition of 5 mM $CaCl_2$ to Xa or Fragment 1 solutions prevents this degradation.

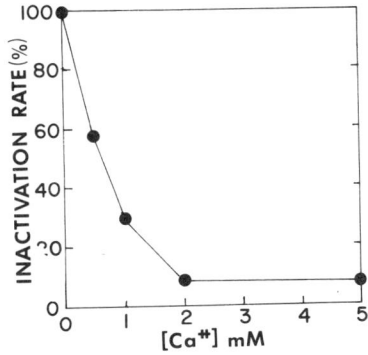

FIGURE 4 The effect of $CaCl_2$ concentration on the inactivation of Xa by α-chymotrypsin. Factor Xa (0.456 mg/ml, 5.5×10^3 unit/ml) was treated with α-chymotrypsin (0.001 mg/ml) at room temperature.

DISCUSSION

The data presented above demonstrate that limited proteolysis of Factor X and Xa by α-chymotrypsin can provide derivatives of Factor X which are extremely useful in investigating the relationship between its molecular structure and its function(s). The requirement for Ca^{2+} for activation of X(-GD) confirms the observations made on activation of acarboxyfactor X (9) and suggests that Ca^{2+} binding by Factor X exists which is distinct from that related to the Gla domain. Such sites, which are postulated here on the basis of activation experiments, may account for the excess of Ca^{2+} binding site observed in Factor X, i.e. 20 (5) over the number of Gla residues available, viz. 12. Participation of the Gla domain in the activation process is suggested however because of the markedly reduced activation rate of X(-GD). Direct Ca^{2+} interaction with X-CP might also explain these observations, but this has been investigated (10) and Ca^{2+} found not to bind to X-CP.

The indistinguishability of Xa and Xa(-GD) in their ability to catalyze prothrombin activation in the absence of phospholipid, and in the presence of Factor Va clearly establish the independence of the phospholipid binding region (the Gla domain) and the Va binding region or site. Comparison of these observations with those made with prothrombin suggest that the Va sites are likely to be derived from the remaining portion (96 residues), of the light chain.

The rapid cleavage of Tyr 44-Lys 45 by chymotrypsin implies that this region of the light chain must be on the surface of the Factor X molecule. Similar observations on the cleavage of Tyr 45-Thr 46 in Prothrombin Fragment 1 by chymotrypsin (see Carlisle, T., Morita, T. and Jackson, C.M., "Gla Region Secondary Structure in Prothrombin and Factor X") suggest that this segment of polypeptide may act as a link between the Gla domains of prothrombin and Factor X and the remainder of Fragment 1 and Factor X, respectively. Ca^{2+} inhibition of this cleavage in both these molecules suggests that the net charge in this region which will be markedly altered by Ca^{2+} binding, a Ca^{2+}-induced conformational change (11), or the Ca^{2+} induced dimerization which occurs in Prothrombin Fragment 1 (12,13) can prevent access to or cleavage of the linkage region Tyr-X peptide bond. Such Ca^{2+} inhibition is exploitable for stabilization of Factor X, Xa and Fragment 1 during long-term storage.

ACKNOWLEDGMENTS

This work was supported by a grant from the National Heart, Lung and Blood Institute (HL 12820). The work was performed while CMJ held an Established Investigatorship from the American Heart Association.

REFERENCES

1. Suttie, J.W. and Jackson, C.M. (1977) Physiological Rev. 57, 1-69.
2. Enfield, D.L., Ericsson, L.H., Walsh, K.A., Neurath, H. and Titani, K. (1975) Proc. Nat. Acad. Sci. USA 72, 16-19.
3. Lindhout, M.J., Kop-Klaassen, B.H.M., Kop, J.M.M. and Hemker, H.C. (1978) Biochim. Biophys. Acta 533, 302-317.
4. Lindhout, M.J. and Hemker, H.C. (1978) Biochim. Biophys. Acta 533, 318-326.
5. Henriksen, R.A. and Jackson, C.M. (1975) Arch. Biochem. Biophys. 170, 149-159.
6. Aronson, D.L. and Mustafa, A.J. (1971) Proc. Soc. Exp. Biol. Med. 137, 1262-1266.
7. Milstone, J.H., Oulianoff, N., Saxton, T. and Milstone, V.K. (1971) Yale J. Biol. Med. 43, 223-235.
8. Dombrose, F.A., Gitel, S.N., Zawalich, K. and Jackson, C.M. (1979) J. Biol. Chem. 254, in press.
9. Lindhout, M.J., Kop-Klaassen, B.H.M. and Hemker, H.C. (1978) Biochim. Biophys. Acta 533, 327-341.
10. Furie, B.C. and Furie, B. (1975) J. Biol. Chem. 250, 601-608.
11. Nelsestuen, G.L. (1976) J. Biol. Chem. 251, 5648-5656.
12. Prendergast, F.G. and Mann, K. (1977) J. Biol. Chem. 252, 840-850.
13. Jackson, C.M., Peng, O.W., Brenckle, G.M., Jonas, A. and Stenflo, J. (1979) J. Biol. Chem. 254, in press.

C-REACTIVE PROTEIN:
A FRUITLESS SEARCH FOR GLA

R. M. IAMMARINO, G. BLANK, and W. DIVEN

Department of Pathology
University of Pittsburgh School of Medicine
Pittsburgh, PA 15261

INTRODUCTION

C-reactive protein (CRP) is a plasma protein found in man (1) and other animal species (2, 3) which is present normally in trace quantities. Its concentration increases up to a thousandfold under diverse stimuli, including infections, collagen diseases, surgery, trauma, and malignancy (4). This stimulus is called the acute phase response and is shared by many plasma proteins which include fibrinogen, alpha-1 antitrypsin, haptoglobin, C3, and transferrin (5). In this latter group of proteins the increase is generally no greater than two- to threefold. Ultrastructural studies reveal that CRP is a pentameric protein which assumes a cyclic configuration. The five identical subunits are held together by electrostatic charges. It shares these properties with a newly designated group of proteins, the "pentraxins", which include the plasma or "P component" of amyloid, and the complement component C1t (6). The isolation of CRP in pure form was reported in 1941 (7) and it was originally recognized as a protein with cell surface binding properties. The name "C-reactive" was adopted because of a characteristic reaction which occurred with the C-polysaccharide coat of the pneumococcus (8). The active component of the C-polysaccharide binding to CRP was later shown to be phosphoryl choline (9). Despite considerable work that has gone on for the last 50 years, a definitive biologic role for CRP and most other proteins of the acute phase response remains unknown. However, when CRP binds to certain ligands, new functional properties can be demonstrated such as:
a) inhibition of platelet agglutination, which has been induced by aggregated IgG, thrombin (10), and other substances (11)
b) activation of complement (12)
c) inhibition of the response of the T-lymphocytes to specific antigens (13)
d) increased phagocytosis of bacteria by polymorphonuclear leucocytes (14).
CRP and the other pentraxins share many of the properties of the vitamin-K-dependent clotting factors, such as calcium-dependent phospholipid binding, calcium-dependent changes in electrophoretic mobility, and isolation by barium sulfate adsorption and citrate elution (15). Since these properties of the vitamin-K-dependent clotting factors are believed to be due to the presence of gamma carboxy glutamic acid (Gla), we undertook a search for Gla in CRP.

MATERIALS AND METHODS

Effusion fluid, a known rich source for CRP, was harvested from pleural or peritoneal cavities of patients with malignancies who were tapped for symptomatic relief. One hundred milliliter aliquots of effusion fluid were mixed with 3.0 grams of barium sulfate. The barium sulfate was washed exhaustively with 0.9% saline to remove contaminating proteins and finally washed with 0.02 molar sodium citrate to elute the bound protein enriched for CRP. The citrate eluate still contained trace quantities of albumin and transferrin. The citrate eluate was then dialyzed against 0.9% saline and retreated with barium sulfate, washed, and eluted again in 0.02 molar sodium citrate, rendering a product which appeared homogenous when analyzed by SDS electrophoresis. The molecular weight corresponded to that of the CRP subunit using appropriate standards. Functional tests for prothrombin activity were negative. Electrophoresis was carried out at pH 8.6 in a barbital buffer, 0.075 ionic strength, made up to 2.0 mM with calcium lactate in 1% agarose. To show the calcium binding effect, we carried out electrophoretic separations in an identical buffer with 2.0 mM EDTA used in place of calcium lactate.

Amino Acid Analysis - Approximately 1 mg of purified CRP was hydrolyzed in 2 M KOH by heating for 22 hours at 110°C, and then chilled in ice. Sixty milligrams of solid $KHCO_3$ was added and the preparation was then brought to pH 7.0 with 70% perchloric acid. A positive control of a Gla containing protein was performed by taking 45 micrograms of Konyne (Cutter Laboratories, Berkely, CA 94710), a commercially available product of vitamin-K-dependent clotting factors, which was hydrolyzed by the same procedure. Following removal of precipitates by centrifugation, suitable aliquots of the supernatant of each fraction was applied to an Aminex A-28 Resin Column (0.9 x 12.5 cm) in the acetate form (16). The resin had been washed to remove "fines" and final particle size was estimated at 9 ± 2 micra. Analysis was performed in a Beckman 120-C amino acid analyzer using 0.3 M acetate buffer, pH 4.6 with flow rate adjusted to 50 ml/minute at 53°C. An authentic Gla standard was generously provided by J. W. Suttie. Under these conditions, a Gla concentration of 1-5 nanomoles would have been detected equivalent to approximately one Gla residue per CRP subunit.

Since Gla containing proteins underwent profound calcium binding electrophoretic changes during the course of dicoumarol therapy, we analyzed a group of patients during treatment with dicoumarol. CRP was detected by direct immunofixation, post-electrophoresis by the application of suitably diluted monospecific antiserum against CRP along the course of the electrophoretic channel according to the method of Johnson (17). This method was also applied for the analysis of β-lipoprotein and C3.

RESULTS

The electrophoretic results are shown below, and document a striking calcium dependent electrophoretic change in CRP. There are similar but less marked changes noted in two other plasma proteins, β-lipoprotein and C3. These results show a striking alteration of electrophoretic mobility of CRP and a more modest alteration of two other plasma proteins, β-lipoprotein and C3. In each case, when EDTA replaces calcium in the buffer system the protein migration becomes more anodal. Not illustrated are the results on patients undergoing dicoumarol therapy. They showed CRP in the usual cathodal position when calcium was in the buffer with no shift noted during the course of dicoumarol therapy. The amino acid chromatographic results show the expected Gla peak of the standard at 66 minutes elution time and a Gla peak in the positive control, but no Gla peak in the CRP sample.

C-Reactive Protein   131

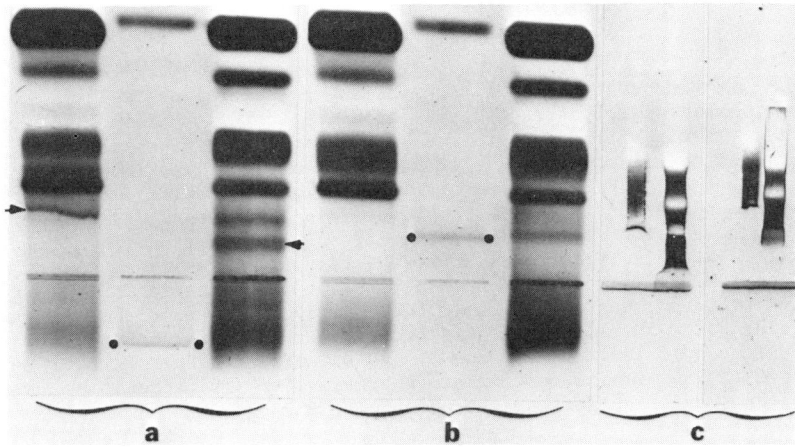

FIGURE 1. Parts "a" and "b" are illustrations of the electrophoretic separation of identical samples sets. The anode is at the top. Whole human serum samples flank the purified CRP in each. Marker albumin has been added to CRP. Part "a" has been run with calcium in the buffer, part "b" with EDTA replacing calcium. The CRP, shown with dots, undergoes a striking calcium dependent electrophoretic change. The arrows in part "a" reflect two other serum proteins showing calcium - EDTA shifts. Note the absence of these proteins in part "b". Part "c" shows the immunofixed β-lipoprotein and C3. At the left side of each channel in "c" is β-lipoprotein and at the right C3. The calcium - EDTA change is shown with calcium in the buffer of the left pair and EDTA replacing calcium in the right pair. Less marked anodal changes are noted in these proteins as contrasted to CRP.

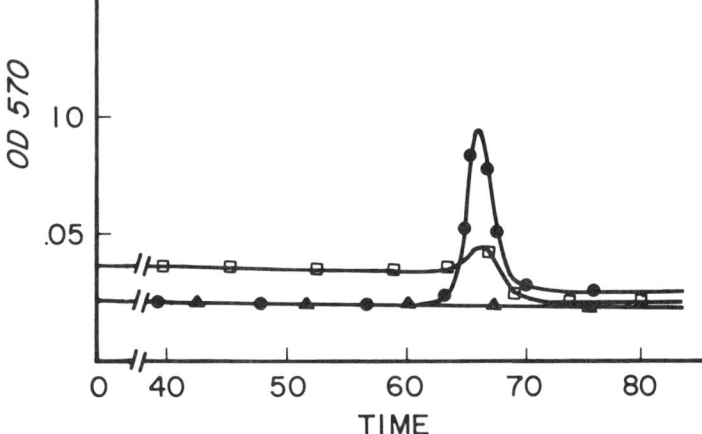

FIGURE 2. The chromatographic results of the amino acid analysis utilizing the Aminex A-28 resin column are shown. The line with the squares is the elution profile of the positive control protein containing Gla. The line with the solid circle markings is the elution profile of the authentic Gla standard, and the line with the solid triangle markings is the elution profile of CRP. The Gla standard and the Gla containing protein each have peaks at 66 minutes which peak is lacking in CRP.

DISCUSSION

The calcium dependent physical and membrane properties of CRP were the phenomena which first attracted our attention to this protein, and analysis for Gla was carried out to see if this modified amino acid could account for these properties as it has for the vitamin-K-dependent clotting factors and other proteins. After we began our work, the complete amino acid sequence of CRP was reported (18). The subunit is a 21,500 dalton single amino acid chain containing no carbohydrate with a loop generated by a disulfide bond between half cysteine residues. Our studies were restricted chemical analysis for the detection of Gla containing proteins, and we believe, conclusively demonstrate the absence of Gla. The study involving patients undergoing dicoumarol therapy was performed to see if the biosynthesis of CRP was affected by this agent which is known to inhibit the carboxylase enzyme system (19). No such changes were found, again supporting the absence of Gla.

The elucidation of the role of Gla containing proteins in blood clotting and bone formation is adding a new chapter in the molecular biology of calcium binding proteins. The similarities of the properties of CRP and the Gla containing proteins made such a study seem worthwhile. Although the search proved fruitless, we have asked what can be learned? It appears to us that two points can be made which are not mutually exclusive. If the Gla regions of the protein are _directly_ involved in calcium binding, then other proteins such as CRP with very similar properties can assume Gla type conformations when suitably folded or combined in unusual subunit configuration. All three cyclic pentameric proteins (pentraxins) bind calcium. If, on the other hand, calcium binding to Gla initiates a protein transition state, work supported by Nelsesteuen et al (20), then other residues are exposed which may then be capable of binding to ligands and producing biologic activity. These transition states can be induced in non-Gla containing proteins. As to this latter point, studies involving circular dichroism and optical rotary dispersion for both prothrombin fragment 1 (21) and recently for CRP and a group of related myeloma proteins (22) has been reported. Based on these data, it has been suggested that tyrosine and certain exposed histidine residues may be located at or near the calcium binding sites for both proteins.

It was hoped that Gla would be found in CRP and this would help define a role for this protein, for in spite of certain ligand associated properties _in vitro_, the function of CRP in host defense remains enigmatic. For those continuing to work with proteins now conclusively shown to contain Gla, we believe this study has proven worthwhile to illustrate that Gla properties can be found in non-Gla containing proteins. Caution is therefore urged in ascribing excessive functional properties to Gla.

ACKNOWLEDGEMENTS

The excellent services of Ellie Ferketic, Sandi McNair, and Linda Shab are gratefully acknowledged for technical, secretarial, and photographic services respectively.

REFERENCES

1. Claus, D. R., Osmand, A. P., and Gewurz, H. (1976) J. Lab. Clin. Med. 87, 120-128.

2. Kushner, I., and Volanakis, J. S. (1976) J. Lab. Clin. Med. 87, 617-623.

3. Baldo, B. A., and Fletcher, T. C. (1973) Nature 246, 145-146.

4. Hedlund, P. (1961) Acta Med. Scand., Suppl. 361, 1-71.

5. Fischer, C. L., Gill, C., Forrester, M. G., and Nakamura, R. (1976) Am. J. Clin. Pathol. 66, 840-846.

6. Osmand, A. P., Friedenson, B., Gewurz, H., Painter, R. H., Hofmann, T., and Shelton, E. (1977) Proc. Nat. Acad. Sci. 74, 739-743.

7. MacLeod, C. M., and Avery, O. T. (1941) J. Exp. Med. 73, 183-190.

8. Tillett, W. S., and Francis, T. (1930) J. Exp. Med. 52, 561-571.

9. Volanakis, J. E., and Kaplan, M. H. (1971) Proc. Soc. Exp. Biol. Med. 136, 612-614.

10. Fiedel, B. A., and Gewurz, H. (1976) J. Immunol. 116, 1289-1294.

11. Fiedel, B. A., and Gewurz, H. (1976) J. Immunol. 117, 1073-1078.

12. Osmand, A. P., Mortensen, R. F., Siegel, J., and Gewurz, H. (1975) J. Exp. Med. 142, 1065-1077.

13. Mortensen, R. F., Osmand, A. P., and Gewurz, H. (1975) J. Exp. Med. 141, 821-839.

14. Kindmark, C. O., (1971) Clin. Exp. Immunol. 8, 941-948.

15. Ganrot, P. O., and Kindmark, C. O. (1969) Biochim. et Biophys. Acta 194, 443-448.

16. Tabor, H., and Tabor, C. W. (1977) Anal. Biochem. 78, 554-556.

17. Johnson, A. M. (1978) Ann. Clin. & Lab. Sci. 8, 195-200.

18. Oliveira, E. B., Gotschlich, E. C., and Liu, T. Y. (1979) J. Biol. Chem. 254, 489-502.

19. Shah, D. V., and Suttie, J. W. (1974) Biochem. Biophys. Res. Commun. 60, 1397-1402.

20. Nelsestuen, G. L. (1978) Fed. Proc. 37, 2621-2625.

21. Gabriel, D. A., Schaefer, J., Roberts, H. R., Aronson, D. L., and Koehler, K. A. (1975) Thromb. Res. 7, 839-846.

22. Young, N. M., and Williams, R. E. (1978) J. Immunol. 121, 1893-1898.

CHEMISTRY OF γ-CARBOXYGLUTAMIC ACID

CHEMISTRY OF PEPTIDES CONTAINING
γ-CARBOXYGLUTAMIC ACID RESIDUES

H. C. MARSH, N. T. BOGGS, III, P. ROBERTSON, JR.,
M. M. SARASUA, M. E. SCOTT, P. B. W. TEN KORTENAAR,
J. A. HELPERN, L. G. PEDERSEN, K. A. KOEHLER‡,
and R. G. HISKEY

Departments of Chemistry and Pathology‡
The University of North Carolina at Chapel Hill
Chapel Hill, NC 27514

INTRODUCTION

In 1974 Stenflo et al. (1) reported the isolation and characterization of γ-carboxyglutamic acid (Gla) from a tetrapeptide (residues 6-9) of bovine prothrombin. Independently, Nelsestuen et al. (2) isolated and characterized Gla from a dipeptide (residues 33-34) of the same protein. The presence of ten Gla residues in the fragment 1 region of prothrombin (residues 1-156) is required for maximum efficiency of calcium ion and phospholipid binding by the protein (3). In the event of substitution of glutamyl residues for some or all of the Gla residues both calcium ion binding and phospholipid binding decrease (4,5). It is intriguing that metal ions other than calcium cannot effectively subsume the role of calcium ions.

Binding of various metal ions to fragment 1 leads to fluorescence quenching (6). The interaction of both calcium and magnesium ions with fragment 1 at neutral pH has been characterized via fluorescence quenching by a K_{diss} of approximately 0.4 mM (7,8). Fluorescence quenching has been shown to be related to fragment 1-phospholipid binding to the extent that fluorescence quenching is observed to have occurred prior to fragment 1-phospholipid binding. However metals such as magnesium induce fluorescence quenching in fragment 1 without imparting phospholipid binding properties to the fragment 1-metal ion complex (6).

A considerable effect, different from simple competition, of magnesium ions on the calcium binding behavior of fragment 1 has been reported (8). At millimolar levels of magnesium ions, the apparent cooperativity of calcium ion binding is increased compared with those values obtained in the absence of magnesium ions. Bloom and Mann (9) concluded from circular dichroism studies on fragment 1 in the presence of calcium, magnesium, or manganese ions that essentially the same secondary structural change occurred in the presence of any of these ions. Despite these similarities phospholipid binding data indicate that processess specific and non-specific for calcium ions occur. The obvious difficulty involves defining the difference between the equilibrium state resulting from a metal ion such as magnesium which does not support phospholipid binding to phospholipid. In an effort to clarify the structural response of fragment 1 to metal ion binding we have utilized model Gla-containing peptides and compared our results in certain cases to similar studies on fragment 1. Since we applied several different spectroscopic techniques to the problem we will discuss the results in terms of the "spectroscopic window" from which the observation is made.

RESULTS AND DISCUSSION

A. Metal Ion Mediated Quenching of Fragment 1 Intrinsic Fluorescence

1. Nature of the Transition. In 1976 Nelsestuen reported the fluorescence of fragment 1 in the presence of calcium ions (6). At equilibrium fragment 1 fluorescence is 40% quenched in the presence of calcium ions at neutral pH. Upon the addition of calcium ions, it was observed that following a rapid initial fluorescence decrease of 25% of the total equilibrium quenching a relatively slow first order decay of fluorescence to an equilibrium level occurred. The magnitude of the 25% fast fluorescence decrease was unaffected by the calcium ion concentration in the range 0.2 - 20 mM. Nelsestuen further demonstrated that the phospholipid binding behavior of bovine prothrombin and fragment 1 paralleled the observed fluorescence behavior of fragment 1. Immediately upon addition of calcium ions, approximately 25% of the fragment bound to phospholipid. The remaining fragment 1 bound to phospholipid in a manner described by precisely the same kinetic and thermodynamic parameters as those which described the slow fragment 1 quenching by calcium ions.

The rate of the slow fluorescence quenching and the activation energies determined in the presence of Mg^{+2}, Ca^{+2}, and Ba^{+2} were all identical within experimental error (7). Nelsestuen (6) suggested that this biphasic fluorescence quenching rate behavior is due to either two sequential protein transitions or to the presence of two populations of fragment 1 molecules.

It is possible to distinguish the possibilities suggested by Nelsestuen by examining both the forward and reverse rates of the slow conformational change. Implicit in such a study is the belief that the "immediate" reversal of the metal ion-mediated quenching of fragment 1 fluorescence by EDTA (Nelsestuen 1976) does not reflect the true reverse of the slow forward quenching process. Thus the reverse process is observed by addition of an excess of calcium ions to the system at various times after addition of EDTA. The rates obtained, k_{+1} and k_{-1}, the equilibrium constants characterizing the distribution of fragment 1 between isomers A and B, and determined thermodynamic parameters characterizing the process are all fully consistent with the model shown in

$$A \underset{k_{-1}}{\overset{k_{+1}}{\rightleftarrows}} B \underset{-Ca^{2+}}{\overset{+Ca^{2+}}{\rightleftarrows}} C \qquad (1)$$
$$\text{slow} \qquad \text{fast}$$

equation 1 (10) where A and B are conformational isomers of fragment 1. Calcium ions interact only with the B isomer to produce the in vivo conformation C which is capable of binding to the phospholipid surface. In view of the absence of a rate dependence on the calcium ion concentration (6) the conversion of A to B is rate limiting. Further supporting this contention are our preliminary stopped-flow studies which indicate that the $t_{1/2}$ for the fast fluorescence quenching step [B to C in (1)] is less than 10 milliseconds at 10°C.

We have speculated (10) that the trigger for the conversion of A ⟶ B may involve the trans- to cis-isomerization of a single proline residue, Pro^{22}, located in the 18-23 cystine loop of the bovine prothrombin sequence. We suggest Pro^{22} is implicated in this process since bovine factor X and human prothrombin which do not exhibit slow conformational changes when metal ion induced fluorescence is examined (8,11) contain substitutions of alanine and threonine, respectively at position 22.

Thus we suggest that the trans- to cis-isomerization of Pro^{22} may limit the rate of an otherwise very rapid calcium ion-fragment 1 interaction which leads to a conformation capable of interacting with a phospholipid surface (C in equation 1).

2. pH Effects on Intrinsic Fragment 1 Fluorescence. The study of the effect of pH on the intrinsic fluorescence of the calcium ion-fragment 1 system was undertaken to deduce the nature of the functional groups involved in the protein's response to added calcium ion (12). A significant dependence of fragment 1 fluorescence on pH was observed involving the ionization of groups with apparent pK$_a$'s of 5.0 and 7.4. Also a significant pH dependence of calcium binding was seen, reflecting the ionization of a group(s) with an apparent pK$_a$ above 7.5. The average affinity of calcium ions for fragment 1 and the Hill coefficient describing that process decrease as the pH is lowered from 8 to 6 (Table I) (13). As noted previously (12) the tight binding of calcium ion to fragment 1 shows a dependence on groups with apparent pK$_a$'s of approximately 7.5. Calcium binding to fragment 1 is an order of magnitude less tight as the pH is lowered from 8 to 5.9; magnesium ion binding however exhibits much less of a change over this pH range.

TABLE I The pH Dependence of Calcium and Magnesium Ion Binding To Fragment 1 Based On Fluorescence Quenching.

pH	Metal ion	n	Midpoint (M)
7.93	Ca^{2+}	2.3	8.9×10^{-5}*
7.41	Ca^{2+}	1.3	2.0×10^{-4}
6.89	Ca^{2+}	1.0	6.6×10^{-4}
5.92	Ca^{2+}	0.8	1.6×10^{-3}
8.04	Mg^{2+}	1.3	7.8×10^{-5}
7.49	Mg^{2+}	1.2	7.8×10^{-5}
6.94	Mg^{2+}	1.2	1.6×10^{-4}
5.85	Mg^{2+}	1.2	1.7×10^{-4}

*At pH 7.93, the limiting slope (0.8) at high occupancy yields an extrapolated value of K$_{diss}$ of 3.7×10^{-5} M.

At calcium ion concentrations below 2 mM the degree of quenching of fluorescence of fragment 1 increases with increasing pH from 4.98 to 7.93. However above 2 mM calcium ion the pH dependence of the calcium ion induced quenching describes a minimum at pH 6 (12). In contrast to calcium ion at magnesium ion concentrations of 0.2-3 mM the degree of quenching increases from pH 6 to maximum at pH 7.5 which falls off by 20% at pH 8.0.

From these studies we conclude:

i. Tight binding of calcium ion to fragment 1 is pH dependent and cooperative (n = 2.3). Tight calcium ion binding involves groups with apparent pK_a's of about 7.5.

ii. Protonation of ionizing groups with apparent pK_a's of 4.5 reduces the affinity of fragment 1 for both calcium and magnesium ions.

iii. Groups with apparent pK_a's of 4.5 appear to be critical for cooperative calcium binding and thus for the establishment of the calcium binding conformation C (equation 1).

B. Circular Dichroism Studies

Studies by Bloom and Mann (9) and ourselves (13) using circular dichroism to evaluate the secondary structure of fragment 1 indicate that the final equilibrium structure, as assessed by CD, is insensitive to the nature of the divalent cation. Calcium ions induce changes in secondary structure of fragment 1 as seen by transitions at 208 and 220 nm. These changes are cooperative (n = 2.1) (Table II) and yield average binding data similar to that obtained via Hill plots of fluorescence quenching

TABLE II CD Fragment 1 Metal Ion Binding Data

pH	Metal	Wavelength (nm)	n	Midpoint (mM)
7.5	Ca^{2+}	208	2.1	0.19
7.5	Ca^{2+}	220	2.0	0.22
7.5	Mg^{2+}	208	1.2	0.23
7.5	Mg^{2+}	232	2.0	0.19
6.0	Ca^{2+}	208	2.1	0.38

data. Magnesium ions also induce changes in secondary structure but in a much less cooperative manner (n = 1.2). The positive cooperativity of the effect of calcium on secondary structure does not change from pH 7.5 to 6.0 (208 nm). Thus the affinity of fragment 1 for calcium ion is related to groups with apparent pK_a's of 7.5 but the cooperativity of calcium binding is not. We note however that the affinity of fragment 1 for calcium ions decrease from 0.2 mM at pH 7.5 to 0.5 mM at pH 6.0. We may conclude that:

i. Cations induce changes in the secondary structure of fragment 1. These changes are cooperative and maximal in the range 0.5 - 1.0 mM calcium ion. At these concentrations 3-4 moles of calcium ion are bound per mole of fragment 1 according to the equilibrium dialysis data of Bajaj and Mann (14).

ii. The peptide representing the sequence of bovine prothrombin 1-39 has been obtained by incubation of fragment 1 with S. aureus protease (strain UV). The peptide contains all of the 10 Gla residues in the protein and exhibits substantial changes in the far UV when examined by circular dichroism as a function of pH with 2.0 mM calcium ion. As with fragment 1 major changes in secondary structure were noted as the pH was lowered 6.5 to 1.9 (15).

C. Metal Ion Nuclear Magnetic Resonance Spectrometry

1. Studies on Peptide Models. In order to characterize the metal ion/protein interaction it was desirable to first describe metal binding to smaller models of the prothrombin system including γ-carboxyglutamic acid and peptides containing this amino acid. With the development of appropriate methods for the chemical synthesis of Gla peptides and a source of chiral Gla intermediates (16) we studied the possible utilization of metal ion NMR as a tool for evaluation of the metal ion-protein interaction. Because ^{43}Ca and ^{25}Mg have nuclear spins of greater than 1/2 (7/2 and 5/2 respectively) and, therefore, have quadrupolar moments we believed that even in rather unstable complexes with small molecules the quadrupolar contributions to the relaxation of the metal nucleus would permit quantitation of the extent of metal ion binding through signal broadening. Our early studies (17) established that both ^{43}Ca^{2+} and ^{25}Mg^{2+} could be used with simple Gla peptides.

In the case of ^{25}Mg^{2+} the addition of an equimolar amount of N-benzyloxycarbonyl-D-γ-carboxyglutamyl-D-γ-carboxyglutamic acid α-methyl ester (1) caused substantial line broadening (to $\sim$ 40 times the line width of "free" ^{25}Mg^{2+}). Although there may also be small changes in the metal ion's chemical shift upon complexation, these changes are obliterated by the extent of line-broadening induced. Calculation of the $K_{Diss}^{25Mg^{+2}}$ (Table III) from these data makes the assumption (apparently valid in these cases) that the exchange between bound and unbound states is fast on the NMR time scale. The calculated $K_{Diss}^{25Mg^{+2}}$ for the 1:Mg^{+2} complex (1:1 ratio) was 0.64 and 0.58 mM in two separate sets of binding experiments. The peptide N-benzyloxycarbonylglycyl-D,L-γ-carboxyglutamyl-glycine ethyl ester (2) containing a single Gla residue, exhibited a much weaker interaction with ^{25}Mg^{2+} ($\sim$ 20 mM).

TABLE III. Interaction of ^{43}Ca^{+2} And ^{25}Mg^{+2} With Gla-Peptides (17)

Peptide	pH	Ratio M^{+2}/peptide	$K_{Diss}^{25Mg^{+2}}$	$K_{Diss}^{43Ca^{+2}}$	^{a}log K_{Assoc}^{Ca}
Z-D-Gla-D-Gla-OMe (1)	6.5	1:1	0.58, 0.64 mM	0.6 mM	3.2 + 0.2
Z-Gly-D,L-Gla-Gly-OEt (2)	6.5	1:1	$\sim$ 20 mM		

^{a}Determined for the H-Gla-Gla-OH/Ca^{++} complex. The mononuclear form (1:1) was observed to predominate above pH 4 (18).

In the case of ^{43}Ca^{2+} which has a small nuclear electric quadrupole moment the line broadening of the ^{43}Ca signal on addition of 1 is very slight. However the resonance peak shifts downfield by 2 ppm between the free and totally complexed states. The $K_{Diss}^{43Ca^{2+}}$ calculated from these data is 0.6 mM in good agreement with the association constant for

L-γ-carboxyglutamyl-L-γ-carboxyglutamic acid determined potentiometrically by Marki et al. (18). Thus ^{25}Mg and ^{43}Ca NMR are complementary methods for the determination of divalent metal binding constants.

We noted that the Gla residues in fragment 1 occur in pairs (or nearly so) and that in at least three groupings the nearest neighbors are basic amino acids, arginine or lysine. In order to establish whether nearest neighbor interactions could influence metal ion binding the model systems N-benzyloxycarbonyl-N$^\epsilon$-nitro-L-argininyl-D-γ-carboxyglutamyl-D-γ-carboxyglutamic acid α-methyl ester (3) and L-argininyl-D-γ-carboxyglutamyl-D-γ-carboxyglutamic acid α-methyl ester (4) were studied using ^{25}Mg^{2+} NMR (Table IV) (19).

TABLE IV pH Dependence of ^{25}Mg^{2+} Binding To Peptides Containing γ-Carboxyglutamic Acid (19).

Peptide	$\frac{M^{2+}}{Peptide}$	pH	^{25}Mg^{2+} K_{Diss}	^{25}Mg^{2+} pH$_{Inflect.}$
Z-L-Arg(NO$_2$)-D-Gla-D-Gla-OMe (3)	1:1	6.8	0.54 mM	4.6 - 4.8
L-Arg-D-Gla-D-Gla-OMe (4)	1:1	6.5	0.60 mM	4.6 - 4.8
Fragment 1	-	-	-	4.2, ~ 7.5

Both the blocked peptide, 3, and the peptide-containing the basic guanidino group, 4, exhibited similar dissociation constants. The line width increases markedly as the pH is increased; the resulting titration curves with 3 and 4 are the same with inflections in the pH range 4.6 - 4.8.

Marki et al. (18) established that the fourth ionization constant of H-L-Gla-L-Gla-OH is 4.7. Thus ionization of the third side chain γ-carboxyl group of a Gla-Gla pair appears to be necessary for the ligand system with ^{25}Mg^{2+} to be established and for significant metal binding to occur. In view of this conclusion we wondered if any combination of oxygen ligands would lead to a peptide: magnesium complex with comparable K$_{Diss}$ to that of 2, 3, 4. Stated another way is the Gla^{33}-Ser^{34} sequence in bovine prothrombin equivalent to a Gla-Gla sequence? In order to evaluate the requirements of the third oxygen ligand we have studied L-phenylalanyl-L-leucyl-L-γ-carboxyglutamyl-L-glutamyl-L-leucine methyl ester (5) and N-benzyloxycarbonyl-L-γ-carboxyglutamyl-L-serine methyl ester (6) (Table V) (20).

TABLE V ^{25}Mg^{2+} Binding To γ-Carboxyglutamic Acid Peptides Containing A Single Gla Residue

Peptide	$\frac{M}{Peptide}$	pH	^{25}Mg^{2+} K_{Diss}	^{25}Mg^{2+} pH$_{Inflect.}$
H-Phe-Leu-Gla-Glu-Leu-OMe (5)	1:1	7.0	0.7 mM	5.1 - 5.2
Z-Gla-Ser-OMe^a (6)	1:1.5	7.0	~ 1 mM	~ 4.8

^{a}Addition of Ca^{2+} to a 2:1 peptide: ^{25}Mg^{2+} solution to a final concentration of 1:1 peptide to metal ion did not change the ^{25}Mg^{2+} line width.

Chemistry of Gla-containing Peptides   143

The value obtained for $K_{Diss}^{25Mg^{2+}}$ in a solution containing 5 and $^{25}Mg^{2+}$ (1:1) is similar to the value obtained for peptides 1, 3, 4 and quite different from either 2 or the dipeptide Z-L-Glu-L-Glu-OMe (~20 mM). Furthermore a sigmoidal titration curve for the extent of magnesium ion binding to 5 as a function of pH reveals a slightly higher inflection point but otherwise a shape similar to peptides 1, 3, 4.

Studies involving 6 indicate that while the serine hydroxyl can apparently serve as a third ligand the plot of $^{25}Mg^{2+}$ line width vs. peptide concentration does not fit a simple 1:1 complex. Furthermore $K_{Diss}^{25Mg^{2+}}$ is somewhat weaker than 2-5 and the pH dependence has shifted more nearly to that observed with peptides containing adjacent Gla residues. Nevertheless a serine residue adjacent to a γ-carboxyglutamic acid unit clearly contributes to the stability of the metal ion complex although the stoichiometry changes.

2. Studies on Fragment 1. The $^{25}Mg^{2+}$ binding to fragment 1 as a function of pH from 2.77 to 8.28 could be studied by similar methods. As with the peptide models no magnesium binding to fragment 1 was apparent at low pH values. However a sharp increase in binding occurs as the pH is raised above 3.8 with a major inflection in the titration curve at pH 4.2 (Table IV). Thus the basic shape of the titration curve is similar to those of the peptide models up to pH 7. At about pH 7 a second increase in magnesium ion binding occurs suggesting a dependence on a protein pK_a of at least 7.5. A similar pH dependence of calcium ion was noted by fluorescence quenching studies (12); the calcium affinity of fragment 1 increased about twenty-fold from pH 6 to 8 while magnesium binding by fragment 1 increased only two-fold over the same range of pH. Presumably $^{25}Mg^{2+}$ NMR is detecting the same set of side chain interactions.

Utilization of $^{43}Ca^{2+}$ and $^{25}Mg^{2+}$ NMR allows the direct monitoring of the relationship between calcium and magnesium ion binding to fragment 1. The ability of calcium ions to displace $^{25}Mg^{2+}$ ions from fragment 1 at various pH values is recorded in Table VI. At high calcium concentrations all magnesium ions are not displaced and the leveling of the $^{25}Mg^{2+}$ line width occurs when about 75% of the originally bound magnesium ions have been displaced. The converse experiment, the displacement of

TABLE VI Calcium: Magnesium Competition for Binding to Fragment 1
(Hill Parameters and Fractional Displacement)

MAGNESIUM-25 DISPLACEMENT FROM FRAGMENT 1 BY CALCIUM			
pH	n	Midpoint (M)	% Not Displaced
8.2	1.96	7.1×10^{-4}	24[a]
7.0	1.37	6.9×10^{-4}	27[a]
6.0	0.93	4.3×10^{-4}	27[a]
CALCIUM-43 DISPLACEMENT FROM FRAGMENT BY MAGNESIUM IONS			
7.0	0.82	5.5×10^{-3}	40[b]

[a]Fraction not displaced was constant above 5 mM calcium chloride. [b]Fraction not displaced at 30 mM magnesium chloride.

$^{43}Ca^{2+}$ bound to fragment 1 by magnesium ions is also given in Table VI. This experiment demonstrates that calcium ions are more persistently bound than magnesium ions; no distinct leveling off in $^{43}Ca^{2+}$ line width was observed in the reciprocal experiment (13). The ease of displacement of $^{25}Mg^{2+}$ by calcium ions is pH dependent. Hill plots (Table VI) show greater cooperativity as the pH increases from 6.0 to 8.3. The displacement of $^{43}Ca^{2+}$ by magnesium ions is not cooperative at pH 7.0

Investigation of the pH dependence of $^{25}Mg^{2+}$ ion (20.2 mM) binding to fragment 1 (0.11 mM) in the presence of calcium ions (19.5 mM) allows one to examine the pH dependence of magnesium ion binding to only those sites from which calcium ions cannot displace magnesium ions. An increase in binding of $^{25}Mg^{2+}$ was observed in the pH range 3 - 4.5 with an inflection point in the titration curve at pH 3.8. Binding at pH > 7.5 was suppressed. Thus the metal ion binding response at a pK_a of approximately 7 - 7.5 is peculiar to a site that binds calcium ion with high affinity.

Investigation of $^{43}Ca^{2+}$ binding to fragment 1 in the presence of magnesium ion reveals a broad pH dependence between pH 4-7 and the expected inflection as pH increases above 7. Thus greater fragment 1 affinity for calcium ion at pH values above 7 is apparent from the fluorecence, circular dichroism, and NMR studies. Benarous et al. (21) have observed an increase in calcium binding to human prothrombin over the pH range 6.7 to 9.0. An apparent dependence on a protein pK_a of 7.3 was noted.

D. Europium (III) Laser-Induced Luminescence

1. Studies on Model Peptides. Horrocks and Sudnick (22) have developed a potentially useful technique for the study of metal ion binding to biomolecules. The method involves the use of laser excitation of certain lanthanide ions in solvents containing varying ratios of water to deuterium oxide and measurement of the subsequent decay rates of luminescence. The rate constant for luminescence decay of the ion, k, (equal to the reciprocal of the excited state lifetime) is sensitive to the constitution of the metal ion coordination sphere. While O-H oscillators are effective in causing deexcitation by energy transfer, O-D oscillators are not, due to the lower vibrational energy of the O-D bond. A plot of k vs X_{H_2O} can be directly related to the number of water molecules in the coordination sphere of the europium (III) ion. Since aquo europium ion is nonahydrated the value of k_{obs} for $X_{H_2O} = 1.0$ corresponds to a coordination number, N, of nine. The value of $k_{obs}^{D_2O}$ for europium (III) ion in deuterium corresponds to N = 0. A quantity ΔN is defined as $N(aquoEu^{+3})$ - N (ligand-Eu^{+3} complex) and can be interpreted as the number of water molecules displaced from the europium (III) coordination sphere by complexation with ligands. The results of our studies (20) with various model peptides are given in Table VII.

The values for K_{Diss} for the experiment using γ-carboxyglutamic (Gla) were calculated in two ways. Weber-Young analysis (24) which assumes a noninteracting model, yielded values of 42.0 μM (n=2.01) in close agreement with the results of Sperling et al. (23). Alternatively, a standard thermodynamic analysis involving the assumption of n (not necessarily identical) binding sites, each having a unique K_{Diss}, was employed. Expressions for the n thermodynamic dissociation (equilibrium) constants were developed and an equation was derived from these expressions for the fraction of sites bound divided by the concentration

TABLE VII. Eu^{3+} Complexes With Peptides Containing γ-Carboxyglutamic Acid Residues

Peptide	ΔN	Std Equilibrium Analysis		Weber-Young Analysis (24)	
		M/L	K_{Diss}	M/L	K_{Diss}
Z-Gly-D,L-Gla-Gly-OEt (2)	5	1:1	43 μM	1:1.02	33 μM
Z-Gla-Ser-OMe (6)	4	1:1	45 μM	1:1.11	44 μM
Z-D-Gla-D-Gla-OMe (1)	4	-	-	-	-
H-Phe-Leu-Gla-Glu-Leu-OMe (5)	2.5	2:1	96 μM		
H-Phe-Leu-Gla-Gla-Leu-OMe (7)	4	2:1	75 μM		
H-Gla-OH	2	1:2	33 μM	1:2.01[a]	42 μM

[a] Sperling et al. (23) report a value of K_{Diss} = 55 μM (1:2.1) for the complex formed between Gla and terbium (III) ion.

of free metal ion. The equation was rearranged and plotted in a form from which binding constants could be extracted. For an assumed stoichiometry of 2:1, Gla:Eu^{3+}, a K_{Diss} of 33 μM resulted. The thermodynamic analysis and the Weber-Young treatment are not equivalent (except for the 1:1 case). It is interesting, however, that the values of K_{Diss} found by the two methods are similar. The affinity of Eu^{3+} for Gla is approximately 10^3-fold greater than that of Mg^{2+}.

The rate constant vs peptide: Eu^{3+} ratio plot for the peptide 2 containing a single Gla residue indicates 1:1 stoichiometry and a constant ΔN of 5 above a 2:Eu^{3+} ratio of 1.2:1. Calculation of K_{Diss} by either Weber-Young analysis or the standard thermodynamic analysis, assuming a 1:1 complex, yielded similar values. Studies involving the dipeptide derivative 6, also containing a single Gla, yielded a linear Weber-Young plot with values of K_{Diss} 44.4 μM similar to 2. The ratio of peptide:Eu^{3+} leveled off at 1:1.11; similar results were obtained from the thermodynamic analysis assuming a 1:1 6:Eu^{3+} complex. The ΔN value of 4 was also comparable to the results obtained with 2. Thus, if we utilize 2 or 6 as models for the interaction of a single protein-bound Gla residue with a single Eu^{3+} ion, such an interaction will involve the loss of 4-5 water molecules from the metal ion coordination sphere.

In contrast to calcium or magnesium which form 1:1 complexes with peptides containing two adjacent Gla residues (1,7), the titration of Eu^{+3} ions with both peptides 1 and 7 indicate higher order complexes of more than one Eu^{+3} binding to a single peptide molecule. The standard equilibrium analysis of the pentapeptide 7 data yielded a stoichiometry of 2:1 Eu^{+3}: peptide with a value for the first (smallest) of K_{Diss} = 74 μM. A non-linear Weber-Young plot was obtained indicating that the two binding sites are highly interactive. The ΔN=4 obtained for peptide 7 is consistent with the loss of 4-5 water molecules per Eu^{+3} bound to a single Gla moiety. Each molecule of 7 thus binds two Eu^{+3} ions with a subsequent loss of 4 water molecules on the average from the coordination sphere of each Eu^{+3} ion. Using peptide 1 with adjacent Gla residues in preliminary studies neither the Weber-Young plot nor the thermodynamic equilibrium analysis gave linear plots indicating that the K_{Diss} values for the Eu ions are apparently different (interactive) but not widely separated in value. From the fact that the titration curve levelled off well below a 1:1 peptide:Eu^{+3} molar ratio and the value of $\Delta N=4$ obtained in the level portion of the titration curve, it can be postulated that peptide 1 is also forming a 1:2 peptide:Eu^{+3} complex. The pH-dependence of a 1:1 mixture of 1 and Eu^{3+} indicates that ΔN changes from 0 to 4.8 as the pH is adjusted from 2.0 to 7.5. An inflection occurs at pH 3.8, approximately 0.5 pH unit lower than with magnesium binding. This pH dependence suggests ionization of the second γ-carboxy group.

The pentapeptide 5 containing adjacent Gla and Glu residues also produced a 1:2 peptide:Eu^{+3} complex with the smallest K_{Diss} = 96 μM. The lower value of ΔN = 2.5 is reasonable since the replacement of Gla (2 γ-CO_2^-) with Glu (1 γ-CO_2^-) would be expected to reduce the amount of coordination to Eu^{+3}. The ΔN value of 4 could represent an average of ΔN 4 for a Eu^{+3} bound to the Gla residue and a ΔN = 1 or 2 for a Eu^{+3} bound to a Glu residue.

The pH titration curve of Eu^{3+} and 5 exhibited an inflection point at pH 4.6. This value corresponds to ionization of a second side chain carboxyl group in the pentapeptide. These results suggest that despite the similar size and coordination levels of Eu^{3+} and Ca^{2+} the former ion does not discriminate between formation of a malonate or an acetate type complex. Thus Eu^{3+} binds to individual Gla or Glu residues. A comparison of Mg^{2+} and Ln^{3+} ion binding to acetate, Gla, and Gla-Gla support this view (Table VIII).

TABLE VIII K_{Diss} For Magnesium and Lanthanide Ion Complexes

Ligand	Mg^{2+}, K_{Diss}	Ln^{3+}, K_{Diss}
$CH_3CO_2^-$	50 mM	12 mM[25]
$CH_2(CO_2^-)_2$	20 mM	42 μM
-Gla-Gla-	0.6 mM	74 μM[a]

[a]Using peptide 7 (Table VII)

2. Studies on Fragment 1. Extension of the Eu^{3+} laser luminescence experiment to fragment 1 yield interesting results which are quite different from those data obtained with peptide models. A plot of k, the rate constant of Eu^{3+} luminescence decay, vs the ratio of the concentration of Eu^{3+} ions to fragment 1 is given in Fig. 1. During the early stages of the titration 2-3 Eu^{3+} ions appear to bind tightly losing approximately 8 water molecules from the inner coordination shell of each ion. Since the equilibrium dialysis of Bajaj et al. (14) suggest 2-3 tight Ca^{2+} binding sites on fragment 1, it is possible that Eu^{3+} has occupied the calcium tight ion binding sites. Further addition of Eu^{+3} from ratios of 6:1 to 30:1 yield a plateau corresponding to ΔN values of about 5.5 water molecules. Clearly Eu^{3+} ions in this region interact with the many combinations of oxygen ligands present on the protein side chains.

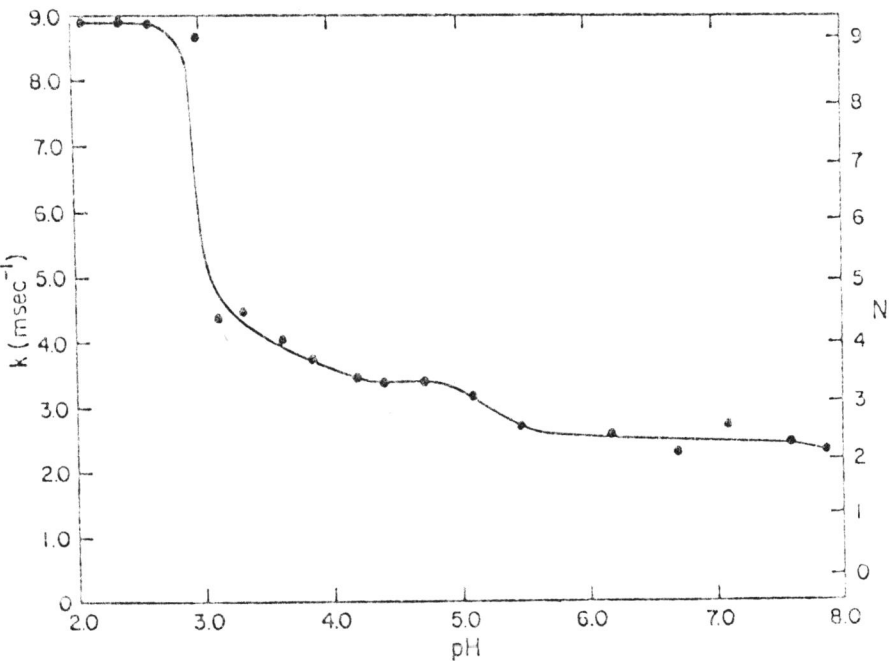

Fig. 1 Eu³⁺ luminescence decay rate and hydration as a function of Eu³⁺/fragment 1 ratio.

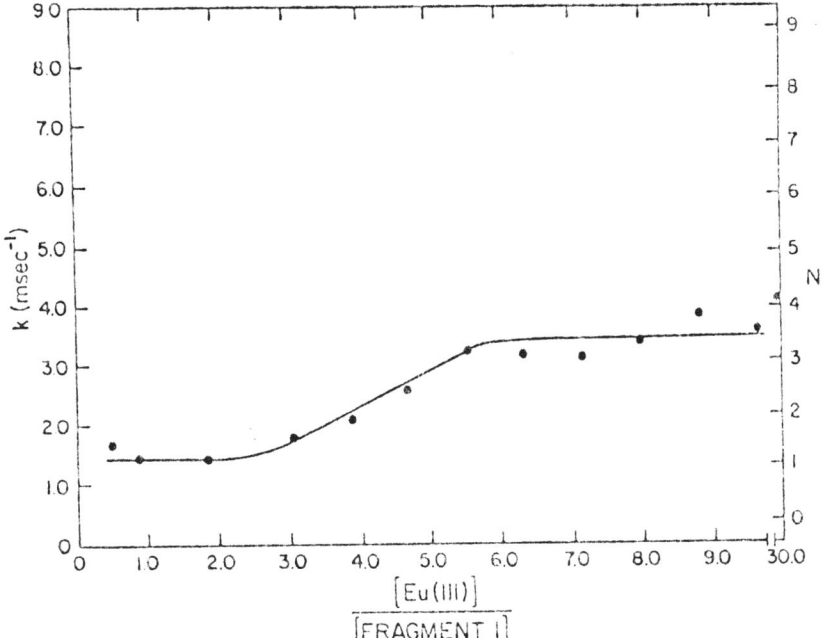

Fig. 2 Effect of pH on Eu³⁺: F1 luminescence decay rate and hydration.

The pH titration curve of the fragment 1:Eu^{3+} complex (4:1 Eu^{3+}/fragment 1) is shown in Fig. 2. In the region pH 8 to 6 ΔN of 7 was observed; from pH 6.0 to 4.7 k increased (ΔN decreased) and leveled to a plateau ($\Delta N=4.6$) from pH 4.7 to 4.4. From pH 4.4 to 3.1, ΔN gradually decreased to a ΔN of 4.5; but from pH 3.1 to 2.5 a dramatic decrease of ΔN to a value of nearly zero water displacement was observed. Thus the pH region from pH 6.0 to 2.0 resembles an ionization region for multiple carboxyl groups; as the carboxyl groups are protonated the ability to bind Eu^{+3} is lost. The first ionization constant corresponding to a pK_a value of 2.8-3.0 is therefore critical to binding of Eu^{3+} to fragment 1. This observation is contrasted with the pH dependence of calcium ion binding (pK_a 7.5) observed by Scott et al. (12) and Benerous et al. (21) for both bovine and human fragment 1.

ACKNOWLEDGEMENT

This investigation was supported in part by grants HL20161, HL18245, and HL23881 from the National Institutes of Health. NTB, III was supported as a postdoctoral trainee, grant HL07255; KAK was an Established Investigator of the American Heart Association. Purchase of the NMR instrument at UNC-CH was made possible by NSF Instrument Grants GU-2059-Amendment I and GP-37602 and by National Institutes of Health award 5S05RR07072. Purchase of the Nicolet 18 mm probe was made possible through funds from the Department of Anesthesiology at UNC-CH.

The authors are particularly grateful to Professor Horrocks and his associates and Mr. Al Schultz for ther assistance in the early stages of the europium (III) laser luminescence work. The technical assistance of Ms. M.W. Pendergraft, Dr. David Harris, and Mr. W.S. Woodward are gratefully acknowledged.

REFERENCES

1. Stenflo, J., Fernlund, P., Egan, W and Roepstorff, P. (1975) Proc. Nat. Acad. Sci. U.S., 71, 2730-2733.

2. Nelsestuen, G.L., Zytokovics, T.H., and Howard, J.B. (1974) J. Biol. Chem., 249, 6347-6350.

3. Esmon, C.T., Suttie, J.W., and Jackson, C.M. (1975) J. Biol. Chem., 250, 4095-

4. Friedman, P.A., Rosenberg, R.D., Hauschka, P.V., and Fitz-James, A. (1977) Biochem. Biophys. Acta 494, 271-276

5. Esnouf, M.P. and Prowse, C.V. (1977) Biochem. Biophys. Acta 490, 471-476.

6. Nelsestuen, G.L. (1976) J. Biol. Chem., 251, 5648-5656.

7. Nelsestuen, G.L., Broderius, M., and Martin, G. (1976) J. Biol. Chem., 251, 6886-6893.

8. Prendergast, F.G. and Mann, K.G. (1977) J. Biol. Chem., 252, 840-850.

9. Bloom, J.W. and Mann, K.G. (1978) Biochemistry, 17, 4430-4438.

10. Marsh, H.C., Scott, M.E., Koehler, K.A., and Hiskey, R.G. (1979) Biochem. J.

11. Nelsestuen, G.L. (1977) in Calcium-Binding Proteins and Calcium Function (Wasserman, R.H., Corradino, R.A. Carafoli, E., Kretsinger, R.H., MacLenna, D.H., and Siegel, F.L., Eds.) North Holland, New York, p 323-332.

12. Scott, M.E., Koehler, K.A., and Hiskey, R.G. (1979) Biochem. J. 177, 879-886.

13. Marsh, H.C., Robertson, Jr., P., Scott, M.E., Koehler, K.A., and Hiskey, R.G. (1979) J. Biol. Chem.

14. Bajaj, S.P., Butkowski, R.J., and Mann, K.G., (1975) J. Biol. Chem., 250, 2150-2156.

15. Marsh, H.C. unpublished studies.

16. Boggs, III, N.T., Goldsmith, B., Gawley, R.A. Koehler, K.A., and Hiskey, R.G. (1979) J. Org. Chem., 44, 0000.

17. Robertson, Jr., P., Hiskey, R.G., and Koehler, K.A. (1978) J. Biol. Chem., 253, 5880-5883.

18. Marki, W., Oppliger, M., Thani, P., and Schwyzer, R. (1977) Helv. Chim. Acta, 60, 798-806.

19. Robertson, Jr., Koehler, K.A., and Hiskey, R.G. (1979) Biochem. Biophys. Res. Commun., 86, 265-270.

20. Robertson, Jr., P., Sarasua, M.M., Scott, M.E., Helpern, J.A., Ten Kortenaar, P.B.W., Boggs, III, N.T., Pedersen, L.G., Koehler, K.A. and Hiskey, R.G. (1980) J. Am. Chem. Soc., submitted.

21. Benarous, R., Elion, J., and Labie, D. (1976) Biochemie, 58, 391-394.

22. Horrocks, Jr., W. De W. and Sudnick, D.R. (1979) J. Am. Chem. Soc., 101, 334-340.

23. Sperling, R., Furie, B.C., Blumenstein, M., and Keyt, B. (1978) J. Biol. Chem., 253, 3898-3906.

24. Weber, G. and Young, L.B. (1964) J. Biol. Chem., 239, 1415-1423.

25. Sherry, A.C., Yoshida, C., Birnbaum, E.R., and Darnall, D.W. (1973) J. Am. Chem. Soc., 95, 3011-3014.

DETECTION OF
γ-CARBOXYGLUTAMIC ACID BY DANSYLATION

MARGARET LOW, JOHN J. VAN BUSKIRK, and WOLFF M. KIRSCH

Division of Neurosurgery,
University of Colorado Medical Center,
Denver, CO 80262

INTRODUCTION

The recognized method of determination of γ-carboxyglutamic acid (γCGlu) has been alkaline hydrolysis of the protein of interest followed by use of an amino acid analyzer, a process which may require 0.1 mg to mg quantities of protein. This paper describes a procedure which requires only pmole quantities of amino acid, or nmole amounts of protein. The highly fluorescent sulfonamide derivatives of dansyl chloride (DNS-Cl) which can be separated by thin layer chromatography have been used for N-terminal analyses of peptides and proteins for many years (1).

MATERIALS AND METHODS

Proteins of interest were hydrolyzed in alkali (2), neutralized to pH 7.5 with HCl, and made to 100mM $NaHCO_3$: amino acids alone or in combination were likewise neutralized and made to 100mM $NaHCO_3$. Solutions were mixed with equal volumes of 750 μg/ml DNS-Cl, which for some experiments included 50 μCi/ml (methyl-^{3}H) DNS-Cl (New England Nuclear), and left 4 hours at room temperature. Frozen samples were then dried under vacuum. Dansyl amino acids were adsorbed onto Porapak Q, mesh 80-100 (Waters Associates, Inc.) in 100mM HCl (3), washed with 100mM acetic acid to remove salts and most of the dansyl hydroxide, and eluted with acetone: ethanol: H_2O (4:5:1). After evaporating to dryness, the dansyl amino acids were dissolved in 10 μl ethanol, and aliquots spotted on 15 X 15 cm polyamide sheets (BDH Chemicals Ltd.). Resolution was achieved by thin layer chromatography, in the first direction with 1.35% formic acid for 1 hour and in the second direction with n-butanol: n-heptane: glacial acetic acid (3:3:1) for 3.5 hours. Better separation of dansyl γCGlu from dansyl hydroxide could be obtained by repeating development in the second direction. The fluorescent dansyl amino acid spots were located under UV-light.

To measure the extent of reaction of amino acids with (methyl-^{3}H) DNS-Cl, spots were scraped from the plates into vials, mixed with 0.5 ml ethanol: acetone: 0.68% formic acid (5:4:1) and 10 ml Aquasol (New England Nuclear) and the ^{3}H measured by liquid scintillation counting.

E. coli ribosomal proteins L 7 and L12 were partially purified from whole ribosomes using ice-cold ethanol (4), and further purified using column chromatography (5). The location and purity of the proteins were checked by an adaptation of the tube electrophoresis method of Li and Subramanian (6) to slab gels, using a water cooled apparatus (Hoefer Instruments).

RESULTS AND DISCUSSION

As can be seen (Fig. 1) this method achieved good separation of dansyl γCGlu from the other amino acid derivatives.

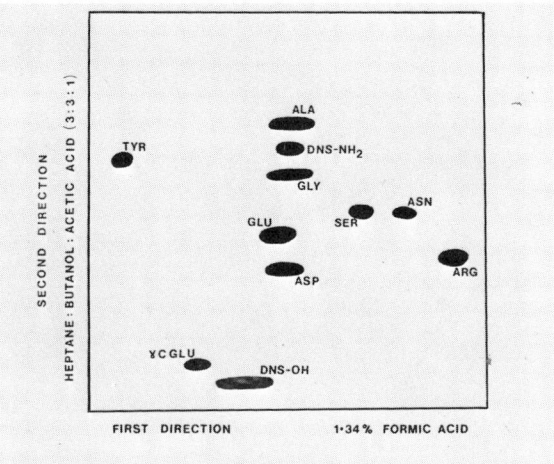

FIGURE 1 Two dimensional thin layer chromatogram. Spots represent the major dansyl amino acids, dansyl γCGlu, and the reaction products, dansyl hydroxide and dansyl amine.

This holds true for all the additional amino acid derivatives not illustrated, as we have always seen dansyl γCGlu as a separate entity, even when we have overloaded a plate with dansyl derivatives from hydrolyzed proteins.

TABLE 1 Detection of γCGlu	Dansyl Derivative	
Source	γCGlu	Glu
Total Ribosomal Proteins		
a) Mid Log Phase	Yes	Yes
b) Stationary Phase	Yes	Yes
Acid Hydrolyzed Ribosomal Proteins	No	Yes
Protein Eluted from Polyacrylamide Gel Bands	No	Yes
Log Phase L7/L12 Protein	Yes	Yes
Stationary Phase L7/L12 Protein	Yes	Yes
γCGlu Eluate from Amino Acid Analyzer	Yes	No
Commercial γCGlu	Yes	Trace
Acid-treated γCGlu	No	Yes

That this fluorescent spot does indeed correspond to dansyl γCGlu is proven by results summarized in Table 1. Clear fluorescence at this location when starting with proteins hydrolyzed in alkali or commercially synthesized γCGlu (Calbiochem) is completely absent if the material has been heated in acid, a treatment known to decarboxylate γCGlu to Glu (7,8). This conversion was demonstrated by our method.

This technique is suitable for use as a screen for the presence of γCGlu in a wide variety of purified proteins. Four thin layer chromatography plates can be run using the dansyl derivatives from only 5-10 nmoles protein. We demonstrated this using the purified E. coli B ribosomal proteins L7/L12. Thus only pmole levels of each amino acid are necessary for detection. Further advantages for screening purposes are that this method is fast and equipment is inexpensive and readily available. Also, developed plates can be filed as permanent visible records. The disadvantage of the technique is that so far we have been unable to use it quantitatively. It was hoped that incorporation of (methyl-^{3}H) DNS-Cl would achieve this goal but while equivalent ratios of isotope could be recovered reproducibly from the majority of dansyl amino acids, this was not so with γCGlu. This is probably due to steric hindrance, or ionic properties of the carboxylated molecule. Further work is in progress to resolve this problem using protein decarboxylation, and the formation of derivatives other than dansyl amino acids.

ACKNOWLEDGEMENTS

This work was supported by NIH Grant #2-5-35440 and V.A. Project #4960-02.

REFERENCES

1. Wang, K. R., and Wang, K-U. (1967) Biochem. Biophys. Acta, 133, 369-370.
2. Van Buskirk, J. J., Low, M., and Kirsch, W. M. (1979) This Volume.
3. Macnicol, P. K. (1978) Anal. Biochem., 85, 71-78.
4. Hamel, E., Koka, M., and Nakamoto, T. (1972) J. Biol. Chem., 247, 805-814.
5. Möller, W., Castleman, H. and Terhorst, C. P. (1970) F.E.B.S. Letters, 8,192-196.
6. Li, K., and Subramanian, A. R. (1975) Anal. Biochem., 64, 121-129.
7. Price, P. A., Otsuka, A. S., Poser, J. W., Kristanopis, J. and Raman, N. (1976) Proc. Nat. Acad. Sci. USA, 73, 1447-1451.
8. Hauschka, P. V., Lian, J. B., and Gallop, P. N. (1975) Proc. Nat. Acad. Sci. USA, 72, 3925-3929.

A NEW METHOD FOR THE DETECTION OF γ-CARBOXYGLUTAMIC ACID AT THE NANOMOLE LEVEL

C. M. GUNDBERG, J. B. LIAN and P. M. GALLOP

Harvard Schools of Medicine and Dental Medicine,
Children's Hospital Medical Center,
Boston, MA 02115

INTRODUCTION

The measurement of urinary γ-CG excretion can supply useful clinical information on various metabolic states related to acute or chronic conditions in which the synthesis or breakdown of vitamin K-dependent proteins is effected. (See R. Levy et al., this volume) Since whole urine contains many interfering components, direct automated amino acid analysis of free γ-CG in urine while possible, is often not convenient. A two-step procedure employing a preliminary anion exchange column separation followed by a high resolution cation exchange column was developed in our laboratory which also employed isotope dilution to facilitate γ-CG quantitation in urine (1). In order to facilitate more rapid γ-CG analysis, we wish to communicate our newest isotope dilution procedure, which employs a simple, single small anion exchange column coupled with a selective buffered magnesium chloride elution of γ-CG. The eluted γ-CG is measured by fluorescence upon reaction with the o-pthalaldehyde (2).

MATERIALS AND METHODS

Samples, Chemicals and Reagents

Twenty-four hour urines were collected from individuals of both sexes ranging in age from 12 to 65, consisting of normals, patients on anticoagulation drugs, and those with a variety of clinical disorders in order to obtain a wide range of urinary γ-CG excretion. Urines were stored frozen at -20°C. All results were normalized to creatinine excretion (3). An Aminco-Bowman 768F spectrophofluorometer equipped with a Schoeffel M460 photometer was used for the fluorescent detection of γ-CG and other amino acids.

Hepes (n-2-hydroxyethyl piperazine-N'-2-ethane sulfonic acid) was obtained from Research Organics, Inc. o-phthalaldehyde was purchased from Eastman Kodak Co. Dowex-1 was purchased from BioRad Laboratories as AG 1 X8 minus 400 mesh, chloride form. [^{14}C]γ-CG labelled in the γ-carboxyl groups was prepared by New England Nuclear (Boston, MA) using N-benzoyl β-chloroalanine ethyl ester and ^{14}C-carboxyl labelled malonate diethylester for the synthesis of [^{14}C]N-benzoyl γ-CG α,γ,γ triethylester. A stock solution of [^{14}C]γ-CG was prepared for hydrolysis in 2N KOH for 24 hours at 100°C. The hydrolysate was neutralized as previously described. After quantitation of the γ-CG by amino acid analysis (4) and measurement of the radioactivity, the stock solution was stored frozen at neutral pH. The specific activity of a typical stock solution was 1.6 mCi/mM.

Chromatography of Urine

Before analysis an aliquot of urine was adjusted to pH 11.5 with 10N NaOH and rapidly centrifuged to remove any precipitate. 1.1 ml of the clarified urine was combined with 2 nanoCi [^{14}C]γ-CG. A 0.1 ml aliquot was counted for ^{14}C radioactivity. The remainder was applied to a 6 x 0.7 cm Dowex-1 X8 (<400) previously equilibrated with a 0.02M Hepes buffer at pH 10.0 (Buffer A). Forty ml of 0.02M Hepes buffer, pH5.0 (Buffer B), was passed through the column at a flow rate of 25 ml/hr and discarded. Twenty-five ml of 0.020M Hepes, 0.02M $MgCl_2$, pH 4.5 (Buffer C) was then passed through the column and also discarded. An additional 25 ml of Buffer C was subsequently collected in five 5 ml fractions. A 0.5 ml aliquot of these fractions was removed for determination of radioactivity and the percent of γ-CG recovery in each fraction calculated.

The quantitation of γ-CG in the latter column fractions which is free of other amino acids (see below) was performed by either one or both of two methods:

1. A 25 μl aliquot of each γ-CG-containing fraction (as determined by the presence of radioactive γ-CG) was adjusted to pH2.2 with 6N HCl and subjected to automated amino acid analysis employing a Beckman-Spinco 121-M automated amino acid analyzer (4).

2. Alternatively, a 0.5 ml aliquot of all final column fractions was combined with 0.5 ml 6.0 mM o-phthalaldehyde in 0.40M boric acid, pH 9.7 (2). Fluorescence was determined by excitation at 340 nm and emission at 455 nm. Concentration was determined by comparison to a standard curve of γ-CG from 0.1 to 10 nM/ml which ranged from 2.3 to 244 nAmperes intensity. Fluorescence was linear up to 100 nM γ-CG/ml. Relative fluorescence of γ-CG and glutamic acid were found to be equal. Urinary γ-CG excretion was calculated from γ-CG concentration in the column fraction, correcting for γ-CG recovery. (The contribution of [^{14}C]γ-CG to fluorescence was usually < 2%.)

Direct Automated Amino Acid Analysis of Urine

To 1 ml of whole urine was added 50 μl of 10% sulfosalicylic acid to precipitate protein. The urine was centrifuged and the supernatant diluted 1:2 or 1:4 with 0.2M sodium citrate buffer, pH 2.2. The pH was checked on indicator paper (pH 1.4-2.8) and further adjusted to pH 2.2 if necessary. The sample was subjected to automated amino acid analysis in the programmed system described by Hauschka (4).

RESULTS

This study was undertaken to develop a rapid, simple and sensitive quantitative procedure for the determination of free γ-CG in urine. An aliquot of urine is subjected to chromatography on Dowex-1 and eluted with the buffer system described. Buffer B immediately removes neutral and basic amino acids. When the pH is lowered and magnesium chloride is added to the elution buffer, the acidic components of the urine are eluted rapidly. Marker [^{14}C]γ-CG is, however, eluted later usually after 40 ml of this buffer (Buffer C) has been passed through the column. (see Figure 1) A peak of material reacting with the fluorophore occurs coincident with the elution of the marker [^{14}C]γ-CG. Figure 2 illustrates the amino acid analysis on the Beckman 121-M of this radioactive fraction, clearly indicating γ-CG as the only ninhydrin positive component.

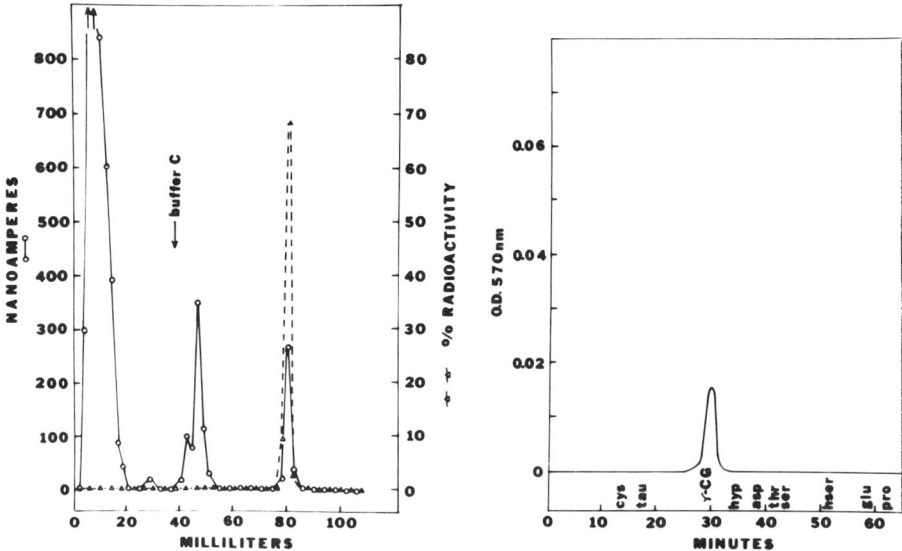

FIGURE 1 Dowex anion exchange chromatography. A typical elution profile of urine shows γ-CG eluting after 40 ml of 0.020M Hepes, 0.020M $MgCl_2$, pH 4.5. Peak $[^{14}C]$γ-CG recovery was 89.7%.

FIGURE 2 Beckman Spinco 121-M amino acid analyzer run of peak γ-CG region of a urine aliquot after Dowex-1 anion exchange chromatography and selective $MgCl_2$ elution.

26 urines of normal and clinical cases to cover a wide range of γ-CG excretion were analyzed for γ-CG content by (a) the described anion exchange chromatographic system coupled with fluorescent quantitation, (b) the described anion exchange chromatographic system with analysis of the γ-CG peak fraction by the ninhydrin reaction carried out on the Beckman 121-M automated amino acid analyzer, and (c) direct amino acid analysis of the diluted urines on the appropriately programmed Beckman 121-M. The correlation coefficient for the methods are $r = .95$ (method a to method b); $r = .98$ (method a to method c) and for method b to method c, $r = .94$.

DISCUSSION

Simple anion exchange chromatographic techniques, such as those described by Tabor and Tabor (5) are useful for relatively simple mixtures containing γ-CG. We have found that for complex mixtures, such as are found in urines from both normal and diseased individuals, a more selective elution of γ-CG from anion exchange columns was necessary. We have developed a buffer system employing a first elution of basic and neutral components, a second elution with early removal of acidic components, and later selective elution of γ-CG from a Dowex-1 column. The γ-CG so obtained is free of other amino acids and other ninhydrin or o-phthalaldehyde reacting components, even if one starts the analysis with mixtures as complex as clinical urine samples. Since the final column fractions containing γ-CG are free of other o-phthalaldehyde reactive components, fluorescent detection can be employed for quantitation which allows the technique to be sensitive in the nanomole range. This method can also be adapted for the determination of γ-CG in alkaline hydrolysates of proteins (6).

We have successfully assayed many urine samples by the methods described in this paper. Figure 3 shows the levels of excretion of γ-CG in healthy individuals ranging in age from 3 to 40. Children excrete relatively higher levels of γ-CG which decline and stabilize at about age 15 through maturity. The normal range of urinary γ-CG for adults (male and female) is 44 ± 11 μm γ-CG/gm Creatinine. Higher free γ-CG excretion appears to be found in cases of active osteoporosis. It also appears significantly elevated in situations where there is extensive ectopic calcifications such as found in certain cases of dermatomyositis and scleroderma. (See R. Levy et al, this volume)

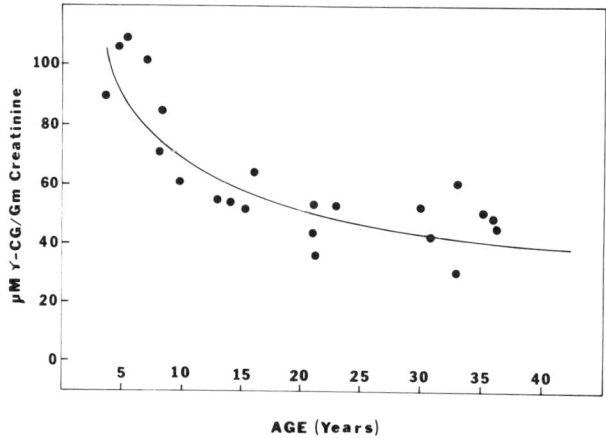

FIGURE 3 Excretion of γ-CG versus age in a normal population. Values are given as μM γ-CG/gm Creatinine.

ACKNOWLEDGEMENTS

The authors wish to thank Drs. Robert Levy and Peter Hauschka for helpful discussions, and Dr. Lauren Pachman for contributing samples of urines from normal children. Supported by NIH grants AG 00376 and HL 20764.

REFERENCES

1. Levy, R. J. and Lian, J. B. (1979) Clin. Pharmacol. Ther., 25, 562-567.
2. Benson, J. R., and Hare, P. E. (1975) Proc. Natl. Acad. Sci. USA 72, 619-622.
3. De Giorgio, J. (1974) in Clinical Chemistry Principles and Techniques (Henry, R. J., Cannon, D. C. and Winhelman, J. W., eds.), pp. 543-548, Harper and Row, Hagerstown, Maryland.
4. Hauschka, P. V. (1977) Anal. Biochem. 80, 212-223.
5. Tabor, H., and Tabor, C. W. (1977) Anal. Biochem. 78, 554-557.
6. Gundberg, C. M., Lian, J. B. and Gallop, P. M. (1979) Anal. Biochem., in press.

A NEW SYNTHESIS OF
γ-CARBOXYGLUTAMIC ACID AND ITS DERIVATIVES

ROBERT K. Y. ZEE-CHENG and ROBERT E. OLSON

Edward A Doisy Department of Biochemistry,
St. Louis University School of Medicine,
St. Louis, MO 63104

INTRODUCTION

Ever since γ-carboxyglutamic acid (GLA) (1-3) was discovered in the N-terminal region of prothrombin and other vitamin K-dependent factors, several reports (4-11) describing the synthesis of this amino acid have appeared. These methods (IA) all involved the alkylation of malonic ester with derivatives of 3-haloalanine or the corresponding unsaturated derivatives, in the presence of base, followed by removal of the protecting groups. The many steps and the low overall yield of these schemes prompted us to search for a more convenient method to prepare this amino acid and its derivatives for further studies.

In microsomal membranes, γ-carboxylation of peptide-bound glutamic acid residues (GLU) including GLU in synthetic pentapeptides (12,13) is catalyzed by a vitamin K-dependent enzyme complex. Several roles of vitamin K in promoting the carboxylation of a microsomal precursor to prothrombin have been suggested (12,14). The failure of synthetic carbonates of vitamin K hydroquinone to yield GLA from peptide substrates in microsomal systems suggests that vitamin K is not a CO_2 carrier (14). CO_2, itself, is the primary substrate for the enzymatic reaction (15) in the relatively anhydrous lipid membrane. Recent work indicates that vitamin K may act through a hydroperoxide intermediate (16) to generate base and remove a γ-proton from peptide-bound glutamate. The activated glutamic acid then makes a nucleophilic attack on CO_2 to yield GLA.

```
        HOOC—CH—COOH              HOOC—CH—COOH
            --+--                       |
             CH2                        CH2
              |                          |
           HC—NH2                    H—C—NH2
              |                          |
            COOH                       COOH

             IA                          IB
```

MATERIALS AND METHODS

To mimic the possible biological pathway, our approach (IB) to obtain a γ-carboxyglutamic acid derivative involved removing the γ-hydrogen of the protected glutamic ester II (17,

18) to γ-carbanion by means of a non-nucleophilic base (19-21), such as lithium diisopropylamide (LDA) in tetrahydrofuran (THF) at low temperature (-78°C). On treatment of the lithium salt of the ester III with benzyl chloroformate or other electrophilic agents in THF at the same temperature, γ-benzyloxycarbonyl derivative derivative of glutamic ester IV was obtained.

The bulky triphenylmethyl (trityl) group was selected to protect the amine nitrogen in order to decrease the chances for formation of lithium salt at the α-carbon and at the amine nitrogen of the glutamic ester, therefore chances of subsequent formation of carbonyl compounds at these places were greatly reduced. In addition, self-condensation of γ-C of III and γ-carbonyl of II was minimized.

On hydrogenation of the resulting N-trityl tribenzyl ester of 3-amino-1,1,3-propanetricarboxylic acid IV in the presence of palladium on charcoal catalyst, all protecting groups were removed in one single step to give the desired γ-carboxyglutamic acid I in 40-50% yield based on II used (or 50-70% in considering the recovered glutamic acid) (22). The product showed the identical physical properties (TLC on Silica gel, R_f=0.36, A; R_f=0.10,B) (23), and the results on the amino acid analyzer (19 minutes for I, 47 minutes for GLU)(24), as that of GLA prepared by the known procedure (4,10) and that of the natural GLA (1). Acid hydrolysis (24 hours, 6 N HCl, 100°C) of I yield glutamic acid (TLC on Silica gel, $R_f=0.65$, A; $R_f=0.35$, B) (23).

RESULTS AND DISCUSSION

This convenient technique is useful for the preparations of not only the γ-carboxyglutamic acid I itself in good yield, but also of the mixed protected ester and amino functions for synthesis of GLA-containing peptides. For example, trifluoroacetic acid treatment (r.t., 2 hours) for the N-trityltribenzyl ester of GLA IV gave the tribenzyl ester of the amino acid V (TLC on Silica gel, $R_f=0.90$, B) which can be used for N-substituted peptide synthesis containing this amino acid. Selective base hydrolysis (35°, 1 hour, pH=8.5, $CuSO_4$) (25) of V yielded α-free carboxylic acid of the amino acid VI (TLC on Silica gel, $R_f=0.84$, B, $C_{20}H_{21}NO_6$ m/e. 371 (M+)). Hydrogenation or base hydrolysis under more drastic conditions of V and VI both gave I. Reprotecting of the amino acid function of VI by other groups such as t-BOC-azide can also be done accordingly.

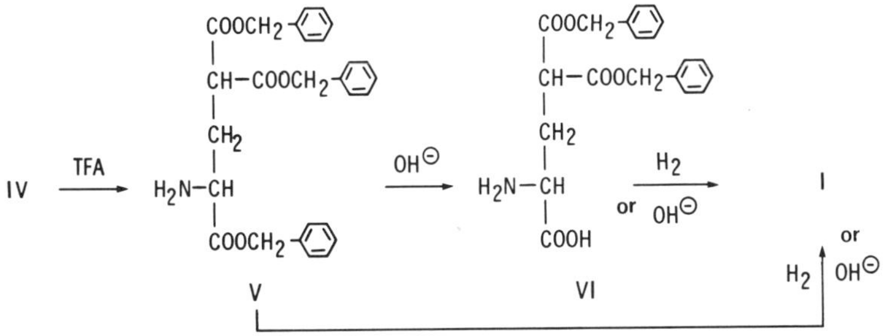

$$IV \xrightarrow{TFA} \begin{array}{c} COOCH_2-Ph \\ | \\ CH-COOCH_2-Ph \\ | \\ CH_2 \\ | \\ H_2N-CH \\ | \\ COOCH_2-Ph \end{array} \xrightarrow{OH^-} \begin{array}{c} COOCH_2-Ph \\ | \\ CH-COOCH_2-Ph \\ | \\ CH_2 \\ | \\ H_2N-CH \\ | \\ COOH \end{array} \xrightarrow[or\ OH^-]{H_2} I$$
V   VI

(V and VI both → I via H_2 or OH^-)

ACKNOWLEDGEMENT

This investigation was supported by Grant AM-09992 from the National Institutes of Health. The authors thank Dr. J. Stenflo for providing us an authentic sample of γ-carboxyglutamic acid. We also thank Mr. Thomas Hooyman and Mr. Scott Hellrung for expert technical assistance, and Mr. Richard Pinkston for the amino acid determinations.

REFERENCES

1. Stenflo, J., Fernlund, P., Egan, W., and Roepstorff, P. (1974) Proc. Natl. Acad. Sci. USA 71, 2730-2733.

2. Magnusson, S., Sottrup-Jensen, L., Peterson, T.E., Morris, H.R., and Dell, A. (1974) FEBS Lett. 44, 189-193.
3. Nelsestuen, G.L., Zytokovicz, T.H., and Howard, J.B. (1974) J. Biol. Chem. 249, 6347-6350.
4. Morris, H.R., Thompson, M.R., and Dell, A. (1975) Biochem. Biophys. Res. Commun. 62, 856-861.
5. Fernlund, P., Stenflo, J., Roestorff, P., and Thomsen, J. (1975) J. Biol. Chem. 250, 6125-6133.
6. Marki, W., and Schwyzer, R. (1975) Helv. Chim. Acta 58, 1471-1477.
7. Bogg, N.T., 3rd, Gawley, R.E., Koehler, K.A., and Hiskey, R.G. (1975) J. Org. Chem. 40, 2850-2851.
8. Bajusz, S., and Juhasz, A. (1976) Acta Chim. Sci. Hung. (1976) 88, 161.
9. Marki, W., Oppliger, M., and Schwyzer, R. (1976) Helv. Chim. Acta 59, 901-902.
10. Weinstein, B., Watrin, K.G., Loie, H.J., and Martin, J.C. J. Org. Chem. (1976) 41, 3634-3635.
11. Marki, W., Oppliger, M., Thanei, P., and Schwyzer, R. (1977) Helv. Chim. Acta 60, 798-806.
12. Suttie, J.W., Hageman, J.M., Lehrman, S.R., and Rich, D.H. (1976) J. Biol. Chem. 251, 5827-5830.
13. Houser, R.M., Carey, D.J., Dus, K.M., Marshall, G.R., and Olson, R.E. (1977) FEBS Lett. 75, 225-230.
14. Olson, R.E., and Suttie, J.W. (1977) Vit. and Horm. 35, 59-108.
15. Jones, J.P., Gardner, E.J., Cooper, T.G., and Olson, R.E. J. Biol. Chem. 252, 7738-7742.
16. Larson, A.E., and Suttie, J.W. (1978) Proc. Natl. Acad. Sci. USA 75, 5413-5416.
17. Amiard, G., Heymès, R., and Vellz, L. (1955) Bull. Soc. Chim. 97-101.
18. Zervas, L., Winitz, M., and Greenstein, J.P. (1957) J. Org. Chem. 22, 1515-1521.
19. Reiffers, S., Wynberg, H., and Strating, J. (1971) Tetrahedron Lett. 3001-3004.
20. Rathke, M.W., and Deitch, J. (1971) Tetrahedron Lett. 2953-2956.
21. Brocksom, T.J., Petragnani, N., and Rodrigues, R. (1974) J. Org. Chem. 39, 2114-2116.
22. The use of excess reagents (about 3-fold of the theoretical as the protected glutamate) was required for better results.
23. Solvent system for A: 70% EtOH; B: EtAc, 40; HOAc, 8; H_2O, 16; EtOH, 16. Developed with ninhydrin spray.
24. Amino acid analyzer, Beckman 120C, Column 0.9cm x 58cm, Beckman Resin AA 15, 54°C, pH 3.5, Buffer 70ml/hr, ninhydrin 35ml/hr.
25. Prestidge, R.L., Harding, D.R.K., Battersby, J.E., and Hancock, W.S. (1975) J. Org. Chem. 40, 3287-3288.

IDENTIFICATION OF γ-CARBOXYGLUTAMIC ACID DURING AUTOMATED SEQUENATOR DEGRADATION OF PROTEINS

PER FERNLUND and JOHAN STENFLO

Department of Clinical Chemistry,
University of Lund, General Hospital,
S-214 01 Malmö, Sweden

INTRODUCTION

γ-Carboxyglutamic acid (1-3) is formed by vitamin K-dependent postribosomal carboxylation of certain glutamic acid residues in vitamin K-dependent coagulation factors. It has also been found in two other vitamin K-dependent plasma proteins called protein C (4,5) and protein S (6,7); in a low molecular weight protein, osteocalcin, purified from bone (8,9) and in a calcium-binding protein from chick chorioallantoic membrane (10).
   In sequence work γ-carboxyglutamic acid has been identified by NMR-spectrometry (11), mass spectrometry of permethylated peptides (1-4, 11-14) and by a diagonal electrophoretic technique (12). Automated sequenator degradation in conjunction with mass spectrometric identification of the methylesterified phenylthiohydantoin (PTH) derivatives has also been used (4,10). Recently we used high pressure liquid chromatography to identify the thiohydantoin derivative of γ-carboxyglutamic acid from an automated degradation of the light chain of protein C (5). Each of the above methods has inherent drawbacks. The direct mass spectrometric identification of γ-carboxyglutamic acid in permethylated peptides is cumbersome and requires purification of a large number of small peptides. The sequenator approach has suffered from low recoveries of PTH γ-carboxyglutamic acid due to poor extraction of the thiazolinone derivative of γ-carboxyglutamic acid from the sequenator cup. This communication describes an alteration of the thiazolinone extraction procedure employed in the standard Beckman sequenator program for proteins (122974) leading to effective extraction of the thiazolinone derivative of γ-carboxyglutamic acid. The thiohydantoin residues were identified by high pressure liquid chromatography.

MATERIALS AND METHODS

Prothrombin fragment 1 (prothrombin residues 1-156) was prepared from bovine prothrombin and purified by standard methods (15). It was reduced and carboxymethylated as described previously (16). Ethanol (spectrographic grade) was obtained from AB Vin & Spritcentralen and it was used without further purification. Butanol (butan-1-ol, Merck, analytical grade) was freed from aldehydes by stirring with $NaBH_4$, dried over CaO and subjected to fractional destillation under N_2 as described for n-propanol by Edman (17). DL-γ-carboxyglutamic acid was synthesized as described previously (11). Its PTH derivative was synthesized according to the procedure for PTH-serine as described by Edman (17).
   Automated sequenator degradations were performed essentially according to Edman and Begg (18) in a Beckman model 890C sequencer. With

161

the exception for ethanol and n-butanol (see above), Beckman chemicals were used throughout. The Beckman protein Quadrol program 122974 was used either unmodified (with chlorobutane in reservoir S4) or modified with ethyl acetate, ethanol or butanol in reservoir S4 and with the S4 delivery times (steps 43 and 45) appropriately adjusted in order to compensate for the viscosity of the solvent used. The chlorobutane, ethyl acetate, ethanol or butanol extracts were dried under N_2 and the thiazolinones were converted to PTH-derivatives and extracted with the standard procedure (18). The residues were identified with high pressure liquid chromatography (Fig. 1) using a μBondapak C_{18} column and a system with stepwise elution using methanol in phosphate buffers (Waters associates). All the amino acid PTH derivatives (including γ-carboxyglutamic acid) were separated from each other in a single run except methionine and isoleucine which coeluted with valine and phenylalanine respectively (Fig. 1).

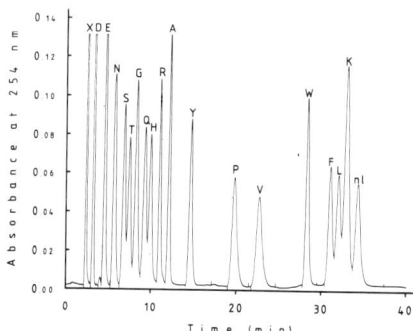

FIGURE 1. High pressure liquid chromatography of standard phenylthiohydantoin (PTH) amino acids. The chromatography was performed at room temperature on a μBondapak C_{18} column (0.39 cm x 30 cm) with stepwise elution (1.6 ml/min) using a system (Waters Associates) with three different solvent mixtures containing a buffer (3 mmol/l sodium phosphate, 3 mmol/l 2|N-morpholino|ethane sulfonic acid, pH 6.6) according to the following schedule: 0-3 min, methanol-buffer (25:75 v/v); 3-20 min, propan-1-ol-methanol-buffer (3:30:67, v/v); 20-33 min, propan-1-ol-methanol-buffer (4:40:56, v/v). Before a new run the column was equilibrated with the first mixture for 12 min. The standard mixture contained approximately 20 nmol of the phenylthiohydantoin derivative of each of the following amino acids: X, γ-carboxyglutamic acid; D, aspartic acid; E, glutamic acid; N, asparagine; S, serine; T, threonine, G, glycine; Q, glutamine, H, histidine; R, arginine; A, alanine, Y, tyrosine; P, proline, V, valine; W, tryptophan; F, phenylalanine; L, leucine; K, lysine; nl, norleucine. Carboxymethylcysteine is eluted between glutamic acid and asparagine (not shown in Figure).

RESULTS AND DISCUSSION

The results of automatic degradation of fragment 1 from bovine prothrombin with the standard Beckman protein Quadrol program were compared with the results obtained using n-butanol instead of chlorobutane in the extraction of the thiazolinone derivatives. The repetitive yields obtained with the standard and modified programs were between 92 and 95 per cent. All of the residues except serine 24 and 34 could be identified up to position 34 with the new program and the overlaps were approximately the same as with the standard (chlorobutane) program. The recovery of PTH γ-

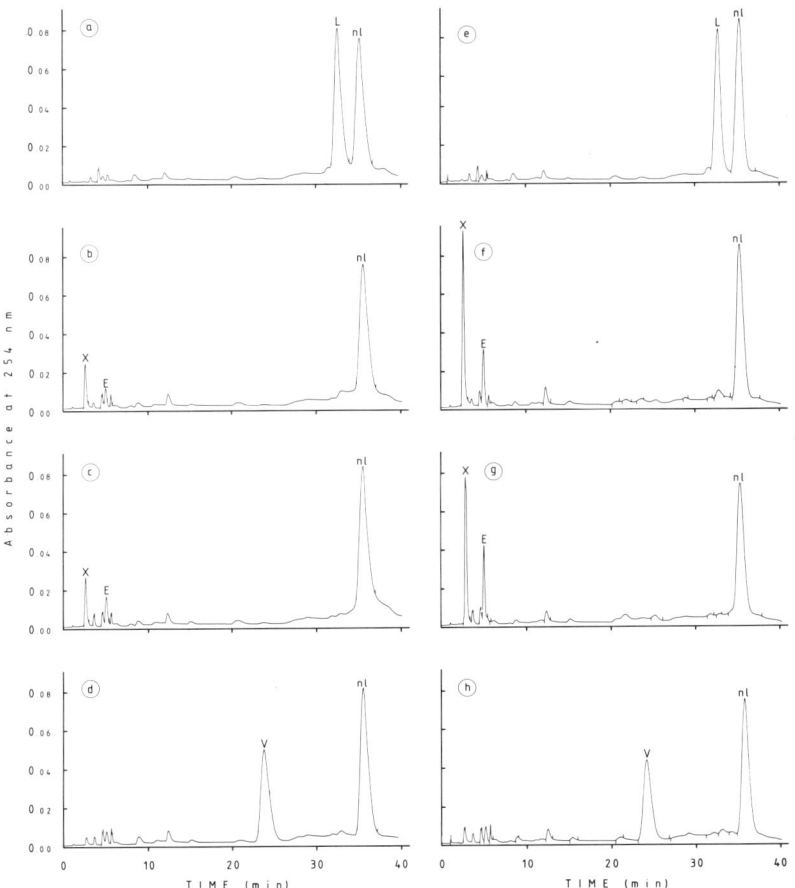

FIGURE 2. High pressure liquid chromatograms of PTH derivatives obtained during sequenator degradation of bovine prothrombin fragment 1 (150 nmol), cycles 6 to 9. a to d, Beckman protein Quadrol program (122974); e to h, modified program with n-butanol extraction of thiazolinone derivatives. Abbreviations: see legend to Figure 1.

carboxyglutamic acid was very low with the standard program (Fig. 2b and c) as previously noted during sequencing of the light chain of protein C (5). With the modified program using butanol extraction, the recovery of PTH γ-carboxyglutamic acid was much better (Fig. 2f and g) and was comparable to that obtained for several of the other amino acids such as Asn, Tyr and Gln. For the thiazolinone to PTH conversion the routine procedure (1 M HCl, 80°C for 10 min) was used for all residues including γ-carboxyglutamic acid. Although γ-carboxyglutamic acid is known to carboxylate to glutamic acid on heating, experiments showed that less than 5 per cent of synthetic PTH-γ-carboxyglutamic acid decarboxylated under these conditions.

All of the ten γ-carboxyglutamic acid residues in prothrombin fragment 1 were identified, the last one in position 33 (Fig. 3). At the positions where γ-carboxyglutamic acid was identified some glutamic acid was also found and the proportion of glutamic acid to γ-carboxyglutamic acid increased during the degradation (Fig. 2f and g and Fig. 3b). This was probably due to partial decarboxylation at the elevated temperature in the sequenator cup.

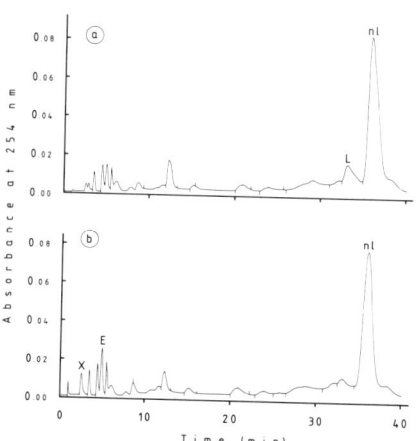

FIGURE 3. Cycles 32 (a) and 33 (b) with modified program (same run as in Figure 2). Abbreviations: see legend to Figure 1.

In preliminary experiments attempts were made to extract the thiazolinone derivatives with ethyl acetate or ethanol instead of chlorobutane. Although ethyl acetate effectively extracted the thiazolinone derivatives of γ-carboxyglutamic acid and the other amino acids as well, its use caused large overlaps between cycles. This was probably due to a partial and reversible blocking of amino groups during the postcleavage extraction with ethyl acetate. With ethanol the material being sequenced was rapidly washed out of the sequenator cup.

γ-Carboxyglutamic acid residues have at present been found only in the aminoterminal part of proteins. The residue furthest away from the amino terminus in any of the proteins studied is in position 39 in bovine factor X (14). In osteocalcin γ-carboxyglutamic acid has been found in positions 17, 21 and 24 (19). This suggests that most or all of the γ-carboxyglutamic acid residues in proteins may be identified by a sequenator run on the intact protein or on a suitable aminoterminal fragment using the modified program.

ACKNOWLEDGEMENT

The expert technical assistance of Mrs Monica Jönsson and Mr Roland Nilsson is gratefully acknowledged. This investigation was supported by grants from the Swedish Medical Research Council (projects no. B79-13X-4487-5C and B79-13X-00581-15B) and by grants from Magnus Bergvalls Stiftelse, Greta and Johan Kocks Stiftelser and Thorsten and Elsa Segerfalks Stiftelse. The sequenator was procured through a grant from the Wallenberg Foundation.

REFERENCES

1. Stenflo, J., Fernlund, P., Egan, W., and Roepstorff, P. (1974) Proc. Natl. Acad. Sci. USA 71, 2730-2733.
2. Nelsestuen, G.L., Zytkovicz, T.H., and Howard, J.B. (1974) J. Biol. Chem. 249, 6347-6350.
3. Magnusson, S., Sottrup-Jensen, L., Petersen, T.T., Morris, H.R., and Dell, A. (1974) FEBS Lett. 44, 189-193.
4. Bucher, D., Nebelin, E., Thomsen, J., and Stenflo, J. (1976) FEBS Lett. 68, 293-296.
5. Fernlund, P., Stenflo, J., and Tufvesson, A. (1978) Proc. Natl. Acad. Sci. USA 75, 5889-5892.
6. DiScipio, R.G., and Davie, E.W. (1979) Biochemistry. In press.
7. Stenflo, J., and Jönsson, M. To be published.
8. Hauschka, P.V., Lian, J.B., and Gallop, P.M. (1975) Proc. Natl. Acad. Sci. USA 72, 3925-3929.
9. Price, P.A., Otsuka, A.S., Poser, J.W., Krislaponis, J., and Raman, N. (1976) Proc. Natl. Acad. Sci. USA 73, 1447-1451.
10. Tuan, R.S., Scott, W.A., and Cohn, Z.A. (1978) J. Biol. Chem. 253, 1011-1016.
11. Fernlund, P., Stenflo, J., Roepstorff, P., and Thomsen, J. (1975) J. Biol. Chem. 250, 6125-6133.
12. Magnusson, S., Petersen, T.E., Sottrup-Jensen, L., and Claeys, H. (1975) in Proteases and Biological Control (E. Reich, D. Rifkin and E. Skaw, eds.), pp 123-149, Cold Spring Harbor Laboratory, Cold Spring Harbor.
13. Morris, H.R., Dell, A., Petersen, T.E., Sottrup-Jensen, L., and Magnusson, S. (1976) Biochem. J. 153, 663-679.
14. Thögersen, H.C., Petersen, T.E., Sottrup-Jensen, L., Magnusson, S., and Morris, H.R. (1978) Biochem. J. 175, 613-617.
15. Mann, K.G. (1976) Methods in Enzymol. 45, 123-156.
16. Stenflo, J. (1974) J. Biol. Chem. 249, 5527-5535.
17. Edman, P., and Henschen, A. (1975) in Protein Sequence Determination (S.B. Needelman, ed.), pp 232-279, Springer Verlag.
18. Edman, P., and Begg, G. (1967) Eur. J. Biochem. 1, 80-91.
19. Price, P.A., Poser, J.W., and Raman, N. (1976) Proc. Natl. Acad. Sci. USA 73, 3374-3375.

β-CARBOXYGLUTAMIC ACID:
AN INTERNAL STANDARD FOR THE QUANTITATION
OF FREE γ-CARBOXYGLUTAMIC ACID IN URINE

PER FERNLUND

Department of Clinical Chemistry,
University of Lund, General Hospital,
S-214 01 Malmö, Sweden

INTRODUCTION

Relatively little is known about what happens with γ-carboxyglutamic acid when proteins containing it are degraded in vivo. It has been shown that a significant amount of γ-carboxyglutamic acid appears in urine (1,2) mainly as the free amino acid (2), and experiments in the rat have shown that γ-carboxyglutamic acid, either in the free or peptide-bound form, is not metabolically degraded but is quantitatively excreted in the urine (3). The urinary excretion of γ-carboxyglutamic acid should therefore reflect the catabolism of γ-carboxyglutamic acid containing proteins and measurements of this amino acid in urine under different experimental conditions and in various disease states might contribute to our understanding of the mechanisms for the catabolism of γ-carboxyglutamic acid containing proteins.

γ-Carboxyglutamic acid is normally present in urine in a rather low concentration (10-50 μmol/l) (1,2) together with a large number of other ninhydrin positive compounds. These two facts make the quantitation of γ-carboxyglutamic acid in urine difficult. A previously described procedure (1) for the measurement of urinary γ-carboxyglutamic acid included a concentration step on an anion exchange resin and separation on the automatic amino acid analyzer at low pH because of these difficulties. The concentration step caused a small but significant error in the quantitation due to a variable yield in that step. An internal standard, added to the urine before the concentration step, would have eliminated that error, but a suitable standard compound was not available at that time.

Several compounds have now been tested and one of the two diastereomers of β-carboxyglutamic acid (1-amino propane-1,2,3-tricarboxylic acid or α-amino tricarballylic acid), a structural isomer of γ-carboxyglutamic acid, appears suitable. This report describes a procedure which uses this compound as an internal standard for the measurement of γ-carboxyglutamic acid in human urine. With this procedure reference values for the daily excretion of γ-carboxyglutamic acid in normal human adults have been determined and the γ-carboxyglutamic acid excretion during anticoagulant treatment has been studied as an example of the application of the procedure.

MATERIALS AND METHODS

D,L-γ-carboxyglutamic acid was synthesized as described previously (4). β-Carboxyglutamic acid was synthesized principally according to Greenstein and Winitz (5). The details of the synthesis and the separation of the two diastereomers will be described elsewhere. The diastereomer that was used as internal standard was the second of the two eluted on the automatic amino acid analyzer under the conditions used for the assay of γ-carboxyglutamic acid. Provisionally, that form is called β-carboxyglutamic acid B.

Urine was collected without any additions, frozen within 16 hours and kept at -20°C until analysis. The reference population consisted of subjectively healthy laboratory personnel with pregnant women excluded.

γ-Carboxyglutamic acid was assayed with the procedure described previously (1) but with a few modifications and with the use of β-carboxyglutamic acid B as an internal standard. Usually one μmol of the internal standard was added to 25 ml of the urine sample prior to the concentration step. The automatic amino acid analysis was performed at 55°C instead of 36°C and the regeneration and equilibration times were changed to 30 and 90 min, respectively.

Urine creatinine concentration was measured by the Jaffe reaction in a Technicon Autoanalyzer. Plasma clotting activity was determined with Simplastin A reagents (General Diagnostics Division, Warner Lambert) and expressed as per cent of a reference plasma. With this method the normal range was 70 to 130 per cent and 15 to 30 per cent was regarded as the optimal range for anticoagulant therapy.

RESULTS AND DISCUSSION

Assay procedure

The urine fraction obtained by the concentration step on the anion exchange resin contains a large number of ninhydrin positive components which are fairly well resolved on the automatic amino acid analyser when the lithium citrate buffer with pH 2.00 is used (Fig. 1, upper). With this system γ-carboxyglutamic acid has a retention time of 76 min (Fig. 1). β-Carboxyglutamic acid B, which has been adopted as an internal standard, has a retention time of 92 min and separates well from other ninhydrin positive components in the concentrate (Fig. 1, lower).

At least two monoamino tricarboxylic acids, γ-carboxyglutamic acid (1,2) and dicarboxyethylcysteine (6,1) are present in human urine, but there has been no evidence for the presence of β-carboxyglutamic acid B. More than twenty urines have been analysed without addition of β-carboxyglutamic acid B and in no case has there appeared any significant peak in the chromatogram in the position for β-carboxyglutamic acid B.

β-Carboxyglutamic acid B is a structural isomer of γ-carboxyglutamic acid and is therefore expected to behave similari-

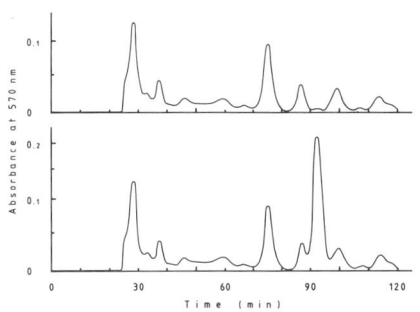

FIGURE 1. Typical chromatograms obtained with normal urine, either without (upper) or with (lower) added (40 μmol/l) β-carboxyglutamic acid B.

ly to the latter in the anion exchange concentration step. That β-carboxyglutamic acid B follows γ-carboxyglutamic acid closely was shown in an experiment with a synthetic mixture made from crystalline γ-carboxyglutamic acid and β-carboxyglutamic acid B. Twentyfive ml of a water solution, which was 40 μmol/l with respect to both γ-carboxyglutamic acid and β-carboxyglutamic acid B, was subjected to the anion exchange concentration step and then run on the automatic analyzer as in the routine assay of γ-carboxyglutamic acid in urine. The recovery of the two amino acids was about 90 per cent and the proportion between the two after the concentration step differed less than 2 per cent from that in the synthetic mixture. The difference is within the experimental error of the automatic analyzer and shows that no significant separation of β-carboxyglutamic acid B from γ-carboxyglutamic acid occurs in the concentration step.

These results show that β-carboxyglutamic acid B fulfills the requirements for an internal standard and can be used for the measurement of γ-carboxyglutamic acid in urine. The precision of the method is 4.7 per cent (coefficient of variation, n=5) according to repeated assay of one urine sample.

Reference values

The daily excretion of γ-carboxyglutamic acid in urine in healthy adults shows a correlation with body weight (Fig. 2) and also with body surface area (not shown). Therefore the normal range becomes narrower and the difference between sexes is eliminated when the γ-carboxyglutamic acid excretion is given in relation to body weight (Table I).

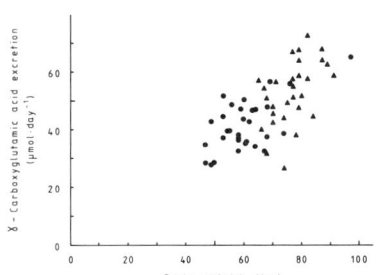

FIGURE 2. Urinary excretion of free γ-carboxyglutamic acid in relation to body weight in healthy human adults. ●, females; ▲, males.

The reference values obtained with the present procedure are somewhat higher than those reported previously using no internal standard and assuming a constant yield of 89 % in the concentration step (1). With an internal standard it was possible to estimate the yield in the concentration step for each individual sample. It was then found that with several urine samples this yield was lower (50-70 %) than had been assumed, indicating a probable underestimation of γ-carboxyglutamic acid excretion in the earlier publication (1).

Effect of anticoagulant therapy on urinary γ-carboxyglutamic acid excretion

The method has been used to quantitate the γ-carboxyglutamic acid excretion in patients on anticoagulant therapy. Patients visiting the laboratory for coagulation assay were randomly selected and asked to leave a urine sample. Most of them were in various stages of dicoumarol or warfarin therapy. As 24 hours urine samples were not obtained from these patients their urinary γ-carboxyglutamic acid excretion was expressed in relation to their urinary creatinine excretion. As seen in Fig. 3, there was a tendency to a positive correlation between the plasma clotting activity

TABLE I

Reference values for urinary excretion of γ-carboxyglutamic acid in healthy human adults (Mean ± 2 S.D.).

γ-Carboxyglutamic acid excretion	Females	Males
Total excretion (μmol/24 hours)	22-61	30-71
Related to body weight (μmol/kg·24 hours)	0.44-0.95	0.44-0.93
Related to creatinine excretion (mmol/mol)	2.4 -5.2	2.0 -4.4
Number of subjects	33	32

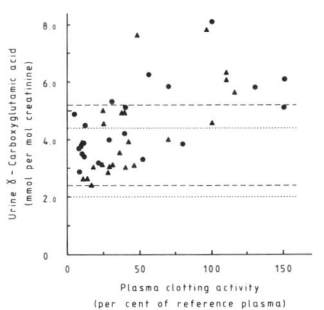

FIGURE 3. Urinary excretion of free γ-carboxyglutamic acid in randomly selected patients on anticoagulant therapy. The normal ranges for females (---) and males (.....) are indicated. ●, females; ▲, males.

and the γ-carboxyglutamic acid excretion in urine. Unexpectedly, however, the value for the γ-carboxyglutamic acid excretion did not decrease below the lower reference limit in the patients with low clotting activity and the tendency was due to the fact that many of the patients with higher plasma clotting activities had an abnormally high excretion of γ-carboxyglutamic acid (Fig. 3). Unfortunately, the individual patients were not examined clinically and the reason for the increased γ-carboxyglutamic acid excrection is not known.

That a short anticoagulant treatment is insufficient to lower the γ-carboxyglutamic acid excretion in urine more than marginally is suggested by the observations obtained with a single healthy male taking dicoumarol for five days and in which the γ-carboxyglutamic acid excretion in urine was measured daily before, during and after the dicoumarol treatment (Fig. 4). Although the plasma clotting activity was lowered into what was considered to be the therapeutic range the γ-carboxyglutamic acid excretion decreased only slightly and remained above the lower normal limit (Fig. 4).

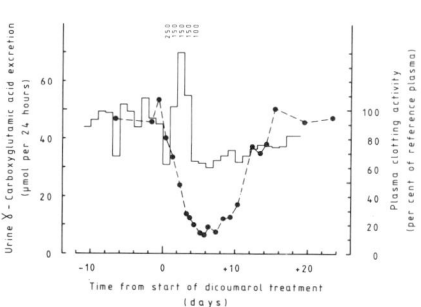

FIGURE 4. Daily urinary excretion of free γ-carboxyglutamic acid in a healthy adult male (body weight 63 kg) before, during and after a short period of dicoumarol treatment. The daily oral dose of dicoumarol given (in mg) is shown on the appropriate day at the top of the figure.———, daily excretion of γ-carboxyglutamic acid; ---●---, plasma clotting activity according to one-stage prothrombin time.

The increased excretion of γ-carboxyglutamic acid that seemed to occur during the first few days after initiation of dicoumarol treatment (Fig. 4) is an interesting observation but cannot be considered seriously until more observations are obtained. It might only be an expression for the rather large daily variation of the γ-carboxyglutamic acid excretion observed in this subject prior to treatment (day -11 to day 0, Fig. 4).

ACKNOWLEDGEMENTS

The expert technical assistance of Mrs Ingegerd Larsson is gratefully acknowledged. This investigation was supported by a grant from the Swedish Medical Research Council (project no. B79-13X-00581-15B) and by grants from Magnus Bergvalls Stiftelse, Greta and Johan Kocks Stiftelser and Thorsten and Elsa Segerfalks Stiftelse.

REFERENCES

1. Fernlund, P. (1976) Clin. Chim. Acta 72, 147-155.
2. Lian, J.B., Glimcher, M.J., and Gallop, P.M. (1977) in Calcium-Binding Proteins and Calcium Function (R.H. Wasserman, R.A. Corradino, E. Carafoli, R.H. Kretsinger, D.H. MacLennan and F.L. Siegel, eds.), pp 379-381, Elsevier North-Holland, New York.
3. Shah, D.V., Tews, J.K., Harper, A.E., and Suttie, J.W. (1978) Biochim. Biophys. Acta 539, 209-217.
4. Fernlund, P., Stenflo, J., Roepstorff, P., and Thomsen, J. (1975) J. Biol. Chem. 250, 6125-6133.
5. Greenstein, J.P., and Winitz, M. (1961) in Chemistry of the Amino Acids, pp 2445-2462, John Wiley and Sons, New York.
6. Kuwaki, T., and Mizuhara, S. (1966) Biochim. Biophys. Acta 115, 491-493.

QUALITATIVE IDENTIFICATION OF GLA BY TWO-DIMENSIONAL HIGH VOLTAGE PAPER ELECTROPHORESIS. PURIFICATION AND AMINO ACID COMPOSITION OF PROTEIN Z, A GLA-CONTAINING PLASMA PROTEIN

TORBEN E. PETERSEN, HANS C. THØGERSEN,
STAFFAN MAGNUSSON, and LARS SOTTRUP-JENSEN

Department of Molecular Biology,
University of Aarhus,
DK-8000 Århus C, Denmark

In addition to the serine protease zymogens, prothrombin, factors X, IX, and VII which have been recognized for many years to be involved in blood clotting and to depend on vitamin K for their biosynthesis (1), two other plasma proteins, protein C (2-7) and protein S (8-10) have recently been discovered and found to contain γ-carboxyglutamic acid (Gla) residues in their N-terminal sequence. Another Gla-containing plasma protein, protein Z was first described as a single-chain factor X (11) later as a separate protein with different properties and containing Gla (12). This report confirms the presence of a Gla-containing plasma protein with an amino acid composition different from those of protein C and protein S, and describe a simple method for the qualitative identification of Gla-residues in proteins, which has been used routinely in our laboratory since 1975 (13). Several Ca^{2+}-binding and other proteins have been investigated in our laboratory to determine whether or not they contained Gla. In some instances, e.g. with smooth muscle myosin from chicken gizzard, Ca^{2+}-ATPase from sarcoplasmic reticulum of rabbit skeletal muscle and with plasma albumin, the alkaline hydrolysates were found to give rise to a ninhydrin-positive peak emerging from the amino acid analyzer column in the same position as Gla. On checking the results with the paper electrophoretic method it became immediately obvious that none of these three proteins contained Gla. These findings and the fact that we have been unable to confirm recent reports (14) stating that ribosomes contain γ-carboxyglutamic acid have indicated to us that it is important to identify Gla not only on the amino acid analyzer but also by an independent method.

EXPERIMENTAL

Alkaline hydrolysis of samples to be analyzed for Gla has been performed by dissolving an amount of protein expected to contain at least 10 nanomole Gla in 200 µl 2 M KOH in a 1 ml Eppendorf polypropylene tube, which is then placed in a Pyrex test tube containing 1 ml 2 M KOH. The neck of the outer tube is then pulled out in a flame leaving a canal wide enough to allow efficient reduction of pressure before sealing the tube. The sealed tube is incubated at 110°C for 16-20 h. The hydrolysate is then treated according to (15) to precipitate K^+. The dried $KClO_4$-supernatant is dissolved in 50 µl pyridine-acetic acid buffer pH 6.5 and applied as two spots to the electrophoresis paper (Whatman 3MM). Electrophoresis for 20-25 minutes at 3 kV at pH 6.5. After the paper is dried at room temperature - 40°C, one sample strip is heated to 150°C for 6 minutes, the other is not heated. Both strips are then stitched to a sheet of Whatman 1 paper and each is subjected to electrophoresis in a formic acetic acid buffer pH 2.1 for 35 minutes at 3 kV. The papers are then dried and stained with Cd^{2+}-ninhydrin (16). On the heated strip Gla will give rise to a spot with the mobility of 1.35 rel. to that of Asp in the first dimension (pH 6.5) and the mobility of Glu (to which it has been converted by the heat decarboxylation) in the second dimension (pH 2.1). On the non-heated strip the mobility 1.35 is again observed in the first dimension; in the second dimension the mobility is the same as for synthetic Gla (slower than Asp). Using this technique no Gla was detected in the three proteins mentioned in the introduction, which had given spurious peaks resembling Gla on the amino acid analyzer. Our conditions for the amino acid analyzer runs have been as follows: A Beckman 121MB instrument, a 2.8 x 170 mm column of LA-28 resin (from Locarte Co., London, U.K.), the buffer has been the common pH 3.29 buffer adjusted with HCl to pH 2.20. The sample has been applied in buffer of pH 2.0, Gla eluting after 21.1 minutes.

On further investigation it turned out that when extreme care was taken to reduce the pressure before sealing the hydrolysis vessel the appearance of the spurious peak could largely be avoided. In practice it is sometimes difficult to be sure how carefully the pressure has been reduced before sealing. Consequently we have been using both methods in combination to avoid false positive conclusions in identifying Gla. We have recently analyzed alkaline hydrolysates of ribosomes isolated from E.coli and from ascites cells of mice with Ehrlich's sarcoma. In contrast to published reports we found Gla neither in the prokaryotic nor in the eukaryotic ribosomes. The lower limit of detection in these experiments was approximately 5 nonomole Gla in one mg og protein.
Protein Z is isolated as a side product (Fig. 1) to our preparations of prothrombin to be used for the crystallization of the A-fragment (fragment 1).For a typical batch 80 lit. bovine blood is collected at slaughter,1.25 lit. 2.85%(w/v) sodium citrate being mixed with 8.75 lit. blood from a single animal. To 45 lit. plasma,obtained with a blood separator is added 2.5 lit. 1 M $BaCl_2$. After 30 min stirring at 4˚ the precipitate is sedimented by centrifugation,washed with 6x250 ml (6 centrifuge cups) 50 mM sodium citrate pH 6.9, containing 1 mM benzamidine. Ten ml 1 M $BaCl_2$ is added before recentrifugation; the washing repeated once; the precipitate"converted"to $BaSO_4$ with 2 lit. 1 M Na_2SO_4 (17), 5 mM benzamidine, 20 min, 4˚, centrifuged. The eluate containing prothrombin is dialyzed against 12.5 mM sodium citrate, 5 mM benzamidine pH 6.9 overnight, then pumped onto a column (5x30 cm) DEAE-Sepharose CL-6B equilibrated with 25 mM sodium citrate, 5 mM benzamidine pH 6.9 and eluted with a linear gradient (2+2 lit.) to 400 mM sodium citrate, 5 mM benzamidine (flow rate 60 ml/h; 4˚). Protein Z elutes after factor X_2 (fractions 260-280 in figure 1). SDS-gel electrophoresis gives a single band (approximate molecular weight 53,000) with or without reduction. Amino acid analysis was performed on material that had been dialyzed against distilled water and then freeze-dried. The results are given in Table 1. A quantitative analysis for Gla indicated approximately 12 residues per mole. A preliminary investigation of peptides from protein Z, isolated from a tryptic and from a chymotryptic digest of reduced, carboxymethylated protein has given a total of 58 sequenced residues in peptides totalling 98 residues. No clear homology with prothrombin or factor X has yet become apparent at this early stage.

DISCUSSION

The presence of a third Gla-containing plasma protein, protein Z, not clearly involved in blood coagulation is confirmed. Its amino acid composition (Table 1) and chromatographic properties are different from those of protein C and protein S (Fig. 1).

It is strongly recommended that the high-voltage paper electrophoretic method described here should be used as an independent means of identifying Gla in proteins and cell organelles in which it has not previously been demonstrated with mass-spectrometric sequence evidence.

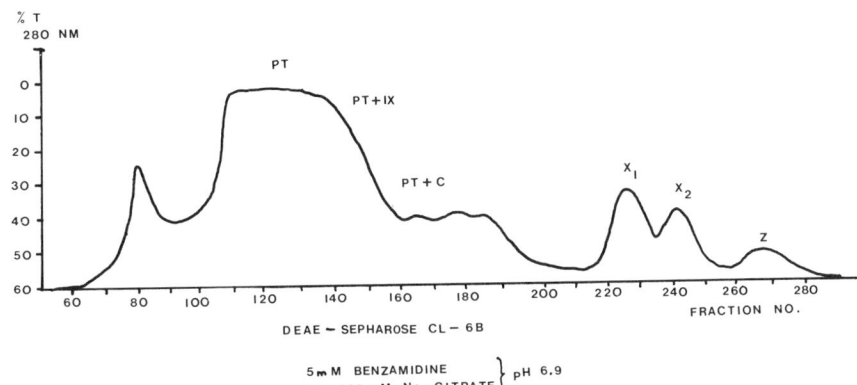

FIGURE 1. Separation of Gla-containing plasma proteins. Conditions in text. PT = prothrombin, IX = factor IX, C = protein C, X_1 = factor X_1, X_2 = factor X_2, Z = protein Z. Protein S is not indicated but is found in the unmarked early peak and the leading edge of the prothrombin peak.

TABLE 1. Amino acid composition of protein C (2), protein S (9) and protein Z.

Residues (mol/mol)	protein Z	protein S	protein C
Cys	20.8[a]	25.9	26.4
Asx	29.7	59.9	41.5
Thr	21.1[c]	25.7	18.9
Ser	21.5[c]	31.3	28.4
Glx	45.0	68.1	52.3
Pro	29.7	24.7	22.2
Gly	37.5	36.4	43.1
Ala	31.4	30.0	23.4
Val	28.5	35.3	34.0
Met	3.9	8.9	7.5
Ile	8.2	27.5	16.9
Leu	35.0	44.5	33.6
Tyr	9.4	19.0	13.1
Phe	11.8	24.1	14.4
Lys	11.0	35.0	19.9
His	10.4	8.8	7.7
Trp	6.9[b]	9.6	13.2
Arg	28.5	17.2	26.0
Total	390.0[d]	531.9[d]	442.5[d]

[a] determined after performic acid oxidation
[b] determined after hydrolysis with mercaptoethanesulfonic acid
[c] uncorrected for hydrolysis loss
[d] molecular weights for the polypeptide part (non-carbohydrate part) of 42,400 , 59,700 and 52,100 were used for the respective proteins

ACKNOWLEDGEMENT

Supported by the U.S. National Institutes of Health (grant HL-16238).

REFERENCES

1. Davie,E.W. and Fujikawa,K.(1975) Ann.Rev.Biochem.44,799-829.
2. Stenflo,J.(1976)J.Biol.Chem.251,355-363.
3. Kisiel,W.,Ericsson,L.H. and Davie,E.W.(1976)Biochemistry 15,4893-4900.
4. Esmon,C.T.,Stenflo,J.,Suttie,J.W. and Jackson,C.M.(1976)J.Biol.Chem. 251,3052-3056.
5. Seegers,W.H.,Novoa,E.Henry,R.L. and Hassouna,H.I.(1976)Thromb.Res.8, 543-552.
6. Fernlund,P.,Stenflo,J. and Tufvesson,A.(1978)Proc.Natl.Acad.Sci.USA 75,5889-5892.
7. Kisiel,W.,Canfield,W.M.,Ericsson,L.H. and Davie,E.W.(1977)Biochemistry 16,5824-5831.
8. DiScipio,R.G.,Hermodson,M.A.,Yates,S.G. and Davie,E.W.(1977)Biochemistry 16,698-706.
9. DiScipio,R.G. and Davie,E.W.(1979)Biochemistry 18,899-904.
10. Stenflo,J. and Jönsson,M.(1979)FEBS Letters 101,377-381.
11. Mattock,P. and Esnouf,M.P.(1973)Nature New Biol. 242,90-92.
12. Prowse,C.P. and Esnouf,M.P.(1977)Biochem.Soc.Trans.5,255-256.
13. Magnusson,S.,Sottrup-Jensen,L.,Petersen,T.E.,Dudek-Wojciechowska,G. and Claeys,H.(1976)Proteolysis and Physiological Regulation.Miami Winter Symposia 11 (Ribbons,D.W. and Brew,K.,eds.)pp.203-238,Academic Press,New York.
14. VanBuskirk,J.J. and Kirsch,W.M.(1978)Biochem.Biophys.Res.Commun. 80, 1033-1038.
15. Hauschka,P.V.,Lian,J.B. and Gallop,P.M.)1975)Proc.Natl.Acad.Sci.USA 72,3925-3929.
16. Heilmann,J.,Barrolier,J. and Watzke,E.(1957)Hoppe-Seyler's Z.Physiol. Chem.309,219-220.
17. Nelsestuen,G.L. and Suttie,J.W.(1973)Proc.Natl.Acad.Sci.USA 70,3366-3370.

NON-MAMMALIAN VITAMIN K METABOLISM

FUNCTIONS OF VITAMIN K_2 IN MICROORGANISMS

H. TABER

University of Rochester
School of Medicine and Dentistry,
Rochester, NY 14642

INTRODUCTION

Within the confines of this communication, I will attempt to review briefly some of the more recent work on menaquinone (vitamin K_2; MK) function in bacteria, including some data on MK involvement in the physiology of <u>Bacillus</u> <u>subtilis</u>, and finally offer some speculations on additional roles that MK might have in bacterial biochemistry. The treatment will necessarily be sketchy in many instances, and I extend my apologies to those whose work may have been passed over hastily.

In prokaryotic cells, menaquinone occurs in the cytoplasmic membrane, either with or without ubiquinone (Q), depending on the species. The general distribution of quinones among many bacterial species was studied by Bishop, Pandya and King (1), and MK was found together with Q only in certain Gram-negative bacteria, but occurred as the sole quinone in Gram-positive species. Demethylmenaquinone (DMK) is often found together with MK, and the MK/DMK ratio can be modified by the degree of aerobiosis during culture (2). MK acts as a low-potential (E'_o = -74mV) reversible redox component of electron transport chains, shuttling between dehydrogenases and iron-sulfur proteins, cytochromes or reductases. As such, MK can participate in aerobic or anaerobic electron transport for energy production, presumably via formation of an electrochemically active gradient of protons (cf. e.g. 3,4,5). The gradient so generated can be utilized for ATP synthesis, active transport of essential nutrients and ions, and cellular motility. MK appears also to play important roles in anaerobic biosynthesis of heme and of uracil; and finally, MK may participate in genetic regulatory events in bacterial cells. Each of these functions will be discussed in more detail below. Comprehensive reviews (6,7) on the oxidation-reduction interactions of MK in bacteria should be consulted for full treatment of earlier work. The discussion which follows will be limited to more recent investigations, particularly those utilizing mutants blocked in quinone biosynthesis (8,9).

ELECTRON TRANSPORT TO FUMARATE AND NITRATE MEDIATED BY MK

Following the establishment of the role of MK and DMK in aerobic electron transfer, particularly through the work of Kröger (cf. 10), Brodie (6), and White (cf. 11) and their collaborators, investigators turned to the redox function in bacteria growing anaerobically. Kröger et al. (12) drew attention to the importance of MK in the anaerobic reduction of fumarate. <u>Proteus</u> <u>rettgeri</u> growing anaerobically with fumarate as sole carbon and energy source forms ATP predominately via fumarate reduction (13), rather than by substrate-level phosphorylation. In agreement with these findings, data of Boonstra et al. (14) suggest that, in <u>E. coli</u> cells growing anaerobically under glycolytic conditions, the electrochemical proton gradient is generated by electron transfer through a MK-dependent fumarate reductase pathway rather than by ATP hydrolysis.

Holländer and Mannheim (15) have developed a system of categorizing Gram-negative bacteria according to their quinone content (DMK/MK, DMK/MK + Q, or Q) and ability to grow anaerobically in the presence of fumarate (summarized and discussed by Kröger (3)). Organisms with Q only will not grow anaerobically with fumarate, a consequence both of the differing structures of the two quinones and of their redox potentials (cf. 3).

On the other hand, quinone-mediated electron transport from formate to nitrate has been shown to utilize either MK or Q, in organisms that possess both quinones. This has been demonstrated in $\underline{E.\ coli}$ by extraction-restoration experiments (16) and by measurements of activity in isogenic strains that are $\underline{men}^+\underline{ubi}^+$ (parent strain), $\underline{men}^-\underline{ubi}^+$ (MK-deficient), $\underline{men}^+\underline{ubi}^-$ (Q-deficient), or $\underline{men}^-\underline{ubi}^-$ (MK- and Q-deficient) (17). In the latter work, the singly-deficient mutants ($\underline{men}^-\underline{ubi}^+$ or $\underline{men}^+\underline{ubi}^-$) exhibited very substantial residual reduction of nitrate in the presence of formate, when compared to the double mutant ($\underline{men}^-\underline{ubi}^-$). Membrane vesicles from anaerobically grown $\underline{E.\ coli}$ are capable of generating a substantial electrochemical proton gradient by nitrate respiration (18,19).

BIOSYNTHETIC REDOX REACTIONS INVOLVING MK

Newton et al. (20) found that an $\underline{E.\ coli}$ $\underline{men}^-\underline{ubi}^-$ double mutant would not grow anaerobically on glucose unless uracil was added. This requirement was traced to a crucial role for MK in the dehydrogenation of dihydroorotate to orotate, coupled to fumarate reduction:

```
    Dihydroorotate          MK           Succinate
                      \    /    \    /
                       \  /      \  /
                        ><        ><
                       /  \      /  \
                      /    \    /    \
    Pyrimidines ←— Orotate   MKH₂    Fumarate ←— Glucose
```

For cultures of $\underline{E.\ coli}$ growing anaerobically on glucose, fumarate is supplied by the activity of the TCA cycle. Membrane preparations from the $\underline{men}^+\underline{ubi}^+$ parent strain were unable to form orotate from dihydroorotate unless fumarate was present, while such preparations from the $\underline{men}^-\underline{ubi}^+$ strain required fumarate and MK. Apparently in vivo, Q could partially replace MK in this reaction, but this replacement could not be duplicated in vitro. The slow growth exhibited by $\underline{ubi}^+\underline{men}^-$ strains growing anaerobically on glucose could be restored completely to normal by addition of uracil to the culture medium. Thus MK may have a crucial role during anaerobic growth in providing precursors for RNA biosynthesis.

Utilizing $\underline{men}^-$ and $\underline{ubi}^-$ $\underline{E.\ coli}$ mutants, Jacobs and Jacobs (21) have demonstrated recently the MK-dependent oxidation of protoporphyrinogen to protoporphyrin, coupled to fumarate or to nitrate under anaerobic conditions. Cytochromes were not involved as electron carriers, since extracts prepared from a heme-deficient (therefore cytochrome-deficient) mutant oxidized protoporphyrinogen normally in the presence of fumarate. These experiments point to an important role for MK in the biosynthesis of heme under anaerobic conditions.

Functions of Vitamin K_2 179

REGULATORY EFFECTS EXHIBITED BY MK

The anaerobic bacterium Bacteroides melaninogenicus has a nutritional requirement for vitamin K, and depletion of the vitamin depresses the growth rate; this response is associated with abnormalities in cell division and in the cell surface (22). Depletion of vitamin K has been found to depress the synthesis of sphingolipids, but not of phospholipids (23). Addition of vitamin K_1 to cell-free extracts of depleted cells did not stimulate 3-ketodihydrosphingosine synthetase activity, but this activity could be detected within 15 minutes after the vitamin was added to slowly growing depleted cultures (24). Synthetase activity increased 7 to 10 fold over a 75 minute period, during which time the growth rate markedly improved. Puromycin and rifampicin prevented the increase in enzyme activity, suggesting that transcription and de novo protein synthesis were required. There was, however, a significant lag in these inhibitory effects. Bacteroides melaninogenicus has the peculiarity of being severely growth-inhibited by monosaccharides, e.g. D-glucose and D-galactose. This inhibition is severe at 1% monosaccharide, but minimal at 0.1%. However, even at the lower concentration, induction of 3-ketodihydrosphingosine synthetase by vitamin K_1 is abolished (25,26). Despite the lack of genetic analysis in Bacteroides, this system shows promise for study of the regulatory effects of vitamin K in enzyme induction.

MK is the only lipophilic quinone species in the aerobic spore-forming bacterium Bacillus subtilis, and takes part in electron transport to oxygen (27,28,29,30,31,32,33). Lowering of the MK level by near-UV irradiation of membrane fragments (27) or of whole cells (34), or by precursor deprivation of a men⁻ auxotroph (30,31) results in loss of electron transfer activity. Experiments with men⁻ strains have shown, however, that more than 90% of the normally regulated concentration of MK must be deleted before significant reduction in electron flow occurs (31). This is exhibited as loss of NADH oxidation and overall lowering of oxygen utilization, but also by a decreased enzymatic reducibility of the cytochromes (Table 1).

TABLE 1. Effect of decreased MK concentration on the enzymatic reduction of cytochromes in B. subtilis strain RB163 (men⁻)*

		Per Cent Enzymatic Reduction	
Strain	Per Cent MK	Cyto $a + a_3$ (605 nm)	Cytos b,c,c_1,o (560 nm)
RB1 (men⁺)	100	92	92
RB163 (men⁻)	100	90	94
	8	81	93
	∿1	60	77
	<1	60	65

* Based on data of Farrand and Taber (31)

Such a severe decrease in MK level (i.e. to <10% of normal) also causes a disturbance in the regulation of cytochrome synthesis (30,31). In wild-type strains of B. subtilis, or in aroD (men⁻) strains made phenotypically Men⁺ by growth with sufficient shikimic acid (shk), cytochromes c_1 (553 nm absorption maximum) and o (557 nm) are synthesized in high concentration during exponential growth, whereas cytochromes $a + a_3$ (602 nm), b (560 nm) and c (549 nm) are synthesized in much lower concentrations. In late exponential and stationary phases, the situation is reversed, with cytochromes $a + a_3$, b, and c present in high concentration, and cytochromes c_1 and o occurring as minor components (29,35). However, in a men^- mutant made phenotypically Men^- by growth in the absence of shk, this regulated change in the cytochrome system does not occur, and stationary cultures retain the spectrum characteristic of exponential cultures (Fig. 1).

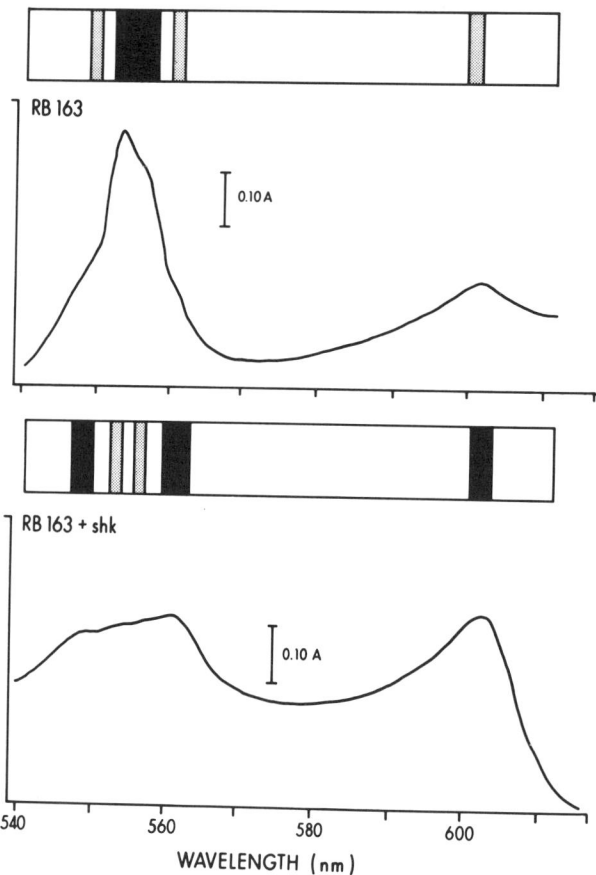

FIGURE 1. Effect of MK on cytochrome synthesis in B. subtilis strain RB163 (men^-). (Above) stationary phase culture, MK-deficient; (below) the same, but grown with shikimic acid to permit normal synthesis of MK. From Farrand and Taber (30), with permission.

It appears, then, that MK in B. subtilis is distributed into at least two functional pools: i) a small pool (<10% of the total) that is directly-- and obligatorily--involved in electron transfer via the cytochromes to oxygen, and (perhaps indirectly) in regulation of cytochrome synthesis; ii) a large pool (>90%) that be deleted without loss of oxidative function. However, this latter fraction is essential for efficient conversion of the vegetatively growing cell to an endospore, as shown in Figure 2. There is close correspondence between the concentration dependence on the MK precursor shikimic acid for MK synthesis, and for formation of heat-resistant spores (31).

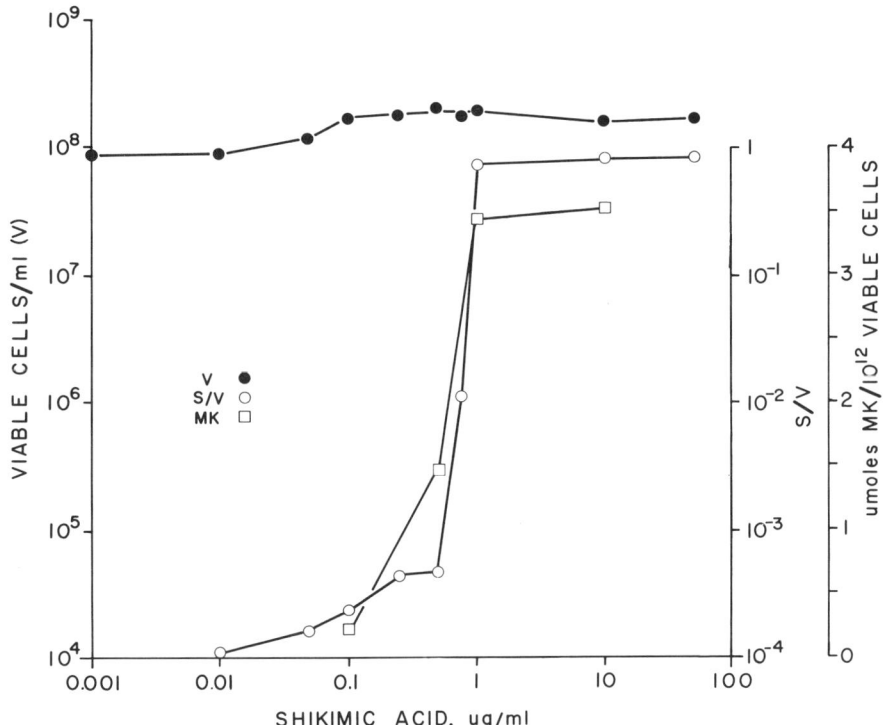

FIGURE 2. Relationship of MK concentration and spore formation to concentration of the MK precursor shikimic acid in B. subtilis strain RB163 (aroD (men$^-$)). V = viable count; S/V = spore fraction. From Farrand and Taber (31), with permission.

The biochemical mechanisms underlying this requirement are not clear; synthesis of a 36 kdal membrane protein is correlated with MK concentration, but the concentration dependence of this change suggests that it is related more to cytochrome regulation than to sporulation (29). It is known (32) that the MK content of men$^+$ B. subtilis cultures rises markedly in the early stages of sporulation, but whether this increase is directly associated with the characteristic cellular developmental events of sporulation, or reflects other complex changes in oxidative metabolism (cf. 36,28) is not known.

REGULATION OF MK BIOSYNTHESIS

The enzymatic steps leading from chorismic acid (in the common aromatic amino acid biosynthesis pathway) to DMK and MK have been the subject of intensive work over the past several years (cf. e.g. 37,38,39,40,41). This effort has been aided by the isolation of mutations affecting these reactions. In E. coli, three men loci have been identified thus far. These appear to be structural genes for enzymes catalyzing the following reactions (38,41):

$$\text{Chorismic Acid} \xrightarrow{menC} \text{2-Succinyl Benzoic Acid} \xrightarrow{menB} \text{1,4-Dihydroxy-2-Naphthoic Acid} \xrightarrow{menA} \text{DMK} \longrightarrow \text{MK}$$

The conversion of DMK to MK apparently involves the participation of S-adenosylmethionine, but this step has not yet been defined by men mutations. The enzymology of this system has been pursued by Young (38,40) and by Bentley (37,39) and their coworkers, and a contribution from the latter group is to be found in this volume (pp. 188-192); a discussion of the enzymes will not, as a consequence, be attempted here.

The growth phase-dependent regulation of MK biosynthesis in B. subtilis discussed in the previous section (32) has prompted a search in our laboratory for mutations in this organism that prevent MK formation. Men mutants of Staphylococcus aureus (42) and of B. subtilis (29) are resistant to the aminoglycoside antibiotics, such as kanamycin, neomycin, streptomycin, and gentamicin. This property allows a ready isolation of mutants; we have used it to select and study more than 20 B. subtilis mutants having the following properties (Taber, H., in preparation): i) resistance to moderate (5-50 µg/ml) concentrations of aminoglycoside antibiotics; ii) very poor growth on broth media not containing glucose; iii) loss of resistance, and stimulation of growth by the addition of 18 µM menadione to broth media, with best growth seen in broth media containing 54 µM menadione and 0.5% glucose; and iv) no requirement for tryptophane, phenylalanine, tyrosine, or p-aminobenzoic acid, showing that mutations in the common aro pathway were not present.

The growth of approximately half of the mutants was stimulated to wild-type levels by 2-succinylbenzoate. Several of these mutations have been genetically mapped by transformation and transduction, and are found to lie extremely close to one another in the B. subtilis genome. These strains are putative menC mutants, blocked in the conversion of chorismic acid to 2-succinylbenzoate. Of the remaining mutants, several have been established as menB mutants because of growth stimulation by 1,4-dihydroxy-2-naphthoic acid, syntrophic cross-feeding of menC mutants, and close linkage to one another by transformation. Those strains not classified as menB or menC mutants map very close to one another, but separate from menB or menC, and are tentatively assigned to the menA class. All men mutants are quite closely linked to one another, are 40-45% cotransducible with the bioB gene, and lie between bioB and sacQ as shown by a series of 2- and 3-factor crosses involving aroG, bioB, sacQ, and ald (see Fig. 3).

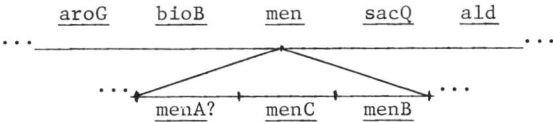

FIGURE 3. Probable fine structure of the men locus in B. subtilis (Taber, H., Lang, T., Rivoire, L., and Tanzi, R., in preparation).

The orientation of the genes has been tentatively established in transformation experiments measuring cotransfer of the bioB gene with men.

In principle, isolation of menA mutants among B. subtilis strains that are growth-stimulated by menadione might seem unlikely, since in order to form MK, menadione must be subject to the polyprenyltransferase reaction that is deficient in menA strains. In support of this, menadione cannot function as a MK precursor in E. coli menA mutants (38). In the present case, growth stimulation of B. subtilis mutants may be due to leakiness of the mutational block. Alternatively, the B. subtilis "menA" mutants may be regulatory mutants affecting menB and menC; however, in this event the strains should show growth stimulation by 1,4-dihydroxy-2-naphthoic acid, and this has not been observed. Studies of the accumulation of biosynthetic intermediates by the mutants are now underway to resolve this question. In either event, the close clustering of genes in B. subtilis controlling the biosynthetic pathway for MK suggests the likelihood of common transcriptional control, and offers a relatively simple system for studying the regulation of a system of enzymes functioning at the interface between cytoplasm and membrane.

ACTIVE TRANSPORT DEPENDENT ON MK

From the fact, discussed previously, of MK participation in electron transport-based generation of the electrochemical proton gradient, it follows that MK will be essential for those transport functions that depend on this gradient. The involvement of MK has been approached in two ways: i) by inactivation of MK with near-UV irradiation, and ii) by use of men mutants made specifically MK-deficient by precursor deprivation.

The use of near-UV irradiation for studying MK-dependent oxidative function in bacteria was pioneered by Brodie and his colleagues in the late 1950's and early 1960's (cf. e.g. ref. 6). Among the early reports of near-UV effects on active transport was that of Hirata, Asano, and Brodie (43), who were able to inhibit proline uptake into membrane vesicles from Mycobacterium phlei by treatment with 360 nm light. MacLeod et al. (44) then showed that glutamate uptake by membrane vesicles prepared from Bacillus licheniformis was inactivated by sunlight or by near-UV irradiation. This inactivation could be reversed by addition of MK. Only lower homologues could function in the restoration of transport. The specificity of quinones for restoration of amino acid transport will be dealt with by Dr. Brodie's group in another contribution to this symposium (pp.193-202). Study of near-UV light effects on transport in E. coli drew Koch et al. (45) to the conclusion that such treatment could in addition to destroying MK or other quinones, also affect transport systems directly, and increase the passive permeability of the bacterial cell. There is also the question of MK photoproducts remaining in the membrane and perhaps interfering with electron and/or proton transfer sequences. In our studies on near UV-induced growth delay in B. subtilis (34), we have found that MK must be present in the membrane at the time of irradiation for substantial growth delay to occur (Men$^+$, Table 2). That is to say,

TABLE 2. Growth delay after near-UV irradiation of B. subtilis strain RB163 (men$^-$)*

MK Phenotype	Near UV Irradiation**	Growth Delay, Min
Men$^+$	−	0
Men$^+$	+	60
Men$^-$	−	0
Men$^-$	+	5-10

* Based on data of Taber et al. (1978)
** "+" Indicates a fluence (at 365 nm) of 325 kJ/m^2

growth delay is associated with disposition of MK photoproducts, rather than with the time required for MK biosynthesis; for if B. subtilis is MK-deficient at the onset of irradiation (Men$^-$), only a very short growth delay period is seen (Table 2).

Bisschop and Konings (46,47) have taken a different approach to examination of the status of MK in bacterial active transport. MK-deficient membrane vesicles could be prepared by depriving a men$^-$ B. subtilis strain (30,31) of the required MK precursor. These vesicles failed to transport amino acids in response to NADH, but would respond to the non-physiological electron donor system ascorbate + phenazine methosulfate. Reconstitution of the vesicles with menadione restored NADH-driven amino acid transport, and this transport responded appropriately to inhibitors. The amount of menadione bound to the vesicles was in excellent agreement with the molecular concentration of MK in B. subtilis, as measured in several different strains (47,32), suggesting that menadione can occupy physiological MK sites in the membrane.* The kinetic relationship observed by Bisschop and Konings between menadione-dependent NADH oxidation and amino acid transport (47) indicated that direct coupling between the respiratory chain and the transport systems was unlikely.

Transport of antibiotics by bacterial cells has received some long overdue attention in recent years. Of particular interest are the aminoglycosides--such as streptomycin, gentamicin, kanamycin, neomycin, etc.-- which must cross the cytoplasmic membrane in order to reach their target of inhibition, the ribosome. In 1976, a men$^-$ mutant of B. subtilis was shown to be deficient in accumulation of kanamycin (48), and a model has been proposed recently (49), which suggests that quinones may participate in a "carrier complex" (perhaps with proteins) to convey aminoglycosides across the cell membrane. In studying the relationship between MK and active accumulation of the aminoglycoside gentamicin by B. subtilis, we

---

* These findings may answer the question raised earlier ("Regulation of MK Biosynthesis") as to why menadione stimulates growth of putative B. subtilis menA mutants. That is, menadione may partially replace MK in the B. subtilis electron transport system, rather than serving only as a MK precursor.

found that MK must be reduced to less than 10% of the normal concentration before restriction of gentamicin uptake occurred (Table 3). This MK level corresponds to that at which loss of electron transfer function

TABLE 3. Gentamicin accumulation by B. subtilis strain RB163 (men$^-$)*

(Shk), µg/ml	(MK), Percent of Normal	Rate of Gentamicin Accumulation, ng/min/mg dry weight
5.0	100	46
1.0	100	50
0.1	8	48
0.05	∼4	20
0	<0.1	0

* Modified from Taber, Halfenger and Sugarman, submitted for publication

occurs (Table 1; ref. 30,31). Therefore, we feel it is likely that aminoglycoside transport responds to the magnitude of the electrochemical proton gradient, as suggested by the work of Bryan and his collaborators (49,50). The decreased uptake of aminoglycosides in MK-deficient strains also provides the rationale for the ready isolation of men$^-$ mutants, and assures us that the MK concentration must be very low before aminoglycoside resistance is expressed.

SUMMARY: PROBABLE AND POSSIBLE ROLES FOR MK IN BACTERIA

A central role for MK in bacterial aerobic energy metabolism has been established for some time, functioning as a mediator between low-potential dehydrogenases and/or iron-sulfur proteins, and cytochromes. Whether DMK, with an E'_o (+ 36 mV) some 110 mV higher, is interchangeable with MK, is not clear (cf. 3); the regulatory significance of the DMK/MK ratio is also unclear (51). More recently, participation of MK in anaerobic electron transfer has been found to be widespread among bacteria, occurring in most anaerobes and anaerobically grown facultative species (52). MK may be involved in a quinone-dependent proton circulation, similar to that envisaged for Q (cf. ref. 5 for a discussion), and assist in the formation of an electrochemical proton gradient to be utilized for active transport of such diverse substances as amino acids and antibiotics, as well as for ATP synthesis.

Relatively uncharted areas include biosynthetic reactions that are dependent on MK (20,21) under anaerobic conditions; these may be important in some species during aerobic growth as well. Possible regulatory roles for MK are undefined; in an effort to explain the greater MK requirement by B. subtilis for sporulation as compared with respiration, we have attempted to demonstrate a possible MK-dependent carboxylase reaction in membrane preparations from this organism, but without success (H. Taber and J. W. Suttie, unpublished). It is, however, possible to state that a bacterial carboxylase, if it exists in B. subtilis, does not have similar properties to the mammalian enzyme. The reported occurrence of γ-carboxyglutamic acid in ribosomal proteins of E. coli (J. Van Buskirk, M. Low, and W. M. Kirsch, this volume, pp. 274-278) may make further search for such an activity extremely important. The possibility that MK may affect expression of the bacterial genome either at the transcriptional or the translational level suggests that, in addition to its several other functions, MK is a versatile molecule indeed.

ACKNOWLEDGEMENTS

The work from my laboratory described in this communication was supported, in part, by research grants PCM-7809217 from the National Science Foundation and AI-09093 from the National Institutes of Health, and by Research Career Development Award 5-K04-AI-70655 from the National Institutes of Health.

REFERENCES

1. Bishop, D. H. L., Pandya, K. P., and King, H. I. (1962) Biochem. J. 83, 606-614.
2. Whitstance, G. R., and Threlfall, D. R. (1968) Biochem. J. 108, 505-507.
3. Kröger, A. (1977) in Microbial Energetics (B. A. Haddock and W. A. Hamilton, eds.), 27th Symp. Soc. Gen. Microbiol., Cambridge U. Press, pp. 61-93.
4. Jones, C. W. (1977) in Microbial Energetics (B. A. Haddock and W. A. Hamilton, eds.), 27th Symp. Soc. Gen. Microbiol., Cambridge U. Press, pp. 23-59.
5. Haddock, B. A., and Jones, C. W. (1977) Bacteriol. Rev. 41, 47-99.
6. Brodie, A. F., and Watanabe, T. (1966) Vitam. Horm. 24, 447-463.
7. Kröger, A., and Klingenberg, M. (1970) Vitam. Horm. 28, 533-574.
8. Cox, G. B., and Gibson, F. (1974) Biochim. Biophys. Acta 346, 1-25.
9. Haddock, B. A. (1977) in Microbial Energetics (B. A. Haddock and W. A. Hamilton, eds.), 27th Symp. Soc. Gen. Microbiol., Cambridge U. Press, pp. 95-120.
10. Kröger, A., and Dadák, V. (1969) Eur. J. Biochem. 11, 328-340.
11. White, D. C. (1965) J. Biol. Chem. 240, 1387-1394.
12. Kröger, A., Dadák, V., Klingenberg, M., and Diemer, F. (1971) Eur. J. Biochem. 21, 322-333.
13. Kröger, A., Schimkat, M., and Niedermaier, S. (1974) Biochim. Biophys. Acta 347, 273-289.
14. Boonstra, J., Downie, J. A., and Konings, W. N. (1978) J. Bacteriol. 136, 844-853.
15. Holländer, R., and Mannheim, W. (1975) Int. J. Sys. Bacteriol. 25, 102-107.
16. Enoch, H. G., and Lester, R. L. (1974) Biochem. Biophys. Res. Commun. 61, 1234-1241.
17. Wallace, B. J., and Young, I. G. (1977) Biochim. Biophys. Acta 461, 84-100.
18. Konings, W. N., and Boonstra, J. (1977) Curr. Top. Membr. Transp. 9, 177-231.
19. Boonstra, J., and Konings, W. N. (1977) Eur. J. Biochem. 78, 361-368.
20. Newton, N. A., Cox, G. B., and Gibson, F. (1971) Biochim. Biophys. Acta 244, 155-166.
21. Jacobs, N. J., and Jacobs, J. M. (1978) Biochim. Biophys. Acta 544, 540-546.
22. Lev, M. (1959) J. Gen. Microbiol. 20, 697-703.
23. Lev, M., and Milford, A. F. (1972) J. Lipid Res. 13, 364-370.
24. Lev, M., and Milford, A. F. (1973) J. Bacteriol. 157, 500-508.
25. Lev, M., and Milford, A. F. (1975) J. Bacteriol. 121, 152-159.

26. Lev., M. (1979) Am. J. Clin. Nutr. 32, 179-186.
27. Downey, R. J. (1964) J. Bacteriol. 88, 904-911.
28. Tochikubo, K. (1971) J. Bacteriol. 108, 652-661.
29. Taber, H., Farrand, S. K., and Halfenger, G. M. (1972) in Spores V (H. O. Halvorson, R. S. Hanson, and L. L. Campbell, eds.) Am. Soc. Microbiol., pp. 140-147.
30. Farrand, S. K., and Taber, H. (1973) J. Bacteriol. 115, 1021-1034.
31. Farrand, S. K., and Taber, H. (1973) J. Bacteriol. 115, 1035-1044.
32. Farrand, S. K., and Taber, H. (1974) J. Bacteriol. 117, 324-326.
33. Weber, M. M., and Broadbent, D. A. (1975) in Spores VI (P. Gerhardt, R. N. Costilow, and H. L. Sadoff, eds.), Am. Soc. Microbiol., pp. 411-417.
34. Taber, H., Pomerantz, B. J., and Halfenger, G. M. (1978) Photochem. Photobiol. 28, 191-196.
35. Taber, H. (1974) J. Gen. Microbiol. 81, 435-444.
36. Taber, H., and Freese, E. (1974) J. Bacteriol. 120, 1004-1011.
37. Bentley, R. (1975) Pure Appl. Chem. 41, 47-68.
38. Young, I. G. (1975) Biochem. 14, 399-406.
39. Bryant, R. W., and Bentley, R. (1976) Biochem. 15, 4792-4796.
40. Shineberg, B., and Young, I. G. (1976) Biochem. 15, 2754-2758.
41. Guest, J. R. (1977) J. Bacteriol. 130, 1038-1046.
42. Sasarman, A., Surdeanu, M., Portelance, V., Dobardzic, R., and Sonea, S. (1971) J. Gen. Microbiol. 65, 125-130.
43. Hirata, H., Asano, A., and Brodie, A. F. (1971) Biochem. Biophys. Res. Commun. 44, 368-374.
44. MacLeod, R. A., Thurman, P., and Rogers, H. J. (1973) J. Bacteriol. 113, 329-340.
45. Koch, A. L., Doyle, R. J., and Kubitschek, H. E. (1976) J. Bacteriol. 126, 140-146.
46. Bisschop, A., de Jong, L., Lima Costa, M. E., and Konings, W. N. (1975) J. Bacteriol. 121, 807-813.
47. Bisschop, A., and Konings, W. N. (1976) Eur. J. Biochem. 67, 357-365.
48. Taber, H., and Halfenger, G. M. (1976) Antimicrob. Agents Chemother. 9, 251-259.
49. Bryan, L. E., and Van den Elzen, H. M. (1977) Antimicrob. Agents Chemother. 12, 163-177.
50. Bryan, L. E., Kowand, S. K., and Van den Elzen, H. M. (1979) Antimicrob. Agents Chemother. 15, 7-13.
51. Alexander, K., and Young, I. G. (1978) Biochem. 17, 4750-4755.
52. Thauer, R. K., Jungermann, K., and Decker, K. (1977) Bacteriol. Rev. 41, 100-180.

ENZYMES INVOLVED IN VITAMIN K BIOSYNTHESIS

R. MEGANATHAN, T. FOLGER, and R. BENTLEY

Department of Biological Sciences,
University of Pittsburgh,
Pittsburgh, PA 15260

INTRODUCTION

The biosynthetic pathway for the production of vitamin K (menaquinone, MK) in bacteria requires the formation of the benzenoid compound, o-succinylbenzoate, OSB, 4-(2'-carboxyphenyl)-4-oxobutyric acid, and its subsequent conversion to the naphthalenoid compound 1,4-dihydroxy-2-naphthoic acid, DHNA (see Fig. 1A). This conclusion derives from tracer experiments with intact organisms (for reviews see refs. 1, 2) and the fact that both compounds replace the usual vitamin K requirement of <u>Bacteroides melaninogenicus</u> (3). Furthermore, the two precursors are accumulated by, respectively, menB$^-$ and menA$^-$ strains of <u>Escherichia coli</u> (4) and OSB promotes normal anaerobic growth of menC$^-$ strains (5). More recently, the enzymatic conversion of OSB to DHNA has been studied in cell free extracts of <u>E. coli</u> and <u>Mycobacterium phlei</u> (6, 7); this conversion is dependent on the presence of coenzyme A (CoA) and ATP. In these experiments, the formation of a spirodilactone derivative of OSB was occasionally observed with <u>E. coli</u> preparations (the spirodilactone is more accurately described as the spirodilactone of 4-(2'-carboxyphenyl)-4,4-dihydroxybutyric acid - see Fig. 1B for the structure).

Hutson and Threlfall (8) have used cell free extracts from <u>Micrococcus luteus</u> to study the utilization of OSB; in a limited number of experiments, <u>E. coli</u> extracts were also examined. In neither case, could they show any conversion of OSB to DHNA. However, with <u>M. luteus</u> preparations there was a consistent formation of the spirodilactone derivative of OSB which was shown to be dependent on the presence of both CoA and ATP. When their preparations were supplemented with membrane fragments and isopentenyl pyrophosphate, OSB was converted to OSB spirodilactone and compounds with thin-layer chromatography properties expected of demethylmenaquinones. Since <u>M. luteus</u> is an organism containing high levels of menaquinones (about four times as much as <u>E. coli</u>, 9) the results of Hutson and Threlfall (8) suggested a possible menaquinone biosynthetic pathway from OSB without DHNA as an intermediate. We have, therefore, reinvestigated OSB utilization in extracts from <u>M. luteus</u>. This was particularly necessary since we recently found that the conversion OSB → DHNA in <u>M. phlei</u> extracts requires the formation of an <u>o</u>-succinylbenzoyl-CoA (OSB-CoA) intermediate and the participation of two enzymes, OSB-CoA synthetase and DHNA synthase (10). Hence the pathway for menaquinone biosynthesis, at least in this organism, is more accurately represented as OSB → OSB-CoA → DHNA → MK. The results reported here provide a rationalization for the production of OSB spirodilactone in enzymatic experiments. A new hypothesis for the biosynthesis of menaquinone in <u>M. luteus</u> is not required.

MATERIALS AND METHODS

<u>Micrococcus luteus</u> ATCC 4698 was grown at 30°, with shaking, in medium containing Bactopeptone 1%, yeast extract 0.1%, and NaCl 0.5%. Cells were collected by centrifugation and were washed with 1/8 volume of 0.02 M

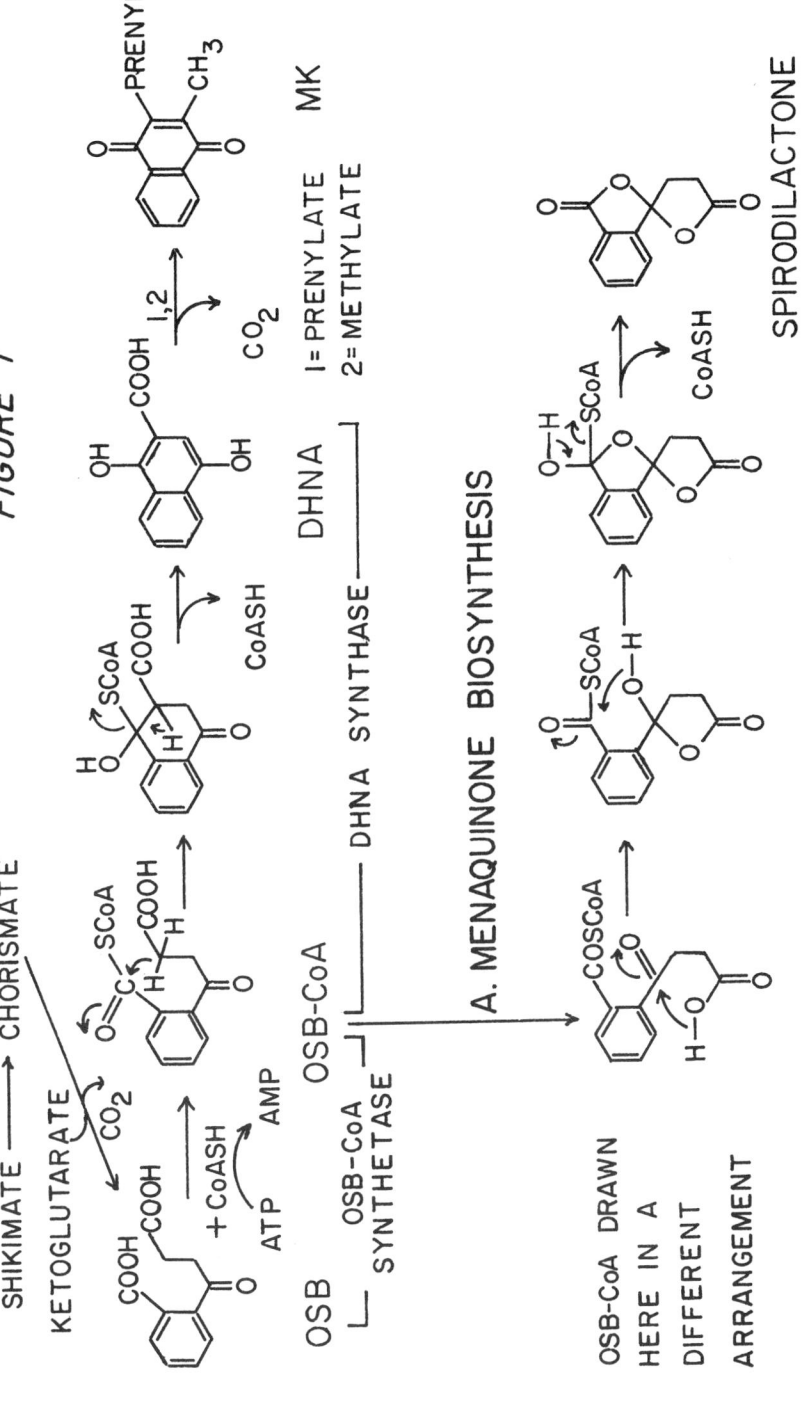

potassium phosphate buffer, pH 6.9, containing 5 mM mercaptoethanol (Buffer A). Extracts were prepared by suspending cells (11 g wet weight) in 22 ml of Buffer A and then adding 1 mg deoxyribonuclease and 22 mg lysozyme; this mixture was incubated at $30°$ for 15 min. After addition of a further 11 ml of Buffer A, the mixture was centrifuged at 27,000 x g for 15 min. The clear supernatant was usually used without further treatment. To determine cofactor requirements for spirodilactone formation, 1 ml portions of the extract were dialyzed against Buffer A at $4°$.

DHNA formation was assayed spectrophotofluorometrically (7) and protein by the method of Bradford (11). Substrates, both non-radioactive and radioactive, were prepared as previously described (6-8).

RESULTS

When the cell free extracts prepared from M. luteus (6.6 mg protein) were incubated under our usual assay conditions with ATP, CoA, OSB, and Mg^{++}, DHNA was easily detected by the spectrophotofluorometric assay. The complete system produced 12.7 nmoles DHNA per tube per 30 min; in the absence of Mg^{++} the yield was reduced to 6.9 and in the absence of ATP, CoA, OSB, or extract, no DHNA formation was observed. The pH optimum of the reaction was between 7.5 and 8.5. The rate of DHNA formation was linear over a 40 min period and was dependent on protein concentration.

Since Hutson and Threlfall had failed to observe this reaction, it was important to characterize the reaction product. For this purpose, the enzyme extract was incubated with the above named cofactors but with [2-^{14}C]OSB (approximately 200,000 total dpm, specific activity 25 mCi/mmole) replacing OSB. After incubation for 30 min at $30°$, a mixture of acetone:benzene:concentrated HCl, 100:100:1 (6 ml) was added. After shaking, 4 ml of the upper layer was withdrawn and 100 µg portions of carrier OSB, OSB spirodilactone, and DHNA were added. Following evaporation to dryness, the residue was subjected to thin-layer chromatography on silica gel GF plates with the solvent system, chloroform:ethyl acetate:formic acid, 135:20:1.5. The dried plates were then examined with the radiochromatogram scanner. This examination revealed three peaks of radioactivity which were identified as OSB (R_f = 0.09), DHNA (R_f = 0.29), and OSB spirodilactone (R_f = 0.49). However, in these experiments, the relative amount of spirodilactone appeared greater than in our previous experiments with extracts of E. coli. In further experiments we therefore added to the M. luteus extracts a preparation of DHNA synthase isolated from M. phlei (10). As expected, the spirodilactone peak was then almost absent, while at the same time, the DHNA peak increased proportionately. DHNA was always present even when the addition of M. phlei DHNA synthase was not made.

Since we knew the DHNA synthase of M. phlei to be unstable to dilute acid under conditions which do not impair OSB-CoA synthetase activity, the M. luteus preparations were examined as follows. Portions of the extract, 0.2 ml, were cooled in ice and 3N HCl was added, along the sides of the tubes, to a concentration of 0.1 N. The contents of the tubes were mixed by swirling, resulting in the formation of a precipitate. After approximately 30 seconds, 0.1 M potassium phosphate buffer, pH 8.0, containing 5mM mercaptoethanol was added to a total volume of 3.0 ml; the precipitate redissolved. When these acid treated extracts were incubated with [2-^{14}C]OSB as just described, only OSB spirodilactone was detected when the chromatograms were scanned for radioactivity. Using dialyzed acid treated extracts, which produced only the spirodilactone, it was possible to show that lactone formation required both ATP and CoA.

Since one difference in our experiments and those of Hutson and Threlfall was our use of freshly grown cells of M. luteus, we have attempted to duplicate their work exactly using spray dried cells of M. luteus (obtained commercially from Miles Laboratories). Using their conditions as precisely as possible we observed DHNA formation in the spectrophotofluorometric assay. The level of DHNA formation we had observed with freshly grown cells was 1.9 nmoles/mg protein/30 min; under identical conditions, spray dried cells produced 1.3 nmoles DHNA/mg protein/30 min. It is worth noting that these spray dried cells had been stored at $-20°$ for approximately five years after purchase.

DISCUSSION

The results described here clearly show the production of DHNA from OSB in extracts from M. luteus. As noted with other microorganisms, the conversion is strictly dependent on the presence of CoA, ATP, and Mg^{++}. The conversion was obtained either with preparations from freshly grown cells or from spray dried cells and is in sharp contrast to the negative results reported by Hutson and Threlfall (8). We have confirmed their observation that OSB spirodilactone is routinely formed from OSB by the extracts from M. luteus and that this process has the same cofactor requirements as DHNA production. In all of our experiments, however, both DHNA and OSB spirodilactone have been formed.

Our earlier experiments have shown that DHNA formation in M. phlei requires two enzyme activities (10). An intermediate, OSB-CoA, is first produced by an OSB-CoA synthetase; ATP is required and is converted to AMP. The OSB-CoA synthetase of M. phlei retained activity after brief exposure to 0.1 N HCl; this concentration of acid, however, destroys the activity of the second enzyme which we have named DHNA synthase. In the present work it was observed that acid treatment of the M. luteus extracts removed the ability to form DHNA, and under these conditions the spirodilactone accumulated. When the acid treated M. luteus extracts were supplemented with DHNA synthase from M. phlei, DHNA production was restored. It appears likely, as suggested by Hutson and Threlfall (8) that the OSB-CoA intermediate is the source of the spirodilactone, probably as a result of a spontaneous conversion (see Fig. 1B). In the presence of DHNA synthase, the non-productive breakdown of the OSB-CoA intermediate to spirodilactone is diminished, and instead the intermediate is converted to DHNA. The relative proportions of dilactone and DHNA in the final product mix depend on the level of DHNA synthase activity which is present.

The relative proportions of OSB-CoA synthetase and DHNA synthase appear to vary considerably from one microorganism to another, but the actual amounts cannot yet be precisely estimated because of the unavailability of the substrate OSB-CoA. In our experience, M. phlei contains a sufficient level of DHNA synthase so that spirodilactone production has never been observed in extracts from this organism - unless the DHNA synthase were first denatured with acid. With E. coli extracts, spirodilactone production was occasionally observed (6) suggesting a lower level of DNNA synthase than in M. phlei. Finally, M. luteus appears to be quite deficient in DHNA synthase activity, since co-production of DHNA and spirodilactone was always observed. Perhaps the failure of Hutson and Threlfall to observe DHNA production was due to an inactivation of the DHNA synthase as a result of a minor operational difference between their laboratory and ours. Much of their work with M. luteus was carried out at pH 6.5, the pH optimum for the formation of spirodilactone. Although DHNA formation was found by us to have a pH optimum of between 7.5 and 8.5, 50%

of the activity was still retained at pH 6.5. Thus, differences in pH are apparently not the reason for the differences between the two groups.

Whatever the reason for the discrepancy, and despite the failure of Hutson and Threlfall to demonstrate DHNA production even in E. coli extracts, we see no reason to postulate any pathway for menaquinone biosynthesis which does not require the participation of DHNA. The following pathway is apparently common to all of the bacterial systems so far investigated (see also Fig. 1A): OSB → OSB-CoA → DHNA → MK. The actual structure of the OSB-CoA intermediate has not yet been determined. We had originally proposed the location of the CoA moiety on the aromatic carboxyl group of OSB (6, 7) and a similar assumption was made by Hutson and Threlfall (8) to account for spirodilactone formation.

ACKNOWLEDGEMENTS

This work has been supported by a grant from the US Public Health Service 5 R01 GM 20053. We are grateful for the excellent assistance of C. Dippold and the undergraduate research participation of S. Galli. Some of this work formed part of the MS thesis of Todd Folger at the University of Pittsburgh. We acknowledge his contribution and mourn his untimely death on May 13, 1979, at age 26.

REFERENCES

1. Bentley, R. (1975) Pure Appl. Chem. 41, 47-68.
2. Bentley, R. (1975) Biosynthesis 3, 181-246. Specialist Periodical Report, The Chemical Society, London.
3. Robins, D. J., Yee, R. B., and Bentley, R. (1973) J. Bacteriol. 116, 965-971.
4. Young, I. G. (1975) Biochemistry 14, 399-406.
5. Guest, J. R. (1977) J. Bacteriol. 130, 1038-1046.
6. Bryant, R. W., and Bentley, R. (1976) Biochemistry 15, 4792-4796.
7. McGovern, E. P., and Bentley, R. (1978) Arch. Biochem. Biophys. 188, 56-63.
8. Hutson, K. G., and Threlfall, D. R. (1978) Biochim. Biophys. Acta 530, 1-8.
9. Bishop, D. H. L., and King, H. K. (1962) Biochem. J. 85, 550-554.
10. Meganathan, R., and Bentley, R. (1979) Fed. Proc. 38, 315.
11. Bradford, M. M. (1976) Anal. Biochem. 72, 248-254.

THE SPECIFICITY OF QUINONES FOR RESTORATION OF ACTIVE TRANSPORT OF SOLUTES AND OXIDATIVE PHOSPHORYLATION

A. F. BRODIE, T. O. SUTHERLAND, and S. H. LEE

University of Southern California,
School of Medicine,
Los Angeles, CA 90033

INTRODUCTION

Mycobacterium phlei contains three major respiratory pathways which are capable of coupling phosphorylation to substrate oxidation. The major respiratory chains include the NAD^+-linked, succinate and malate-vitamin K reductase pathways (1). The succinoxidase pathway does not contain a quinone respiratory carrier. In contrast, the NAD^+-linked and malate-vitamin K reductase pathways contain a menaquinone which plays a subcellular role as a respiratory carrier between the flavoprotein and cytochrome b. The menaquinone has been identified as $MK_9(II-H)$ which contains a methyl group in the C_2-position of the naphthoquinone nucleus, and 9 isoprenoids units in the C_3-position containing a saturated double bond in the second isoprenoid unit (2).

The natural naphthoquinone of M. phlei was destroyed by irradiation with near ultraviolet light (360 nm). Irradiation of the electron transport particles (ETP) or membrane vesicles resulted in a concomitant loss in the capacity of the vesicles to carry out succinate or NAD^+-linked oxidation, coupled phosphorylation (3) and active transport of solutes. Restoration of these activities with NAD^+-linked substrates occurred on the addition of certain specific quinones such as the natural menaquinone from M. phlei, vitamin K_1 (4) or closely related homologues.

Studies of the structural requirements for restoration of oxidation and phosphorylation by quinones following light-treatment have revealed at least three different responses to quinone addition. The nature of the restoration was found to be dependent on the substitutions in the C_2 and C_3 position of the naphthoquinone nucleus. The three patterns were as follows: a) Quinones which restore oxidation and phosphorylation (i.e., vitamin K_1), b) Quinones which restore only oxidation but by the same electron transport pathway as that observed with the natural quinone (such as lapachol) and c) Quinones which restore only oxidation by "bypassing" a segment of the electron transport pathway or by reacting directly with oxygen, such as menadione (5).

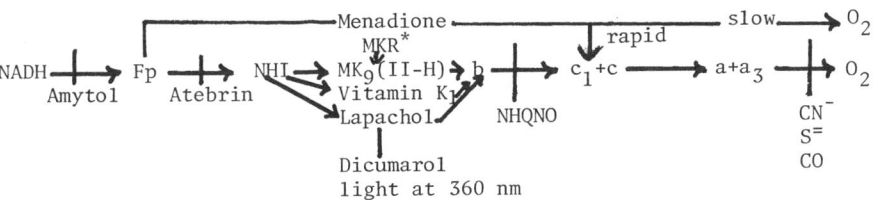

Figure 1. Restoration of Electron Transport by Naphthoquinones in M. phlei Membrane Vesicles (ETP)
*Malate-vitamin K reductase

Active transport of proline and calcium ions have been demonstrated with the membrane vesicles of M. phlei (6-9). The uptake of proline or Ca^{2+} proceeded against a concentration gradient with succinate, generated NADH, exogenous NADH or ascorbate-TPD as substrate. Active transport of proline or Ca^{2+} was inhibited by respiratory inhibitors, uncouplers, anaerobiosis, and various ionophores (6). It has also been shown that the irradiation of membrane vesicles resulted in a loss of the active transport of solutes. However, the restoration of proline or Ca^{2+} transport occurred following the addition of the natural naphthoquinone from M. phlei to the irradiated membrane vesicles (6,9). Thus, it was of interest to determine whether the strict specificity observed for restoration of active transport by quinones in the membrane vesicles was similar to that observed for the restoration of oxidative phosphorylation.

Information concerning the bioenergetic mechanism(s) of membrane related processes, such as, oxidative phosphorylation and active transport of solutes may be obtained by studying the restoration of these phenomena by quinones which differ in structure, degree of restoration of oxidation and in the nature of the respiratory chain utilized. In this paper, we describe the restoration of active transport of proline, proton gradient, and coupled phosphorylation by naphthoquinones (vitamin K_1, menadione and lapachol) in irradiated membrane vesicles from M. phlei and the relationship between these activities.

MATERIALS AND METHODS

Materials

The following materials were purchased commercially: vitamin K_1 and 9-aminoacridine from Sigma Chemical Co.; [^{14}C]proline and [^{14}C]methylamine from New England Nuclear; m-chlorocarbonylcyanide phenylhydrazone from Calbiochem; and menadione and lapachol from Matheson Coleman and Bell. All other chemicals were of reagent grade purity.

Preparation of Membrane Vesicles

Mycobacterium phlei (ATCC 354) was grown as previously described (10) and the electron transport particles or membrane vesicles were prepared by sonic disruption of cells as described by Brodie (11) and suspended in 10 mM $MgCl_2$ at a protein concentration of 10 mg/ml. Irradiated membrane vesicles were prepared by ultraviolet irradiation at 360 nm for 30 min in a cold rotary radiation apparatus using a series of GE lamps (type BLB black light) (12).

Preparation of Quinones

The quinones purified by column chromatography and the purified quinone were suspended by sonication in 5.0 ml of 50 mM Hepes-KOH buffer (pH 7.5) containing 37 mg of partially purified asolectin or phospholipids obtained from M. phlei (13). The preparation was sonicated in a 10 Kc Raytheon Sonic Oscillator for 10 min.

Measurement of Oxidation and Coupled Phosphorylation

Oxygen consumption was measured at 30° with a Yellow Springs Instrument

Model 53 Oxygen Monitor, and coupled phosphorylation was measured manometrically with a Gilson differential respirometer at 30°. Following termination of the reaction with 1.0 ml of 10% trichloroacetic acid, phosphorylation was estimated by the procedure described previously (10).

Measurement of pH Gradient

The pH gradient was measured by the distribution of a weak base, [^{14}C] methylamine, using a flow dialysis apparatus (1.0 ml microsize, BelArt Product, New Jersey) described by Schuldiner et al. (14). The internal pH of membrane vesicles was calculated by the method of Waddell and Butler (15), and the external pH was measured by using a Corning digital pH meter with an expanded scale. The pH gradient was then calculated from the difference between internal and external pH. The concentration gradient for solutes taken up by the membrane vesicles was calculated using the intravesicular volume of 1.7 µl per mg of membrane protein. This volume was obtained from the difference between the total $^{3}H_2O$-permeable space and [carboxyl-^{14}C]dextran-impermeable space (16,17).

Measurement of 9-aminoacridine Fluorescence

A proton gradient was also measured by the method of Schuldiner et al. (18) using 9-aminoacridine (9-AA) as a fluorescence probe. The fluorescence change of 9-AA was measured in 2.5 ml of reaction mixture containing 10 mM Hepes-KOH buffer (pH 7.5), 0.15 M KCl, 10 mM $MgCl_2$, 4 µM 9-AA and 0.5 mg of membrane protein. The quenching of 9-AA fluorescence was monitored with MPF-4 Perkins Elmer Spectrofluorometer equipped with a thermostatic cell holder. Excitation was carried out at 365 nm wavelength while the emission was set at 451 nm. A thermostatic bath was used to control the temperature of the cuvette at 30°.

Assay of Proline Transport

The membrane vesicles (2.0 mg of protein) were suspended in 1.0 ml of reaction mixture containing 50 mM Hepes-KOH buffer (pH 7.5), 10 mM $MgCl_2$, 10 mM NaCl. After 10 min of preincubation at 30° (in the presence and absence of naphthoquinone), the reaction was started by the addition of 25 µM proline (containing [^{14}C]proline, 1.0 µCi/ml) and substrate. At indicated time intervals, 0.1 ml aliquots were removed and immediately diluted in 2.0 ml of 50 mM Hepes-KOH buffer (pH 7.5). The suspension was rapidly filtered on a membrane filter (Millipore 0.45 µM) and the filters were washed twice with 2.0 ml of the same buffer. The filters were removed, dried and the radioactivity retained on the filters was counted in a Nuclear Chicago Liquid Scintillation counter using a scintillation fluor.

Protein Estimation

Protein concentration was determined either by the method of Lowry et al. (19) or by a modification of the biuret method (20) with bovine serum albumin as standard.

RESULTS

Restoration of Proline Transport and Oxidative Phosphorylation in Irradiated Membrane Vesicles

Irradiation of the membrane vesicles with near UV light at 360 nm, a procedure which inactivates the natural naphthoquinones (3), resulted in a loss of oxidation and active transport of proline (Table I).

TABLE 1. Restoration of proline transport in irradiated membrane vesicles by naphthoquinones

Addition	Proline Transport (pmol/min/mg protein)	Oxidation (natom/min/mg protein)
ETP*	136	10.0
ETP + Vitamin K_1	130	9.8
ETP + Menadione	147	11.5
ETP + Lapachol	138	10.2
Irradiated ETP	24	0.2
Irradiated ETP + Vitamin K_1	78	7.0
Irradiated ETP + Menadione	124	16.5
Irradiated ETP + Lapachol	95	10.9

The assay of transport and the measurement of oxidation were similar to those described in "Materials and Methods". Generated NADH system (1.0 mM NAD^+, 20 mM hydrazine, 1 mg of alcohol dehydrogenase and 50 µM ethanol) was used as the substrate. Vitamin K_1 (0.5 mM), menadione (0.4 mM) and lapachol (0.4 mM) were added during the period of 10 min preincubation. The reaction was started by the addition of ethanol as the substrate.

*ETP, electron transport particle or membrane vesicles

The addition of naphthoquinones such as vitamin K_1, menadione or lapachol was found to restore both oxidation and active transport of proline. However, the degree of restoration of active transport with the different quinones varied, menadione restored (91%) of the activity observed with untreated membrane vesicles whereas lapachol and vitamin K restored 70 and 51% of this activity respectively. In addition higher rates of oxidation were obtained with menadione and lapachol than that observed in the untreated or K_1 restored system (Table I & II). The addition of menadione to the untreated membrane vesicles resulted in a slight increase in the uptake of proline (5 to 10%), whereas vitamin K_1 and lapachol had no effect (Table I).

The K_m for proline in the untreated and quinone-reconstituted system was tested, since these lipid soluble quinones may alter the affinity of the proline carrier. The Lineweaver-Burk plots were found to be linear (Fig. 2) and the apparent K_m was 5.7 µM in both systems. It should be noted that restoration of oxidative phosphorylation following irradiation of the membrane vesicles (ETP) occurred only with vitamin K_1 whereas menadione or lapachol only restored oxidation in the irradiated system (Table II). Since menadione, lapachol or the irradiated

TABLE II. Restoration of oxidative phosphorylation by various quinones.

Addition	ΔO₂ (μatoms)	ΔPi (μmoles)	P/O
Unirradiated ETP	6.96	6.00	0.86
Irradiated ETP	0.71	0.00	0.00
Irradiated ETP + Vitamin K$_1$	6.02	3.67	0.61
Irradiated ETP + Menadione	8.75	0.16	0.02
Irradiated ETP + Lapachol	7.23	0.23	0.03
Irradiated ETP + Asolectin	0.89	0.00	0.00

The main compartment of the vessel contained 100 μmoles of Hepes-KOH buffer, pH 7.5, 15 μmoles of MgCl$_2$, 15 μmoles of Pi (potassium salt, pH 7.5), 3 mg of ETP and naphthoquinones in asolectin (0.5 mM of vitamin K$_1$, 0.4 mM of menadione and 0.4 mM of lapachol). After a 10 min preincubation period at 30°, the reaction was started by the addition of the substrate from the side arm. The side arm contained 5 μmoles of ADP, 25 μmoles of KF, 100 μmoles of ethanol, 1 μmole of NAD$^+$, 50 μmoles of hydrazine, 1 mg of alcohol dehydrogenase and sufficient water to bring the total volume to 2.0 ml. The reaction was terminated after 15 min by the addition of 1.0 ml of 10% trichloroacetic acid.

products of the natural naphthoquinone may act as uncoupling agents, the effects of these quinones on oxidative phosphorylation were determined. Ascorbate-TPD has been shown to enter the respiratory chain at the level of cytochrome c and phosphorylation was associated with the oxidation of this electron donor (21). In addition, quinoline-N-oxide which inhibits at the level of cytochrome b was used to assure inhibition of electrons flow which may arise from endogenous substrate oxidation. The addition of menadione or lapachol to the untreated or irradiated system with ascorbate-TPD did not inhibit the phosphorylation associated with the oxidation of this electron donor. Furthermore, it has been found that the analogues of vitamin K$_1$ did not inhibit the membrane bound latent ATPase activity.

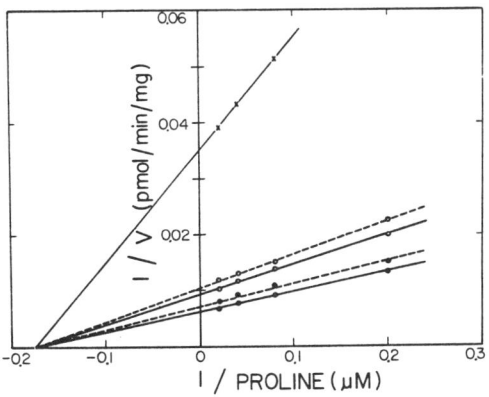

FIGURE 2. Lineweaver-Burk plots for proline transport. The assay of transport and the reaction mixture were similar to those described in Table I except various concentrations of proline were used. x—x, irradiated ETP; o--o, irradiated ETP + vitamin K$_1$ (0.5 mM); o—o, irradiated ETP + lapachol (0.4 mM); •--•, irradiated ETP + menadione (0.4 mM); •—•, ETP.

Restoration of pH Gradient in Irradiated Membrane Vesicles

The pH gradient across the membrane was determined by measuring the distribution of the weak base methylamine or by changes in fluorescence of 9-AA (see Methods). As shown in Fig. 3, the fluorescence of 9-AA was quenched when NADH was used as a substrate indicating the formation of a pH gradient in untreated and quinone-restored vesicles. Further

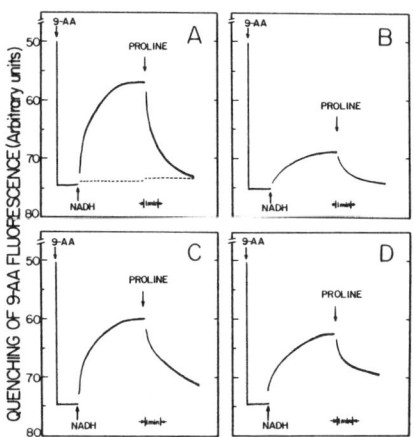

FIGURE 3. Quenching of 9-AA fluorescence
The reaction mixture was similar to that described in "Materials and Methods". At the time indicated NADH (0.5 mM) and proline (25 μM plus 10 mM NaCl) were added. A, non-irradiated ETP (——) and irradiated ETP (- - -); B, irradiated ETP + vitamin K_1 (0.5 mM); C, irradiated ETP + menadione (0.4 mM); D, irradiated ETP + lapachol (0.4 mM).

it was observed that the addition of proline and Na^+ (Fig. 3,A) or the proton conductor CCCP (data not shown) resulted in a dissipation of the pH gradient. Quenching of 9-AA fluorescence did not occur on addition of substrate to the irradiated membrane vesicles unless the specific naphthoquinones were added (Fig. 3,B,C, &D). Similar results were obtained by measuring the distribution of methylamine with a quantitative method such as the flow dialysis technique. The formation of a pH gradient upon substrate addition results in the accumulation of methylamine in untreated (0.5 pH unit) and quinone restored vesicles (Table III). The addition of proline and Na^+ or CCCP resulted in collapse of the proton gradient and the efflux of methylamine.

Effect of Inhibitors

The effect of respiratory inhibitors and uncoupling agents on proline transport was examined with the quinone restored system. As shown in

TABLE III. Restoration by naphthoquinones of a pH gradient in irradiated ETP

Addition	Incubation pH	pH_{ex}	pH_{in}	Gradient mean	range
ETP	7.52	7.62	7.10	0.52	(0.48-0.56)
Irradiated ETP	7.52	7.54	7.33	0.21	(0.20-0.25)
Irradiated ETP + vitamin K_1	7.48	7.57	7.22	0.35	(0.32-0.36)
Irradiated ETP + Menadione	7.52	7.61	7.16	0.45	(0.44-0.48)
Irradiated ETP + Lapachol	7.48	7.61	7.18	0.43	(0.40-0.45)

The pH distribution was determined by the distribution of [^{14}C]methylamine as described in "Materials and Methods". The upper chamber contained 50 mM Hepes-KOH buffer (pH 7.5), 10 mM $MgCl_2$, 10 mM NaCl, substrate (1.0 mM NAD^+, 20 mM hydrazine, 1 mg of alcohol dehydrogenase) and 2.0 mg of membrane protein in a total volume of 0.85 ml. The experiment was started by the addition of [^{14}C]methylamine at a final concentration of 27 µM. The upper and lower chamber were separated by cellulose dialysis tubing and both chambers were stirred continuously by means of small magnetic bars. The dialyzing buffer (Hepes-KOH, pH 7.5) was pumped through the lower chamber at a rate of 6.0 ml/min with a Buchler Multi-Static pump (Model No. 2-6200). Ethanol was added to the upper chamber to give a final concentration of 50 µM. Fractions of 2.0 ml were collected and assayed for radioactivity by liquid scintillation counter using Bray's solution. The mean value represents the average of three experiments. pH_{ex} indicates the external pH at the end of incubation and pH_{in} indicates internal pH.

Table IV, KCN inhibited the uptake of proline, whereas DCCD (an ATPase inhibitor and uncoupler) fail to inhibit the uptake of proline. However, restoration of proline transport by menadione was insensitive to KCN, since menadione can react directly with oxygen. In the presence of KCN under anaerobic conditions proline uptake was inhibited. Dicumarol (quinone analogue) or CCCP (a proton conducting uncoupler) inhibited the uptake of proline in the quinone reconstituted systems independent of the type of quinone used to restore proline uptake.

TABLE IV. The effect of inhibitors on the reconstituted active transport of proline.

Addition	Concentration	ETP pmol/mg	(% of Inh.)	Irradiated ETP + vitamin K_1 pmol/mg	(% of Inh.)	Irradiated ETP + menadione pmol/mg	(% of Inh.)	Irradiated ETP + lapachol pmol/mg	(% of Inh.)
None		227	-	113	-	217	-	161	-
KCN	10 mM	54	(76)	23	(80)	218	(0)	29	(82)
Dicumarol	1 mM	46	(80)	34	(70)	75	(65)	34	(79)
Carbonylcyanide m-chlorophenyl hydrazone	20 µM	54	(76)	53	(53)	50	(77)	29	(82)
N,N'-dicyclohexyl carbodiimide	0.6 mM	216	(5)	104	(8)	169	(22)	134	(17)

The assay of transport and the reaction mixture were similar to those described in "Materials and Methods". The inhibitors were preincubated with vesicles in the reaction mixture at the indicated concentrations for 10 min at 30°. Generated NADH system was used as the substrate. Proline uptake in irradiated membrane vesicles alone was 56 pmol/mg protein.

DISCUSSION

A subcellular role for naphthoquinones in respiration, coupled phosphorylation, pH gradient and active transport of amino acids has been demonstrated. Various quinone analogues appear to act as electron acceptors for different segments of the chain and donate electrons either to oxygen or to the cytochromes. This feature of the quinone bypass of the electron transport chain has permitted the studies on the mechanisms of the bioenergetic processes such as oxidative phosphorylation and active transport of solutes. The structural requirements or the specificity of naphthoquinones for restoration of these activities with the quinone-depleted system from M. phlei has been studied. The structural requirements for restoration of phosphorylation are more strict than those necessary for restoration of the active transport. It was found that the restoration of coupled phosphorylation required the presence of a methyl group in the C-2 position of the naphthoquinone and a β-γ unsaturated isoprenoid side chain.

Although the chemical coupling hypothesis and the chemiosmotic hypothesis have been entertained as possible mechanisms of the bioenergetic processes (22-24), Mitchell's chemiosmotic hypothesis is now well established for the respiration coupled ATP synthesis as well as for active transport. In a number of bacterial systems it has been demonstrated that the electrochemical gradient of protons, the protonmotive force, is a driving force for the active transport of solutes. Although the protonmotive force consists of a membrane potential and a proton gradient, certain transport systems may be driven primarily or solely by the proton gradient, or the membrane potential (25-30).

Attempts have been made to determine relationships between oxidation, pH gradient, proline transport and phosphorylation in membrane vesicles from M. phlei. As shown in Table V, the treatment of membrane vesicles with UV light at 360 nm resulted in photoinactivation of the natural menaquinone and in a loss of oxidation, pH gradient, active transport of proline, Ca^{2+} and phosphorylation. Various analogues of the natural quinone (MK_9(II-H)) of M. phlei such as vitamin K_1, menadione and lapachol can restore oxidation with NAD^+-linked substrate in the irradiated membrane vesicles. Both the pH gradient and proline transport can also be restored by these naphthoquinones, and there appeared to be a correlation between the level of proline uptake into the

TABLE V. Summary of activities restored by naphthoquinones

Addition	Oxidation	pH Gradient	Proline transport	Ca^{2+} uptake	P/O ratio
ETP	+	+	+	+	+
Irradiated ETP	-	-	-	-	-
Irradiated ETP + vitamin K_1	+	+	+	+	+
Irradiated ETP + Menadione	+	+	+	+	-
Irradiated ETP + Lapachol	+	+	+	+	—

restored membrane vesicles and the generation of pH gradient (Fig. 3). Furthermore, the addition of proline and Na^+ results in the collapse of a preformed pH gradient, indicating a direct link between these two processes. A proton gradient-dependent proline uptake has been previously demonstrated with the proteoliposomes prepared from purified proline carrier protein which was isolated from the membrane vesicles of M. phlei (31,32). A proton gradient was generated across the lipid bilayer by the reduction of the entrapped ferricyanide by ascorbate oxidation with benzoquinone serving as a lipid-soluble hydrogen carrier. The uptake of proline in this model system was inhibited by CCCP, and the movement of proline across the artificial membrane resulted in a simultaneous collapse of the proton gradient (32).

Active transport of Ca^{2+} was also inhibited in irradiated membrane vesicles and the restoration or Ca^{2+} occurred following addition of the naphthoquinones (vitamin K_1, menadione and lapachol). The degree of restoration of Ca^{2+} uptake by naphthoquinones was similar to that observed for the transport of proline. Furthermore, it should be noted that ATP driven Ca^{2+} uptake was not inhibited by UV irradiation (9); since the membrane-bound ATPase from M. phlei was found to be insensitive to UV irradiation (33).

Vitamin K_1 was capable of restoring both pH gradient and coupled phosphorylation, whereas menadione and lapachol were capable only of restoring the pH gradient. Therefore, the data presented in this paper showed that in addition to the pH gradient and the intactness of both the membrane and the coupling apparatus, other factors such as the membrane potential may be necessary in providing the driving force for oxidative phosphorylation. It is possible that restoration of coupled phosphorylation requires a conformational change in the membrane-bound coupling factor or other closely associated membrane proteins (34). Vitamin K_1 may restore phosphorylation since the entire respiratory chain may be involved in eliciting such conformational changes, whereas menadione which bypasses the respiratory chain cannot induce the changes in membrane associated proteins. Furthermore, certain naphthoquinones such as lapachol, dihydrophytyl vitamin K_1 or the cis geometric isomer of vitamin K_9(II-H) which utilize the complete respiratory chain and form a pH gradient, but fail to restore phosphorylation;which indicated the importance of the side chain in inducing changes favoring the energy transducing process.

Rottenberg (35) has also discussed proton transport across membranes and the lack of a direct mediation of this phenomena to coupled phosphorylation. As was pointed out by Rottenberg, all methods for the determination of internal pH, as well as of the membrane potential are subject to some question. Nevertheless, accumulated data as shown in this paper and other sources (35) utilizing various techniques, have raised serious doubts about a strict relationship between membrane potential, the proton gradient and energy transduction.

ACKNOWLEDGEMENTS

The authors wich to express their appreciation to Miss Nancy A. Telford for her technical assistance and to Miss Lynne Peschke for the typing of the manuscript. This work was supported by a grant from the National Institutes of Health, Grant # 5 RO1 AI05637-17.

REFERENCES

1. Cohen, N. S. and Brodie, A. F. (1975) J. Bacteriol. 123, 162-173.
2. Dunphy, P. J., Gutnick, D. L., Phillips, P. G. and Brodie, A. F. (1968) J. Biol. Chem. 243, 398-407.
3. Brodie, A. F. and Ballantine, J. (1960) J. Biol. Chem. 235, 226.
4. Brodie, A. F. and Watanabe, T. (1966) Vitamin and Hormones, 24, 447-463.

5. Brodie, A. F., Revsin, B., Kalra, V. K., Phillips, P., Bogin, E., Higashi, T., Krishna, M. C. R., Cavari, B. Z. and Marquez, E. (1970) in Natural substances formed biologically from Melavonic Acid, (Goodwin, T. W., ed) Biochem. Soc. Symp. 29, 119-143, Academic Press, New York.
6. Hirata, H., Asano, A. and Brodie, A. F. (1971) Biochem. Biophys. Res. Commun. 44, 368-374.
7. Hirata, H., Kosmakos, F. C. and Brodie, A. F. (1974) J. Biol. Chem. 249, 6965-6970.
8. Brodie, A. F., Lee, S. H. and Kalra, V. K. (1979) Microbiology 1979, 46-53.
9. Kumar, G. and Brodie, A. F. (1979) Eur. J. Biochem. In press.
10. Brodie, A. F. and Gray, C. T. (1956) J. Biol. Chem. 219, 853-862.
11. Brodie, A. F. (1959) J. Biol. Chem. 234, 398-404.
12. Brodie, A. F. and Ballantine, J. (1960) J. Biol. Chem. 235, 226-231.
13. Asano, A., Kaneshiro, T. and Brodie, A. F. (1965) J. Biol. Chem. 240, 895-905.
14. Schuldiner, S., Weil, R. and Kaback, H. R. (1976) Proc. Natl. Acad. Sci. USA 73, 109-112.
15. Waddell, W. J. and Butler, T. C. (1959) J. Clin. Invest. 38, 720-729.
16. Hunter, G. R. and Brierley, G. P. (1969) Biochim. Biophys. Acta 180, 68-80.
17. Jacobs, A. J., Kalra, V. K., Prasad, R., Lee, S. H., Yankofsky, S. and Brodie, A. F. (1978) J. Biol. Chem. 253, 2216-2222.
18. Schuldiner, S., Rottenberg, H. and Avron, M. (1972) Eur. J. Biochem. 25, 64-70.
19. Lowry, O. H., Rosebrough, N. J., Farr, A. L. and Randall, R. J. (1951) J. Biol. Chem. 193, 265-275.
20. Dowson, R. M. C., Elliot, D. C., Elliot, W. H. and Jones, K. M. (1969) Data for Biochem. Res. 2nd ed., 618, Oxford University Press, New York.
21. Orme, T. W., Revsin, B. and Brodie, A. F. (1969) Arch. Biochem. Biophys. 134, 172-179.
22. Mitchell, P. (1966) Biol. Rev. 41, 445-502.
23. Mitchell, P. and Moyle, J. (1969) Eur. J. Biochem. 7, 471-484.
24. Mitchell, P. (1974) FEBS Lett. 43, 189-194.
25. Simoni, R. D. and Postma, R. W. (1975) Ann. Rev. Biochem. 43, 523-554.
26. Harold, F. M. (1977) Curr. Top. Bioenerg. 6, 83-149.
27. Ramos, S. and Kaback, H. R. (1977) Biochemistry 16, 854-859.
28. Guffanti, A. A., Susman, P., Blanco, R. and Krulwich, T. A. (1978) J. Biol. Chem. 253, 708-715.
29. Lanyi, J. K. (1978) Biochemistry 17, 3011-3018.
30. Wilson, D. B. (1978) Ann. Rev. Biochem. 47, 965-993.
31. Lee, S. H., Jacobs, A. J., Cohen, N. S. and Brodie, A. F. (1979) Biochemistry (in press).
32. Lee, S. H. and Brodie, A. F. (1978) Biochem. Biophys. Res. Commun 85, 788-794.
33. Higashi, T., Kalra, V. K., Lee, S. H., Bogin, E. and Brodie, A. F. (1975) J. Biol. Chem. 250, 6541-6548.
34. Boyer, P. D. (1977) Ann. Rev. Biochem. 46, 957-966.
35. Rottenberg, H. (1975) Bioenergetics 7, 61-74.

VITAMIN K DEPENDENT SPHINGOLIPID SYNTHESIS IN *BACTEROIDES MELANINOGENICUS*

MEIR LEV and ALBERT MILFORD

Department of Microbiology & Immunology
Albert Einstein College of Medicine
Bronx, NY 10461

INTRODUCTION

Strains of B. melaninogenicus isolated from the bovine rumen have an obligate requirement for vitamin K (1). This property was subsequently found for other subspecies isolated from clinical material and the oral cavity (2). Vitamin K supplementation of media is now routine for the isolation of B. melaninogenicus and other fastidious anaerobes, although an obligate requirement for vitamin K is rare among microorganisms.

A microorganism with an obligate requirement for low levels of vitamin K provides an important system for the study of vitamin K mode of action. In practice the use of B. melaninogenicus presents a number of experimental difficulties; it is an obligate anaerobe with complex nutritional requirements, such as a requirement for heme from which a b type cytochrome is made and a peptide requirement (3,4). Thus a defined medium is not available and the genetics of this microorganism are not known. Succinate is important in the nutrition of B. melaninogenicus since with succinate supplementation slow growth can be maintained through serial subculture in the absence of vitamin K. The succinate grown cells respond to added vitamin K by an increase in growth rate.

The lipid content of B. melaninogenicus is unusual in that the cells contain two phosphosphingolipids ceramide phosphorylethanolamine (CPE) and ceramide phosphoryglycerol (CPG) in addition to phosphatidyl ethanolamine (PE) and phosphatidyl serine (PS) (5,6).

We have shown previously that vitamin K depletion results in cell membrane perturbation resulting in elongated cell formation (7). No effect of vitamin K depletion was found on protein, RNA or DNA synthesis. However, a specific defect in lipid synthesis was found in vitamin K depleted cells which was indicated initially be experiments on the uptake of succinate. Succinate was incorporated at 6x the rate in vitamin K depleted cells than in cultures grown with vitamin K and a significantly greater proportion of succinate carbon appeared in the lipid fraction of the cells.

Analysis of the phospholipids of vitamin K depleted cells showed that PS and PE were synthesized whereas synthesis of the phosphosphingolipids CPE and CPG was markedly reduced. The addition of vitamin K to a vitamin K depleted culture resulted in an increased rate of CPE and CPG synthesis before an increase in general cell metabolism as indicated by an increased rate of growth of the culture, whereas the synthesis of PE and PS was unchanged by addition of vitamin K (8). The stage of sphingolipid biosynthesis affected by vitamin K depletion and the mechanism involved are the subject of this paper.

MATERIALS AND METHODS

The microorganism B. melaninogenicus, subspecies levii (ATCC 29147), was that used in all experiments. The growth medium was the pancreatic digest of casein, yeast-extract medium supplemented with lysed red cells, and vitamin K_1 (0.1 µg/ml) (4). Vitamin K depleted cells were maintained in medium supplemented with lysed red cells plus 10^{-2} M sodium succinate. Assay methods for 3-ketodihydrosphingosine (3KDS) synthetase were described previously (9).

RESULTS

To determine which stage in sphingolipid synthesis was inhibited by vitamin K depletion of the culture, we examined the activity of the first enzyme of the sphingolipid pathway 3KDS synthetase which catalyses the formation of 3KDS from palmitoyl CoA + serine (Figure 1).

$$C_{15}H_{31}\overset{O}{\overset{\|}{C}}\text{-CoA} + \text{serine} \rightarrow C_{15}H_{31}\overset{O}{\overset{\|}{C}}\text{-CH-CH}_2\text{OH} + CO_2 + \text{CoA}$$
$$\underset{NH_2}{|}$$

Figure 1. Formation of 3-ketodihydrosphingosine (3KDS) from palmitoyl CoA and serine. The enzyme, 3KDS synthetase, has a cofactor, pyridoxal phosphate.

This enzyme is membrane bound and is solubilized by sonication. The activity was measured in extracts from cells grown with vitamin K, and in extracts of cells depleted of vitamin K by growth in a vitamin K free medium or in a medium supplemented with succinate. Good activity was found in extracts of the cells grown with vitamin K but the extracts of the vitamin K depleted cells showed only trace activity. The addition of vitamin K_1, (0.1 µg/ml) to a vitamin K depleted culture results in a linear increase in enzyme activity. This increase in synthetase activity is prevented by inhibitors of protein synthesis (puromycin) and RNA synthesis (rifampicin) (Figure 2A) indicating an effect of vitamin K on de novo synthesis of the enzyme (9).

This effect of vitamin K on synthetase activity was examined further using washed vitamin K-depleted cells. With these washed cells, addition of vitamin K_1 or menadione alone, does not affect synthetase activity (10). We have shown previously that glutamine is a specific energy source for B. melaninogenicus and is required for the incorporation of 3KDS into the complete sphingolipids, CPE and CPG (4).

When vitamin K_1 or menadione is added to washed vitamin K-depleted cells together with 50 mM glutamine, an increase in synthetase activity occurs (Figure 2B). Glutamine alone does not affect synthetase activity. With this system 1:4 naphthoquinone possessed < 30% the activity of either vitamin K_1 or menadione. Phthiocol (2 methyl-3-hydroxy- 1:4 naphthoquinone) which acts as an anti-vitamin K (11) and phenindione both inhibit the vitamin K_1 or menadione stimulated activity by 70-85%.

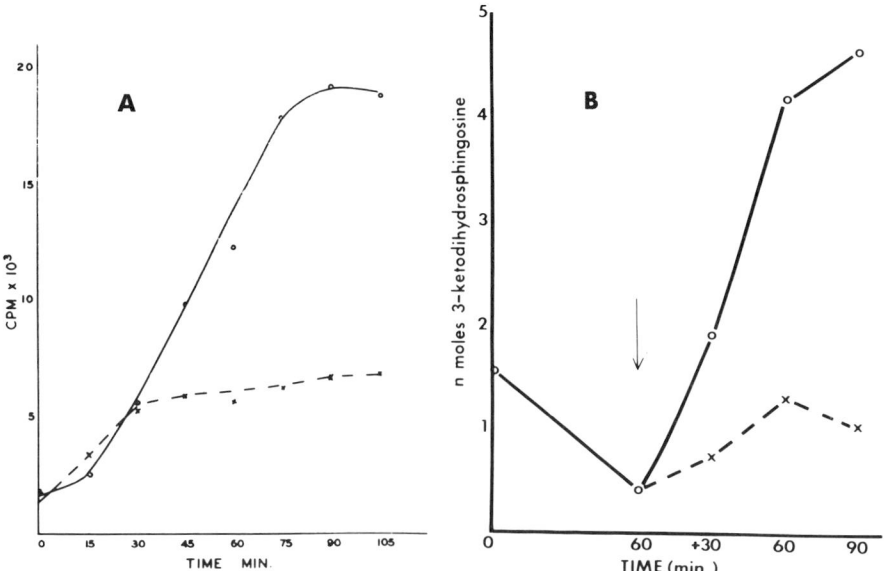

Figure 2A. Activation of 3KDS synthetase following addition of vitamin K to a vitamin K depleted culture 0──0. Inhibition by puromycin (50 μg/ml) x--x-- (9).

Figure 2B. Induction of 3KDS synthetase activity by vitamin K in washed vitamin K depleted cells. Cells are grown without vitamin K in the presence of 2×10^{-2} M succinate, washed, and suspended in phosphate buffer. Vitamin K_1 (20 μg/ml) and glutamine were added as indicated by the arrow. Samples were removed after 30, 60 and 90 min, further incubated and synthetase activity determined 0--0 plus vitamin K and glutamine x--x vitamin K_1 only.

Vitamin K is not a cofactor for 3KDS synthetase and does not enhance activity on incubation with cell-free extracts. Pyridoxal phosphate is a known cofactor for 3KDS synthetase. Earlier experiments had indicated that added pyridoxal phosphate did not affect synthetase activity when added to cell-free extracts (9). However, that the low synthetase activity found in vitamin K-depleted cells is related to a lack of pyridoxal phosphate was shown in two experiments. (1) The incubation of intact vitamin K depleted cells with increasing levels of pyridoxal phosphate resulted in a linear increase in synthetase activity in extracts of these cells and glutamine included with the pyridoxal phosphate enhanced this stimulation (Figure 3A). (2) The incubation of cell-free extracts of vitamin K-depleted cells with pyridoxal phosphate significantly increases synthetase activity and maximum stimulation occurred over the range 0.01 → 1mM (Figure 3B).

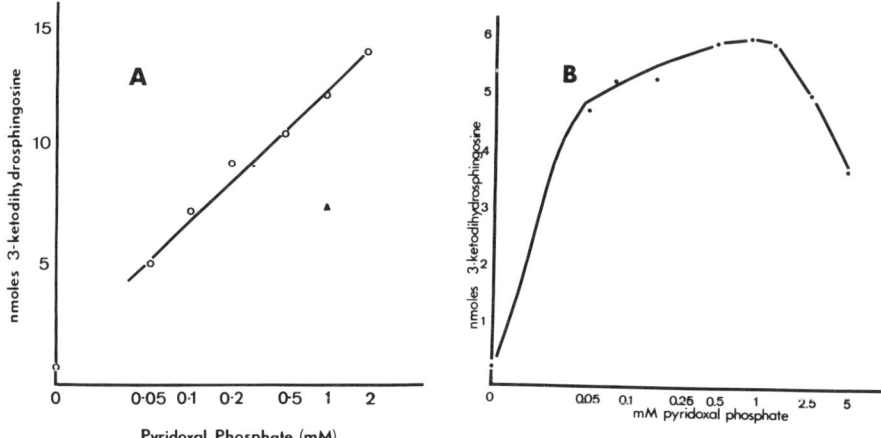

Figure 3A. Stimulation of 3KDS synthetase activity by pyridoxal phosphate. Vitamin K-depleted cells of B. melaninogenicus were washed and incubated with increasing levels of pyridoxal phosphate + 50 mM glutamine. The enzyme activity was then determined in cell-free extracts. A sample incubated with 1mM pyridoxal phosphate only (▲) showed 60% activity of the sample containing 1mM pyridoxal phosphate plus glutamine.

Figure 3B. Stimulation of 3KDS synthetase activity by pyridoxal phosphate in cell-free extracts of vitamin K depleted cells. Following a 60 min. incubation with pyridoxal phosphate, a significant stimulation in synthetase activity occurred between 0.05 and 1mM.

DISCUSSION

The mechanism of vitamin K mode of action in B. melaninogenicus was studied by vitamin K depletion of the cultures. A specific effect on phosphosphingolipid synthesis was found. Sribney (12) has presented evidence for the participation of vitamin K in sphingolipid synthesis in chicken liver.

To determine what stage in the synthesis of these complex lipids is affected by vitamin K depletion, the activity of first enzyme in sphingolipid pathway was examined. In contrast to eukaryotic systems this enzyme, 3KDS synthetase, can be solubilized and the activity determined in the supernatant of sonicated cells. The extracts of cells grown with vitamin K showed good activity, whereas trace activity was found in extracts of vitamin K depleted cells. The induction of enzyme activity by vitamin K was shown by the addition of vitamin K to a vitamin K depleted culture. A linear increase in activity occurred which was prevented by inhibitors of protein or RNA synthesis indicating that vitamin K induces de novo enzyme synthesis.

When vitamin K was added to washed vitamin K depleted cells as opposed to growing cultures, certain differences were found. For example, a specific energy source, glutamine, was required in conjunction with vitamin K_1 or menadione. 1:4 Naphthoquinone was a poor inducer compared with menadione and vitamin K_1, in contrast to what is found with growing cultures (11, 13).

Recent experiments have shown that the effect of vitamin K depletion on 3KDS synthetase activity is related to the pyridoxal phosphate level in the cell. The incubation of pyridoxal phosphate plus glutamine with washed cells or with cell-free extracts results in increased 3KDS synthetase activity. There is some specificity for pyridoxal phosphate since pyridoxal and pyridoxamine are inactive.

Thus, the specific inhibition of sphingolipid synthesis in cells of B. melaninogenicus found following vitamin K depletion is an indirect effect and appears mediated by the cofactor of the first enzyme of the sphingolipid pathway, pyridoxal phosphate.

The inhibition of the vitamin K stimulated synthetase activity found when inhibitors of protein and RNA synthesis are included in the reactions may, therefore, reflect an effect of these inhibitors on an enzyme(s) involved in the biosynthesis of pyridoxal phosphate. Experiments to determine activity of pyridoxal phosphate synthesizing enzymes in vitamin K supplemented and vitamin K depleted cultures are in progress.

REFERENCES

1. Lev, M. (1958) Nature 101, 203-204.
2. Holdeman, L. V., Cato, E. P. and Moore, W. E., Eds. (1977) Anaerobe Laboratory Manual 4th Ed. pp. 30-47. V.P.I. Anaerobe Laboratory. Virginia Polytechnic Institute and State University, Blacksburg, VA.
3. MacDonald, J. B., Socransky, S. S. and Gibbons, R. J. (1963) J. Dent. Res. 42, 529-544.
4. Lev, M. (1977) J. Bacteriol. 129, 562-563.
5. LaBach, J. P. and White, D. C. (1969) J. Lipid Res. 10, 528-534.
6. Rizza, V. A., Tucker, A. N. and White, D. C. (1970) J. Bacteriol. 101, 84-91.
7. Lev, M. (1968) J. Bacteriol. 95, 2317-2324.
8. Lev, M. and Milford, A. F. (1970) J. Lipid Res. 13, 364-370.
9. Lev, M. and Milford, A. F. (1973) Arch. Biochem. Biophys. 157, 500-508.
10. Lev, M. and Milford, A. F. unpublished observations.
11. Lev, M. (1959) J. Gen. Microbiol. 20, 697-703.
12. Sribney, M. (1971) Canad. J. Biochem. 69, 306-310.
13. Robins, D. J., Yee, R. B. and Bentley, R. (1973) J. Bacteriol. 116, 965-971.

BIOSYNTHESIS AND METABOLISM OF VITAMIN K IN INVERTEBRATES

J. F. PENNOCK and V. T. BURT

Biochemistry Department,
The University of Liverpool,
Liverpool, United Kingdom

INTRODUCTION

It is now well established that, in the formation of the four vitamin K-dependent blood clotting proteins, vitamin K is involved in the carboxylation of specific glutamyl residues to form γ-carboxy-glutamyl residues (GLA) so endowing calcium-binding properties to these proteins (1). It would indeed be most surprising if this K-dependent carboxylation system had evolved solely for the formation of four blood clotting proteins and it is much more likely that vitamin K is involved in the formation of many calcium-binding proteins. In the last few years several reports show the presence of GLA-containing protein in bone, kidney, ribosomes and some plasma proteins not associated with blood clotting (2,3,4,5). Prior to the discovery of GLA, work commenced in these laboratories to attempt to discover whether vitamin K had a role in animals other than its well established role in formation of blood clotting proteins. Accordingly a study of vitamin K metabolism was carried out in some invertebrates and particularly in the common shore crab, Carcinus maenas. Invertebrates were selected because blood, where present, is not coagulated by the well established mammalian system, but by a simple gel formation involving only one protein (6) and indeed some of the animals selected contained no blood system.

Initially 2-[^{14}C]methyl-1:4-naphthoquinone was injected into the shore crab Carcinus maenas and the small sea urchin Psammechinus miliaris and later experiments were carried out with [2-^{14}C] mevalonate in the presence of unlabelled menadione (7). In C. maenas radioactivity was incorporated into menaquinone-4 (MK-4) and the 2,3-epoxy derivative (MK-4 oxide) whereas P. miliaris synthesized only MK-4. All other invertebrates studied incorporated radioactivity from [2-^{14}C] mevalonate into MK-4 and some also made MK-4 oxide.

The subject of this communication is the study of the effect of warfarin on biosynthesis of vitamin K in the crab and on the growth of the brine shrimp Artaemia salina. Furthermore, attempts have been made to establish how the crab makes MK-4 in vivo. Menadione is not, as far as is known, a naturally occurring compound and so it must be assumed that the prenylating enzyme is either relatively non-specific with regard to the nuclear precursor or the crab is able to make menadione.

MATERIALS AND METHODS

Animals
C. maenas specimens were obtained from the Marine Biological Station, Millport, Isle of Cumbrae, Scotland, and were maintained in aerated sea-water aquaria at 8°C. Eggs of the brine shrimp A. salina were purchased from King British Aquarium Accessories Co. Ltd., Bradford, Yorkshire, U.K. The eggs were sprinkled on the surface of the sea water (ca 1 inch deep) and hatching occurred after two days at 21°C. After hatching the nauplii were fed on a dilute yeast solution and were used when about three weeks old.

Chemicals

[2-^{14}C]Mevalonate and [^{14}CH$_3$]methionine were obtained from The Radiochemical Centre, Amersham, Bucks., U.K. [2'-^{14}C] O-Succinyl benzoate was a gift from Dr. D. R. Threlfall, Dept. of Plant Biology, University of Hull, U.K. 1:4-Naphthoquinone and menadione were purchased from Hopkin and Williams, Chadwell Heath, U.K., O-succinyl benzoate and 2-carboxy-1,4-naphthoquinol were gifts from Dr. D. R. Threlfall and sodium warfarin was a gift from Ward Blenkinsop and Co. Ltd., Widnes, U.K. Menadione sodium bisulphite was a gift from Roche Products Ltd., Welwyn Garden City, U.K. Other chemicals and synthetic methods are as described by Burt et al (7).

Incorporation Studies

When studying the effect of warfarin on vitamin K biosynthesis in the crab, the animals received an injection of 1mg. of sodium warfarin in 0.1ml sea water at the same time as injection of 5µCi of [2-^{14}C] mevalonate and received further similar doses of warfarin at 5, 10 and 21 h after the initial injection. Menadione (1mg in 10% Tween 80/sea water) was administered by injection 1h before the mevalonate. Alternatively animals were injected with menadione and [2-^{14}C] mevalonate and maintained in sea water containing 0.075% sodium warfarin. The crabs were usually killed 24h after injection of the labelled mevalonate.

In experiments to examine the effect of various nuclear precursors on the biosynthesis of vitamin K in C. maenas, the nuclear precursor (58 nmole, the equivalent of 1mg menadione) was injected 1h before injection of [2-^{14}C]mevalonate (usually 5µCi).

Hepatopancreas tissue incubations were carried out using 1g. portions of C. maenas hepatopancreas (this tissue is very soft and can be converted into a slurry by gentle teasing apart with a scalpel and can then be pipetted with a relatively wide bore pipette). The incubation medium was 0.1M sodium phosphate buffer pH 7.4, containing 2.3% NaCl, 0.075% KCl, 0.1% MgCl$_2$, 0.03M nicotinamide and 0.125M sucrose. Also added were 2.5mM ATP, 0.2mM NADPH, 0.8mM NADP$^+$, 1mM EDTA, 2.5mM DTT and 5mM NaF. A mixture of penicillin/streptomycin was added to prevent bacterial contamination. The incubation was carried out in 5ml of buffer for 3h at 21°C and the reaction was started by the addition of 1µCi of [2-^{14}C]mevalonate in 0.1ml buffer and the required amount of menadione in 100µl ethanol. The reaction was stopped by the addition of 2:1 chloroform/methanol.

Incorporation into terpenoids was determined by extraction of lipids with chloroform/methanol and analysis by t.l.c. using both adsorption and reversed-phase procedures as described previously (7). High performance liquid chromatography (h.p.l.c.) was used in some cases to confirm identifications (8).

RESULTS

Interconversion of Phylloquinone and 2,3-Epoxy-phylloquinone in C.maenas

[1',2'-^{3}H]Phylloquinone (197µCi/mg) was synthesized and the related 2,3-epoxy derivative formed using H$_2$O$_2$ (9). Injection of 5µCi of tritiated phylloquinone into a male specimen of C. maenas resulted in

5% of the recovered radioactivity appearing in 2,3-epoxy-phylloquinone after 24h incubation. Only 2.1% of the recovered radioactivity when given 1.5μCi of tritiated 2,3-epoxy-phylloquinone was found in phylloquinone. Relatively large amounts of radioactivity were found in polar metabolites following administration of tritiated phylloquinone and epoxy-phylloquinone (36% and 21% of the recovered radioactivity respectively). This interconversion was small compared with the conversion of MK-4 to MK-4 oxide during incubation studies using $[2-^{14}C]$ mevalonate and menadione (the radioactivity in MK-4 oxide is usually only slightly less than that in MK-4).

Effect of Warfarin on The Synthesis of MK-4 and MK-4 Oxide in C. maenas

The effect of warfarin on the synthesis of MK-4 and the related MK-4 oxide was examined and the results are shown in Table 1.

TABLE 1. The Effect of Warfarin on Vitamin K Synthesis in the Crab

Sodium warfarin administered	$[2-^{14}C]$MVA (μCi)	Incubation time (h)	Radioactivity (dpm) MK-4	MK-4 oxide
1mg. injected[a]	5	24	36,200	41,730
None	5	24	46,540	30,770
0.075% in sea water[a]	5	24	6,450	20,630
None	5	24	56,050	45,550
0.075% in sea water	10	144	2,645	12,550
None	10	144	2,770	3,830

Each animal was injected with 1 mg menadione prior to injection with $[2-^{14}C]$mevalonate. [a]The warfarin was either injected into the animal or dissolved to 0.075% in the sea water of the incubation aquarium.

As can be seen the action of sodium warfarin is to increase the proportion of MK-4 oxide formed relative to MK-4 in each case. The effect is more dramatic when the animals are maintained in sea water containing sodium warfarin and there appears to be a considerable reduction in synthesis of vitamin K (MK-4 and MK-4 oxide) in the animal maintained in sodium warfarin/sea water compared with that injected with sodium warfarin. After a 6 day incubation the total radioactivity recovered in vitamin K is low but the proportion of MK-4 oxide present has increased even when no sodium warfarin was administered. The action of warfarin on vitamin K metabolism in the crab is thus similar to that found in the rat, i.e. an accumulation of the 2,3-epoxy derivative presumably by inhibition of the epoxide reductase (10).

The Effect of Warfarin and Vitamin K on the Survival of A. salina

During experiments on the effect of warfarin on vitamin K metabolism in C. maenas it was noted that some specimens died after being kept for several days in 0.075% sodium warfarin in sea water. To carry out a controlled experiment on the survival rate of these animals in sodium warfarin would have required large numbers and furthermore, because the crabs were captured from the sea as adults, there would be considerable individual variation. Accordingly large numbers of A. salina were grown and were used to examine the toxic nature of warfarin towards arthropods.

A. salina specimens were placed in sea water containing
concentrations of sodium warfarin from 0.075 - 0.20%. Dead animals were
removed at intervals and the survival measured over 120h. As can be seen
from figure 1 all concentrations proved toxic to the shrimp.

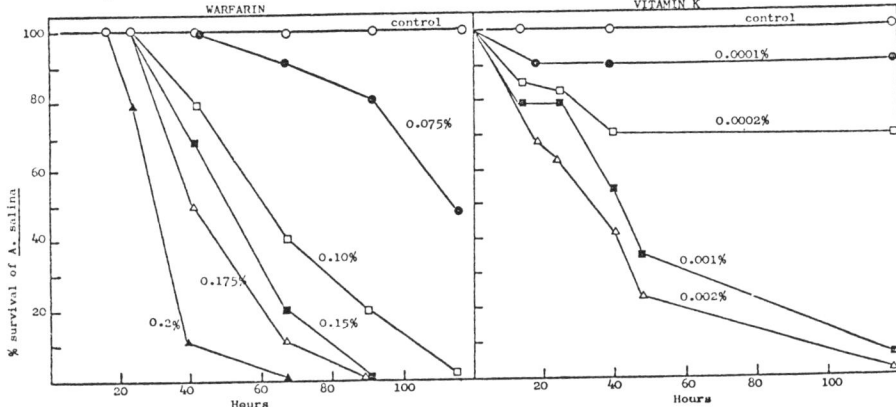

FIGURE 1 The effect of warfarin and vitamin K on the survival of A. salina.

To follow the effect of vitamin K on A. salina, a similar
experiment was carried out using a phylloquinone-phospholipid micelle,
using differing quantities of phylloquinone with a standard quantity of
phospholipid. Surprisingly the phylloquinone was much more toxic than
warfarin, as little as 0.001% proving fatal in the majority of animals
after 48h (Fig. 1). In the case of administration of vitamin K and
warfarin to the crab, C. maenas, it appears that the method of
assimilation is important. For instance, if a specimen is placed in
500 ml of 0.0005% phylloquinone in sea water it dies quite quickly, but
if an equivalent quantity of phylloquinone (2.5 mg) is injected into a
crab there appears to be no adverse effect. Thus it may well be that the
toxic effect is on the gills or perhaps alimentary canal and the latter
significantly turned black when A. salina was placed in either sodium
warfarin or phylloquinone solution.

However, in an attempt to connect vitamin K with warfarin action in
A. salina, a solution of 0.05% sodium warfarin was supplemented with
0.0002% phylloquinone and A. salina specimens added. The rate of
survival was identical with the control animals placed in 0.05% sodium
warfarin in sea water. There was little or no effect on animals placed
in 0.0002% phylloquinone.

The Nuclear Precursor of Menaquinone-4 in C. maenas

In the crab, C. maenas, [2-^{14}C]mevalonate can be incorporated into the
side chain of MK-4 in the presence of menadione as nuclear precursor.
To investigate the effect of menadione concentration on MK-4 synthesis in
C. maenas, varying amounts of menadione were incubated with 1g. portions
of hepatopancreas and 1μCi of [2-^{14}C]mevalonate (see Materials and
Methods). The results are shown in figure 2. As can be seen maximal
vitamin K (MK-4 and MK-4 oxide) production occurred with 250μg
menadione/g of hepatopancreas. Above 500μg of menadione, inhibition of

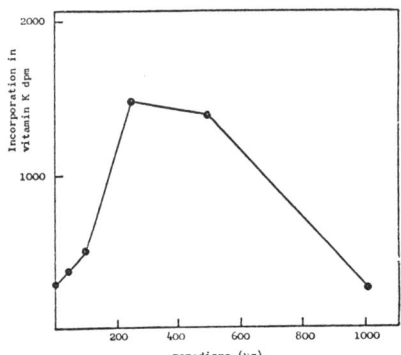

FIGURE 2 Stimulation of vitamin K (MK-4 and MK-4 oxide) biosynthesis in crab hepatopancreas.

vitamin K synthesis occurred. Significantly there was a small but marked synthesis of vitamin K in the absence of any added menadione. This was checked with an intact animal and quite clearly C. maenas synthesizes vitamin K following injection with [2-^{14}C]mevalonate and thus may be regarded as a normal endogenous compound in the animal.

To investigate the nature of the in vivo nuclear precursor of vitamin K in C. maenas, specimens were given equimolar amounts of several possible nuclear precursors together with 5µCi of [2-^{14}C]mevalonate. The two major candidates for the natural nuclear precursor seemed to be phylloquinone (or a menaquinone) or O-succinyl benzoate. Billeter and Martius (11) showed that pigeons and chickens were capable of removing the phytyl side chain of dietary phylloquinone and utilising the resulting menadione for MK-4 synthesis. They further suggested that the cleavage of the side chain might be accomplished by intestinal bacteria. Similarly Duello and Matschiner (12) showed utilization of the nucleus of phylloquinone for MK-4 synthesis in the dog. In bacteria (and plants) the naphthoquinone nucleus is assembled by condensation of an aromatic compound derived from shikimate with a succinyl group precursor to yield O-succinyl benzoate (13,14). Thus it might be possible for the crab to obtain O-succinyl benzoate from its gut flora or even by synthesis from benzoic acid and succinyl CoA.

Other compounds used as possible nuclear precursors were 1:4-naphthoquinone and menadione sodium bisulphite. Neither of these compounds has a natural occurrence but menadione sodium bisulphite has been used as a water-soluble vitamin K and it was of interest to find whether its activity depends on the conversion to MK-4. 1:4-Naphthoquinone is very similar to menadione and may test the specificity of the prenylating enzyme. The results of the experiments are shown in table 2.

TABLE 2. The Effect of Various Nuclear Precursors on the Incorporation of [2-^{14}C]Mevalonate into Vitamin K in C. maenas.

Nuclear precursor given (58µmole)	[2-^{14}C]Mevalonate	Vitamin K* (dpm)
None	5	4000
"	5	2824
"	8	21140
Menadione	5	77310
"	8	64360
"	10	101600
"	10	81200
Menadione sodium bisulphite	5	28600
Phylloquinone	8	7200
O-Succinyl benzoate	5	14300
Carboxynaphthoquinol	5	16260
Naphthoquinone	5	2248
"	10	18820
"	10	5900

* Vitamin K is estimated as MK-4 plus MK-4 oxide.

As can be seen no nuclear precursor stimulated vitamin K synthesis as much as menadione but menadione sodium bisulphite gave appreciable stimulation. This was not unexpected as at the pH of sea water (pH 8) menadione sodium bisulphite is converted to menadione. The experiments with no added nuclear precursor showed that there was a very considerable variation in vitamin K biosynthetic rates between different specimens. As can be seen the amounts of vitamin K synthesized in the presence of phylloquinone, O-succinyl benzoate, carboxynaphthoquinol and naphthoquinone fall within the control range (i.e. no nuclear precursor added).

Clearly the variation was such that it is very difficult to tell whether any stimulation had taken place. However, no precursor showed any stimulation to compare with menadione.

The Formation of Geranylgeranylnaphthoquinone (Demethyl MK-4)

In the experiments with naphthoquinone as a possible nuclear precursor of MK-4 when radiolabelled mevalonate was administered to a crab, a third radioactive material was detected in the 'vitamin K' region of t.l.c. chromatograms in addition to MK-4 and MK-4 oxide. This compound migrated between MK-4 and MK-4 oxide on reversed-phase t.l.c. (paraffin-impregnated Kieselguhr/90% aqueous acetone) with an Rf of 0.72 (MK-4 Rf 0.66, MK-4 oxide Rf 0.81). The amount of radioactivity in this compound varied between experiments but in one experiment when 5µCi of [2-^{14}C]mevalonate was injected with about 1mg of 1:4-naphthoquinone, 2248 dpm were recovered in MK-4 and MK-4 oxide while 28,040 dpm was detected in this compound. Geranylgeranyl naphthoquinone (demethylmenaquinone-4, DMK-4) seemed a likely candidate and synthesis of DMK-4 by standard methods (8) proved its identity. The unknown migrated with DMK-4 on adsorption, argentation and reversed phase t.l.c. and also on h.p.l.c. (8).

To investigate the possibility that the DMK-4, formed in the presence of naphthoquinone, was being converted by methylation with S-adenosyl methionine to MK-4 by C. maenas, a specimen of C. maenas was injected with [^{14}CH$_3$]methionine (25µCi) together with unlabelled naphthoquinone and mevalonate. Although radioactivity was detected in ubiquinone and choline-containing phospholipids (as would be expected) no radioactivity was detected in MK-4. Thus it would appear that DMK-4 formed in the presence of naphthoquinone is not converted to MK-4 in C. maenas.

O-Succinyl Benzoate and MK-4 Synthesis in the Crab

The results using O-succinyl benzoate as a nuclear precursor in the presence of [2-^{14}C]mevalonate proved inconclusive and we were fortunate at this stage to obtain a sample of [2'-^{14}C]O-succinyl benzoate. 3µCi of ^{14}C-labelled O-succinyl benzoate was injected into a crab and following a 20h incubation the lipids were extracted and examined. No radiolabel was detected in MK-4.

DISCUSSION

The data presented in this paper shows clearly that the crab, Carcinus maenas can form MK-4 as indicated by the incorporation of $[2-^{14}C]$-mevalonate and that this incorporation is greatly stimulated by the administration of menadione. Such a conversion had previously been

shown in chickens, rats and invertebrates, but with the use of radio-labelled menadione (7,15,16,17,18). It is much more convenient to use radiolabelled mevalonate to study MK-4 synthesis in the crab that in mammals because in mammals the great majority of injected mevalonate is incorporated into cholesterol. Arthropods such as C. maenas cannot synthesize squalene or cholesterol, there being a block between farnesyl pyrophosphate and squalene. Thus much more of the administered mevalonate is available for synthesis of other relatively minor terpenoids (in terms of amount present in the cell compared with cholesterol) such as ubiquinone, dolichol and vitamin K (19). Attempts in our laboratories to detect MK-4 synthesis in the rat using $[2-^{14}C]$-mevalonate and menadione have not been successful although MK-4 synthesis can be shown during radiolabelled menadione (17).

The formation of MK-4 in the crab encourages the idea that it has a role in this animal, which it must be stressed, has no prothrombin or similar blood clotting protein. Furthermore, the specificity of side-chain length (i.e. C_{20}, geranylgeranyl) used for vitamin K synthesis in all animals so far studied from the primitive coelenterate, Actinia equina through the phyla to mammals, e.g. the rat, is surely not without significance. The specificity of prenylating enzyme is underlined by the fact that the crab incorporates relatively large amounts of radioactivity into geraniol (C_{10}), farnesol (C_{15}) and geranylgeraniol (C_{20}) but only makes MK-4 (i.e. with a geranylgeranyl sidechain). Further evidence suggesting a similar role for vitamin K in crabs to that in mammals comes from the finding of 2,3-epoxymenaquinone-4 in crabs. The recent view that carboxylation of glutamyl residues and epoxidation of vitamin K are coupled, possibly through a common intermediate (20), puts great significance on the occurrence of the epoxide. Another very interesting fact which relates to this idea is that when radiolabelled mevalonate and 1:4-naphthoquinone were injected into a crab, radiolabel was detected in DMK-4 (demethyl menaquinone-4) but not in 2,3-epoxy demethyl menaquinone-4. This suggests that epoxidation of MK-4 to MK-4 oxide is not a non-specific reaction and the lack of epoxidation of DMK-4 is consistent with the finding that demethyl phylloquinone is inactive in a carboxylation system from liver microsomes (21).

The action of warfarin on vitamin K metabolism in the crab is entirely similar to that in the rat, i.e. it brings about an increase in the relative amount of 2,3-epoxy derivative present. This once again points to a common metabolic role in both animals. However, although warfarin is lethal in the invertebrate it was surprising to find that vitamin K was even more toxic. The effect is produced only when warfarin or vitamin K is administered in the immediate environment of the animal and appears not to have any harmful effect when injected. It may well be that the vitamin K presented in a phospholipid micelle is assimilated better than the completely water-soluble sodium warfarin. The brine shrimp in particular may well deliberately ingest these micelles as food. Nevertheless the inability of weak vitamin K solutions to prevent the harmful effects of warfarin suggests a general toxic effect.

The synthesis of MK-4 from menadione and geranylgeranyl pyrophosphate in animals is puzzling. In bacteria and plants the key intermediate appears to be O-succinyl benzoate, a compound formed from a shikimic acid derivative and a succinyl group precursor (13). O-Succinyl benzoate is converted to 2-carboxy-1:4-naphthoquinol (14) and Shineberg and Young (22) found that the carboxynaphthoquinol is prenylated to form demethyl menaquinone, 1:4-naphthoquinol not being an intermediate. Furthermore menadione is not considered to be a normal intermediate in menaquinone biosynthesis (23). The inability of the crab to incorporate O-succinyl benzoate into MK-4 indicates that it does not possess a biosynthetic pathway akin to that in bacteria. Also, although demethyl menaquinone appears to be an intermediate in menaquinone biosynthesis in bacteria (22) it does not appear to be so in the crab although DMK-4 is formed if the animal is supplied with naphthoquinone (see figure 3).

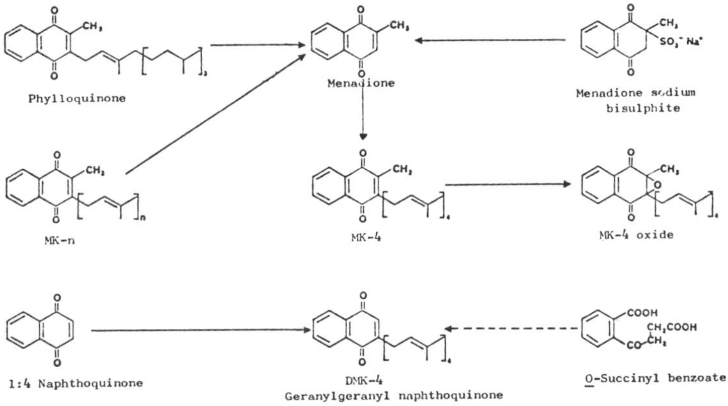

FIGURE 3 Possible interrelationships in vitamin K biosynthesis.

How then does the animal get its nuclear precursor? It seems unlikely that it is being assembled from relatively common metabolites in the crab and at the present time the pathway proposed by Billeter and Martius (11) appears to be the only feasible route. Some dietary vitamin K may have its sidechain removed (by intestinal bacteria according to Billeter and Martius) and the menadione so produced is used by the animal for MK-4 synthesis. Administration of phylloquinone either by feeding or injection has been unable to stimulate MK-4 synthesis in the crab to anything like the level produced by menadione. Perhaps it is impossible to achieve the rates of MK-4 biosynthesis when given menadione, by administration of a 'natural' precursor. If for instance dietary vitamin K is the source of menadione then the rate at which the animal or intestinal flora can deprenylate the ingested vitamin K may be the limiting factor. By-passing this limitation by injection of menadione may produce extremely high rates of synthesis of MK-4 completely unrelated to normal rates.

REFERENCES

1. Stenflo, J., and Suttie, J. W. (1977) Ann. Rev. Biochem. 46, 157-172
2. Hauschka, P. V., Lian, J. B., and Gallop, P. M. (1975) Proc. Natl. Acad. Sci. USA 72, 3925-29
3. Hauschka, P. V., Friedman, P. A., Traverso, H. P. and Gallop, P. M. (1976) Biochem. Biophys. Res. Commun. 71, 1207-1213
4. Van Buskirk, J. J., and Kirsch, W. M. (1978) Biochem. Biophys. Res. Commun. 80, 1033-1037
5. Stenflo, J. (1976) J. Biol. Chem. 251, 355-363
6. Fuller, G. M. and Doolittle, R. F. (1972) Invertebrate Immune Defense Mechanisms, pp 190-202, M.S.S. Information Corp., New York
7. Burt, V. T., Bee, E., and Pennock, J. F. (1977) Biochem. J. 162, 297-302
8. Donnahey, P. L., Burt, V. T., Rees, H. H., and Pennock, J. F. (1979) J. Chromatog. 170, 272-277
9. Tishler, M., Fieser, L. F., and Wendler, N. L. (1940) J. Am. Chem. Soc. 62, 2866-2871
10. Bell, R. G., and Matschiner, J. T. (1972) Nature 237, 32-33
11. Billeter, M., and Martius, C. (1960) Biochem. Z. 333, 430-439
12. Duello, T.J., and Matschiner, J. T. (1971) Int. J. Vitam. Nutr. Res. 41, 180-188
13. Dansette, P., and Azerad, R. (1970) Biochem. Biophys. Res. Commun. 40, 1090-1095
14. Bryant, R. N. and Bentley, R. (1976) Biochemistry, 15, 4792-4796
15. Martius, C., and Esser, H. (1958) Biochem. Z. 331, 1-9
16. Martius, C., Semandeni, E. G., and Alvino, C. (1965) Biochem. Z. 342, 492-494
17. Taggart, W. V. and Matschiner, J. T. (1969) Biochemistry 8, 1141-1146
18. Dialemeh, G. H., Yekundi, K. G., and Olson, R. E. (1970) Biochim. Biophys. Acta 223, 332-338
19. Walton, M. J., and Pennock, J. F. (1972) Biochem. J. 127, 471-479
20. Larson, A. E., and Suttie, J. W. (1978) Proc. Natl. Acad. Sci. USA 75, 5413-5416
21. Friedman, P. A., and Shia, M. (1976) Biochem. Biophys. Res. Commun. 70, 647-654
22. Shineberg, B., and Young, I. G. (1976) Biochemistry 15, 2754-2758
23. Baldwin, R. M., Snyder, C. D., and Rapoport, H. (1974) Biochemistry 13, 1523-1530

NON-PLASMA VITAMIN K–DEPENDENT PROTEINS

STRUCTURE AND FUNCTION OF THE VITAMIN K-DEPENDENT PROTEIN OF BONE

PAUL A. PRICE, DAVID J. EPSTEIN,
JOSEPH W. LOTHRINGER, SATORU K. NISHIMOTO,
JAMES W. POSER, and MATTHEW K. WILLIAMSON

Department of Biology,
University of California at San Diego,
La Jolla, CA 92093

INTRODUCTION

The most abundant non-collagenous protein in bone is a low molecular weight protein which contains three residues of γ-carboxyglutamic acid (Gla). This protein, which we have termed bone Gla protein (1), has also been called osteocalcin based on its binding affinity for calcium (2) (Kd=3mM). We present here a brief review of our earlier work on the structure and biosynthesis of this novel protein (1,3,4) followed by a summary of recently completed investigations which clearly demonstrate that the bone Gla protein is not required for biological mineralization. We also present our recent work with a specific radioimmunoassay for the human Gla protein. This investigation shows that the bone Gla protein is present in human plasma and that the plasma levels are elevated dramatically in human bone diseases characterized by an increased rate of bone resorption.

RESULTS

Structure of Bone Gla Protein

The complete covalent structures of Gla proteins from calf leg cortical bone and swordfish vertebral cancellous bone were determined (3,5). As is evident from the comparison of these structures (Figure 1), each protein has the three Gla residues and single disulfide bond in identical sequence positions. The calf Gla protein also has a second unusual amino acid, 4-hydroxyproline, at position 9. Neither bone Gla protein has any

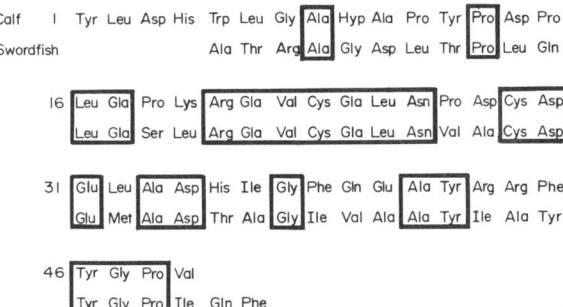

FIGURE 1 Sequence homology between calf and swordfish bone Gla proteins.

sequence homology with the vitamin K-dependent blood coagulation factors. In addition, adjacent pairs of Gla residues which are found in each blood coagulation factor are absent in the bone Gla proteins. The specificity of glutamic acid γ-carboxylation in the bone proteins appears to depend on sequence position; all Glu residues from the N-terminal to Glu_{31} are γ-carboxylated in both proteins. A similar N-terminal location of all Gla residues is found in prothrombin (6).

Biosynthesis in Bone Culture

Direct proof that bone Gla protein is synthesized in bone was obtained through analysis of the proteins labeled with radioactive proline during in vitro culture of calf bone (4). In these experiments, coincident elution of proline label and Gla protein upon DEAE Sephadex chromatography, and comigration of label and Gla protein on gel electrophoresis, and the expected ratio of proline label in the tryptic peptides derived from the labeled proteins (4) confirmed the in vitro synthesis of Gla protein. Thermal decarboxylation of Gla to Glu (see below) resulted in an identical shift in the isoelectric point of both radioactive Gla protein from bone culture and native calf Gla protein. Thus, the labeled protein must be fully γ-carboxylated during synthesis in bone culture.

The bone culture system was also employed to determine the rate of Gla protein biosynthesis and the effect of Warfarin on biosynthesis. As seen in Table 1, Gla protein is synthesized at the same slow relative rate as bone matrix collagen, suggesting that the Gla protein, like collagen, is a component of the slow turnover pool of bone matrix proteins (4). This evidence, combined with the presence of 4-hydroxyproline in both bone Gla protein and collagen, suggests that Gla protein is, like collagen, synthesized in bone by osteoblasts. Addition of Warfarin to the culture medium completely inhibits the biosynthesis of the Gla protein with no effect on the rate of general protein synthesis in bone culture (4). Examination of the bone after Warfarin culture failed to demonstrate even 1 percent of labeled protein in the gel electrophoresis positions characteristic of native or thermally decarboxylated Gla proteins (4).

TABLE 1. Protein Synthesis in Calf Bone Culture.

Trabecular bone was cultured with [^{3}H] proline for 24 h and then fractionated into the three protein components. The specific radioactivity values were determined by amino acid analysis (4).

Protein Fraction	Specific Radioactivity of [^{3}H]-Proline, cpm/μmol Pro + Hyp (x10^{-4})
Collagen	1.0
Gla Protein	1.1
Other Noncollagenous Proteins	88

Role of γ-Carboxyglutamic Acid

In order to probe the role of γ-carboxyglutamic acid in the function of the protein, we have developed a specific thermal decarboxylation procedure to convert Gla to Glu in the bone Gla protein (7). This procedure entails freeze-drying the Gla protein from appropriate buffers followed by heating at 110° in the dry state; control experiments with several enzymes established that this heating procedure does not effect enzymic activity (7).

The thermally decarboxylated protein has been compared with the native Gla protein in several experiments. Ca^{2+} binding to the Gla protein is abolished by thermal decarboxylation (7); this identifies the three Gla residues as components of the binding sites for the three Ca^{2+} atoms which bind weakly to the Gla protein (K_d=3mM)(5). A characteristic property of the Gla protein is its ability to retard the precipitation of calcium phosphate salts from supersaturated solutions at physiological pH (1,7). Thermal decarboxylation also eliminates this ability. Reduction of the disulfide bond which, like the Gla residues, is part of the conserved structure of the protein (Figure 1), also reduces the ability to retard precipitation.

Direct comparison between the binding of native and thermally decarboxylated protein to hydroxyapatite, the mineral phase of bone, is complicated by the high affinity of both species for mineral (7). Titration of protein with mineral, at high concentrations of both, demonstrates that the number of protein binding sites on the crystal is the same for both species (7). To probe the affinity of the native and decarboxylated proteins directly, we have used ^{125}I-labeled calf bone Gla protein. In this way, the concentration of protein can be estimated accurately at levels which are always negligible relative to the number of binding sites on mineral. The titration curves thus obtained for native and decarboxylated Gla proteins are compared in Figure 2. The binding behavior of the iodinated native Gla protein exhibits a simple logarithmic binding isotherm consistent with the interaction of a single species with identical non-interacting binding sites (8). The affinity of the native protein is approximately $10^{-7}M$ (in apatite binding sites) or 0.01 mg/ml (in weight of apatite) at pH 7.4 and 25°. In contrast, the broad binding isotherm of the decarboxylated Gla protein is not consistent with a single class of non-interacting binding sites.

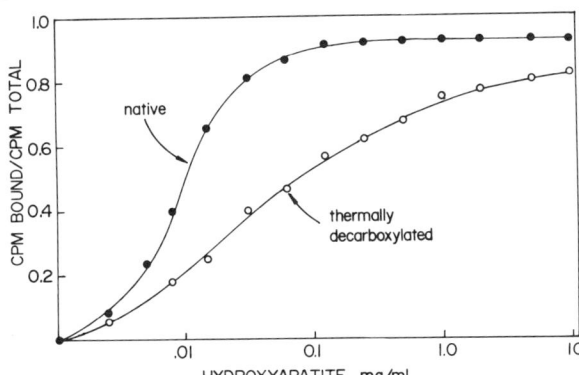

FIGURE 2. Role of γ-Carboxyglutamate in Binding of Bone Gla Protein to Synthetic Hydroxyapatite. ^{125}I-bone Gla protein or ^{125}I-decarboxylated bone Gla protein (7) was incubated with indicated suspension of hydroxyapatite for 1 hr at pH 7.4 and 25°. Extent of protein binding was assayed by monitoring ^{125}I-protein in the supernatant after removal of hydroxyapatite by centrifugation (8).

The mode of native Gla protein binding to hydroxyapatite requires direct association between the side chain carboxyl groups of Gla and the mineral surface, as is shown by the fact that the Gla protein bound to hydroxyapatite is protected from thermal decarboxylation (7). Thus we conclude that γ-carboxyglutamate permits the Gla protein to form a specific, high affinity complex with the mineral surface. This type of complex is clearly required for inhibition of calcium phosphate precipitation and may also be required for other biologically relevant processes.

Effects of Warfarin on Gla Protein Biosynthesis in Rabbits

We have devised a protocol in which young, growing rabbits can be maintained on a high dosage of Warfarin (9). Intravenous administration of purified rabbit clotting factors is a critical aspect of this protocol. In the absence of this procedure, the rabbits invariably died of hemorrhage within three days when given as little as 10 percent of the Warfarin dose employed.

The rabbits on Warfarin increase in body weight at almost the same rate as do control rabbits, about a 3-fold weight gain in the first 21 days of Warfarin treatment. The long bones of the rabbits increase in length, thickness, and mass also at approximately the rate as the bones of control rabbits. By approximately 35 days, the diameter of the marrow cavity exceeds the outer diameter of the original bone shaft. Thus, chemical analysis of the long bones obtained from rabbits maintained on Warfarin for various times should reflect the increasing contribution of bone synthesized during Warfarin treatment.

For chemical analysis, the long bones of rabbits were removed, freed of adhering tissue, dried and ground to a fine powder. The γ-carboxyglutamate content per weight of this bone was determined following alkaline hydrolysis of 25 mg of bone and subsequent amino acid analysis (1). As seen in Figure 3, the Gla content of the rabbit long bones declines rapidly after the initiation of Warfarin treatment, reaching a constant five percent of the control rabbit level after fifty days.

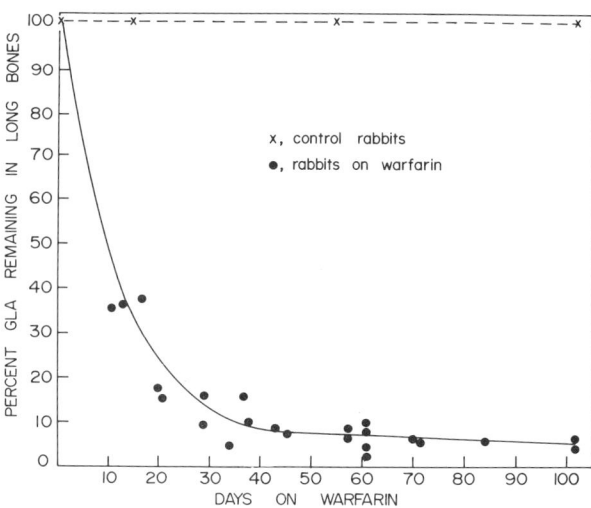

FIGURE 3. Warfarin Inhibition of γ-carboxyglutamate Formation in Growing Rabbit Bones. x, control rabbits; ●, rabbits on warfarin. For details, see text and (9).

The effect of Warfarin on the Gla protein content of rabbit bone is shown in Figure 4. Clearly, the decline in Gla content has been paralleled by a corresponding decline in the level of Gla protein. No non-γ-carboxylated Gla protein is observed in the position expected from studies with the thermally decarboxylated protein. To evaluate the possible presence of a non-γ-carboxylated Gla protein or Gla protein precursor more fully, we developed a specific radioimmunoassay for the rabbit Gla protein. This assay is equally sensitive to native and thermally decarboxylated Gla protein and is not affected by cyanogen bromide treatment, undoubtedly because the protein contains no methionine (9). Samples were prepared by cyanogen bromide digestion, which permitted the simultaneous and complete solubilization of all bone mineral and protein (9). Radioimmunoassays performed on appropriate dilutions of this solubilized bone showed that the Gla protein level was 3% of the control rabbit level in a Warfarin treated rabbit whose Gla content was 5% of the normal level. Thus, we conclude that the Warfarin treated rabbit bones have neither a non-γ-carboxylated Gla protein nor an immunoreactive non-γ-carboxylated precursor.

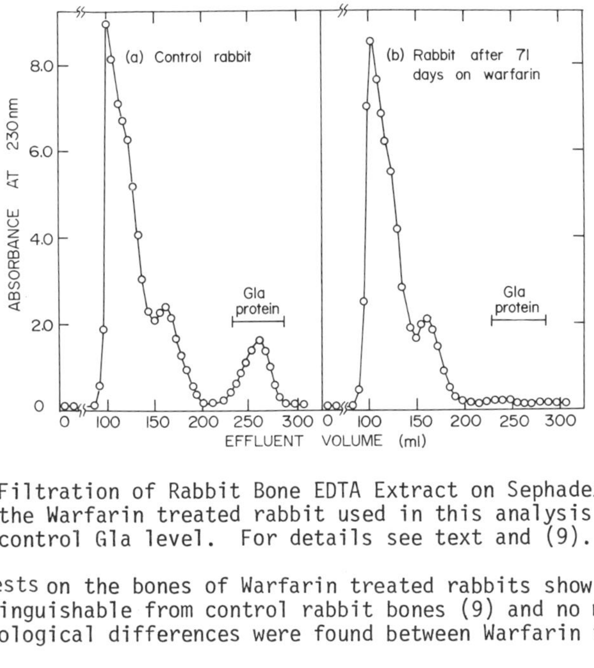

FIGURE 4. Gel Filtration of Rabbit Bone EDTA Extract on Sephadex G100. The bones from the Warfarin treated rabbit used in this analysis had 4 percent of the control Gla level. For details see text and (9).

Strength tests on the bones of Warfarin treated rabbits show that they are indistinguishable from control rabbit bones (9) and no morphological or histological differences were found between Warfarin treated

TABLE 2. Mineralization in Warfarin Treated Rabbits.*

Sample	γ-Carboxyglutamic acid	Proline	Phosphate	Calcium	Calcium/Phosphate
	nm	nm	moles x10^6	moles x10^6	
Warfarin Rabbit	0.07	177.1	4.36	5.97	1.37
Control Rabbit	1.52	179.5	4.30	5.79	1.34

* For details see (9).

rabbits and controls. The mineral and protein content of these bones is also normal (Table 2), and the infrared spectrum (10) of this mineral is identical with that of age-matched control rabbit bones (9). Thus, essentially complete depletion of Gla protein in rapidly growing bone fails to evoke any observable anomalies of mineralization. These data appear to preclude any important role for Gla protein in mineralization.

Absence of Gla Protein in Early Mineralization in the Rat

We have developed a specific radioimmunoassay to the rat bone Gla protein in order to follow its appearance during development (11), and have also established a rapid and quantitative method to extract the Gla protein from bone for direct analysis by this assay (11). Using these procedures we have discovered that negligible amounts of Gla protein are present in rat done during the early stages of mineralization (Figure 4). Fetal limb bones obtained from rat at 20 days of gestation (approximately 1 day before birth) have 41% of the adult bone mineral level and only 0.05% of the adult bone Gla protein content. This result clearly shows that Gla protein is not needed for initial mineralization during rat development. The level of Gla protein per weight of mineral rises over 2 orders of magnitude within 16 days of birth (Figure 4), leading to the conclusion that the biological function of this protein only requires its presence in bone at some time in the first 10 days following birth.

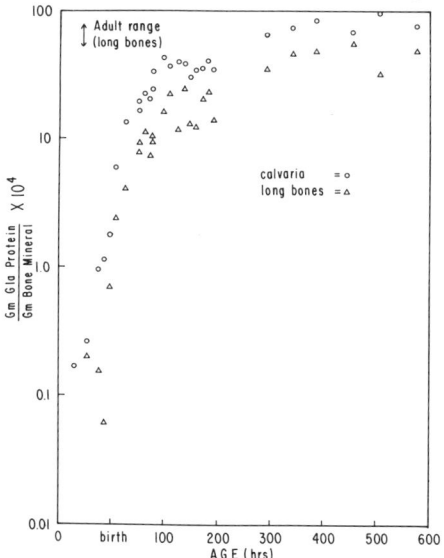

FIGURE 5. Developmental Appearance of Gla Protein in Rat Bone As Determined by Radioimmunoassay (11). o, calvaria; Δ, long bones.

Bone Gla Protein in Human Plasma

Using a specific radioimmunoassay for the detection of human Gla protein, we have shown that this protein is present in human blood plasma and urine (12). The Gla protein found in plasma has the same molecular weight as the bone protein and also appears to be identical by immunological criteria (12). Since the Gla protein is the most abundant non-collagenous bone protein and is not known to occur in significant concentrations in non-calcified tissues, its appearance in plasma suggests that plasma levels may reflect the underlying state of bone metabolism. Analysis of plasma from patients with bone diseases confirms this expectation (Table 3)(12,13). Plasma from patients with bone diseases characterized by increased rates of bone turnover, such as Paget's disease, primary and secondary hyperparathyroidism, and metastatic bone cancer, all have plasma Gla protein levels significantly above normal. Extensive clinical experiments in collaboration with Dr. Leonard J. Deftos of the UCSD Department of Medicine indicate that plasma Gla protein levels may be a more useful measure of some bone diseases than the standard alkaline phosphatase method used to determine bone turnover (13).

TABLE 3. Plasma Levels of Bone Gla Protein in Bone Diseases

Plasma Sample	N	Plasma Gla Protein Average, ng/ml
Normals	69	4.9
Bone Fractures	27	4.7
Paget's Disease of Bone	11	16
Primary Hyperparathyroidism	12	12
Renal Osteodystrophy	10	22
Metastatic Bone Disease	8	26

DISCUSSION

The biological function of bone Gla protein is not known. The experimental data detailed in this paper appear, however, to preclude several functions that have been postulated for the protein (14). The Warfarin treated rabbits have bones essentially free of Gla protein, yet the bones grow normally and appear normal by chemical, histological, and biomechanical criteria (9). These data cannot be reconciled with a proposed structural role for the Gla protein. The absence of Gla protein in rapidly mineralizing fetal rat bone also precludes a critical role for the protein in initial mineralization (11). Indeed, the _in vitro_ effect of Gla protein on supersaturated calcium phosphate is the inhibition of precipitation rather than epitactic nucleation (1,7).

With the body of experimental data weighing against a structural or catalytic role for bone Gla protein, tentative assignment of Gla protein as an informational molecule seems justified. Several characteristics of the molecule are consistent with such a postulate. The relatively low molecular weight is comparable to other peptide hormones. The protein is abundant in its tissue of origin and appears in fairly constant trace quantities in serum, again consistent with behavior of peptide hormones. The calf Gla protein contains the unusual dipeptide Pro-Lys which has been recently postulated as an effector site in several informational proteins (15).

In a role as an informational protein, two speculative modes of action for the Gla protein can be envisioned. In the first, the protein would serve in bone to modulate the localization or activity of osteolytic and osteoblastic cells. The specific binding properties of the protein might target particular bone domains for osteolytic or mineralizing cellular activity. An alternate role for an informational bone Gla protein would be to serve as a humoral messenger, a hormone. Bone Gla protein released upon dimineralization could exert feedback on the calcitonin-PTH system and thus play a role in calcium homeostasis. Experiments are currently underway employing bone cell culture chemotactic assays and pharmacologic manipulation of Ca^{++} homeostasis in intact animals to probe any hormonal or cell effector function of the Gla protein of bone.

ACKNOWLEDGEMENTS

Supported in part by USPHS grant GM 17702.

REFERENCES

1. Price, P.A., Otsuka, A.S., Poser, J.W., Kristaponis, J., and Raman, N. (1976) Proc. Natl. Acad. Sci. USA 73, 1447-1451.
2. Hauschka, P.V., and Gallop, P.M. (1977) in Calcium Binding Proteins and Calcium Function, (Wasserman, R.H. ed) pp. 338-347, Elsevier, Amsterdam.
3. Price, P.A., Poser, J.W., and Raman, N. (1976) Proc. Natl. Acad. Sci. USA 73, 3374-3375.
4. Nishimoto, S.K., and Price, P.A., (1979) J. Biol. Chem. 254, 437-441.
5. Price, P.A., Otsuka, A.S., and Poser, J.W. (1977) in Calcium Binding Proteins and Calcium Function, (Wasserman, R.H. ed.) pp. 333-337, Elsevier, Amsterdam.
6. Stenflo, J., and Suttie, J.W. (1977) Annu. Rev. Biochem. 46, 157-172.
7. Poser, J.W., and Price, P.A. (1979) J. Biol. Chem. 254, 431-436.
8. Price, P.A., and Epstein, D.J. (submitted for publication)
9. Price, P.A., and Williamson, M.K. (submitted for publication)
10. Termine, J.D., and Posner, A.S. (1966) Science 153, 1523-1525.
11. Price, P.A., and Lothringer, J.W. (submitted for publication)
12. Price, P.A., and Nishimoto, S.K. (submitted for publication)
13. Price, P.A., and Deftos, L.J. (submitted for publication)
14. Lian, J.B., Hauschka, P.V., and Gallop, P.M. (1978) Fed. Proc. 37, 2615-2620.
15. Tzehoval, E., Segal, S., Stabinsky, Y., Fridkin, M., Spirer, Z., and Feldman, M. (1978) Proc. Natl. Acad. Sci. USA 75, 3400-3404.

OSTEOCALCIN IN DEVELOPING BONE SYSTEMS

PETER V. HAUSCHKA

Children's Hospital Medical Center and
Harvard School of Dental Medicine,
Boston, MA 02115

INTRODUCTION

Osteocalcin is an abundant Ca^{2+}-binding protein of bone which is distinguished by its high content of γ-carboxyglutamic acid (Gla). Chicken bone osteocalcin, which was first isolated from neutral EDTA extracts of bone powder (1), has a molecular weight of 6500, contains 4 Gla residues / 57 total amino acid residues, and binds 2 Ca^{2+} ions with high specificity at K_d = 0.8mM (2). Each mg of dry mineralized adult chicken long bone diaphysis contains about 3 μg of osteocalcin, accounting for about 1.2% of the total protein. After collagen, osteocalcin is the next most abundant protein in bone; numerically there is one molecule of osteocalcin for every one or two molecules of bone tropocollagen (2). Many papers have addressed osteocalcin properties such as: purification and characterization (1-3), Ca^{2+} binding (2), inhibitory action in calcium phosphate mineral transitions (2,3), sequence (4), biosynthesis by bone microsomes (5,6), and the vitamin K-dependence (7) and developmental aspects of its biosynthesis (8).

Interaction between Ca^{2+} ions and solid phases of calcium phosphate with protein and phospholipid constituents of the organic matrix of bone is a key element in control of bone mineralization and turnover. Osteocalcin first appears in developing bone coincident with the onset of mineralization (8). Vitamin K and osteocalcin have been implicated in the fetal warfarin syndrome affecting bone mineralization, as well as in other aspects of Ca^{2+} metabolism (6,7,9). Recently, a strong correlation has been established in our laboratory between osteoporosis and elevated levels of urinary Gla excretion (Gundberg and Gallop, unpublished results). Presumably this results from abnormal catabolism of osteocalcin in the rapidly resorbing bone.

This report presents further studies of osteocalcin in developing bone and provides some initial evidence of a complex pathway of osteocalcin biosynthesis.

MATERIALS AND METHODS

Chick embryos were incubated, dissected, stained with alizarin red for examination of skeletal mineralization, and assessed for Hamburger-Hamilton developmental stage as before (8). Day-old chicks were raised on standard diets at 28° in constant light (7,8). 17 d chick embryo long bones were dissected free of adhering tissue and frozen immediately in liquid N_2. After homogenization in 50% pyridine at 0° to destroy latent protease activity, the bone fragments were washed with water, acetone, ether, and dried before pulverization to a fine powder in liquid N_2 (100 mesh). Adult (10 wk Penobscot) chicken long bone (metatarsal), 6 mo fetal calf mandible, 2 yr cow tibia, and 6 wk rat tibia were prepared as previously described (1,2). Amino acid analysis for Gla and other amino acids was carried out as described (5,8,11). Osteocalcin was purified as before and the concentration determined by A_{276} nm , where ε = 3800 $M^{-1}cm^{-1}$ (2).

Demineralized bone matrix prepared from rat diaphyses was transplanted subcutaneously in the thoracic region of 6 wk male rats (Long-Evans strain) in bilateral sites (10). On designated days after transplantation, the plaques were dissected free of adhering muscle, washed in ice cold 0.15M NaCl, and lyophilized.

Bone powders were demineralized at 0° to 4° in 0.5M EDTA, pH 8, 12.5% trichloroacetic acid (TCA), or 0.65M HCl. The TCA procedure was followed by extraction with 1M triethylamine-phosphate (TEAP), pH 4.4, for high pressure liquid chromatography (HPLC). To study trypsin-catalyzed release of osteocalcin from bone powder, further exhaustive washing of the TEAP-extracted bone was performed with 0.1M borate buffer, pH 8.6, using 20 ml per g bone (4 times, 4 hr at 23°).

HPLC of osteocalcin and bone protein extracts (12) was done with a Waters liquid chromatograph using a 4.4x300 mm µBondapak-CN column operated at 1200 p.s.i.g., 23°, and 2.0 ml/min. The mobile phase was 0.1M TEAP, pH 4.40, with increasing amounts of acetonitrile (13). Protein was monitored by absorbance at 210 nm. Osteocalcin concentration in complex mixtures was determined by peak areas relative to standard samples of pure osteocalcin. Radioactivity in 1 ml fractions of the effluent stream was counted by liquid scintillation at an efficiency for tritium of 34.6%.

Specific tritium labeling of Gla residues in osteocalcin and complex protein mixtures was achieved by in vacuo decarboxylation of acidified protein after equilibration with tritiated 0.05M DCl (12). Greater than 99% of the incorporated tritium is in glutamic acid residues after acid hydrolysis of the washed, dialyzed protein (12). Because the decarboxylation is carried out in the absence of water, no changes are introduced in the protein, save for the substitution of γ-tritiated glutamic acid residues at all positions formerly occupied by Gla (12).

RESULTS

Appearance of Gla in the chick embryo skeleton is first measureable in mandible and long bones on the 8th day (Stage 33) of development (Fig. 1). At this point the Gla concentration rises significantly above the Stage 29 (6 d) whole embryo value of 1.7 residues of Gla/10^5 amino acid residues. Gla in the calvaria does not begin to increase until days 11-13. Gla continues to increase in developing bones until well beyond hatching, but levels off after about 3-6 wk. Gla in the long bone diaphysis of 9 wk chickens is only 10% higher than at 3 wk.

Interestingly, each type of bone exhibits its own reproducibly distinct kinetics of Gla accumulation. In the calvaria Gla appears several days later than in long bone, and the final Gla content is only 55-60% as great at all stages of development (Fig. 1). These differences may derive from the presence of endochondral vs. membranous patterns of mineralization.

The first observable mineral in these embryonic bones coincides with the time of onset of Gla (osteocalcin) accumulation (Fig. 2). Alizarin red

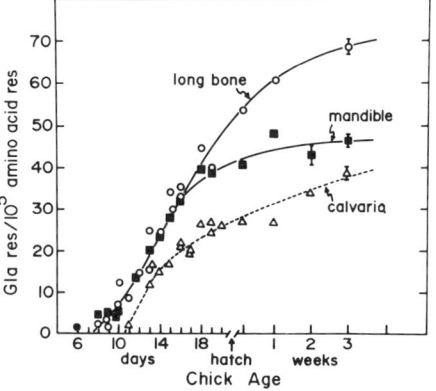

Figure 1. Kinetics of Gla appearance in developing bones of the chick. Long bone diaphysis (O), mandible (■), calvaria (△), and whole 6-day embryo (●). Bars represent the standard error of the mean. Developmental stage correlation is shown in (8).

staining is characteristic of bone mineral and commences at about day 8 (Stage 31-33) in the perichondral region of the tibiotarsus. Bone is formed by the perichondrium on the surface of the cartilaginous rudiment. The bony ring which is barely evident in the 8-day tibiotarsus gradually lengthens as a hollow cylinder and extends toward the ends of the cartilage model. The ratio of alizarin-stained length/overall length is ∼ 0.7 at day 10, dropping abruptly to 0.1 at day 8 and extrapolating to zero (i.e., no mineralized ring) at about 7.5 days or Stage 30-32 (Fig.2).

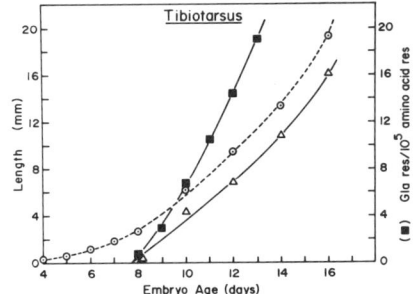

Figure 2. Correlation of tibiotarsus growth with mineralization and Gla content. Overall length of alcohol-fixed bone, including unmineralized cartilage (◎); axial shaft length stained by alizarin red (△); Gla content of midshaft (■).

Correlation of longitudinal growth of the tibiotarsus with mineralization and Gla accumulation is shown in Fig. 2. Starting at 7-8 days both the Gla content and the axial length of the mineralized ring increase steeply, in contrast to the whole bone rudiment length which has been growing steadily since about the 4th day of development. Earlier histological studies of the timing of initial long bone mineralization corroborate the 7-8 day onset observed here (14,15). We have sampled only the midshaft portion of these developing long bones for amino acid analysis. The preponderance of nonmineralized cartilage in early samples (before day 12) masks the true onset of Gla appearance. Thus osteocalcin may be formed even slightly earlier than the

TABLE I

γ-Carboxyglutamic Acid in the 10 Day Chick Embryo Tibiotarsus

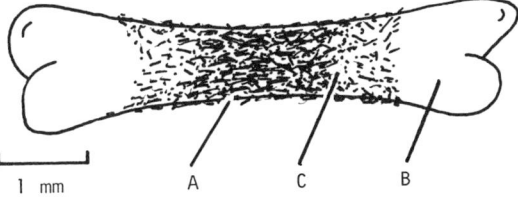

	Anatomical Region	res Gla 10^5 amino acid res	% Osteocalcin
A	Perichondral zone of initial mineralization	28.8 ± 1.4	0.41
B	Cartilaginous epiphyseal ends	3.9 ± 0.4	<0.06
C	Cartilaginous rudiment core	4.0 ± 0.7	<0.06
	Adult diaphyseal bone	78.6 ± 0.8	1.12

Stage 31-33 estimated in Fig. 2.

This problem was further investigated by microdissection of the 10-day (Stage 36) chick embryo tibiotarsus. When the newly mineralized perichondral shaft is freed of other tissue (Table I), it shows a greatly enhanced Gla and osteocalcin content (28.8 res Gla/10^5 amino acid res) compared with the whole 10-day midshaft studied in Figs. 1 and 2 (7-11 res Gla/10^5 res). Thus the initiation of osteocalcin formation at 7-8 days is more abrupt and dramatic than previously reported (8).

Studies were performed on matrix-induced endochondral bone using the rat implant system elegantly described by Reddi and Huggins (10). In this system a strict temporal sequence of histological changes (10,16) follows subcutaneous implantation of demineralized bone powder at day 0: transient inflammatory response (day 1), fibroblast proliferation (day 3), chondroblasts (day 5), chondrocyte hypertrophy and cartilage calcification (days 7-9), osteogenesis (day 10), ossicle remodeling (days 12-18), and bone marrow formation (day 18).

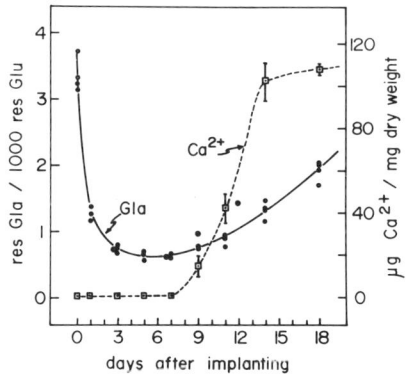

Figure 3. Changes in the Gla and Ca^{2+} content of demineralized rat bone matrix after subcutaneous implantation in 6 wk rats. Gla content of plaques from two separate experiments (O,●) was determined after 2M KOH hydrolysis; Ca^{2+} was measured in the alkali-insoluble residue (----). All implants for this study were prepared and kindly provided by A. H. Reddi (NIDR).

Numerous individual 20-30 mg powder implants were studied for Gla and Ca^{2+} content (Fig. 3). Compared to rat bone diaphysis (7-9 res Gla/1000 res glutamic acid), the demineralized powder used for implantation retained about 50% of its Gla (osteocalcin) content. Most residual Gla is rapidly removed from the implanted matrix by inflammatory processes during the first day. Then, in keeping with the developing long bone, the Gla content of the implant begins to rise coincident with the onset of mineralization at 8-9 days (Fig. 3). This initiation of Gla (or osteocalcin) biosynthesis may in fact be more dramatic than depicted in Fig. 3 because our measurements have included large amounts of inert matrix collagen in the plaque samples.

In order to investigate in greater detail the pathway of biosynthesis, deposition, and degradation of osteocalcin and other Gla-proteins, a method was developed for specific radioactive labeling of Gla residues by <u>exchange decarboxylation</u> [Fig. 4; (12)]. The efficiency of labeling by this procedure using tritiated DCl is very nearly 100%: 0.95 atoms T incorporated per Gla residue decarboxylated (Table II). Equilibration with tritiated HCl yields only 0.69 atoms T incorporated/Gla decarboxylated. Thus, there is a primary (kinetic) isotope effect k_T/k_D ÷ k_T/k_H of about 1.4 (12). The high specificity for labeling Gla residues has been documented elsewhere (12). This procedure can be performed on pure peptides or complex mixtures of proteins, and the labeled material so produced can be chromatographed by various procedures to follow the fate of Gla-containing substances. No significant degradation of osteocalcin or other proteins is caused by the dry heating at $110°$ (12,17).

TCA-demineralized bone powders from embryonic and adult chicken, cow, and rat were tritium labeled by the above procedure. The TCA step is very useful in this regard because it does not solubilize osteocalcin or other matrix proteins while removing all bone mineral. HPLC of the labeled pro-

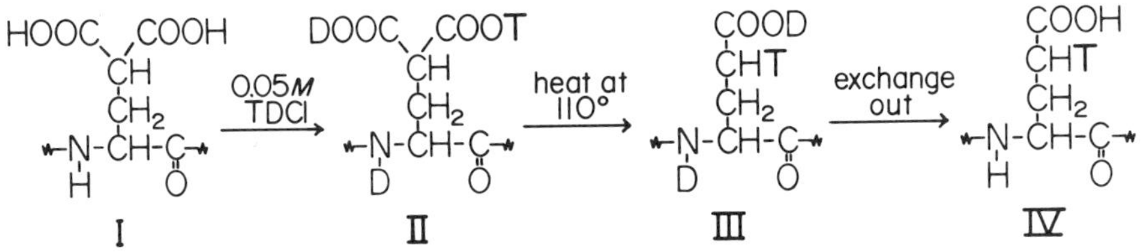

$$\underset{I}{\overset{HOOCCOOH}{\underset{H}{\overset{}{\underset{\leftarrow N-CH-C\rightarrow}{\overset{CH}{\underset{}{\overset{|}{\underset{}{\overset{|}{CH_2}}}}}}}}}} \xrightarrow{0.05M\;TDCl} \underset{II}{\overset{DOOCCOOT}{\underset{D}{\overset{}{\underset{\leftarrow N-CH-C\rightarrow}{\overset{CH}{\underset{}{\overset{|}{\underset{}{\overset{|}{CH_2}}}}}}}}}} \xrightarrow{\text{heat at }110°} \underset{III}{\overset{COOD}{\underset{D}{\overset{}{\underset{\leftarrow N-CH-C\rightarrow}{\overset{CHT}{\underset{}{\overset{|}{\underset{}{\overset{|}{CH_2}}}}}}}}}} \xrightarrow{\text{exchange out}} \underset{IV}{\overset{COOH}{\underset{H}{\overset{}{\underset{\leftarrow N-CH-C\rightarrow}{\overset{CHT}{\underset{}{\overset{|}{\underset{}{\overset{|}{CH_2}}}}}}}}}}$$

Figure 4. Reaction scheme for tritium (T) incorporation by <u>exchange decarboxylation</u> of Gla. Proteins and peptides containing Gla (I) are equilibrated briefly with high specific activity tritiated 0.05M DCl and then lyophilized. Approximately 10^{-4} to 10^{-5} of the exchangeable hydrogens indicated by D are actually T. The tritium-labeled deuterated material (II) is heated in vacuo at 110° for up to 6 hr, during which time Gla decarboxylation occurs with transfer of T to the γ-carbon of the newly formed glutamic acid residue (III). Back exchange of other hydrogens is achieved by dialysis or repeated lyophilization, yielding the specifically labeled product (IV). Hydrolysis of IV shows that all of the T (>99%) is in glutamic acid (12).

teins (Fig. 5) shows several important new features regarding the state of osteocalcin in bone: 1) there is <u>heterogeneity</u> of osteocalcin in normal bone, with at least two isomeric forms obvious in embryonic bone and up to four or more species in adult bone; 2) a much larger fraction of osteocalcin is extractable as the 6500 dalton form from adult bone compared with embryonic bone; and 3) Gla is not restricted to the 6500 dalton osteocalcin peaks at 34-41 min, but is also found in peaks at 27 and 32 min and in a large peak at the column front. This front peak is reduced but <u>not</u> eliminated by dialysis (membrane retention >3000 daltons; Spectrapor 3) prior to HPLC; thus it appears to be a highly polar Gla-containing species in bone. Results with tritium-labeled proteins from embryonic and adult cow

TABLE II

Specific Labeling of Gla Residues in Osteocalcin

Treatment[+]	mole Gla / mole protein	mole T* / mole protein	mole T** / mole Gla → Glu
Untreated (D)	3.63 ± 0.16	0.008 ± 0.005	--
6 hr, 110° (D)	0.95 ± 0.13	2.16 ± 0.08	0.95 ± 0.14
6 hr, 110° (H)	0.78 ± 0.12	1.68 ± 0.05	0.69 ± 0.09

[+]Triplicate samples of osteocalcin were exchanged in vacuo for 3 hr at 23° with 0.05M TDCl (D) or 0.05M THCl (H) before heating 6 hr at 110° to promote decarboxylation of Gla to glutamic acid.
*After removal of all exchangeable T.
**Corrected for 15% exchange loss of T from the γ-carbon which results from 24 hr hydrolysis in 6M HCl at 100°. All values are ± standard error of the mean.

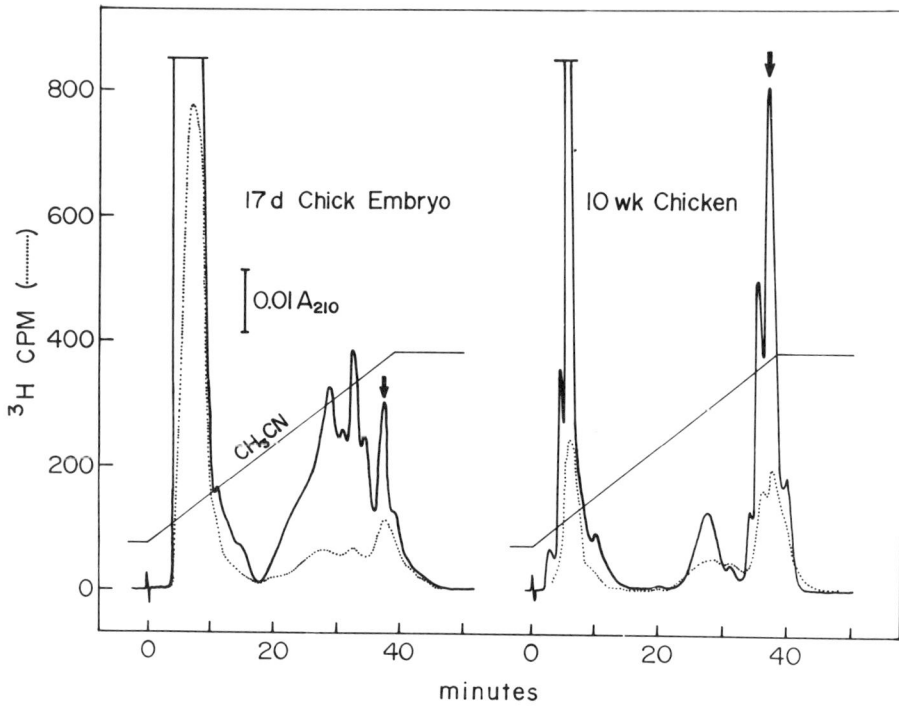

Figure 5. HPLC profiles of proteins extracted from bone powders of 17 d embryonic (left) and 10 wk adult (right) chicken long bone. Tritium labeling (----) of Gla residues preceded extraction with TEAP buffer. Elution required a linear gradient of 14-35% acetonitrile. The principal 6500 dalton species of osteocalcin elutes at 37 min (↓), while closely related forms of the protein appear between 34 and 41 min.

bone and rat bone are similar to those in Fig. 5. Particularly noteworthy is the complex mixture of peptides eluting slightly before osteocalcin. This mixture includes some Gla-containing protein species and is much more abundant in embryonic than adult bone (Figs. 5 and 6). It was earlier observed that a small fraction of the Gla extractable from adult chicken bone chromatographed with the high molecular weight fraction (>40,000 daltons) on Sephadex G-100 (2). Correlation of the HPLC-resolved Gla-protein peaks with this and other Gla-containing fractions purified from bone by other procedures is in progress.

Numerous experiments in our laboratory have shown that most, but not all of the Gla-containing proteins of bone are extractable by demineralization in 0.5M EDTA or 0.65M HCl. The fraction of Gla which is nonextractable generally decreases with increasing bone age and shows variation between species. Could this nonextractable Gla be present in proteins with a higher molecular weight than osteocalcin? Might these larger Gla proteins be intimately entangled with, or a part of, the collagenous organic matrix, thus preventing their solubilization by demineralization? In an effort to explore these questions, adult chicken bone was thoroughly demineralized and washed with several buffers until no further osteocalcin was extractable, yet about 20% of the original Gla content still remained. At this point, addition of small quantities of trypsin rapidly released most of the remaining Gla, much of it in the form of osteocalcin and its

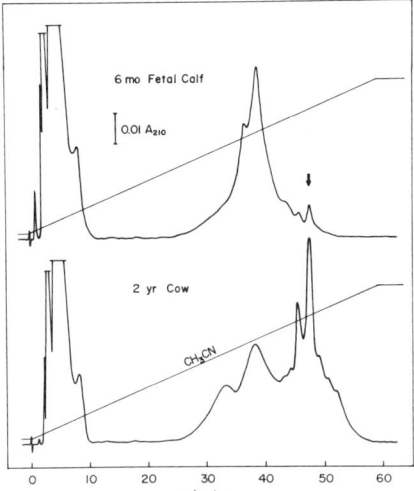

Figure 6. HPLC profiles of proteins extracted from bones of fetal (upper) and adult cow (lower). Elution required a 0-50% acetonitrile gradient. A variety of Gla-rich osteocalcin species elute at 45-51 min, with the major species at 47 min (↓).

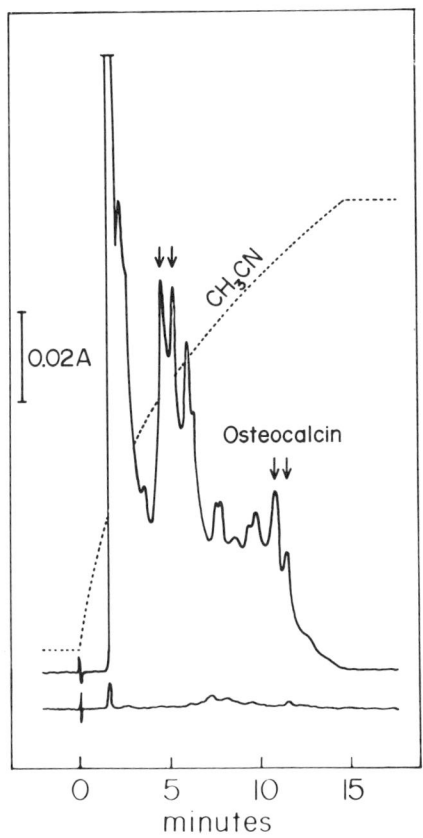

Figure 7. Trypsin-catalyzed release of osteocalcin from adult chicken bone after prior demineralization and extraction of all soluble protein. HPLC elution with a 0-50% acetonitrile gradient (---). Bone powder (230 mg) was suspended in 1 ml 0.1M borate buffer, pH 8.6 at 37° after exhaustive extraction in 12.5% TCA, 0.1M TEAP, pH 4.4, and 0.1M borate. Lower trace, 5 μl borate buffer supernatant after 40 min at 37°. Upper trace, 5 μl of borate supernatant 40 min after adding TPCK-trypsin (1/100, enzyme/substrate, w/w) at 37°. Osteocalcin and its trypsin-resistant core (∼3.3 μg total protein) elute at 11-12 min (arrows), while characteristic tryptic peptides of osteocalcin elute at 4.6 and 5.4 min (arrows).

major trypsin-resistant core (Fig.7). Thus it is apparent that for both the chicken and rat bone powders studied, trypsin quantitatively releases osteocalcin peptides which are otherwise unextractable by conventional procedures.

DISCUSSION

The coincidence of mineralization onset and Gla accumulation in the developing bone is of great interest and must certainly relate in some fashion to the function of the Gla-rich protein osteocalcin. Since most of the Gla in bone resides in the osteocalcin molecule (1,2), Gla measurements are a reasonably precise and specific index of the quantity of osteocalcin. In chick embryo long bone, osteocalcin increases about 30-fold from 0.02% of the total protein at 8 d to 0.57% at 18 d. Most of the protein in mature bone (80-90%) is collagen.

The makeup of the remaining noncollagen proteins changes dramatically during development. Osteocalcin rises from a mere 0.02% contribution to the total noncollagen proteins at 8 d to 3.4% at 18 d, a 100- to 200-fold increase. Later, in adult chicken bone, osteocalcin comprises up to 10% of the noncollagen protein (8).

The observed disproportionate increase in osteocalcin relative to other noncollagen bone proteins is a clear biochemical reflection of a differentiation process. Osteocalcin formation coincides with histologically detectable mineralization both temporally and topologically in two quite distinct systems studied here (Figs. 2 and 3; Table I). From these correlations and from the apparently unique association of osteocalcin with osseous tissues (1,9,11), an inescapable inference may be drawn: osteocalcin is a specialized molecular product of one or more cell types differentiated with respect to bone formation. Whether or not osteoblasts are the source of osteocalcin awaits further experimentation.

What factors might be responsible for turning on the biosynthesis of osteocalcin? Obviously there is the temporal appearance of a competent cell population. Competence to produce functional macromolecules assumes a new dimension for osteocalcin, however, because of the essential post-translational modification characteristic of this Ca^{2+}-binding protein—namely, vitamin K-dependent carboxylation resulting in four Gla residues per osteocalcin molecule (2,5,6). This study has utilized direct measurements of Gla as an index of osteocalcin concentration. Thus it is possible that the initiation processes seen at about 8 days in the long bone (Fig. 2) and at 8-9 days in the matrix induction system (Fig. 3) represent either (i) development of the vitamin K-dependent protein carboxylase enzyme complex, or (ii) de novo formation of osteocalcin precursor, or both of these events simultaneously. Conceivably, osteocalcin is formed even earlier than day 8, but the protein is not sequestered in the bone until sufficient hydroxyapatite has been deposited in the matrix. Interestingly, the vitamin K-dependent proteins of blood plasma are not found until day 11 in the developing chick (18), well after the first appearance of osteocalcin at day 8.

An important feature of proteins containing Gla is their ability to

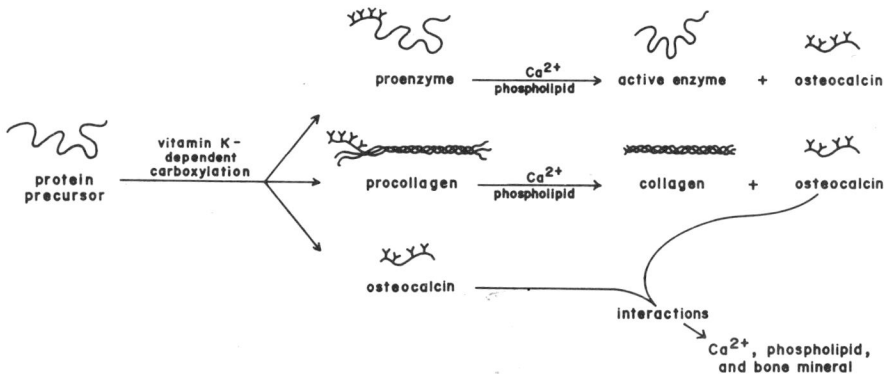

Figure 8. Possible biosynthetic pathways for osteocalcin in developing bone. Vitamin K-dependent carboxylation of a precursor protein could lead to: (i) (upper) a Gla-containing proenzyme; (ii) (middle) Gla in procollagen; or (iii) (lower) direct formation of osteocalcin with a molecular weight of 6500. Ca^{2+}- and phospholipid-dependent cleavage could release osteocalcin from larger proteins in the first two schemes. Gla residues are indicated by the symbol " Y."

interact with Ca^{2+} ions in a reversible fashion at physiological (plasma) concentrations of calcium (2,19). Narrow fluctuations in plasma $[Ca^{2+}]$ will titrate the Ca^{2+} binding sites, and this may lead to protein conformational changes, proteolytic activation, etc. Furthermore, bound Ca^{2+} promotes adsorption of Gla-containing proteins to phospholipid micelles and membrane surfaces (19,20).

Acidic phospholipids (21) and phospholipid-rich matrix vesicles (22, 23) are especially abundant in the epiphyseal regions of growing bone and may regulate the cartilage matrix calcification which immediately precedes true bone formation. We have demonstrated that osteocalcin is present in the epiphyseal region of chicken bones (8). By analogy to the prothrombin system, perhaps osteocalcin or some higher molecular weight Gla-containing precursor is adsorbed to exposed phospholipid surfaces in the epiphysis during the endochondral ossification process. Such adsorption would likely be Ca^{2+}-mediated and may result in the Ca^{2+}-dependent proteolytic cleavage of a Gla-containing protein or proenzyme in bone. Figure 8 schematically indicates this and other possibilities.

It is clear from Figures 5 and 6 that heterogeneity of osteocalcin exists in normal bone and that this is not merely an artifact of the extraction and purification procedure. Earlier observations corroborate the present findings, since undercarboxylated and other isoelectric and sequence-distinct forms of osteocalcin are present in the EDTA extracted protein purified from normal chicken bone (2,7). Thus there is strong suggestion of protease processing in the normal life cycle of osteocalcin.

Trypsin is found to release otherwise unextractable, cryptic forms of osteocalcin from exhaustively demineralized and washed bone powder (Fig. 7). This release may be comparable to the liberation of residual Gla from demineralized bone matrix during the first day after implantation (Fig. 3). The transient inflammatory response accompanying implantation involves invasion by polymorphonuclear leukocytes (10,16). Proteases associated with these cells apparently cleave osteocalcin sequences in the matrix, thereby accounting for the rapid initial decline in Gla content (Fig. 3).

The possible existence of higher molecular weight protein species containing the osteocalcin sequence is supported by the above observations, as well as by recent labeling studies with $^{14}CO_2$ in cultured bones and bone microsomes (24).

ACKNOWLEDGEMENTS

The author is indebted to P. M. Gallop and J. Levy for helpful discussions, and to M. Reid and J. Komar for technical assistance. A.H. Reddi (NIDR) kindly prepared the rat bone matrix implants (Fig. 3), and A.I. Caplan (Case-Western Reserve) generously provided some of the Stage 36 chick embryo limbs used for data in Table I. This work was supported by The National Foundation-March of Dimes, by NIH grants AM 16754 and AM 15671, and by GRS funds of the Children's Hospital Medical Center. The author is the recipient of a Research Career Development Award from the NIDR, K04-DE00049.

REFERENCES

1. Hauschka, P.V., Lian, J.B., and Gallop, P.M. (1975) Proc. Nat. Acad. Sci. USA 72, 3925-3929.
2. Hauschka, P.V. and Gallop, P.M. (1977) In "Calcium Binding Proteins and Calcium Function"(R.H. Wasserman et al., eds.), pp. 338-347. Elsevier

North Holland, Amsterdam and New York.
3. Price, P.A., Otsuka, A.S., Poser, J.W., Kristaponis, J., and Raman, N. (1976).Proc. Nat. Acad. Sci. USA 73, 1447-1451.
4. Price, P.A., Poser, J.W., and Raman, N. (1976) Proc. Nat. Acad. Sci. USA 73, 3374-3375.
5. Lian, J.B. and Friedman, P.A. (1978) J. Biol. Chem. 253, 6623-6626.
6. Lian, J.B., Hauschka, P.V., and Gallop, P.M. (1978) Fed. Proc. 37, 2615-2620.
7. Hauschka, P.V. and Reid, M.L. (1978) J. Biol. Chem. 253, 9063-9068.
8. Hauschka, P.V. and Reid, M.L. (1978) Develop. Biol. 65, 426-434.
9. Hauschka, P.V., Lian, J.B., and Gallop, P.M. (1978) Trends in Biochem. Sci. 4,75-78.
10. Reddi, A.H. and Huggins, C.B. (1972) Proc. Nat. Acad. Sci. USA 69, 1601-1605.
11. Hauschka, P.V. (1977) Anal. Biochem. 80, 212-223.
12. Hauschka, P.V. (1979) Biochemistry (In Press).
13. Rivier, J.E. (1978) J. Liq. Chromatog. 1, 343- 355.
14. Fell, H.B. (1925) J. Morphol. 40, No. 3.
15. Anderson, H.C. and Reynolds, J.J. (1973) Develop. Biol. 34, 211-227.
16. Reddi, A.H. and Anderson, W.A. (1976) J. Cell. Biol. 69, 557-572.
17. Poser, J.W. and Price, P.A. (1979) J. Biol. Chem. 254, 431- 436.
18. Kane, R.E. and Sizer, I.W. (1953) Anat. Rec. 117, 614.
19. Esmon, C.T., Suttie, J.W., and Jackson, C.M. (1975) J. Biol. Chem. 250, 4095-4099).
20. Nelsestuen, G.L., Broderius, M., Zytkovicz, T.H., and Howard, J.B. (1975) Biochem. Biophys. Res. Commun. 65, 233-240.
21. Irving, J.T. and Wuthier, R.E. (1968) Clin. Orthop. 56, 237-260.
22. Anderson, H.C. (1976) J. Cell Biol. 35, 81-101.
23. Bonucci, E. (1967) J. Ultrastruct. Res. 20, 35-50.
24. Lian, J.B., Friedman, P.A., Heroux, K.M., and Gallop, P.M. (1979) Eighth Steenbock Symposium-Vitamin K, Madison, Wisconsin.

OSTEOCALCIN CONTENT IN NORMAL, RACHITIC AND VITAMIN K ANTAGONIZED BONE

JANE B. LIAN, BARRY REIT, ALBERT H. ROUFOSSE,
MELVIN J. GLIMCHER and PAUL M. GALLOP

Departments of Orthopaedic Surgery and Biological Chemistry,
Harvard Medical School,
Children's Hospital Medical Center,
Boston, MA 02115

INTRODUCTION

A unique vitamin K dependent calcium-binding protein, named osteocalcin (1), has been characterized in normal bone. The calcium binding properties of osteocalcin are conferred by the presence of γ-carboxyglutamic acid (Gla) which is synthesized in a vitamin K-dependent and CO_2-requiring enzymatic carboxylation reaction of glutamic acid residues. The specific function of Gla residues in the vitamin K dependent blood coagulation factors is the binding of calcium to promote protein-phospholipid interaction which mediates conversion of proenzyme factors to active proteins in the cascade sequence of the intrinsic clotting pathway (2). Although the function of osteocalcin is unknown, it has been postulated that Gla residues can similarly act in bone to promote a calcium ion-protein-phospholipid interaction (3). This highly specialized interaction may mediate the mineralization process of bone since high concentrations of acidic phospholipids are observed in the mineralization front of endochondral bone and in dentin (4). Further implication of a vitamin K dependent process in bone development and perhaps in the initial events of mineralization arises from the warfarin embryopathy (5) in which mothers receiving anticoagulants during the first trimester of pregnancy give birth to neonates with stippled epiphyses and hypoplasia of the nasal bridge (6). In addition γ-carboxyglutamic acid containing proteins have also been found in pathologically mineralized tissues, namely calcium-containing renal calculi (7), atherosclerotic plaque (8) and the subcutaneous calcifications observed in scleroderma and dermatomyositis (8). Such findings strongly implicate Gla proteins as having a role in calcification of tissues.

Further insight into the role of osteocalcin in mineralization might be gained by examination of the distribution of Gla as a function of the degree of mineralization in normal bone. In this study the most recently synthesized bone is separated from maturing bone at progressively increasing stages of mineralization, measuring Gla in each fraction. Richelle et al. (9) and Roufosse et al. (10) have shown that cortical bone powder can be fractionated into various densities by differential density centrifugation in bromoform-toluene mixtures. Russell et al. (11) utilized this technique to demonstrate a defect in mineralization of bone from uremic rats. In the bone density fractionation method, advantage is taken of the fact that the density of microscopic portions of bone tissue is a direct function of the amount of mineral present. Since collagen (density = 1.35 g/cm^3) constitutes 90% of the organic matrix and fully mineralized whole bone has a density of approximately 2.2 g/cm^3, the separation of bone powder into various fractions as a function of density, partitions the bone tissue according to its mineral content or degree of maturation (age of the bone). In the present study, we have also taken advantage of this separation technique to determine if vitamin K deficiency produces defects in bone mineralization. Such a phenomenon would be revealed by the distribution of particles fractionating at the densities between 1.5 and 2.2 g/cm^3. The fractionation of vitamin K deficient bone is compared not only to control bone but also to vitamin D deficient bones in which the mineralization defect, histologically, is recognized. In rachitic bone, wide osteoid seams are observed; although new bone matrix is synthesized, mineralization of matrix does not follow. As a result, the histogram representing the distribution of bone tissue as a function of density is displaced towards lower densities. Mineralization defects should be detected in the newly synthesized, non-mineralized bone tissue which is represented by the lowest density fractions. It is of interest to determine if osteocalcin synthesis, as measured by Gla content in the various bone density fractions, is altered in vitamin D deficient bone.

MATERIALS AND METHODS

White Leghorn male chicks were obtained at 1 day (Lawton Poultry Farm, Foxboro, MA) and raised in wire bottom brooders with a constant heat (light) source in a room at 28°C for 6 weeks. Chicks had free access to fresh water and Purina No. 5070 chow. Vitamin K deficiency was induced by the addition of dicoumarol (Sigma Chemical Co., St. Louis, MO) 800 mg/kg diet (12). Vitamin K antagonism was produced in chick embryos by injection of 200 μg of sodium warfarin per diem into the allantoic sac from day 13 to day 16. Vitamin K deficiency in the embryonic and 6-week bones was assessed by the decreased Gla content. Vitamin D deficiency was produced by vitamin D deficient and low calcium diets. Chicks were raised in brooder cages shielded from fluorescent and day lighting. The extent of vitamin D deficiency was measured by plasma 25 hydroxylase activity and kidney 1,25 hydroxylase activity. In vitamin D deficient birds, the average body weight was 60% of the control, whereas in vitamin K deficient birds, the average body weight did not vary significantly from controls.

Preparation of Bone

Animals were sacrificed by etherization and dissected one at a time. The tibia and femur bonds were removed, cleaned free of muscle and periosteum and after longitudinal splitting, the marrow removed by gentle scraping. It is critical that no water is in contact with bone tissues as this will change the structure of their mineral components. Each individual bone was immediately frozen in liquid nitrogen after cleaning and lyophilized. After lyophilizing, the dried bones were ground in a liquid nitrogen bath hammer mill (Spex Industries, Model 6700 freezer mill, Metuchen, NJ) for a total time of approximately 1 minute, using short grinding pulses of about 3-4 seconds. The bone powder was sieved using the U.S. standard sieve series (Newark Wire Cloth Co., Hoboken, NJ), and grinding continued until most particles ranged from 1 to 10 microns in diameter with an average particle size of 5 microns. The bone particles were then dispersed in ethanol by sonication (Ultrasonic Industries, Inc., Albertson, NY) several times to eliminate colloidal particles. After drying the bone particles are ready for density fractionation.

Differential Density Centrifugation Technique

Eleven different mixtures of bromoform (density 2.88 g/cm^3) and toluene (density 0.8 g/cm^3) are prepared to span from the ranges 1.4 to 2.2 g/cm^3 with a 0.1 g/cm^3 interval. The fluid densities were measured with an 0.02 g/cm^3 accuracy by using hydrometers and sink float standards (R.P. Cargille Labs Inc., Cedar Grove, NJ). Rather than using a gradient column, a batch technique was used to provide sufficient amounts of bone particles for the physical and biochemical analyses. For batch preparations approximately 0.4 g of whole bone powder are suspended by sonication in 35 ml of polyallomer centrifuge tubes (Beckman, #326823) partially filled with a bromoform-toluene solution equal to 1.8 g/cm^3 density and centrifuged in a swinging bucket rotor SW 27 in a Beckman L2-65B ultracentrifuge at room temperature for 30 minutes at 10,000 rpm. The density of the supernatant was modified to 1.7 g/cm^3 made by the addition of toluene and the new solution recentrifuged as above. The precipitate obtained initially from the 1.8 g/cm^3 density solution was resuspended in a solution of density 1.9 g/cm^3. Successive centrifugations (30 min; 10,000 rpm) at progressively increasing (0.1 g/cm^3 steps) densities provided higher density fractions. All isolated fractions were washed several times with 100% ethyl alcohol to remove organic solvents and then dried to constant weight under vacuum at room temperature. From weight determinations, the percent distribution of the various bone density fractions in a sample of whole bone powder was calculated.

Amino Acid and Mineral Analysis

Analysis was performed on 8-10 mg quantities of dried bone powder, particles from the density fractions. For Gla determination the samples were hydrolyzed in 2M KOH at 110°C for 22 hours as previously described (13). The Gla is expressed as either residues per 1000 glutamic acid or 10^5 amino acid residues. Complete amino acid analysis was determined after 6N HCl hydrolysis at 110°C for 24 hours, from which protein and and collagen content were calculated. The calcium contents of each fraction were obtained from 6N HCl hydrolysates. An aliquot was diluted 100-fold in 0.3M HCl, 0.586% lanthanum oxide for determination of calcium by atomic absorption spectroscopy. A Perkin Elmer model 603 was calibrated with calcium solutions prepared from a calcium phosphate standard (No. 120B) of the National Bureau of Standards.

RESULTS

Normal Bone

Differential density centrifugation was performed on mid-diaphyseal bone from embryos, 5-6 week chicks, and 1 and 2 year chickens. For embryonic chicks, a 17 to 18 day age was chosen in order to obtain a sufficient amount of material from only the mid-diaphyseal regions. Histological evaluation of several dissected samples with Safranin O stain showed the absence of calcified cartilage. In embryonic bone, density fractions from 1.5 to 2.0 g/cm^3 are obtained and at age 5-6 weeks, the bone particles fractionate between 1.8-2.3 g/cm^3, whereas in 1-2 year chicken bone only 2.1 to 2.3 g/cm^3 fractions are obtained. The Gla content as a function of density fraction is plotted in Figure 1 for the four animal ages. A linear correlation is observed over the range of fractions from 1.4 to 2.3 g/cm^3. It is interesting that for a given density, although obtained at different ages, the Gla content is approximately similar; for example, density fractions 1.6 and 1.7 in the embryo and 6-week bone. Thus a fraction is not only defined by a constant calcium, collagen and protein content, but by a constant Gla content. In a whole bone analysis Gla content is lower in the embryo than a 6 week bone because 50% of the bone particles are between 1.9-2.0 g/cm^3 and at 6 weeks, 60% of the bone is of a 2.1-2.2 g/cm^3 density.

Vitamin K Antagonized Bone

In both warfarin-treated embryonic and dicoumarol fed chick diaphyseal bone, Gla content was decreased 62-65% of the controls indicating inhibition of Gla synthesis. In Table 1 and Figure 2 the distribution of mid-

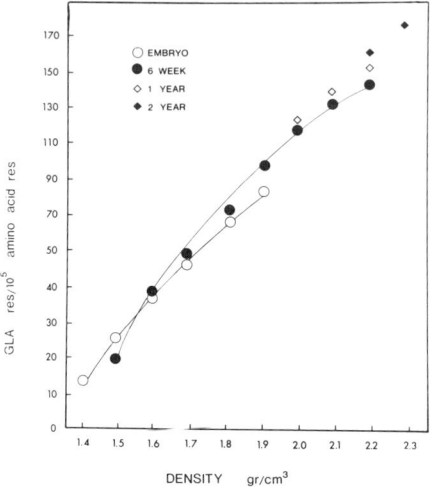

FIGURE 1 Gla content in bone density fractions obtained from mid-diaphyseal bone from 17 day embryos, 6 week, 1 and 2 year old chickens.

diaphyseal bone powder particles in control and warfarin-treated chick embryos is compared. In the warfarin treated chicks, a total of 27% of the particles is below 1.8 g/cm^3, whereas 11.5% fractionates below this density in the control. In the heavier density fractions, the distribution is reversed with a striking decrease of 20.5% of the particles in the 2.0-2.1 g/cm^3 range in warfarin treated bone. It is interesting to note that when the average weighted density is computed from the percent at each density (Table 1), the warfarin samples calculate to 1.91 g/cm^3 and the control to 1.97 g/cm^3. Thus it would be extremely difficult to measure significant differences between warfarin or control bone density or calcium content in whole, unfractionated bone specimens. As expected from the differential density centrifugation procedure, the fractions at each density in warfarin and control samples have approximately the same calcium content in each fraction. In separate fractionation experiments, and in different chick preparations, the percent distribution of particles between 1.5 and 1.9 g/cm^3 was variable, but the net effect was consistently a 12-15% increase in the lower density fractions in warfarin treated bones and an 18-20% decrease in the 2.0-2.1 g/cm^3 fraction.

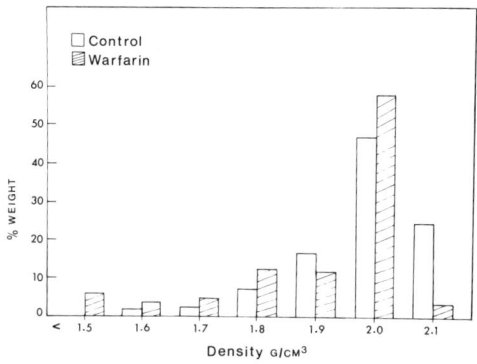

FIGURE 2 Distribution of mid-diaphyseal bone density fractions obtained from 17-18 day normal and warfarin-treated chick embryos.

TABLE 1. Embryonic bone fractionation by mineral densities (% distribution by weight)

Density g/cm^3	Control	Warfarin-treated
< 1.5	0	6.5
1.5-1.6	1.8	3.5
1.6-1.7	2.5	4.5
1.7-1.8	7.2	12.5
1.8-1.9	16.5	12
1.9-2.0	47.5	58
2.0-2.1	24.5	3.5
Average weighted	1.968	1.9135

The distribution of density fractions of mid-diaphyseal bone powder obtained from 5-6 week control and dicoumarol fed chickens for 5-6 week was also examined. In normal bone of this age group, less than 4% of the particles are found in densities lower than 2.0 g/cm^3, and most of the

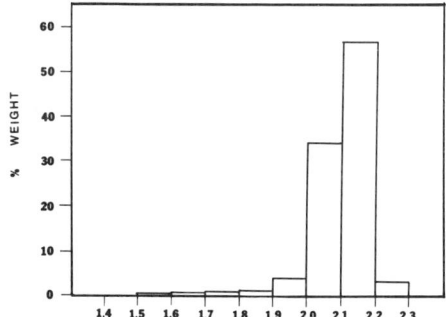

FIGURE 3 Bone density distribution in <u>normal</u> 5-6 week chicks.

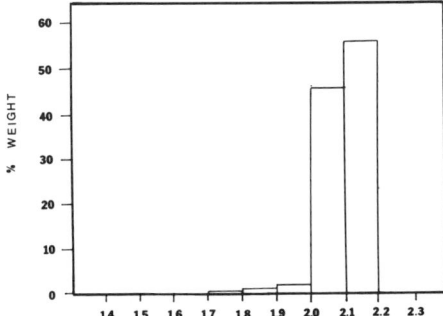

FIGURE 4 Bone density distribution in <u>vitamin K antagonized</u> 5-6 week chicks.

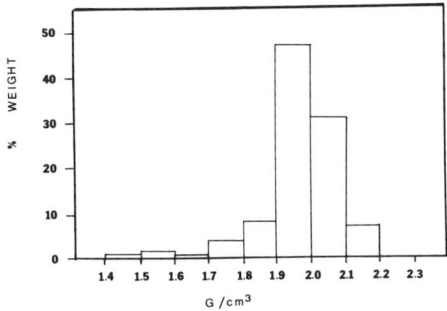

FIGURE 5 Bone density distribution in <u>vitamin D deficient</u> 5-6 week chicks.

bone partitions between 2.0 and 2.2 g/cm^3. The histogram from the control and dicoumarol fed chick bone (Figs. 3 and 4) reveals only a small difference in the percent distribution between 2.1 and 2.3 g/cm^3. In the 6-week vitamin K deficient bone a 3% decrease is evident in the 2.2-2.3 g/cm^3 fraction, the most mature portion of the bone, and approximately 10% more of the particles fractionate between 2.0 and 2.1 g/cm^3.

Vitamin D Deficiency

Since this technique of differential density centrifugation has not been previously utilized for the demonstration of mineralization defects in vitamin D deficient bone formation, we have examined the partitioning of bone particles from 5-6 week old rachitic chicks. The results (Fig. 5) show a dramatic shift of the bone powder to the lower densities. Fifty percent fractionates at 1.9-2.0 g/cm^3 in rachitic bone as compared to 5% in normal bone. A comparison of the histogram in vitamin D deficiency to the vitamin K deficient bone at the same age, suggests that the defect in mineralization in vitamin K deficiency is not at the level of mineralization of osteoid. In vitamin D deficiency, <u>no mineralization</u> of newly synthesized bone matrix occurs as evident by the bone density profile, while in vitamin K deficiency, mineralization of newly synthesized osteoid occurs, however the maturation of the mineral components could be altered since the 2.3 g/cm^3 fraction is absent.

It was of interest to compare the Gla content for each bone density fraction representing bone tissue at all levels of maturation, from most recently synthesized matrix to most mature bone in rachitic and normal bone. These results are illustrated in Figure 6 which shows a marked elevation of Gla content in the rachitic bone fractions, especially at the lower densities. In the 1.5-1.6 g/cm^3 fraction a 187% increase in Gla is calculated, 70% in fraction 1.6-1.7 but only 2.9% in the 2.1-2.2 g/cm^3 fraction. The results of duplicate analyses from four experiments showed a significance of 0.010 by the student t-test. Thus the greatest change in the Gla content is observed in the most "rachitic" bone (lower densities) which is being separated from the more normal bone (higher densities).

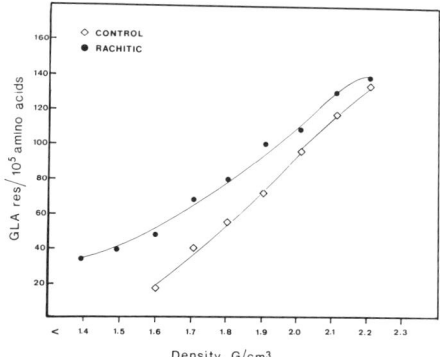

FIGURE 6   Gla content in bone density fractions from normal and vitamin D-deficient 5-6 week chick.

DISCUSSION

Although anatomically, a homogeneous sample of tissue, i.e. the midshaft, is taken, the density fractionations separate such a sampling into even more homogeneous fractions. This technique also offers the advantage of examining the recently synthesized bone at any animal age and the bone tissue at various stages of maturation to completely mineralized bone.

An examination of the distribution of Gla at varying densities in normal embryonic, 5-6 week and 1-2 year bone (Fig. 1) demonstrates that the percent of protein in bone which is osteocalcin is related to the degree of mineralization. This distribution suggests that the vitamin K dependent calcium binding protein of bone may function in the regulation of bone mineral. If osteocalcin played a role in nucleation of the mineral phase in bone, one would expect to find a higher distribution of Gla in the low density fractions, which represent newly mineralized bone and a lower Gla content in the mature bone. However, if Gla residues are involved in earliest interactions between organic, phospholipid and inorganic components, due to their specific calcium binding properties osteocalcin could perhaps remain embedded in the mineral components. Osteocalcin may be the Gla-rich peptide of a pro-enzyme, which functions in the development of bone, or osteocalcin itself may play an active role in the maintenance of bone mineral after nucleation events have occurred.

Some insight into the potential function of osteocalcin in bone mineralization is derived from the effect of vitamin K antagonism on the density fractionation in the embryo. Our results with chick embryo bone show that with about 50% inhibition of the Gla synthesis in bone there is only about 10% less mineralization; however, there is a significant decrease in the most highly mineralized osteoid (2.0-2.1 g/cm^3) from 24.5% in the control to 3.5% in the warfarinized animal. Also there is a significant increase in the lowest density fractions from 11.5% in the control to 27% in the warfarin-treated (Table 1). An increased proportion of the bone particles fractionate at the lower densities when compared to control in embryonic bone suggesting that mineral maturation processes are inhibited. In 5-6 week vitamin K-deficient bone, it is again apparent that the normal sequence of bone maturation is slightly altered by a decrease in 2.2-2.3 g/cm^3 fraction. Clearly however vitamin K antagonism does not result in the absence of mineralization of new bone matrix as observed in vitamin D deficiency. In normal 5-6 week bone the percent of new bone synthesis relative to the whole is very small, less than 2%; thus, it may be difficult to assess the defect at this age.

In vitamin D deficient bone, the Gla content does increase with the degree of mineralization as in normal bone (Figure 6). However for any given density, the Gla content relative to total protein (residues/10^5 amino acids) is higher in rachitic bone. This could be the result of a decreased amount or the absence of a non-collagenous protein component, thus making the Gla residues per total residues of amino acids in the rachitic appear higher; however the absolute amount of osteocalcin in the rachitic bone would be comparable to normal bone. On the other hand, if osteocalcin functions in the regulation of bone mineral deposition, its net synthesis could be increased to compensate for the defect in mineralization in vitamin D deficiency which is the lack of mineral deposition in newly synthesized osteoid. In the 2.0-2.1 g/cm^3 and 2.1-2.2 g/cm^3 fractions of rachitic bone the Gla content is closer to normal bone than in the lower density fractions, thus alternatively, it may be that osteocalcin is not being utilized in its normal biosynthetic pathway in the lower density fractions because of the lack of sufficient mineral components. Since rachitic bone is so deficient in the 2.1-2.2 g/cm^3 fraction (60% loss), osteocalcin could be accumulating in the lower density fractions, perhaps even in a possible pro-enzyme form (3). Experiments are in progress to examine the extracted osteocalcin from each fraction in normal, vitamin D and vitamin K deficient bone, to determine the relative quantities of a proenzyme form and the osteocalcin peptide. Evidence from in vitro studies of osteocalcin synthesis in chick bone cultures indicates a higher molecular weight form of osteocalcin occurs (14).

In summary, these experiments have demonstrated 1) the correlation of increasing Gla content with the degree of mineralization in normal bone, 2) a change in the rate of maturation of bone to its most mineralized state but not a defect at the level of mineralization of newly synthesized osteoid in vitamin K deficiency, and 3) in vitamin D deficiency, an increased distribution of Gla towards the lower density fractions. These data suggest that a vitamin K dependent synthesized protein "prepares" a matrix for the action of vitamin D on bone tissue. We postulate a process whereby a precursor matrix is converted to "osteoid" by the deposition of osteocalcin or osteocalcin precursor. This osteoid matrix can accept deposited mineral if enough calcium and phosphate ion or organic phosphate is supplied to the site containing osteocalcin which then interacts with the mineral components. If too little osteocalcin is present as in warfarin treatment, the content of precursor matrix is increased until enough osteocalcin can be deposited to regulate mineral deposition. Once nucleation is started mineral will deposit although the process in some instances can not be as well controlled as in a normal situation where the "osteoid matrix" is properly prepared by vitamin K dependent osteocalcin. Hence there are situations where the calcifications will appear punctate and somewhat erratic in deposition as in the "stippled" epiphysis of fetal warfarin syndrome (5). In the rachitic embryo "osteocalcinized" osteoid accumulates as if awaiting the delayed or "reduced content" of the mineral components. Hence it appears that osteocalcin precursor prepares the pre-osteoid matrix for mineralization. The sequence of events for the actions of vitamin K and D which may occur in the formation of bone can be represented as follows:

$$\text{precursor matrix} \xrightarrow{\text{vit K}} \text{osteoid matrix} \xrightarrow[\text{vit K}]{\text{Ca}\downarrow \text{vitamin D}} \text{calcified matrix.}$$

ACKNOWLEDGEMENTS

The authors acknowledge the expert technical assistance of J. Blech, K. Heroux and D. Seaman. This work was supported by NIH grants DE 04651 and AM 15671.

REFERENCES

1. Hauschka, P.V., Lian, J.B., and Gallop, P.M. (1975) Proc. Natl. Acad. Sci. USA 72, 3925-3929.
2. Suttie, J.W., and Jackson, C. (1977) Physiol. Rev. 57, 1-70.
3. Lian, J.B., Hauschka, P.V., and Gallop, P.M. (1978) Fed. Proc. 37, 2615-2620.
4. Irving, J.T., and Wuthier, R.E. (1968) Clin. Orthop. 56, 237-260.
5. Pettifor, J.M., and Benson, R. (1975) J. Pediatrics 86, 459-462.
6. Warkany, J. (1975) Am. J. Dis. Child. 129, 287-288.
7. Lian, J.B., Prien, E.L., Glimcher, M.J., and Gallop, P.M. (1977) J. Clin. Invest. 59, 1151-1157.
8. Lian, J.B., Skinner, M.S., Glimcher, M.J., and Gallop, P.M. (1976) Biochem. Biophys. Res. Commun. 73, 349-355.
9. Richelle, L.J. (1964) Clin. Orthop. 33, 211.
10. Roufosse, A.H., Landis, W.J., Sabine, W.K., and Glimcher, M.J. (1979) J. Ultrastruct. Res., in press.
11. Russell, J., Termine, J.D., and Avioli, L. (1975) J. Clin. Invest. 56, 548.
12. Hauschka, P.V., and Reid, M.L. (1978) J. Biol. Chem. 253, 9063-9068.
13. Hauschka, P.V. (1977) Anal. Biochem. 80, 212-223.
14. Lian, J.B. (1979) Eighth Steenbock Symposium, Madison, Wisconsin.

IN VITRO STUDIES OF OSTEOCALCIN BIOSYNTHESIS IN EMBRYONIC CHICK BONE CULTURES

J. B. LIAN and K. M. HEROUX

Departments of Biological Chemistry and Orthopaedic Surgery,
Children's Hospital Medical Center,
Harvard Medical School,
Boston, MA 02115

INTRODUCTION

Bone contains a small protein, rich in the vitamin K-dependent calcium binding amino acid γ-carboxyglutamate (Gla) (1). This protein, named osteocalcin, is extractable by neutral EDTA demineralization and contains 80% of the total Gla found in bone. Osteocalcin is distinctly different from the vitamin K-dependent blood coagulation factors by molecular weight, amino acid composition (2) and sequence (3). Gla synthesis has been demonstrated to occur in isolated chick bones, calvarium, mandible and long bones in organ culture, in the presence of ^{14}C sodium bicarbonate containing medium. In addition, it has been established that the vitamin K-dependent carboxylase enzyme system occurs in microsome preparations from embryonic chick bones (5) and shares many of the characteristics of the liver microsomal vitamin K-dependent carboxylase enzyme system characterized in rat (6,7). Recently, numerous reports of vitamin K carboxylase enzyme activity in a variety of tissues including kidney (8), pancreas, lung (9) and placenta (10) has raised the question as to the nature of the Gla containing proteins synthesized in a specific tissue. It is important then to establish that the synthesis of the Gla protein which occurs in bone tissues is osteocalcin.

In the vitamin K-dependent blood coagulation factors Gla synthesis regulates the conversion of proenzyme to activated enzymes (11). To gain some understanding of the vitamin K-dependent carboxylation reaction in non-hepatic tissues, as a potential proenzyme regulator, it is of interest to determine if Gla peptides from various tissues arise from larger molecules or are synthesized directly. This laboratory has studied the biosynthesis of osteocalcin in bone cultures and in microsome preparations from embryonic chick bone to determine if a proenzyme pre-osteocalcin molecule occurs in bone tissue.

METHODS

Treatment of Animals

Fertile eggs were purchased from Spafas Co. (Norwich, CT) and kept at 38°C in a commercial incubator with a humid atmosphere. Vitamin K deficiency was produced in the embryos by injection with sodium warfarin (Endo Laboratories, Garden City, NJ) into the allantoic sac as follows: 100 micrograms per egg on days 11, 12 and 13, and 200 micrograms/egg on days 14 to 16; eggs were killed at either 16 or 17 days. The effect of the warfarin was assessed in each batch of embryos by measuring the Gla content in several bones after alkaline hydrolysis and amino acid analysis.

Vitamin K-dependent Labeled Microsomes

A fraction greatly enriched in microsomes was prepared from homogenates of pooled calvarium and limb bones (femur and tibia dissected from cartilaginous ends), following the differential centrifugation procedure described by Peterkovsky et al for embryonic chick bone (12). The subcellular fractions and aliquots of the microsomes were assayed for marker enzyme activities as previously described (5). Fresh microsomal suspensions were incubated in a 1 ml volume which included 100 µg of vitamin K_1, 50 µC [^{14}C] $NaHCO_3$, 100 mg cycloheximide, and 0.3 mg diethiothreitol for one hour at 30°C with constant shaking. The reaction was stopped by the addition of 4N acetic acid to pH 6.0 and dialyzed exhaustively against .05M $NaHCO_3$. The microsomal proteins were examined by SDS slab gel electrophoresis described below.

Bone Cultures

Calvarium, mandible and long bones were dissected from chick embryos at various ages and cultured in either tightly capped roller tubes for short pulses (from 1 to 8 hours) or on stainless steel grids for long term incubation (from 1 to 8 days). For vitamin K-dependent incorporation of [^{14}C] $NaHCO_3$, Dulbecco's modified Eagles medium, supplemented with HEPES (25 mM) glutamine (2 mM), aspartic acid (.15 mg/ml), glutamic acid (.15 mg/ml), ascorbic acid (.5 mg/ml) and 5 mg/ml of powdered bovine serum albumin was utilized. In cultures of normal bones 10 µCi/ml of [^{14}C] $NaHCO_3$ bicarbonate was included in the medium and no vitamin K; however bone incubations from warfarin-treated animals included 100 µg/ml of vitamin K_1 in the form of aquaMEPHYTON (Merck, Sharp and Dome, W. Point, PA). For long periods of bone culture, a modified BGJ medium (13) supplemented with glutamine (2 mM), ascorbic acid (.5 mg/ml), powdered bovine serum albumin (5 mg/ml), penicillin (100 units/ml), streptomycin (100 µg/ml) and Fungizone (0.25 µg/ml) was utilized. Labeling was performed with uniformly labeled [^{14}C] glutamic acid (New England Nuclear, Boston, MA) by applying 10 µC directly to the bone. For short pulse labeling with [^{14}C] $NaHCO_3$, bones were transferred to roller tubes containing Dulbecco's MEM as described above.

Identification of [^{14}C] Gla

Following the appropriate incubations, bones were rinsed gently with water and lyophilized. For each analysis, 4 bones were alkaline hydrolyzed as described by Hauschka (14) and the samples analyzed for both radioactive and ninhydrin amino acid components on a Beckman 121M amino acid analyzer. Radioactivity was detected by means of a Packard flow scintillation counter which monitored the analyzer eluante in Instagel (Packard Instruments). An aliquot of the same hydrolyzate used for radioactive analysis was also analyzed for amino acids by ninhydrin detection to allow for the quantitation of counts in Gla per nanomole of Gla or glutamic acid. Proof of the putative [^{14}C] Gla structure was performed by isolation of the compound on a Dowex-1 anion exchange column as described by Gundberg et al (15). An aliquot of the isolated ^{14}C Gla was treated with strong acid (6N HCl) for 6 hours at 108°C. Radioactive amino acid analysis demonstrated the purified [^{14}C] Gla and its conversion to [^{14}C] glutamic acid.

Characterization of ^{14}C Gla-containing Proteins

Soluble non-collagenous proteins from labeled bones were extracted by

0.2M EDTA demineralization at pH 8.0 for 18 hours at 5°C, dialyzed and chromatographed on Sephadex G-100 as previously described for the characterization of osteocalcin (1). The labeled fractions were pooled and Gla detected after alkaline hydrolysis. The total of bone proteins were examined by the following procedure. Following incubation, bones were treated with 12.5% trichloroacetic on ice, gently homogenizing for 10 min. which serves to both demineralize the bone and leave precipitated the bone proteins, including osteocalcin (16). The TCA precipitate was washed with acetone, dried and 2 mg dissolved in 1 ml 1% sodium dodecyl sulfate .05M TRS buffer, pH 6.8 with .01% β-mercaptoethanol for gel electrophoresis. Slab gel electrophoreses using a gradient gel as described by Laemmli (17) was performed to identify the labeled protein fraction(s). Following electrophoresis, the gels were frozen, sliced in 1 mm portions and solubilized by hydrogen peroxide treatment at 50°C for 8 hours. The solubilized gel slices were taken up in Instagel and counted in a Packard tricarb scintillation counter. Osteocalcin obtained from 10 week adult metatarsal bone, chromatographed on Sephadex G-100 and DEAE chromatography as previously described (2), was used as standard osteocalcin marker for disc gel electrophoresis and column chromatography.

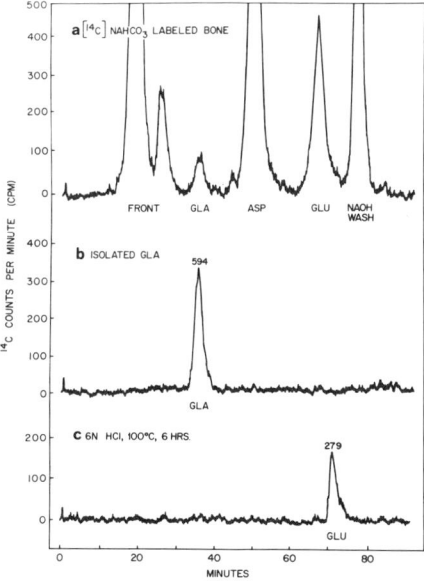

Figure 1. Synthesis of [^{14}C]γ-carboxyglutamic acid (Gla) in 15 day embryonic chick calvaria (a) radioactive elution profile from Beckman 121M analyzer of alkaline hydrolyzed [^{14}C] NaHCO$_3$ labeled bone; (b) after isolation of the bone-synthesized ^{14}C Gla by anion exchange chromatography (c) conversion of [^{14}C] Gla to [^{14}C] glutamic acid with loss of 53% of the original radioactivity.

RESULTS

Synthesis of Gla in Bone Cultures

When chick calvarium or mandible bones are pulsed for at least 1 hour in [^{14}C] NaHCO$_3$-containing medium, rinsed, alkaline hydrolyzed and applied to the amino acid analyzer, a radioelution profile is obtained as shown in Fig. 1. In this system of normal bone growth bicarbonate label is utilized for the formation of aspartic and glutamic acids as well as the post-translational vitamin K-dependent synthesis of Gla. The structure of the putative Gla component was proven by isolation of Gla on a preparative Dowex-1 column. Equal aliquots of the isolated Gla component, one acid hydrolyzed, were re-applied to the Beckman 121M analyzer (Fig. 1b) which demonstrated conversion of γ-carboxyglutamic acid to glutamic acid (Fig. 1c). Forty-seven percent of the counts in Gla were recovered in glutamic acid as expected, since random decarboxylation of either equivalent γ-carboxyl group can occur.

The rate of incorporation of [^{14}C] NaHCO$_3$ label into a growing bone and the percent of the counts which are utilized in Gla formation is dependent upon the age and type of bone and duration of the pulse. Figure 2 shows the age dependent incorporation of [^{14}C] NaHCO$_3$ for a chick calvarium bone incubated from 1 to 8 hours. For a young embryonic bone (between 12 and 13 days), the total incorporated counts found in Gla within one hour are higher than observed in older bones which suggests that at this age more endogenous precursor substrate is immediately available. In 14-16 day bones Gla synthesis is seen to increase steadily, accounting for some 5 to 3% of the total bicarbonate label. From ages 17-19 day lower levels of radioactivity are found in Gla as well as in other amino acids. Although bone Gla content is 2-3 times greater at 19 day than at 12 day (14), the rate of synthesis of Gla is not increased 2-fold as measured by ^{14}C Gla formation.

The post-translational synthesis of Gla was demonstrated by the formation of ^{14}C Gla from ^{14}C glutamic acid in 14 day mandible bones cultured on grids for over 60 hours. Bones were cultured for 15 hours in

Table 1. Post-translational synthesis of γ-carboxyglutamic from ^{14}C-glutamic acid in 14 day chick embryo mandible bone.

		CPM/10 mg	
	Gla	Glu	Asp
Pulsed 24 hours	428	60,146	40,550
Chased 24 hours	919	52,510	33,704

BGJ medium, pulsed for 24 hours with ^{14}C glutamic acid, and then label chased with fresh medium. The bones were analyzed for ^{14}C Gla at each 24 hour point after alkaline hydrolysis. As shown in Table 1, ^{14}C Gla increased as the pool of labeled amino acids decreased.

Isolation of Osteocalcin

An examination of the medium obtained from chick mandible bones cultured on stainless steel grids for 24 hours in [^{14}C] NaHCO$_3$ supplemented medium revealed that no Gla protein is found in the culture medium, as shown in Fig. 3. It appears that osteocalcin remains with the intact bone tissue. Osteocalcin was extracted by EDTA demineralization from batch preparations of 15 day calvarial bones which were [^{14}C] NaHCO$_3$ labeled for 8 hours. The extracted labeled proteins were fractionated over Sephadex G-100 and radioactive osteocalcin separated (Fig. 4). Forty percent of the total eluted radioactivity was found in the osteocalcin fraction. This peak as well as the void volume fraction contained ^{14}C Gla following alkaline hydrolysis and detection on the Beckman 121M. The radioactive fraction eluting with

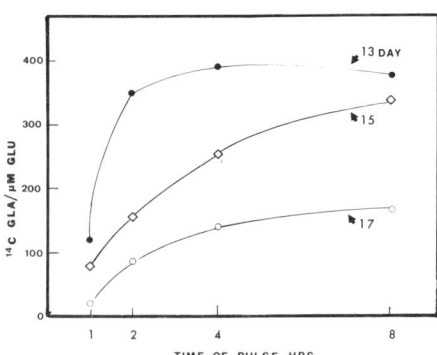

Figure 2. Age dependent formation of [^{14}C] γ-carboxyglutamic acid in embryonic chick calvaria. Each point represents the average of 3 determinations which varied less than 10%.

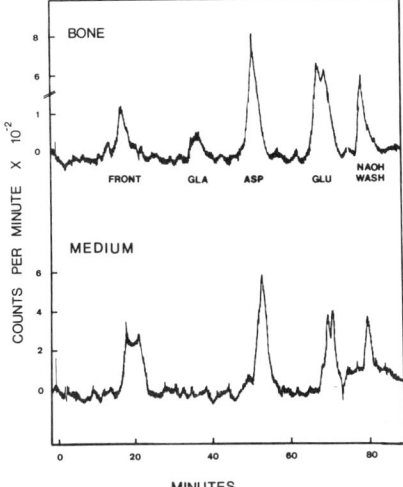

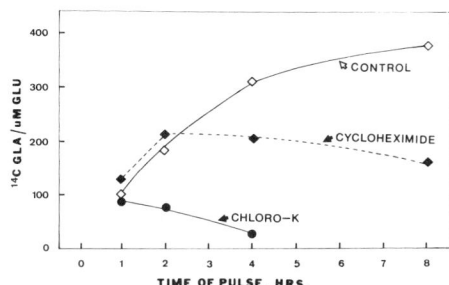

Figure 5. Formation of $[^{14}C]\gamma$-carboxyglutamic acid in 15 day chick calvaria bones incubated in $[^{14}C]$ NaHCO$_3$ supplemented medium containing 200 μg cycloheximide/ml and 20 μg Chloro vitamin K/ml. Each point is the average of 2 determinations.

Figure 3. Amino acid analyzer radioelution profiles of the alkaline hydrolysates of (a) chick mandible bone cultured for 24 hrs. in $[^{14}C]$ NaHCO$_3$ supplemented medium and (b) the culture medium.

the salt contained labeled amino acids but no Gla. Alkaline hydrolysis of the labeled bone residue remaining after EDTA extraction revealed that 90% of the bone Gla had been extracted.

Vitamin K dependency of Gla Synthesis in Bone Cultures

The bone organ culture system can be manipulated such that γ-carboxyglutamic acid accounts for some 60-70% of the bicarbonate incorporated label. If 15 day normal bones are cultured in medium which contains cycloheximide, (Fig. 5), no net increase in the counts incorporated into Gla is observed after 2 hours indicating that protein synthesis has ter-

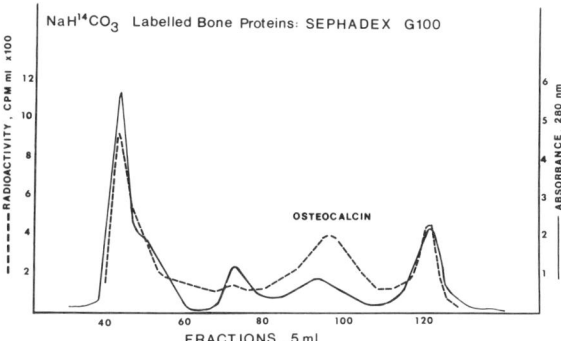

Figure 4. Fractionation of EDTA soluble proteins from 15 days calvaria pulsed 8 hrs. The dialyzed and lyophilized extract was applied to a column 2.5 x 100 cm eluting with 0.1M NH$_4$HCO$_3$, pH 8.0 at 12 ml/hr at 5°C.

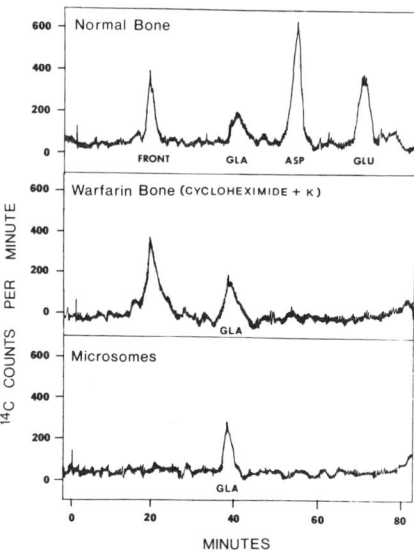

Figure 6. Trichloroacetic acid precipitated bone proteins from [^{14}C] NaHCO$_3$ labeled 15 day calvaria pulsed 4 hrs. (a) normal bone (b) bones removed from warfarin-treated embryos and cultured with the addition of cycloheximide (200 μg/ml) and vitamin K$_1$ (100 μg/ml). (c) The lower profile demonstrates that [^{14}C] Gla is the only labeled product resulting from the incubation of bone microsomes in the presence of vitamin K$_1$ and [^{14}C] NaHCO$_3$ as described in methods.

minated and endogenous substrate for Gla synthesis is no longer available. When 2 chloro vitamin K$_1$, a direct inhibitor of vitamin K, is included in the medium at a concentration of 20 μg/ml, rapid inhibition of Gla synthesis is achieved also at 2 hours. The counts per minute at each point are normalized to the glutamic acid content in the hydrolysate. It is apparent from this type of experiment that approximately 2 hours are required for the inhibitors to be completely effective. Having established these conditions Gla synthesis can be specifically achieved in organ culture by suitable incubation of bones from a warfarin-treated embryo incubated in the presence of cycloheximide and vitamin K. A bone excised from a warfarin-treated embryo presumably has endogenous precursor substrate accumulated. Shown in Fig. 6 are the [^{14}C] NaHCO$_3$ pulsed normal calvarial bones and warfarin-treated calvarial bones after a 2 hour pre-incubation period in medium without bicarbonate of vitamin K but including cycloheximide. The bones were alkaline hydrolyzed after 12.5% TCA treatment which removed labeled pools of amino acids which were not protein bound. The percent of the counts found in Gla in normal bone prepared in this way is increased to 20% as compared to 3% when the bone is analyzed directly as shown in Fig. 1a. In the warfarin bones, 62% of the incorporated counts are found as Gla with the remainder found in the front peak resulting from CO$_2$ reaction products. Thus, the labeling of bone from a warfarin-treated embryo in the presence of cycloheximide and vitamin K$_1$ is much more specific in that protein bound ^{14}C aspartic and glutamic acid formation does not occur. The radioelution profile is compared to that obtained after alkaline hydrolysis of a labeled microsomal preparation (Fig. 6c). in which Gla is the only ^{14}C labeled component.

Characterization of Osteocalcin in Warfarin-treated Bones

The labeled TCA precipitated proteins from normal and warfarin-treated bone and labeled microsomal proteins obtained from warfarin-treated embryo were examined by slab gel electrophoresis as shown in Fig. 7. Radioactive analysis of the electrophoretically separated proteins revealed several protein bands in the samples. In a normal bone culture, it is seen that the collagen α chains are labeled due largely to the formation

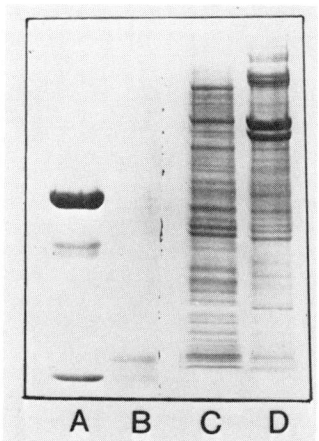

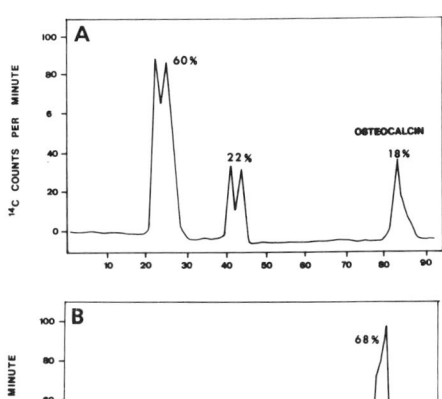

Figure 7. Slab gel electrophoresis (Laemmli system) of (a) albumin, pepsin and lysozyme (b) osteocalcin standard (c) SDS solubilized bone microsomal proteins (d) TCA extracted proteins from embryonic chick calvaria.

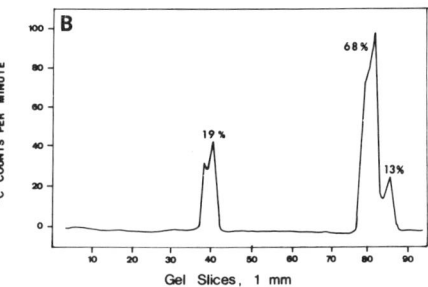

Figure 8. Distribution of radioactivity in TCA extracted proteins from (a) normal 15 day calvaria bone incubated in [^{14}C] $NaHCO_3$ containing medium and (b) warfarinized bones incubated in [^{14}C] $NaHCO_3$ containing medium supplemented with cycloheximide (200 μg/ml) and vitamin K_1 (100 μg/ml). In normal bones, the radioactive bands at 22 and 25 mm correspond to collagen α chains.

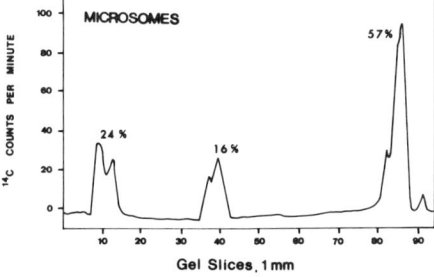

Figure 9. Radioactive proteins found in labeled bone microsome preparations. The fraction at 10 mm is in the 200,000 dalton range and at 40 mm approximately 71,000 daltons. The peak at 84 mm coincides with osteocalcin standard as shown in Fig. 7.

of [^{14}C] aspartic and glutamic acids (Fig. 8a). An additional radioactive peak is observed in the molecular weight range of 70–75,000 daltons and approximately 20% of the radioactive protein is seen to migrate to the position of osteocalcin standard. In the extracted proteins from a warfarin culture (Fig. 8b), in which protein synthesis has been inhibited by cycloheximide, label is found in two fractions; one, eluting in the 70–75,000 dalton range and a large percentage (58%) of the labeled proteins in bone microsome preparations (Fig. 9) also showed the same two radioactive fractions as observed in the proteins from warfarin bone cultures. In addition, in microsomal proteins, a third radioactive fraction of extremely high molecular weight in the range of slightly over 200,000 daltons was evident.

DISCUSSION

Explanted chick embryonic bones of various types, cultured under bone growth conditions, have the capacity to synthesize γ-carboxyglutamic acid. We have previously shown that over long periods of culture not only does collagen synthesis increase as measured by hydroxyproline, but Gla synthesis is also increased; removal of bones during an 8 day culture period at specific time intervals for incubation in the presence of ^{14}C sodium bicarbonate has demonstrated that the bone is capable of de novo synthesis of Gla(18). Thus the possibility of labeling a precursor osteocalcin which had accumulated in the bone from circulating proteins before removal from the chick for culture studies is remote. In this study, it is clearly evident that Gla synthesis occurs post-translationally in bone on protein bound [^{14}C] glutamic acid side chain residues. The results of this study indicate that osteocalcin is clearly the product of Gla synthesis in the cultured chick bones. Extraction of the labeled proteins in neutral demineralizing salts followed by chromatography on Sephadex G-100 indicates that approximately 40% of the labeled protein is found as the osteocalcin component. Alkaline hydrolysis of the void volume radioactive fraction revealed the presence of [^{14}C] Gla. It was of interest therefore to examine not only the noncollagenous soluble proteins of bone but the entire matrix of bone synthesized proteins by electrophoresis to determine the distribution of Gla labeled-protein. For this purpose we developed a more specific labeling for Gla in cultures of bones from warfarin-treated animals in which endogenous precursor has presumably accumulated. Incubations were carried out in the presence of vitamin K_1 which overcomes warfarin inhibition and cycloheximide to inhibit the synthesis of new protein which would be labeled as a result of [^{14}C] glutamic and aspartic acid incorporation. Alkaline hydrolysis of the incubated warfarinized bone revealed that the majority of amino acid labeling was found only in Gla (Fig. 6). The bone matrix proteins from warfarin-treated bone cultures showed two labeled components identical to those found in labeled bone microsomes, one in the 70-75,000 molecular weight range and the majority of the label in the osteocalcin region. In microsomal proteins, however, additional label is found in a very high molecular fraction in the range of 200,000 daltons. It is possible that the small osteocalcin molecule could be absorbed onto membrane fragments or ribosomal proteins or that a higher molecular weight form of osteocalcin occurs in microsomal preparations. This form of 200,000 daltons may not be observed in the warfarin-treated bones incubated in the presence of cycloheximide due to the fact that protein synthesis of a 200,000 molecular weight form has been inhibited. This form may be accumulated in the warfarin-treated bone which when carboxylated is rapidly converted to osteocalcin molecule. The labeled component of 71,000 daltons may represent an intermediate in the formation of osteocalcin. Other studies (16) of osteocalcin characterization have revealed that heterogeneity of the molecule occurs (isoelectric and sequence distinct forms) which is not merely an artifact of the isolation procedure. Thus there is a strong suggestion of proteolytic processing of the osteocalcin peptide.

It appears from the labeling studies in both microsomal and in whole bone culture that higher molecular forms of osteocalcin occur at least in

the range of 70-75,000 daltons. At this point it is too premature to
to say that the 70-75,000 or 200,000 molecular weight forms are proenzyme
forms of osteocalcin. Such a statement requires isolation of the high
molecular weight forms and their conversion to osteocalcin demonstrated
in chicken bone. In previous pulbications (18,19) the possible origin
of osteocalcin biosynthesis has been discussed in detail. The data of
these experiments appears to have limited the potential choices which
included 1) direct synthesis of osteocalcin, 2) a Gla-containing proenzyme, or 3) arising from pro-collagen peptides. Although a close association of collagen biosynthesis with osteocalcin biosynthesis occurs in
chick (19) and bovine (20) bone, it appears unlikely from the labeled
microsomal products that a pro-collagen α chain is formed. The labeled
product of 70-75,000 daltons is too small to account for a pro-collagen
species (21). It appears that osteocalcin does arise from a higher molecular protein form and is not synthesized directly. Further experimentation is required to determine if an active enzyme is also produced
along with the osteocalcin peptide by proteolytic conversion analogous
to prothrombin conversion or if the osteocalcin peptide plays an active
role in bone function by mediating Ca^{++}-phospholipid-bone mineral interactions.

ACKNOWLEDGEMENTS

The authors wish to thank Drs. P.M. Gallop, M.J. Glimcher and P.V.
Hauschka for helpful discussions. This work was supported by grants
DE 04651 and AM 15671. J.B.L. is a Senior Investigator of the Arthritis
Foundation.

REFERENCES

1. Hauschka, P.V., Lian, J.B. and Gallop, P.M. (1975) Proc. Natl. Acad. Sci. USA 72, 3925-3929.
2. Hauschka, P.V. and Gallop, P.M. (1977) in Calcium Binding Proteins and Calcium Function (Wasserman et al, eds.) pp. 338-347, Elsevier North Holland, Inc. Amsterdam.
3. Price, P.A., Poser, J.W. and Roman, N. (1976) Proc. Natl. Acad. Sci. 73, 3373-3375.
4. Lian, J.B., Hauschka, P.V., Glimcher, M.J. and Gallop, P.M. (1976) Trans. Orthop. Res. Soc. 1, 176.
5. Lian, J.B. and Friedman, P.A. (1978) J. Biol. Chem. 253, 6623-6626.
6. Esmon, C.T., Sadowski, J.A. and Suttie, J.W. (1975) J. Biol. Chem. 250, 4744-4748.
7. Friedman, P.A. and Shia, M. (1976) Bioch. Biophys. Res. Commun. 72, 647-654.
8. Hauschka, P.V., Friedman, P.A., Traverso, H.P. and Gallop, P.M. (1976) Bioch. Biophys. Res. Commun. 71, 1207-1213.
9. Bell, R.G. (1979) Eighth Steenbock Symposium, Madison, Wisconsin.
10. Friedman, P.A., Hauschka, P.V., Shia, M. and Wallace, J.K. (1979) Bioch. Biophys. Acta 583, 261-283.
11. Suttie, J.W. and Jackson, C. (1977) Physiol. Rev. 57, 1-70.
12. Peterkovsky, B. and Assad, R. (1976) J. Biol. Chem. 251, 4770-4777.
13. Ascher, M.A., Sledge, C.B. and Glimcher, M.J. (1974) J. Clin. Endocrin. Metab. 38, 376-389.
14. Hauschka, P.V. (1977) Anal. Biochem. 80, 212-223.
15. Gundberg, C., Lian, J.B. and P.M. Gallop (1979) Eighth Steenbock

Symposium, Madison, Wisconsin.
16. Hauschka, P.V. (1979) Eighth Steenbock Symposium, Madison, Wisc.
17. Laemmli, U.K. (1970) Nature 222, 680.
18. Lian, J.B., Hauschka, P.V. and Gallop, P.M. (1978) Fed. Proc. 37, 2615-2620.
19. Hauschka, P.V. and Reid, M.L. (1978) Develop. Biol. 65, 426-434.
20. Nishimoto, S.K. and Price, P.A. (1979) J. Biol. Chem. 254, 437-441.
21. Sherr, C.J., Taubman, M.B. and Goldberg, B. (1973) J. Biol. Chem. 248, 7033-7040.

POSSIBLE PHYSIOLOGICAL ROLE OF THE VITAMIN K-DEPENDENT BONE PROTEIN

S. REDDY and J. W. SUTTIE

Department of Biochemistry
College of Agricultural and Life Sciences
University of Wisconsin-Madison
Madison, WI 53706

INTRODUCTION

The vitamin K-dependent bone protein discovered by Hauschka (1) and Price (2,3) and their collaborators has been isolated and characterized and studies of its physiological role have begun. Although it has been shown that this protein is synthesized in the bone rather than being synthesized elsewhere and transported to the bone (4,5), and significant decreases in the amount of this protein can be demonstrated following long-term coumarin administration (6,7), a physiological role for this protein has yet to be established. Coumarin therapy (8,9) has been reported to affect calcifying tissues during fetal development, and vitamin K has been reported to influence the development of osteoporosis in the human (10). Vitamin K deficiency has also been reported to increase the width of the osteoid seam in growing chick bones (11). However, no direct involvement of the vitamin K-dependent bone protein has been shown in any of these cases. We have considered the possibility that the lack of any observation of a significant effect of vitamin K deprivation on calcified tissue metabolism has been due to the inability to affect enough of the total bone pool to observe an effect. We are, therefore, reporting an effect of coumarin administration on calcium metabolism in two rapidly mineralizing tissue systems.

METHODS

Two systems have been studied. The developing rat fetus began to calcify at 17 days, and the short period between this and the normal 21-day term delivery therefore represents a perid of very rapid calcification. Pregnant Holtzman rats were given an injection of 5.0 mg/kg Warfarin i.p. at various times after conception, and then given a 1 mg i.m. injection of vitamin K_1 after 36 h. This dose of Warfarin will completely block the action of vitamin K for this time period, and the injection of vitamin K at 36 h overcomes the action of the antagonist and prevents hemorrhage due to low levels of the plasma vitamin K-dependent clotting factors. The rats were killed at the time periods indicated in Figures 1 and 2, the fetuses were removed, weighed, dried, ashed, and the ash analyzed for Ca, P, and Mg. The second model studied was that of the developing rat incisor. The rat incisor grows continuously at a rate of about 0.5 mm/day and 200 g male Holtzman rats were again given a 5 mg/kg Warfarin injection followed by 1 mg of vitamin K 36 h later. These animals were killed after 30 days, the incisors were embedded in plastic and the Ca and P content of the enamel determined by electron microprobe analysis and the Knoop number by a microhardness apparatus. Additional details of the experimental procedure will be presented elsewhere.

RESULTS

In an initial study, pregnant rats were injected with Warfarin at various times between 17.5 and 19 days of pregnancy, administered vitamin K 36 h later, and killed at 21 days. This treatment did not have any consistent,

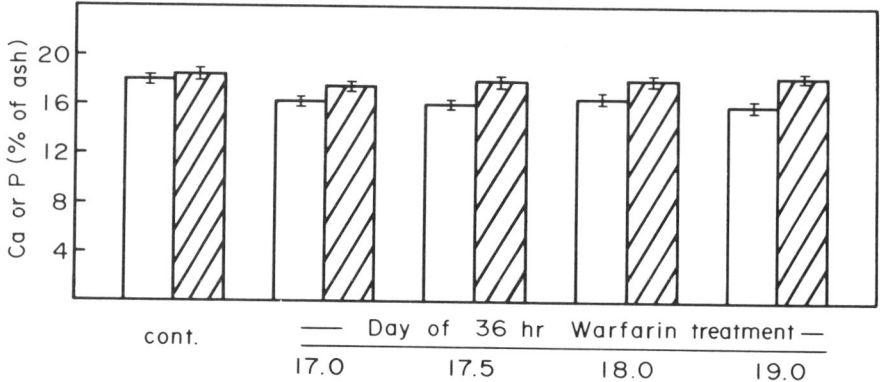

FIGURE 1. Effect of Warfarin administration on fetal mineralization. At the various days after conception which are indicated, pregnant rats were given warfarin for 36 h. The Ca (open bars) and P (hatched bars) content of the ash of 21-day fetuses is shown. The Ca content at all time periods was significantly different (p < .001) than the controls (saline injection). From 6-10 fetuses were removed from five pregnant rats per group and analyzed.

statistically-significant effect on fetal weight (control = 6.0 g/pup, treated 5.5-6.0 g/pup) or the percentage of the dried fetal weight which was ash (control = 12.8%, treated = 12.1-12.5%). However, as shown in Figure 1, this treatment did significantly decrease the percent of calcium in the ash of the Warfarin-treated pups. There was no effect of warfarin administration on the content of P or Mg in the ash. In a second experiment, pregnant rats were treated at 17.5-19.5 days with Warfarin and killed 36 h later. Again, this treatment had no effect on pup weight or the calcification of the fetus but again did (Fig. 2) influence the percent of calcium in the ash. This effect was most pronounced in the pups from dams given Warfarin at 17.5 days where the treated pups had only 77% as as much Ca in the ash as did the controls treated with saline at the same time. Again, the phosphorus content of the ash was not influenced by Warfarin treatment.

The data in Figure 3A illustrate the concentration of Ca in the incisor enamel of rats given Warfarin for a 36 h period 30 days before they were killed and of the concentration observed in control (saline injected) animals. In normal rats, there was a sharp increase in Ca content from the immature enamel at the growing base of the incisor to the mature enamel at the tip. This same general pattern of calcium concentration was seen in the Warfarin-treated rats with the exception of a sharp dip in enamel calcium content which was observed at the point that would be expected to correspond to the previous 36 h Warfarin treatment. The exact point along the incisor where the lowered Ca concentration was seen varied

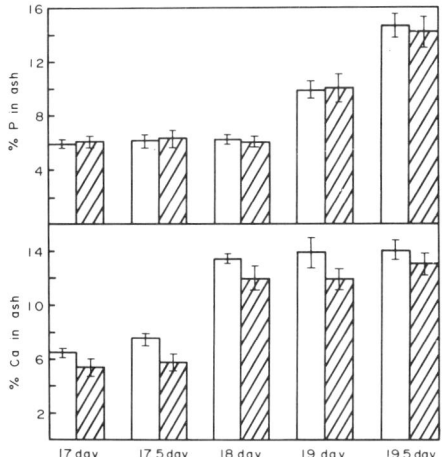

FIGURE 2. Effect of Warfarin administration on fetal mineralization. Pregnant rats were given Warfarin at the various times after conception indicated, and then killed and pups removed 36 h after the Warfarin treatment. Fetal ash was analyzed for phosphorus (top) and calcium (bottom). The Ca content of the Warfarin-treated pups (hatched bars) differed significantly ($p < 0.01$ at 17.5 days; $p < 0.1$ at other days) from the saline treated controls (open bars). Phosphorus content was not altered. From 6-10 fetuses were removed from five pregnant rats per group and analyzed.

somewhat from one animal to another as might be expected from normal variations in incisor growth rate. The phosphorus content of the enamel was not influenced. The data in Figure 3B show that the hardness of the enamel, as measured by the Knoop number, was not affected by this treatment.

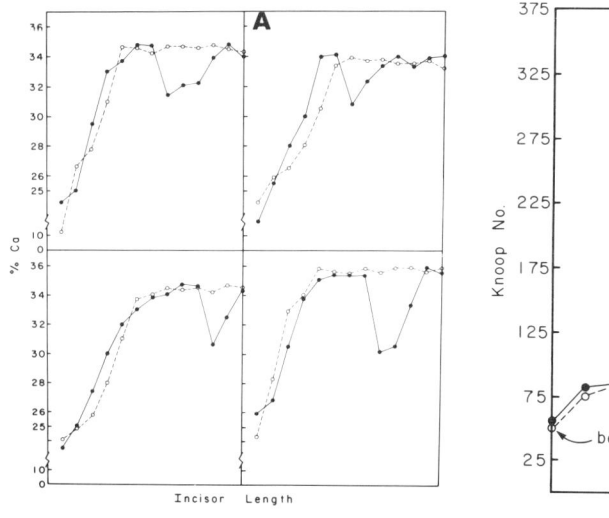
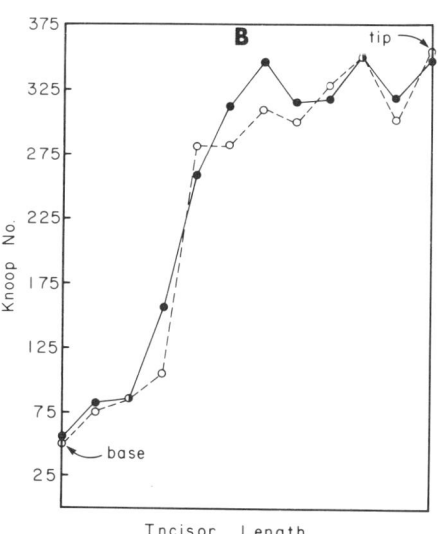

FIGURE 3. (A) Effect of Warfarin treatment on enamel calcium content. The values shown are data from individual incisors of four Warfarin-treated (closed circles) and four saline injected (open circles) animals. The position along the incisor at which a drop in Ca was seen, and extent of the drop in Ca content is typical of that seen for 13 other animals. The P content of the enamel was not affected by Warfarin treatment. (B) Effect of Warfarin treatment on enamel hardness. Hardness of the enamel at various points was measured and expressed as a Knoop number. The values shown are the averages of 17 Warfarin-treated (closed bars) and 17 control (open bars) incisors.

DISCUSSION

These data appear to represent the first conclusive demonstration of a defect in mineralized tissue caused by the lack of action of vitamin K. Whether the alterations seen are a result of the lack of synthesis of the vitamin K-dependent bone protein described by others, or represent an as of yet unknown action of the vitamin cannot be determined. Placental tissue contains a vitamin K-dependent protein (12), and lack of synthesis of this protein could have been involved in the fetal rat effect. It is also possible that the enamel forming organ contains an unrecognized vitamin K-dependent protein that could mediate the response seen. It is possible however, that these effects might be related to the physiological role of the vitamin K-dependent bone protein and if so, it suggests that this protein is in some manner involved in determining the type of bone mineral which is formed in mineralizing tissue. Unless it is determined that some normal component of mineralized tissue is greatly increased in these tissues, the change in Ca/P ratio would seem to imply a change in type of bone salt which is present. Preliminary data on the total fetal ash composition (data not shown) by emission spectroscopy did not reveal any substantial alteration resulting from Warfarin treatment. Alterations in the compositon of mineralized tissue has not been reported in patients or experimental animals subjected to long term coumarin treatment. In the present study, action of vitamin K was completely blocked for 36 h, and the models studied were such that this represented a significant part of the total mineralization which was investigated. It may be that severe conditions such as these were required before the effect of vitamin K on mineralization can be observed.

ACKNOWLEDGEMENTS

This research was supported by the College of Agricultural and Life Sciences of the University of Wisconsin-Madison and in part by a Public Health Service Grant from the National Institutes of Health (AM-14881) and a postdoctoral training grant in nutrition from the National Institute of Dental Research (DE-07031).

REFERENCES

1. Hauschka, P. V., Lian, J. B., and Gallop, P. M. (1975) Proc. Nat. Acad. Sci. USA 72, 3925-3929.
2. Price, P. A., Otsuka, A. S., Poser, J. W., Kristaponis, J., and Raman, N. (1976) Proc. Nat. Acad. Sci. USA 73, 1447-1451.
3. Price, P. A., Poser, J. W., and Raman, N. (1976) Proc. Nat. Acad. Sci. USA 73, 3374-3375.
4. Lian, J. B., and Friedman, P. A. (1978) J. Biol. Chem. 253, 6623-6626.
5. Nishimoto, S. K., and Price, P. A. (1979) J. Biol. Chem. 254, 437-441.
6. Lian, J. B., Hauschka, P. V., and Gallop, P. M. (1978) Fed. Proc. 37, 2615-2620.
7. Hauschka, P. V., and Reid, M. L. (1978) J. Biol. Chem. 253, 9063-9068.
8. Pettifor, J. M., and Benson, R. (1975) J. Pediatr. 86, 459-462.
9. Warkany, J. (1975) Am. J. Dis. Child. 129, 287-288.
10. Tomita, A. (1971) Clin. Endocrinol. (Tokyo) 19, 731-736.
11. Taylor, D. N., Crenshaw, M. A., and Bawden, J. W. (1977) J. Dent. Res. 56, 9 (abstract)
12. Friedman, P. A., Hauschka, P. V., Shia, M. A., and Wallace, J. K. (1979) Biochim. Biophys. Acta 583, 261-265.

MACROMOLECULAR INHIBITORS OF CALCIUM PHOSPHATE PRECIPITATION IN BONE

AUSTIN G. DIAMOND and WILLIAM F. NEUMAN

Department of Radiation Biology and Biophysics,
University of Rochester School of Medicine and Dentistry,
Rochester, NY 14642

INTRODUCTION

How the rate and location of calcium exchange between the mineral phase of bone and the extracellular fluids is controlled remains an unanswered question. Although the exact composition of the bone fluid is difficult to determine, it probably is metastable with respect to the major mineral present, hydroxyapatite ($Ca_{10}(PO_4)_6OH_2$). That is, mineral crystals in contact with such a phase should grow at the expense of the constituent ions in the solution. However, bone in contact with such a solution is capable of maintaining it at a higher level of Ca^{2+} and P_i than would be expected for mineral alone (1). One possible reason is that macromolecules secreted by the cells interact with the crystals to modify the reactivity of the mineral surface. Various macromolecules present in bone cause or inhibit nucleation of mineral formation from metastable solutions or affect the interconversions of the various mineral phases that have been postulated to exist in the tissue (2). Recently, the discovery of a unique gamma-carboxyglutamic acid-containing protein in bone and the fact that it has action in such systems has lead to speculation that it may have an important role in the regulation of bone mineral homeostasis (3,4). The assay described here tests the ability of macromolecules isolated from bone to interact with hydroxyapatite crystals to inhibit their growth under similar ionic conditions to those expected in bone.

MATERIALS AND METHODS

Assay

The assay buffer was 50mM PIPES, 130mM NaCl, 10mM KCl, 1.6mM $MgCl_2$, pH 7.4. Stock solutions of buffer containing either 4mM $CaCl_2$ or 6mM KH_2PO_4 were prepared. Fractions to be assayed were dissolved in the P_i buffer at appropriate concentrations (usually 0-2mg/ml). For assay, 0.25ml of the Ca^{2+} solution and 0.25ml of the P_i (containing test substances at a range of concentrations) were pipetted into 17mm diameter polypropylene tubes (Final Ca^{2+} 2mM; P_i 3mM). Hydroxyapatite crystals (0.5mg; Matheson, Coleman and Bell) in 0.01ml buffer, or buffer alone, were added, the tubes capped, and shaken for 6 hrs at 25°C. The contents were transferred to 1.5ml polypropylene conical centrifuge tubes and centrifuged (7000 x g, 5 min). The supernatants were analysed for calcium content with a Calcette (Precision Systems Inc.) EGTA-titrator. In some cases the ionic calcium was determined with a Ca-selective electrode. The inorganic phosphate measured colorimetrically.

Preparation and EDTA-Extraction of Rat Bone

Cortical sections of long bones of adult (150-250 g) rats were cleaned of soft tissue and powdered in a liquid nitrogen-cooled mill (Spex Industries). The bone powder was placed in a dialysis sac (Spectrapore 3) with 2 ml/g 4M NaCl and dialysed against several changes of 0.5M EDTA pH 8.0 (with 1mM PMSF, 1mM PCMB, 0.02% NaN$_3$) for 7-10 days at 4°C. Both the contents of the sac and the diffusate were stirred continuously. The sac contents were then centrifuged (2000 x g, 20 min) and the supernatant dialysed against water and freeze-dried.

Chromatography of EDTA-Extract

A 100mg portion of the extract was dissolved in 10 ml 0.05M NH$_4$HCO$_3$ and applied to a 2.5 x 100 cm column of Sephadex G100 at 4°C. Elution was at a rate of 22ml/hr and 4.5ml fractions were collected. For DEAE-cellulose chromatography 50mg of extract was applied to a 1.6 x 4 cm column (Whatman DE52) equilibrated with 0.05M Tris/HCl pH 7.4. A gradient (200ml) of 0-0.6M NaCl in the same buffer was used for elution which was at a flow rate of 36 ml/hr with 2ml fractions collected.

Amino acid analysis.

Amino acid analysis was performed on samples hydrolysed in 2M KOH for 24 hr at 110°C using a Beckman 120C analyser with a 0.9 x 22 cm column. The elution position of Gla was determined with a synthetic sample.

RESULTS

The assay of the total material extracted by EDTA is shown in Figure 1. The final Ca value falls from 2mM to 0.75mM in the absence of any added protein (0% inhibition). In the presence of increasing amounts of EDTA-extract the final Ca drops only to 1.8mM at the higher concentrations representing an 84% inhibition of precipitation. Analysis of ionic Ca gave similar results. No change in Ca was seen in the presence of increasing concentrations of extract when no hydroxyapatite seed was added. The change in P$_i$ (not shown) mirrored that of Ca with a drop from 3mM initial to 2.3mM at zero protein, with an identical inhibition curve.

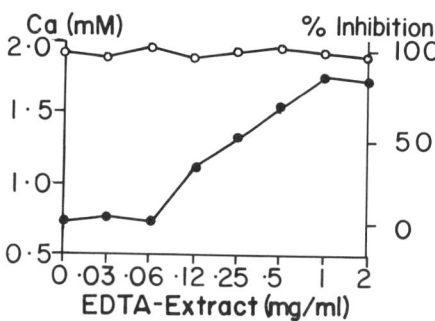
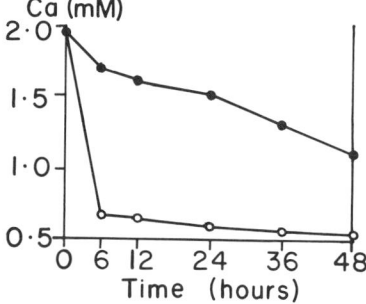

Fig. 1. Effect of Bone Protein on Assay
(●--● With, o--o Without Apatite)

Fig. 2. Time course of Calcium Phosphate Precipitation
(●--● With, o--o Without Protein)

With a fixed concentration of extract (1 mg/ml) it is seen that over a 48 hr period the Ca continues to fall slightly in the absence of added protein but that the extract is capable of delaying the reaction over this period (Fig. 2).

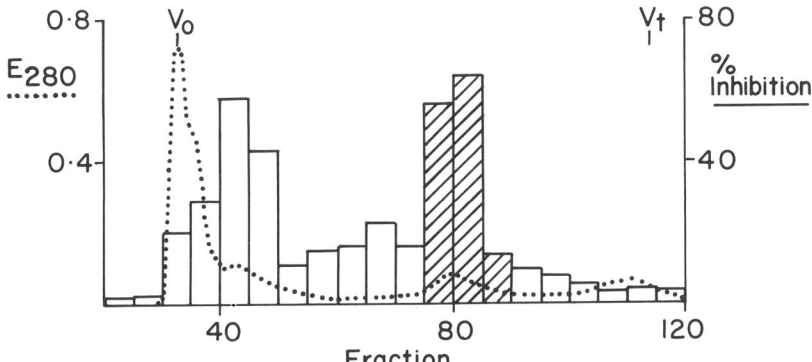

Fig. 3. Activity of Sephadex G 100 Fractions of Rat Bone EDTA-Extract (Fractions where Gla was detected are indicated by cross-hatching)

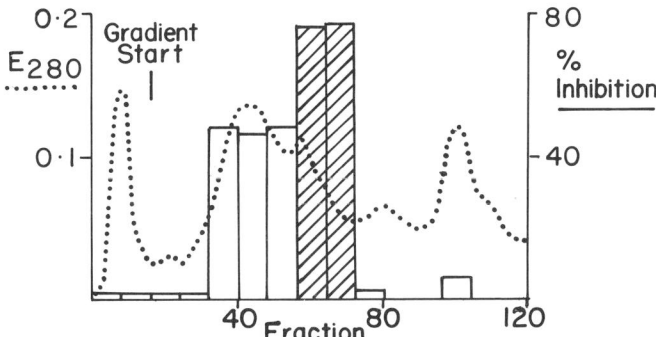

Fig. 4. Activity of DEAE-Cellulose Fractions of Rat Bone EDTA-Extract (Fractions where Gla was detected are indicated by cross-hatching)

When the extract was fractionated on either Sephadex G100 (Fig. 3) or DEAE-cellulose (Fig. 4) the inhibitor-activity was associated with more than one fraction. The profile was obtained by pooling the lyophilized fractions from the column and dissolving in a fixed amount of buffer prior to assay and thus shows the relative contributions of the individual fractions to the total activity. When the fractions were incubated with papain and pronase prior to assay the inhibitory activity of all of them was destroyed. Analysis of the pooled fractions for Gla content showed detectable amounts only in one major fraction from each column. In both cases this fraction had the highest activity in the assay both as a part of the total and on an activity per unit weight basis.

DISCUSSION

The inhibitory activity demonstrated by the assay represents the ability of macromolecules to interact with the hydroxyapatite crystal surface in such a way as to render it less able to sequester ions from the solution to continue crystal growth. An action by binding of calcium ions in solution is ruled out by the observation that the ionized calcium content does not change appreciably in the initial solution with changing macromolecular content. Furthermore, the extent to which macromolecules are able to inhibit crystal growth depends on the amount of hydroxyapatite added to the solution - the amount used in these experiments was chosen to give a conveniently measurable change in calcium over the assay period. The activity is not just a reflection of binding to the crystal surface since some macromolecules (e.g. serum albumin) that bind to apatite do not show inhibitory activity.

The presence of a number of components in bone that possess this activity is clearly shown by both gel and ion-exchange chromatography. Of course, the number of active components demonstrated is a minimum since the separations are relatively crude and the resultant fractions are far from homogeneous. Despite this, there is a variation of activity between the different fractions. Although the fraction richest in Gla has the highest activity, it contributes less than half of the total. Inability to detect Gla in the other active fractions probably means that it is not required for this activity or that it is present but the molecules containing it are only there in small amounts in which case they would have to be extremely active.

This action of bone components to reduce the rate of crystal growth may be significant in controlling the rate and position of mineral deposition within the tissue. The secretion of such components by the cells would enable them to regulate these events at a site removed from their own location. The actual concentrations of the active components are probably much higher in the tissue than was possible to test in the assay, so that the contribution of even the lesser active fractions could be significant in controlling mineral homeostasis. When the function of bone macromolecules in the regulation of solution-mineral homeostasis is considered, the contribution of the Gla-containing protein should be recognized, but not overemphasized.

ACKNOWLEDGEMENTS

The authors wish to thank Dr. J. W. Suttie for his gift of Gla standard. This work was supported in part by U.S. Public Health Service Grant, NIH #AM-17074 and in part by a contract with the U.S. Dept. of Energy, was performed at the University of Rochester and has been assigned Report No. UR-3490-1547.

REFERENCES

1. Neuman, W. F. (1977) Calcif. Tiss. Res. Suppl. to 22, 169-178.

2. Urist, M. R. in Bourne, G. H. (1976) The Biochemistry and Physiology of Bone, Vol IV pp. 2-60, Academic Press, New York.

3. Price, P. A. et al. (1976) Proc. Natl. Acad. Sci. 73, 1447-1451.

4. Lian, J. B., Hauschka, P. V. and Gallop, P. M. (1978) Fed. Proc. 37, 2615-2620.

THE OCCURRENCE OF γ-CARBOXYGLUTAMIC ACID IN ELASMOBRANCH ENDOSKELETON

J. B. LIAN, J. A. GLOWACKI and M. J. GLIMCHER

Departments of Biological Chemistry, Surgery, and Orthopedic Surgery,
Children's Hospital Medical Center,
Harvard Medical School,
Boston, MA 02115

INTRODUCTION

The characterization of osteocalcin, the γ-carboxyglutamic acid (Gla)-containing protein in normal bone tissues (1,2), has raised questions as to the potential role of this vitamin K-dependent calcium-binding protein in bone. The Gla content of bone diaphysis is the highest of any tissue in the body and correlates with the degree of mineralization (3,4). The Gla level in calcified cartilage is 23% of the value in bone; thus, osteocalcin has been implicated in the mineralization process of bone. On the other hand, osteocalcin may function only in the initial events of bone formation and secondarily be associated with the mineral (5). A third possibility for osteocalcin function may be the homeostatic regulation of calcium exchange in bone (5). To further document the distribution of Gla in relation to mineralized tissues, and/or its possible function in calcium mobilization, it is of interest to examine the focally-calcified cartilage in the endoskeleton of elasmobranchs. Sharks are devoid of bone tissue throughout the endoskeleton. Calcification in the spinal column occurs in the centers of the vertebral bodies in a highly species-specific and constant pattern (6). The cartilage of sharks is a homogeneous tissue with respect to the connective tissue and cellular components, unlike mammalian epiphyseal cartilage, in which chondrocytes undergo degeneration and are replaced by bone cells ("provisional calcification"). Although the chondrocytes in both calcified and uncalcified parts of the shark skeleton appear similar, the matrix of the calcified regions differs from uncalcified areas in that calcified cartilage has a higher collagen content (7), shows elevated alkaline phosphatase activity (8), and contains a greater proportion of chondroitin sulfate-A (9) although less total mucopolysaccharides. Although sharks possess hydroxyapatite (as in bone), the deposition of calcium in their cartilage is not regulated by the mechanism of other vertebrates. They do not display hypercalcemia during the reproductive cycle, nor do they respond to injections of either estrogen, vitamin D or parathyroid hormone (7). Sharks do not synthesize parathyroid hormone but do produce large amounts of calcitonin in ultimobranchial glands.

The present study was undertaken to determine whether γ-carboxyglutamic acid, which has a presumed role in the maintenance of mineralized bone tissue, might be present in the calcified cartilage of elasmobranchs.

METHODS

Tissue Specimens

Dogfish sharks (Squalus acanthias) from Long Island waters, approximately 2-3 feet long, were obtained fresh-frozen. Specimens of muscle, skin, dorsal fin cartilage, calvarium and vertebrae were dissected free of surrounding tissue. Pieces of calcified centra and of uncalcified spiny processes of vertebrae were sharply dissected free of each other and other contaminating tissues (Figs. 1 and 2). Portions for acid and alkaline hydrolysis and histological evaluation were taken from adjacent regions. Specimens for histology were fixed in formalin and stained with Safranin O or von Kossa stain, counterstained with nuclear fast red. The specimens were defined as either calcified or uncalcified by histological stains, as well as by percent ash weight.

Gla Determination

2N KOH hydrolyses of lyophilized tissue samples were performed as described by Hauschka (10). Gla content was determined by automatic amino acid analysis on a Beckman 121M automatic amino acid analyzer and expressed as residues Gla/Glutamic acid residues. For complete amino acid analysis, samples were hydrolyzed in 6N HCl, 108°C, 22 hours. Proof of γ-carboxyglutamic acid content in the various shark tissues was obtained by preparative isolation of Gla from 10 mg alkaline hydrolyzed samples on Dowex-1 (<400 mesh, Bio-Rad), eluting with pH 5.0, 0.02M Hepes buffer, followed by pH 4.5, 0.02M Hepes in 0.02M Mg Cl_2 (Buffer C) (11). [^{14}C]-Gla (synthesized by New England Nuclear, Boston, MA) of specific activity 2000 cpm/nmole, was included in the samples before chromatography to serve both as a marker for the Gla fraction and to quantitate recovery. The radioactive fractions were pooled, lyophilized and reconstituted in 0.01N HCl. Aliquots of the sample were taken for measurement of radioactivity, for Gla determination and for its conversion to glutamic acid by 6N HCl hydrolysis, 108°C, 6 hours. Gla and glutamic acid were identified by the amino acid analyzer quantitating Gla as nm/mg dry weight of the hydrolyzed sample, which was applied to the Dowex-1 column.

RESULTS

The uncalcified and calcified portions of the endoskeleton were confirmed histologically by von Kossa staining, as shown in Figures 1-4. The dorsal fin cartilage and calvarium from a pup (fetus) were totally uncalcified in the pup as well as in adult specimens. The Gla content per 10^5 residues of total amino acids in various shark tissues is presented in Table 1, and compared to the Gla content of other vertebrate bone and cartilage tissues. In shark cartilage, two features of Gla content are striking: 1) The uncalcified regions of the cartilaginous vertebrae contain abundant quantities of Gla and this is not true of mammals and birds; 2) The elasmobranch calcified cartilage regions contain Gla equivalent to

TABLE 1. Gla content of several vertebrate tissues. Gla residues/10^5 amino acids.

Species	Calcified Tissue		Uncalcified Tissue	
Bovine	Bone Diaphysis	67	Articular Cartilage	0.9
	Bone Metaphysis	74		
Chick	Bone Diaphysis	74	Articular Cartilage	2.0
			Sternum	1.7
Shark	Skin and scales	0	Muscle	0
	Vertebra, Centrum	71	Vertebra Spiny process	170
			Dorsal Fin	161
			Calvarium (fetus)	95

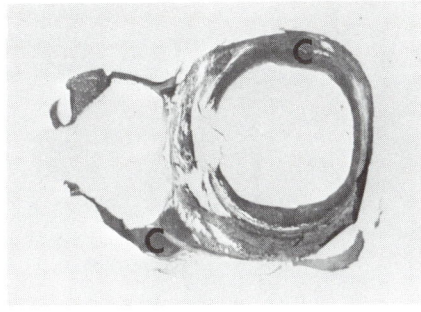
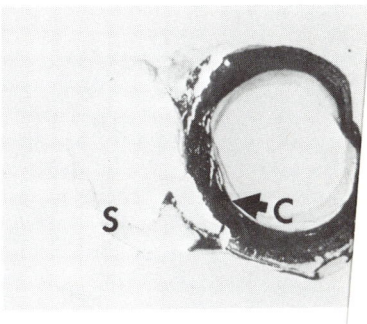

FIGURE 1 Mid-body vertebra cartilage (C). Safranin O.

FIGURE 2 Mid-body vertebra, Kossa, showing the calcified trum (C) and non-calcified process (S).

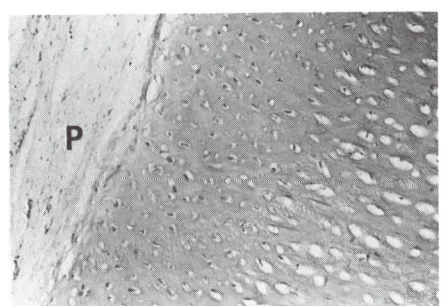
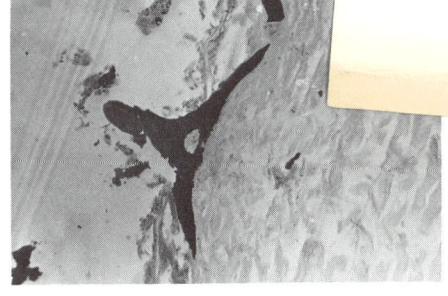

FIGURE 3 Dorsal fin cartilage densely populated with chondrocytes and perichondrium (P). Safranin O.

FIGURE 4 Skin, von Kossa, showing calcified placoid scale.

the level found in bovine and chick bone. There is no correlation then to mineralization nor an obvious correlation to collagen content; dorsal fin is 25%, uncalcified vertebra 43% and calcified centrum 70% collagen.

Alkaline hydrolysis of cartilaginous tissues produces several acidic components which were resolved on the Beckman 121M analyzer in the Gla region (Fig. 5). To prove the structure of Gla in the shark tissues, pure Gla was isolated from the alkaline hydrolysate by anion exchange chromatography (Fig. 6) as described in the Methods. The Dowex-Gla fraction was analyzed for Gla on the Beckman 121M (Fig. 7) and shown to be free of amino acids. An aliquot of the fraction which was acid hydrolyzed converted the Gla to glutamic acid (Fig. 7) quantitatively. Using these procedures which employ [^{14}C]-Gla for quantitating recovery, the nanomoles of Gla/mg dry weight of an alkaline hydrolyzed sample calculated after Dowex-1 chromatography was in agreement with the direct analysis for Gla on the Beckman 121M (Fig. 5).

DISCUSSION

The analysis of calcified and uncalcified elasmobranch tissues for Gla has revealed a surprising distribution of the vitamin K dependent calcium-binding amino acid with more Gla found in uncalcified cartilages. In the

FIGURE 5 Beckman 121M automatic amino acid analyzer profile of alkaline hydrolyzed uncalcified vertebra.

FIGURE 6 Dowex-1 chromatography of 10 mg uncalcified vertebra, alkaline hydrolyzed and adjusted to pH 10 by perchloric acid precipitation.

FIGURE 7 Radioactive fraction from the Dowex-1 column, lyophilized and applied to the Beckman 121M analyzer in citrate buffer, pH 2.2 (left). An aliquot of the fraction hydrolyzed 6 hrs, 6N HCl, 100°C converted to glutamic acid (right).

calcified regions of the vertebra, the Gla content is similar to that of various cortical bones. It remains to be established if the Gla-containing protein(s) in the shark's calcified cartilage is of similar origin and function as osteocalcin is in bone. During endochondral bone formation Gla content is extremely low in articular cartilage and in other uncalcified cartilages (Table 1) which suggests a certain degree of specificity for Gla in the functioning of mineralized bone. However in uncalcified cartilage tissues of the sharks, some of which never became calcified, e.g. the dorsal fin , the Gla content is 2-fold greater than in the calcified centrum. The lower level of Gla in the fetal calvarium tis-

TABLE 2. Comparison of the ion concentrations of elasmobranch serum and its ocean habitat.

Ion (MMoles/l.)	Sea Water	Shark Serum
Na	509	235
K	30	10
Mg	48	3
Ca	10	5
Cl	540	230
HCO_3	2	5
PO_4	0	1.2
SO_4	30	0.5
Total Ions	1169	489
	Urea	338

sue is most likely a reflection of the embryonic state. In the chick for example, lower Gla content is observed in the embryo than in adults (12).

To search for a function of a Gla-containing calcium binding protein in the elasmobranch endoskeleton, which is not exclusively associated with calcification, the physiology of the shark should be examined. The most distinguishing feature of the shark serum is a total ion concentration of 480 millimoles per liter supplemented by levels of urea sufficient to sustain osmotic equilibrium with respect to the sea water (Table 2). Bony fishes have a total serum ion concentration of 300-350 millimoles/liter of urea (9). The elasmobranch species presumably controls calcium through membrane mechanisms, their gills and kidneys. Man stores calcium and phosphate and regulates calcium with great precision by ion exchange in calcified tissues regulated by vitamin D and parathyroid hormone action upon kidney and bone cells, whereas the shark is endowed only with calcitonin. Could a vitamin K-dependent calcium-binding protein participate in the shark's calcium homeostatic regulation throughout its cartilaginous tissues? Perhaps the Gla-protein in the uncalcified tissues serves a function which is akin to vitamin D and parathyroid hormone regulation in other vertebrates.

The absence of Gla in the shark skin, which is highly calcified by a covering of acellular placoid scales (dermal denticles) (Fig. 4) and the presence of Gla in uncalcified vertebral regions, as well as the negative finding of Gla in the jaw by Price et al. (2), clearly implies that the Gla-protein in the endoskeleton is not exclusively associated with mineralized tissues. Neither is there a correlation between collagen content and Gla content as observed in chick (13) and bovine (14) bone. We therefore propose Gla-proteins in elasmobranchs may function in regulating calcium movement throughout the skeleton.

ACKNOWLEDGEMENTS

The authors thank Drs. P.V. Hauschka and P.M. Gallop for helpful discussions and Ms. K. Heroux for expert technical assistance. This work was supported by NIH grants DE 04651 and AM 15671.

REFERENCES

1. Hauschka, P.V., Lian, J.B. and Gallop, P.M. (1975) Proc. Natl. Acad. Sci. USA 72, 3925-3929.
2. Price, P.A., Otsuka, A.S., Poser, J.W., Kristaponis, J. and Raman, N. (1976) Proc. Natl. Acad. Sci. USA 73, 1447-1451.

3. Hauschka, P.V., Lian, J.B. and Gallop, P.M. (1978) Trends in Bioch. Sci. 3, 75-78.
4. Lian, J.B., Reit, B., Roufosse, A. and Glimcher, M.J. in this volume.
5. Lian, J.B., Hauschka, P.V. and Gallop. P.M. (1978) Fed. Proc. 37, 2615-2620.
6. Moss, M.L. (1977) Amer. Zool. 17, 335-342.
7. Urist, M.R. (1961) Endocrinology 69, 778-801.
8. Urist, M.R. (1962) Perspectives in Biol. and Med. 6, 75-115.
9. Mathews, M.B. (1966(Clin. Orthop. and Rel. Res. 48, 267-283.
10. Hauschka, P.V. (1977) Anal. Bioch. 80, 212-213.
11. Gundberg, C.M., Lian, J.B. and Gallop, P.M. (1979) Anal. Biochem., in press.
12. Lian, J.B., Reit, B., Roufosse, A., Gallop, P.M. and Glimcher, M.J. (1979) Eighth Steenbock Symposium, Madison, Wisconsin.
13. Hauschka, P.V. and Reid, M.L. (1978) Develop. Biol. 65, 426-434.
14. Nishimoto, S.K. and Price, P.A. (1979) J. Biol. Chem. 254, 437-441.

γ-CARBOXYGLUTAMIC ACID AND ATHEROSCLEROTIC PLAQUE

ROBERT J. LEVY, JANE B. LIAN, and PAUL M. GALLOP

Departments of Cardiology, Orthopaedic Surgery and Biological Chemistry,
Harvard Medical School,
Children's Hospital Medical Center,
Boston, MA 02115

INTRODUCTION

Atherosclerosis progresses pathologically from early fatty streak lesions to fibrous plaque, and finally to complex calcified plaque. The mechanisms by which this pathologic progression occurs are incompletely understood (1). Previous work has suggested that regulation of plaque mineralization may be associated with proteins and ultrastructural components similar to those found in normal bone (2-6). Our laboratory has demonstrated the presence of the vitamin K dependent, Ca^{++} binding amino acid, γ-carboxyglutamic acid (Gla), in calcified atherosclerotic plaque, as well as in other pathologic calcifications including calcium containing renal stones, and subcutaneous calcifications (7). These findings suggest that Ca^{++} binding proteins containing Gla may be involved in events leading to plaque mineralization perhaps through Ca^{++} binding interactions analogous to those of other Gla containing proteins, such as the vitamin K dependent clotting factors, which exhibit a unique Ca^{++} phospholipid interaction (8) and the Gla containing bone protein, osteocalcin (9,10). In the present study Gla content is quantitated in atherosclerotic plaque development, relative to progression of severity, and the Gla containing protein(s) of atherosclerotic plaque are isolated and partially characterized.

METHODS

Tissue Preparation

Aortic tissue from twenty-two aortas was obtained at autopsy and dissected over ice. Atherosclerotic lesions were rinsed with cold saline to remove blood, and then pooled as either fatty streak, fibrous plaque, or calcified plaque. In addition, several normal aortas were stripped of adventitia, and minced over ice for control tissue. The tissue pools were freeze dried, and then milled to a coarse powder under liquid nitrogen. The calcified plaque powder preparation was then extracted in 0.5M EDTA (pH 8.2) as previously described (9). The extracts were extensively dialyzed with Spectropor 3, and then freeze dried.

Amino Acid Analysis

Automated amino acid analysis to quantitate Gla was performed on 2N KOH hydrolysates of the tissue preparations, and purified extracts by the method established in our laboratory (11). Gla content was confirmed by 6N HCl decarboxylation of hydrolysates to convert the putative Gla peak to glutamic acid (9). Amino acid analysis was performed on 6N HCl hydrolysates using a Beckman-Spinco 121M amino acid analyzer as previously described (11).

Protein Purification Procedures

Gel filtration chromatography of EDTA extracts was carried out on Sephacryl S-200 Superfine Columns (2.5 x 100 cm) eluting with 0.1M ammonium acetate (pH 7.1) in 0.7 mM dithiothreitol at a flow rate of 8.0 ml/hr. Ion exchange chromatography of Gla rich pools was carried out with a DEAE cellulose column (1.5 x 25 cm) run at 60 ml/hr with a buffer containing 20 mM imidazole, 2 mM EDTA, 20 mM $CaCl_2$ at pH 7.0 and with a NaCl gradient as shown in Figure 2. Column fractions were assayed for protein concentration using the procedure of Bradford (12). Extracts and column pools were dialyzed with Spectropor 3.

Electrophoresis

SDS disc-gel electrophoresis was performed at 14°C with 15% acrylamide vertical slab gels using a modification of the procedure of Neville and Glossmann (13). Isoelectric focusing was done at 2°C on a BioRad 1415 horizontal slab apparatus using 4% acrylamide gels and pH 4-6 Ampholine (LKB) maintaining constant power at 80 watts for three hours. The electrofocusing gels were stained using 0.05% Coomassie blue according to the procedure of Righetti and Drysdale (14).

RESULTS

Protein-bound Gla is present in atherosclerotic tissue, at all levels of pathologic severity, and is also found at low levels in "normal" aorta (Table 1). Of interest is the markedly increased Gla levels found in calcified plaque. Also of importance is the finding of an almost constant ratio of Ca^{++}/Gla in disease tissue pools of various levels of pathologic severity. The EDTA extract of calcified plaque (after dialysis) yielded 5.7% of the total tissue Gla. The residue after EDTA extraction contained only 12.5% of the original Gla content with the remainder lost, presumably as low molecular weight peptides.

TABLE 1. Aortic Gla and calcium content.

Tissue	Gla/ 1000 Glu	Gla nm/ mg protein	Ca nm/ mg protein	Ca nm/ Gla nm
Normal aorta	0.54	0.39	295.0	756.3
Fatty streak	0.44	0.37	1190.0	3215.0
Fibrous plaque	0.40	0.31	1237.5	3992.5
Calcified plaque	8.64	8.47	30075.0	3550.0

Column chromatography of the EDTA extract of calcified plaque with Sephacryl S-200 yielded two Gla rich regions (Figure 1): a peak occurring at 240-260 ml (Peak II, Fig. 1) and a peptide fraction eluting between 280 and 400 ml (Peak III, Fig. 1). DEAE cellulose chromatography of Peak II resulted in three protein peaks, only one of which (Peak D, Fig. 2) contained Gla (Table 2).

SDS Disc gel electrophoresis of the DEAE peak pools reveals peaks B and C to have similar molecular weight bands of about 68000 Daltons, while the Gla containing peak D has a molecular weight of approximately 80000. The amino acid composition and isoelectric point of DEAE peak D is presented in Table 3 in comparison to some other selected Gla containing proteins. As can be seen there are 19 Gla/1000 amino acid residues, or approximately 12.0 per molecule. Peak D (Figure 2) was found to have a pI of 4.3-4.45, while peaks B and C both focused at a pI of 4.40-4.5.

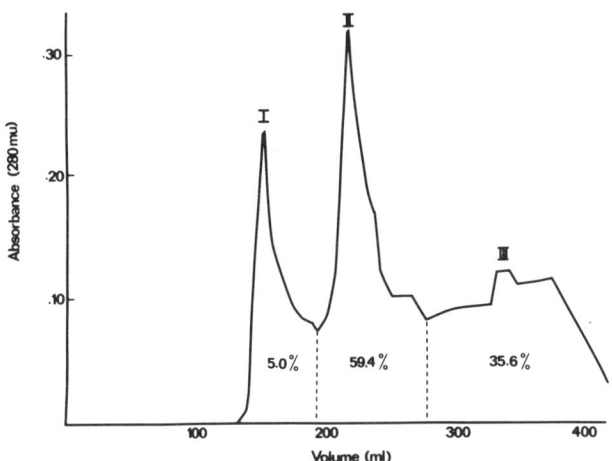

FIGURE 1   Sephacryl S-200 profile of EDTA-plaque extract, % Gla distribution.

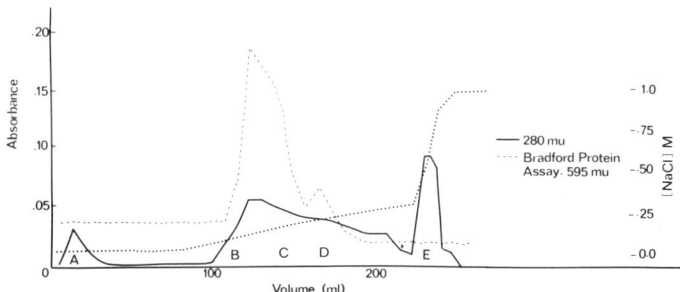

FIGURE 2   DEAE cellulose profile of S-200 Peak II.

DISCUSSION

We have demonstrated for the first time, the presence of a unique Gla containing protein in atherosclerotic plaque, which we have named atherocalcin. Partial characterization of the Gla protein isolated from calcified plaque reveals it to be a very acidic protein according to both amino acid composition and by isoelectric focusing. Table 2 presents a comparison of a number of Gla containing proteins of human origin with atherocalcin. Only prothrombin and protein S have a molecular weight approximating the atherocalcin, and they differ significantly in amino acid composition and charge. The amino acid composition of the protein described in the present paper is consistent with other work, which has

TABLE 2. Gla protein amino acid compositions.

	Atherocalcin	Prothrombin[*]	Protein C[*]	Protein S[*]
Asp	153	101	94	116
Thr	62	50	43	52
Ser	69	68	64	76
Glu	164	106	133	92
Pro	50	61	50	47
Gly	59	80	97	68
Ala	68	57	53	69
Cys	19	36	60	37
Val	63	59	77	63
Met	10	14	17	9
Ile	38	33	38	56
Leu	68	77	76	90
Tyr	17	31	30	28
Phe	36	35	33	34
His	21	18	17	20
Lys	50	56	45	75
Arg	36	72	59	35
Trp	N.D.[**]	27	–	–
Gla	19	18	23	17
Molecular Weight	80000	71500	56100	69000
PI	4.3–4.45	4.7–4.9	4.4–4.8	5.0–5.5

[*]DiScipio and Davies, 1979 (8).   [**]Not determined

demonstrated that cold alkali or EDTA extracts of calcified plaque show a population of proteins rich in acidic amino acids (2-4); these studies, however, were not aware of the presence of Gla containing proteins.

The functional significance of the association of Gla containing proteins with the development of atherosclerotic plaque calcification may be of great importance. The deposition of calcium in the atherosclerotic lesions is well recognized as a complex phenomena. Many investigators feel that calcification of atherosclerotic lesions is related to a sequence of events involving thrombosis and necrosis (1). However, the deposition of mineral in developing atherosclerotic plaque may well represent a highly complex developmental step, in which calcium binding proteins, such as the Gla containing protein described in the present work, play an integral role in the pathogenesis. This hypothesis is supported by our finding that the Gla content increases with pathologic severity. Also, the finding that demineralization results in extraction of 87% of the Gla protein points to a strong association of Gla containing proteins with the mineral phase. It may be that calcified plaque is very similar metabolically to bone, and this view is further supported by the finding of enrichment of Type I collagen (of bone) in mineralized plaque (15), as well as the presence of matrix vesicles (5,6). It may well be that the Gla containing atherosclerotic protein described in this paper is normally found in bone, and/or is present in plasma as well. Preliminary attempts in our laboratory to obtain an antibody to this protein have been successful, and these important questions are currently being addressed. Circulating levels of the Gla atherosclerotic protein (if measurable by radioimmunoassay) might correlate with disease status, and would therefore be a valuable clinical parameter. Furthermore, it may be that a calcium-Gla interaction occurs in the lipid rich plaque resulting in mineralization, that is similar to the phospholipid - Ca^{++} - Gla interaction established for prothrombin (8). If Gla containing proteins facilitate plaque progression, then one obvious approach to the prevention of "hardened" plaque formation would be vitamin K antagonism using warfarin and related drugs.

ACKNOWLEDGEMENTS

The authors thank Mr. John Zenker for expert technical assistance, and Mr. Mark Knowlton of the Peter Bent Brigham Hospital for obtaining pathologic specimens. This work was supported by NIH grants DE 04641, AG 00376, and HL 05606

REFERENCES

1. Ross, R., and Glomset, J.A. (1976) N. Engl. J. Med. 295, 420-425.
2. John, R., and Thomas, J. (1972) Biochem. J. 127, 261-269.
3. Spina, M., and Garbin, G. (1976) Atherosclerosis 24, 267-279.
4. Keeley, R.W. (1977) Biochim. Biophys. Acta 494, 384-394.
5. Kim, K.M., and Trump, R.F. (1975) Calcif. Tiss. Res. 18, 155-160.
6. Kim, K.M. et al. (1976) Human Path. 7, 47-60.
7. Lian, J.B., Skinner, M., Glimcher, M.J., and Gallop, P.M. (1976) Biochem. Biophys. Res. Commun. 71, 349-355.
8. DiScipio, R.G., and Davies, E.W. (1979) Biochemistry 18, 899-904.
9. Hauschka, P.V., Lian, J.B., Gallop, P.M. (1975) Proc. Natl. Acad. Sci. USA 72, 3925-3929.
10. Price, P.A., Otsaka, A.S., Poser, J.W., Kristaponis, J., Raman, N. (1976) Proc. Natl. Acad. Sci. USA 73, 1447-1451.
11. Hauschka, P.V. (1977) Analyt. Biochem. 80, 212-223.
12. Bradford, M.M. (1976) Anal. Biochem. 72, 248-254.
13. Neville, D.M., and Glossmann, H. (1971) J. Biol. Chem. 246, 6339-6346.
14. Righetti, P.G., and Drysdale, J.W. (1974) J. Chromatogr. 98, 271-318.
15. McCullagh, K.A., and Balian, G. (1975) Nature 258, 74-75.

GROWTH-RELATED CHANGES IN THE CARBOXYLATION OF *E. COLI* RIBOSOMES

JOHN J. VAN BUSKIRK, MARGARET LOW, and
WOLFF M. KIRSCH

Division of Neurosurgery,
University of Colorado Medical Center,
Denver, CO 80262

INTRODUCTION

We have reported the identification and estimation of γ-carboxyglutamic acid (Gla) in the ribosomes of mammals (rat, mouse, man, cultured cells), wheat germ, and E. coli (1,2). Thus, Gla-containing ribosomes and carboxylating enzymes are widely distributed in nature, and may be common to all species. The presence of Gla in mammalian ribosomes has been confirmed by Olson and colleagues, who also showed that rat liver ribosomes can be carboxylated in vitro (3). The possible role(s) of Gla in ribosome synthesis or function and the biological significance of CO_2 fixation by pre-existing ribosomes are not yet known. These questions have been approached in our laboratory by studying the carboxylation of E. coli ribosomes during the aerobic growth cycle and also under conditions of oxygen deprivation.

MATERIALS AND METHODS

E. coli (strains B or PA 340) were grown in rich broth containing 1.0% bactotryptone (Difco), 0.5% yeast extract (Difco), 0.25% NaCl, 0.5% glucose, adjusted to pH 7.0. Cultures were incubated in large spinner flasks with constant and vigorous aeration; or in conical flasks which were equilibrated in air, tightly sealed after inoculation, and agitated in a rotary water bath. Growth curves were plotted from A_{540} of serial aliquots (spinner flasks) or of the entire contents of sealed flasks. Cells were harvested at times indicated (Fig. 1), or at points for which doubling times were computed (Table 1). When cytosol was required, cells were resuspended in 10 mM $MgCl_2$, 50 mM KCl, 10 mM Tris·HCl, pH 7.5, and recentrifuged.
 Ribosomes were prepared by the method of Staehelin and Maglott (4), then washed in 1 M NH_4Cl as described by Subramanian, et al (5). Ribosomal or cytosol proteins were separated from RNA with LiCl Urea, precipitated by TCA, washed in ethanol, and analyzed for Gla and protein, as previously described (1), except: (i) TCA precipitates were hydrolyzed immediately, never stored. (ii) Samples were hydrolyzed at 107-108° for 22 hours by air-free 2 N NaOH in teflon-lined aluminum tubes with teflon disks in screw caps. The tubes were sealed under N_2 in a glove box. Preparation of ribosomal proteins L7 and L12 is described in (6). L12/L7 ratios were calculated from A_{592} of bands eluted from gels, prepared as in (7).

RESULTS AND DISCUSSION

The quantity of Gla in E. coli ribosomes is not constant, but undergoes changes of considerable magnitude. Although the mechanism and significance of these changes are not yet clear, our present studies show that there is an increase in the Gla content of E. coli ribosomes at times of (a) rapid growth and (b) excessive accumulation of CO_2. These relationships are illustrated in Table 1.

TABLE 1 VARIABLE GLA CONTENT OF E. COLI RIBOSOMES

Strain, Temperature	Phase of Growth	Doubling Time (Min)	γ-carboxyglutamic Acid (nMoles/mg Protein)	
			RIBOSOMES	CYTOSOL
(Constant aeration)				
(1) PA 340 26°	Logarithmic Stationary	75	57.1 20.0	– –
(2) Type B 26°	Logarithmic Stationary	60	46.6 31.3	– –
(3) Type B 37°	Logarithmic Stationary	30	112.1 75.9	18.9 10.5
(Limited air supply)				
(4) PA 340 37°	Logarithmic Stationary	–	104.4 149.6	– –
(5) PA 340 37°	Logarithmic Stationary	35	125.6 161.4	–

For experiments 1-3, E. coli were cultured aerobically and harvested in late logarithmic or stationary phases of the growth cycle. The comparative growth rates of the log phase cells are expressed as doubling times. These were estimated from slope of the growth curve at the points where E. coli were harvested in each experiment. Differing combinations of temperature and strain resulted in a wide range of growth rates, but the higher levels of Gla always appeared in ribosomes isolated from log phase (growing) cells, rather than stationary (non-growing) cells. The results of experiments 2 and 3 also show that the concentration of Gla in ribosomes from the same strain of E. coli increased 2.4 fold when the growth rate was doubled. Interestingly a proportionate increase occurred in the ribosomes of the stationary cells, though net growth was not detectable. It seems probable that this increase was due in part to more rapid turnover of stationary cells at the higher temperature of experiment 3. Still another indication that growth rate is reflected by the Gla content of the ribosomes is the pattern of Gla concentrations in the cytosol proteins, which closely resembles that in the corresponding ribosomes. We regard this as evidence that nascent ribosomal proteins are carboxylated prior to assembly of the E. coli ribosome.

A different type of change occurs when E. coli are grown with limited air supply. In this case the ribosomes of stationary cells acquire excessive amounts of Gla, as shown in experiments 4,5. These cultures were not aerated, but were tightly sealed immediately after inoculation. O_2 was therefore continually replaced by CO_2 during the growth cycle. Under these conditions stationary phase is attained at cell densities 30-35% lower than in aerated cultures; but rapid growth resumes if air is admitted to the flasks, indicating that termination of growth is due to depletion of oxygen, rather than nutrients. Approximately 50% of the ribosomal Gla in these prematurely stationary E. coli appears to be in excess, judging from the results of experiment 3. Acquisition of this additional Gla is not easily explained by carboxylation of nascent ribosomal proteins, since formation of new ribosomes is comparatively slow in stationary cells even under fully aerobic conditions. But a relatively high concentration of CO_2 was available, and the ribosomes may well have been carboxylated by direct fixation of CO_2 without intervention of ribosome synthesis. This reaction could be analogous to the in vitro fixation of CO_2 by rat liver ribosomes described by Olson, et al (3).

Fluctuations in the carboxylation level of E. coli ribosomes which reflect (a) growth rate and (b) high CO_2 concentrations can be observed as separate events in the growth cycle, as revealed by Figure 1.

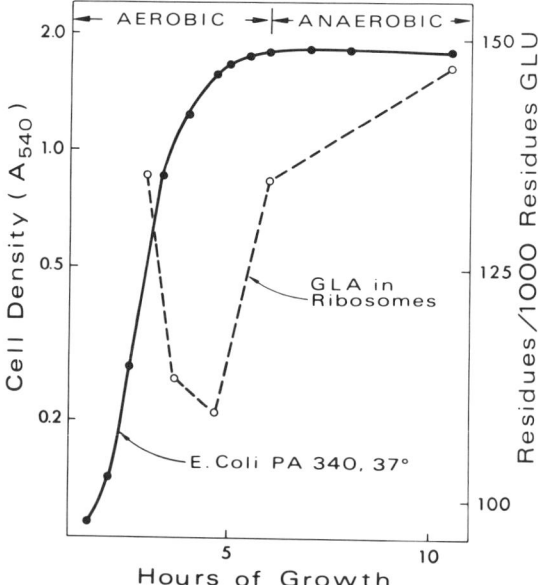

FIGURE 1 Changes in the carboxylation level of E. coli ribosomes during a growth cycle with limited air supply

In this experiment E. coli grown with limited air supply (sealed flasks) were harvested at 5 points, from approximately mid-logarithmic to late stationary phases. The Gla content of the ribosomes is seen to be high in mid-log phase, the time of maximum growth rate. Thereafter it drops with the decreasing growth rate as the culture traverses most of late log phase. But when the ratio of CO_2/O_2 becomes critical and premature stationary phase is imminent, ribosomal Gla rises sharply and then continues to increase for several hours in the absence of net growth. Apart from providing a kinetic picture which fits the results in Table 1, this figure shows that the carboxylation of E. coli ribosomes increases under two highly dissimilar sets of conditions, as described earlier. Thus the two types of carboxylation are likely to arise from different causes, and to play different roles in the synthesis or function of ribosomes.

The carboxylation that reflects growth rate appears to be coordinated with changes in the proportions of E. coli ribosomal proteins L12 and L7, described by Ramagopal and Subramanian (7). These authors showed that the ratio of these proteins, expressed as L12/L7, increases during early logarithmic growth and reaches a maximum in mid-log phase. It then decreases, arriving at a low plateau in stationary phase. Determination of L12/L7 ratios in several of our experiments revealed that L12 predominated in ribosomes from log phase cells, whereas L12 and L7 were nearly equal in ribosomes from stationary cells. In experiment 3, Table 1, for example, L12/L7 ratios in the ribosomes assayed for Gla were found to be: 3.7 (log phase ribosomes) and 1.1 (stationary phase ribosomes). Although these confirmatory results apply only to widely separated points in the growth cycle, they strongly suggest that growth reflecting changes in the carboxylation level of E. coli ribosomes occur synchronously with changes in the relative amounts of proteins L12 and L7. In view of this relationship it was exciting to discover that Gla is present in proteins L12,L7 (6). The number of Gla residues in this important pair of ribosomal proteins may be found to vary during the growth cycle.

ACKNOWLEDGEMENTS

We are grateful to Miss Virginia Sweeney for her expert performance of the amino acid analyses.
This work was supported by NIH Grant #2-5-35440 and V.A. Project #4960-02.

REFERENCES

1. Van Buskirk, J.J., and Kirsch, W.M. (1978) Biochem. Biophys. Res. Comm., 80, 1033-1038.
2. Van Buskirk, J.J., and Kirsch, W.M. (1978) Biochem. Biophys. Res. Comm., 82, 1329-1331.

3. Olson, R.E., Houser, R.M., Searcey, M.T., Gardner, E.J., Scheinbuks, J., Subba Rao, G.N., Jones, J.P., and Hall, A.L. (1978) Federation Proc. 37, 2610-2614.
4. Staehelin, T., and Maglott, D.R. (1971) Methods Enzymol., 20C, 449-456.
5. Subramanian, A.R., Haase, C., and Giesen, M. (1976) Eur. J. Biochem. 67, 591-601.
6. Low, M., Van Buskirk, J.J., and Kirsch, W.M. (1979) This Volume.
7. Ramagopal, S., and Subramanian, A.R. (1974) Proc. Nat. Acad. Sci. USA, 71, 2136-2140.

THE PRESENCE OF γ-CARBOXYGLUTAMIC ACID IN NASCENT POLYPEPTIDES AND RIBOSOMAL PROTEINS FROM RAT LIVER

J. SCHEINBUKS

Edward A. Doisy Department of Biochemistry,
St. Louis University School of Medicine,
St. Louis, MO 63104

INTRODUCTION

Vitamin K, in the presence of CO_2 and O_2, affects the post-translational carboxylation of selected glutamyl residues in prothrombin precursor proteins to produce γ-carboxyglutamyl (GLA) residues (1-3). The precursor proteins which accumulate in the endoplasmic reticulum of vitamin K-deficient rats have the same molecular weights as prothrombin (4) and the translation product of preprothrombin mRNA in a reticulocyte system also appears to have a similar molecular weight. Although clearly post-translational, the question of whether the vitamin K-dependent carboxylation under physiological conditions occurs during elongation of the nascent peptide or after its completion has remained open. There is good evidence that glycosylation of some proteins occurs on nascent chains (5,6). We have examined the vitamin K-dependent modification of glutamyl residues released from purified rat liver polysomes by puromycin and determined that not only are nascent polypeptide chains carboxylated, but a fraction of ribosomal proteins are also modified. Buskirk and Kirsch previously reported the presence of GLA in ribosomal proteins from a variety of sources (7,8).

MATERIALS AND METHODS

Microsomes, prepared as described elsewhere, (9) from vitamin K-starved (10) male Sprague Dawley (ARS: Madison, Wisconsin) rats were incubated together with 10 mM cycloheximide 10 µCi/ml $NaH^{14}CO_3$ (New England Nuclear), 45 µg/ml PMSF and 1 mM benzamidine either in the presence or absence of 100 µg/ml reduced menaquinone-2 (MK-2) at 37°C for 10 min. Following the incubation, aliquots were removed and vitamin K-dependent carboxylation was determined as described elsewhere (9). All determinations of vitamin K-dependent, $^{14}CO_2$ fixation were corrected for radioactivity fixed in the absence of the vitamin.

Microsomes are solubilized in 1.0% sodium deoxycholate after adjusting the ionic concentrations to 10 mM Mg^{2+} and 0.5 M K^+. Samples were layered onto discontinuous sucrose gradients containing the same ionic environment. Polysomes were washed through the 0.5 M and 1.85 M sucrose layers twice.

Purified ribosomal subunits (11-13) were prepared and extracted with 2 M urea prior to their isolation. Protein was extracted from ribosomal particles by the LiCl-urea procedure

(14) and then GLA was determined according to Hauschka (15). Protein was determined according to Bradford (16). Analysis of ribosomes by CsCl bouyant density centrifugation has been described elsewhere (17).

RESULTS AND DISCUSSION

Rat liver microsomes from vitamin K-deficient animals were incubated with 100 µg/ml reduced MK-2, 10 mM cycloheximide, 10 µCi/ml $NaH^{14}CO_3$ for 10 min at 37° C. Under these conditions $^{14}CO_2$ was fixed into membrane proteins only in the presence of MK-2 (Table 1). We have previously shown that most

TABLE 1. Distribution of $^{14}CO_2$ incorporated between ribosomes and membranes during vitamin K-dependent carboxylation by microsomes

	^{14}C Incorporated cpm	%
Microsomes	225,964	100
DOC Solubilized Supernatant	189,540	83
Polysomal Fraction:	7,175	3
1. Heavy Polysomes	4,731	2.1
2. Polysomes Pelleted	1,200	0.5

vitamin K-dependent ^{14}C incorporated was recoverable as GLA (18). Three percent of the total radioactivity, fixed into TCA precipitable protein, segregated into purified polysome derived from the microsomal fraction. Polysomes so isolated and fixed with either 4% formaldehyde or glutaraldehyde showed a correspondence between absorbance and TCA precipitable radioactivity tracings when analyzed by CsCl buoyant density centrifugation (Fig. 1). This suggested a close interaction between those radiolabeled proteins and the ribosome. By contrast, the high speed solubilized supernatant possessed a radioactive peak with buoyant density 1.35 characteristic of proteins alone. The peak at 1.54, characteristic of RNP particles was absent from these samples.

MK-2 dependent carboxylation of microsomes appeared to be enhanced with increasing temperatures up to 37° C. The membrane fraction at 4° C and 25° C labelled more readily than did the polysome fraction compared to the incorporation of $^{14}CO_2$ into protein at 37° C (Fig. 2). The differences in the labeling pattern observed at the temperatures studied might be due to a difference in constraints in the enzymatic reaction. As the temperature was elevated, an increase in the fluidity of membranes was possible and a decrease in con-

γ-Carboxyglutamic Acid Present in Rat Liver   281

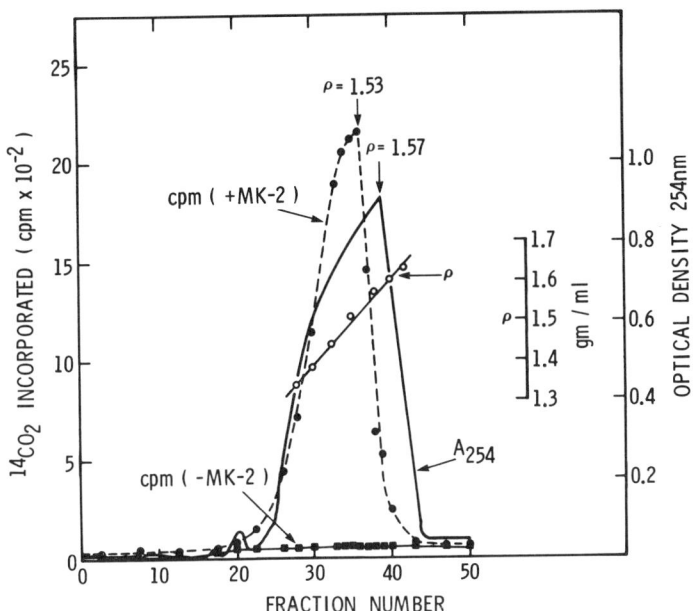

FIGURE 1. Equilibrium sedimentation in CsCl of rat liver ribosomes. Radiolabeled ribosomes were prepared as described in METHODS AND MATERIALS and analyzed as described elsewhere (19). Each of 5 gradients contained 20 units (A_{260}) ribosomes. Gradients were fractionated into 0.25 ml fractions. ^{14}C incorporated in the presence of MK-2 (●---●) and in the absence of MK-2 (■---■). Density determinations (ℓ) in gm/CM^3. (o---o), absorbance at 254 nM (——). From (22)

straints was probably imposed upon polysomal interactions with the carboxylase. By contrast the membrane proteins appeared to have relative freedom to interact with the carboxylase at most temperatures.

Ribosomal proteins were extracted from labeled polysomes using the LiCl-urea technique. Ninety percent of the ^{14}C label segregated into the protein fraction. Following basic hydrolysis, 80% of the remaining label was recovered from the amino acid analyzer in a peak which resembled GLA. Analysis of the acidic hydrolysate of the same protein fractions recovered 35% of the label co-eluting from the amino acid analyzer with glutamic acid.

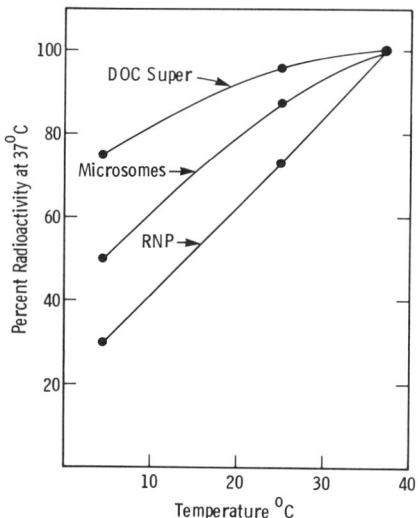

FIGURE 2. The effect of temperature on $^{14}CO_2$ uptake by various fractions. 5 ml liver microsomes were incubated at each of the above temperatures. Values obtained at 37° C for microsomes (10,055 cpm/ml), DOC solubilized supernatant (7,239 cpm/ml) and RNP (2,807/100 A_{260} units) represented 100%.

A radioimmune assay (RIA) was employed to detect the presence of prothrombin antigens on the purified polysome. The assay detected a minimum of 23 ng prothrombin/15 A_{260} units ribosomes or 1 prothrombin molecule per 1,000 ribosomes. Table 2 demonstrates the requirements for stripping and extracting the nascent carboxylated peptide chain (presumably prothrombin) from polysomes. The reaction was dependent upon a low concentration of puromycin, EF-2 and 0.2 mM GTP (20). Proteolytic inhibitors had been added to the reaction mixture since the partially purified EF-2 preparation had slight protease contamination. Following the incubation of polysomes with puromycin, the reaction mixture is adjusted to 2 M urea before sedimenting stripped ribosomes or ribosomal subunits through high salt (0.88 M KCl) gradients. Stripped ribosomes or ribosomal subunits remain active in polyphenylalanine synthesis in response to a poly U template. The supernatant contained 25-30% of the ^{14}C label presumably in the form of released puromycin derivatized polypeptides. The remaining label was associated with the sedimented stripped 80S or derived 40S and 60S preparations. A second stripping procedure was ineffective in removing fixed $^{14}CO_2$ from the sedimented particles.

TABLE 2. Requirement for stripping carboxylated nascent chains from ribosomes

RNP $^{14}CO_2$, EF-2, 02 mM GTP[a]	TCA Soluble Supernatant cpm	TCA Precipitable Supernatant cpm	RNP cpm	% Release
+2 M urea	0	0	1590	0
+ 0.1 mM Puromycin	16	0	1668	1.0
+0.1 mM Puromycin + 2 M urea	20	9	1630	1.8
+ 0.1 mM Puromycin + 45 µg/ml PMSF + 1 mM Benzamidine + 2 M Urea	368	181	1258	30.4

[a] 100 units (A_{260}) of carboxylated ribosomes were incubated as above for 30 min at 37°C. Following the stripping reaction, appropriate samples were treated with 2 M urea on ice for 1 hr. The particles were centrifuged through a 0.5 M sucrose cushion in high salt at 10°C.

Van Buskirk and Kirsch (7,8) reported that GLA is present in ribosomes prepared from mammalian cells, wheat germ and E. coli. Amino acid analysis of ribosomal proteins from highly purified mammalian and wheat germ sources contained approximately 40 residues of GLA/ribosome. Similarly we have detected the presence of GLA in rat liver ribosomes and ribosomal subunits (TABLE 3) although the amounts detected were somewhat less. We also detected GLA in ribosomal proteins

TABLE 3. The GLA content of ribosomes and ribosomal subunits

	cpm/mg protein	pmol ^{14}C Incorporated/ pmol particle	in vivo GLA content nmol GLA/nmol particle
Polysomes	390	0.019	10
d40S	358	0.006	1.3
d60S	312	0.007	5.3

labeled in vitro using vitamin K starved rats in a reaction dependent upon the presence of vitamin K. The low degree of labeling was most likely due to either the high initial GLA content of the ribosome or to inherent difficulties related to the in vitro reaction.

The presence of several residues of GLA per ribosome might be related to specific binding sites for either metal cations transitory factors involved in the steps of protein synthesis, or sites related to the processing or assembly of mature ribosomal particles as Buskirk and Kirsch (21) suggest. Other modifcations of ribosomal proteins have been reported such as acetylation, phosphorylation and methylation; however, none of these have been shown to possess a unique functional role even though they have been related to specific proteins. We are currently attempting to localize GLA to specific ribosomal protein(s) so the study of its functional significance can be advanced.

ACKNOWLEDGEMENTS

I would like to thank John Wagner for his technical assistance and contributions to the experiments presented and Richard Pinkston for his expert amino acid analyses. This work was supported by a research grant from NIH AM-09992 and a NIH training grant, HL-07050.

REFERENCES

1. Stenflo, J., Fernlund, P., Egan, W. and Roepstorff, P. (1974) Proc. Natl. Acad. Sci. USA 71, 2730-2733.

2. Magnussen, S., Sottrup-Jensen, L., Peterson, T.E., Morris, H.R. and Dell, A. (1974) FEBS Lett. 44, 189-193.

3. Esmon, C.T., Sadowski, J.A., and Suttie, J.W. (1975) J. Biol. Chem. 250, 4744-4748.

4. Nardacci, N.J., Jones, J.P., Hall, A.L. and Olson, R.E. (1975) Biochem. Biophys. Res. Commun. 64, 51-58.

5. Robinson, G.B. (1969) Biochem. J. 115, 1077-1078.

6. Kiely, M.L., McKnight, G., and Schimke, R.T. (1976) J. Biol. Chem. 251, 5490-5495.

7. Van Buskirk, J.J. and Kirsch, W.M. (1978) Bioch. Biophys. Res. Commun. 80, 1033-1038.

8. Van Buskirk, J.J. and Kirsch, W.M. (1978) Biochem. Biophys. Res. Commun. 82, 1329-1331.

9. Houser, R.M., Carey, D.J., Dus, K.M., Marshall, G. and Olson, R.E. (1977) FEBS Lett. 75, 226-230.

10. Matschiner, J. and Doisy, E.A. Jr. (1966) J. Nutr. 90, 97-100.

11. Martin, T.E. and Wool, I.G. (1968) Proc. Natl. Acad. Sci. USA 60, 569-574.

12. Sherton, C.C. and Wool, I.G. (1972) J. Biol. Chem. 247, 4460-4467.

13. Gasior, E. and Moldave, K. (1970) J. Mol. Biol. 66, 391-402.

14. Leboy, P.S., Cox, E.C. and Flaks, J.G. (1964) Proc. Natl. Acad. Sci. USA 52, 1367-1371.

15. Hauschka, P.V., Lian, J.B. and Gallop, P.M. (1975) Proc. Natl. Acad. Sci USA 72, 3925-3929.

16. Bradford, M. (1976) Anal. Biochem. 72, 248-254.

17. Hirsch, C.A., Cox, M.A., Van Venrooij, W.J.W. and Henshaw, E.C. (1973) J. Biol. Chem. 248, 4377-4385.

18. Jones, J.P., Gardner, E.J., Cooper, T.G. and Olson, R.E. (1977) J. Biol. Chem. 252, 7738-7742.

19. Thompson, H.A., Sadrik, I., Scheinbuks, J. and Moldave, K. (1977) Biochemistry 16, 2221-2230.

20. Moldave, K., Galasinski, W. and Rao, P. (1971) in Methods in Enzymology XX, K. Moldave and L. Grossman, eds., pp. 337-348, Academic Press, N. Y.

21. Van Buskirk, J.J. and Kirsch, W.M. (1973) Biochem. Biophys. Res. Commun. 52, 562-568.

22. Olson, R.E., Houser, R.M., Searcy, M.T., Gardner, E.J. Scheinbuks, J., Subba Rao, G. N., Jones, J.P., and Hall, A.L. (1978) Fed. Proc 37, 2610-2614

VITAMIN K DEPENDENT CARBOXYLATION IN LUNG MICROSOMES

ROBERT G. BELL

Department of Biochemistry and Biophysics
University of Rhode Island,
Kingston, RI

INTRODUCTION

The first indication that vitamin K might have a role other than in the synthesis of clotting proteins in liver came from the discovery of γ-carboxyglutamic acid (Gla) in bone protein (1,2). Shortly afterwards, this new tricarboxylic amino acid, which depends on vitamin K for its formation, was found in proteins of kidney and atheromatous plaques (3,4). Vitamin K stimulated the carboxylation of glutamic acid (Glu) residues in proteins when kidney and bone microsomes were incubated with $NaH^{14}CO_3$ (3,5).

Vitamin K is taken up and metabolized by a number of extra-hepatic tissues (6,7). Although liver accumulates the highest amount of vitamin and metabolites per gram of tissue, spleen, bone and lung approach the hepatic levels (TABLE 1).

TABLE 1. Tissue distribution of ^3H-vitamin K_1

Tissue	dpm/mg of tissue[a]	Vitamin K-dependent carboxylation
Liver	174	Present
Spleen	163	Present
Sternum	119	Present
Lungs	104	Present
Xyphoid Cartilage	94	?
Kidney	69	Present
Testes	58	?
Heart	56	Not detected
Adipose	34	?
Brain	32	?
Skeletal Muscle	20	Not detected
Blood	19	?
Placenta		Present
Intestines		Not detected

[a]The results are taken from Matschiner (6).

Since the vitamin may have a function in tissues where it accumulates, we tested a number of organs for vitamin K dependent carboxylation of Glu residues. We detected the activity in lung, as described below, and in spleen (8). Carboxylase activity was not detected in heart, skeletal muscle or intestines.

MATERIALS AND METHODS

Male Sprague-Dawley rats (10-15 weeks old) from Charles River Laboratories were used. ^{14}C Sodium carbonate (58.9 mCi/mmole) was obtained from Amersham. Menaquinone-3 was a generous gift from Dr. Peter Hauschka, Dept. of Oral Biology, Harvard University.

Vitamin K Dependent Protein Carboxylation

A 25% homogenate of lungs from 3-6 rats in 0.25M sucrose, 0.005M Mg acetate, 0.1M KCl, 0.025M imidazole buffer, pH 7.2 was prepared with a Potter-Elvejhem homogenizer. The homogenate was centrifuged for 10 min at 15,000 x g and the supernatant was centrifuged at 100,000 x g for 1 hr. The microsomal pellet was resuspended in the above buffer containing 0.2% Triton. One ml of the microsomal suspension (10-30 mg microsomal protein per ml) was incubated with 1 mg of NADH, 1 mg of dithioerythritol (DTE), 5 x 10^7 dpm of $Na_2{}^{14}CO_3$ and 50 µg of vitamin K_1 for 30 min at 27°. ^{14}C Protein was determined by precipitation with trichloroacetic acid (TCA) according to Esmon and Suttie (9).

Vitamin K Dependent Peptide Carboxylation

The incubation mixture was the same as for protein carboxylation except that 0.5 mg of pyridoxal phosphate and 1 mg of the peptide phe-leu-glu-glu-leu (Vega Corp.) were added. After incubation for 30 min at 27°, the ^{14}C in the TCA supernatant was determined according to Suttie et al. (10).

RESULTS

Vitamin K Dependent Carboxylation in Lung Microsomes

Lung tissue from Warfarin-treated rats was homogenized and the 15,000 x g supernatant, which presumably contained the microsomal and cytosolic fractions of the cell, was prepared. This fraction was inactive in catalyzing vitamin K dependent protein carboxylation. However, if the microsomal fraction (the 100,000 x g pellet) was incubated with NADH, DTE and $Na_2{}^{14}CO_3$, vitamin K_1 stimulated the formation of ^{14}C protein as compared to controls without vitamin (TABLE 2). If microsomes were obtained from vitamin K deficient rats, the ^{14}C protein formation was almost 4 times as great as that observed in anticoagulant-treated animals. In contrast, there was very little carboxylation with microsomes from untreated rats fed a normal diet. This suggests that a precursor(s) accumulates during vitamin K antagonism or deficiency which can be carboxylated in vitro upon addition of the vitamin.

TABLE 2. Vitamin K-dependent protein carboxylation in lung microsomes[a]

	cpm in TCA precipitate		cpm/g of lung
Microsomes from:	No K	K_1 added	
Warfarin-treated[b]	361	993	994
Vitamin K deficient[c]	362	2680	3805
Normal[d]	225	298	125

[a]See Materials and Methods
[b]Rats were injected with Warfarin (1 mg/kg body wgt) 16 hr before microsomes were prepared. The results are the averages for 5 preparations of microsomes.
[c]Rats were fed vitamin K deficient diet for at least 10 days. The results are the averages for 2 preparations of microsomes.
[d]Rats were fed Purina rat chow. The results are the averages for 2 preparations of microsomes.

Hydrolysis of ^{14}C Protein and Identification of ^{14}C Gla

To determine the nature of the carboxylated product, a large-scale incubation with the microsomes from 6 Warfarin-treated rats was carried out. The ^{14}C protein produced was dialyzed extensively against 0.5M NH_4HCO_3 and lyophilized. The ^{14}C protein (800 dpm/mg) was analyzed by Dr. Peter Hauschka of the Dept. of Oral Biology, Harvard University, Boston (11). After alkaline hydrolysis and analysis with an amino acid analyzer, 83% of the ^{14}C was found in a peak corresponding to Gla and the remainder in 2 small peaks which corresponded to pyroglutamic and pyro-γ-carboxylglutamic acids. To establish the identity of ^{14}C Gla another sample of the alkaline hydrolysate was heated with 4N HCl for 14 hr to decarboxylate ^{14}C Gla. Forty-five percent of the ^{14}C was lost and the remainder all eluted in a peak corresponding to glutamic acid. Theoretically 50% of ^{14}C in Gla should be lost when it is decarboxylated to Glu.

Requirements for Vitamin K Dependent Carboxylation in Lung

Vitamin K_1 required a reducing agent in order to stimulate carboxylation (TABLE 3). Both NADH and DTE were required for optimal activity. However, vitamin K_1 hydroquinone stimulated carboxylation without added reducing agents (TABLE 4). This indicates that the vitamin must be reduced to the hydroquinone form for activity. Further evidence that vitamin K_1 hydroquinone is the active form is that it had almost twice the carboxylating activity of vitamin K_1 at the same concentration. Menaquinone-3 was also more active than vitamin K_1 at a lower concentration. The concentration of vitamin K_1 required for maximal carboxylating activity appears to be between 2 and 20 µg/ml.
    Tetrachloro-4-pyridinol, an inhibitor of vitamin K dependent carboxylation in liver microsomes, also inhibited carboxylation in lung preparations (TABLE 3). A relatively low concentration of Warfarin also inhibited carboxylation by 76%.

TABLE 3. Requirements for vitamin K-dependent protein carboxylation

Incubation mixture	cpm in TCA precipitate % control[a]
Omit NADH	36
Omit DTE	63
Omit NADH and DTE	0
Add 1 mM tetrachloropyridinol	20
Add 0.1 mM Warfarin	26
Incubate at 17°	82
Incubate at 32°	68
Incubate at 37°	43

[a] The control is the complete incubation mixture as described in Materials and Methods. The results are averages for 2 or 3 preparations of microsomes from rats treated with Warfarin or fed a vitamin K deficient diet.

TABLE 4. Vitamin K requirements for protein carboxylation in lung microsomes

Vitamin	Concentration µg/ml	cpm in TCA precipitate % control[a]
Vitamin K_1	250	95
Vitamin K_1	20	87
Vitamin K_1	2	76
Vitamin K_1	0.2	37
Vitamin K_1 Hydroquinone	50	182
Vitamin K_1 Hydroquinone with omission of DTE and NADH	50	82
Menaquinone-3	20	263

[a] The control is the complete incubation mixture as described in Materials and Methods. The results are averages for 2 or 3 preparations of microsomes from rats treated with Warfarin or fed a vitamin K deficient diet.

The temperature optimum for carboxylation in lungs was around 27° (TABLE 3).

Increase in Vitamin K Dependent Carboxylation with Time After Warfarin

Vitamin K dependent protein carboxylation was very low with microsomes from untreated rats but increased rapidly over the first 2 hr after injection with Warfarin (Fig 1). The degree of carboxylation was similar from 2 to 16 hr and increased slowly to a maximum at 48 hr. However, the extent of carboxylation in microsomes from vitamin K deficient rats was over twice as high as the maximum obtained with anticoagulant treated animals.

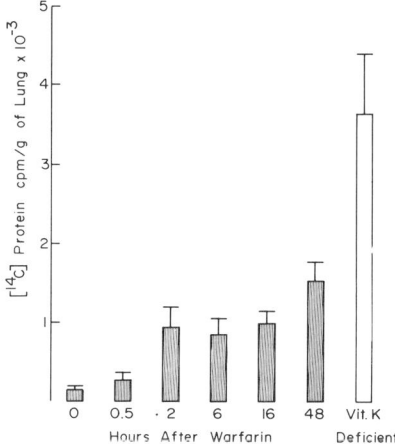

FIGURE 1. Increase in vitamin K dependent carboxylation with time after Warfarin. Rats were injected with Warfarin (1 mg/kg body wgt) and sacrificed at the times indicated. The vitamin K deficient group were fed a vitamin deficient diet for at least 10 days. Vitamin K_1 dependent protein carboxylation was determined as described in Materials and Methods. The results are the average for 3 or more preparations of microsomes with the S.E. shown.

Vitamin K Dependent Peptide Carboxylation

To determine if lung microsomes would catalyze the carboxylation of Glu residues in a synthetic peptide substrate, they were incubated with the pentapeptide phe-leu-glu-glu-leu. Vitamin K_1 clearly stimulated peptide carboxylation in lung microsomes from both vitamin K deficient and Warfarin-treated rats (TABLE 5). For comparison, peptide carboxylation with liver microsomes from the same animals were determined. The vitamin K dependent carboxylase activity of lung microsomes was 4-13% of the activity in liver microsomes per mg of microsomal protein. The requirements for peptide carboxylation were similar to those for protein carboxylation except that 2 mM pyridoxal phosphate stimulated the peptide carboxylation 3-fold.

DISCUSSION

Vitamin K dependent carboxylation of Glu residues in endogenous proteins of lung microsomes has now been demonstrated. The characteristics of the carboxylating system are very similar to that observed in liver microsomes except that the activity in liver was much higher. In both lung and liver, vitamin K_1 requires a reducing agent (NADH or DTE) for activity

TABLE 5. Vitamin K dependent peptide (phe-leu-glu-glu-leu) carboxylation in lung and liver microsomes[a]

		cpm in TCA supernatant		cpm per mg of microsomal protein
Microsomes from:		No K	K_1 added	
Vitamin K-deficient[b]	lung	1,010	6,540	4,700
	liver	609	63,000	37,000
Warfarin-treated[c]	lung	938	3,440	2,300
	liver	630	89,600	52,800

[a]See Materials and Methods.
[b]Rats were fed vitamin K deficient diet for at least 10 days. The results are for lung and liver microsomes taken from the same 3 animals.
[c]Rats were injected with Warfarin (1 mg/kg body wgt) 16 hr before microsomes were prepared. The results are for lung and liver microsomes taken from the same 3 animals.

and the hydroquinone is much more active than the vitamin (12). Also menaquinone-3 is more active than vitamin K_1 (13). The concentration of vitamin K_1 necessary for optimal activity is between 2 and 20 µg/ml which is similar to that found with liver microsomes (9). Tetrachloropyridinol, an antagonist of vitamin K in vivo, (14) inhibits carboxylation in both lung and liver preparations. Warfarin, also an antagonist of vitamin K in vivo, is inhibitory at a lower concentration than tetrachloropyridinol.

Protein carboxylation in lung microsomes increases with time after Warfarin administration as observed with liver microsomes (15). Maximum carboxylation is found in liver or lung microsomes from vitamin K deficient rats. In liver the increase is partly due to a build-up of substrate for carboxylation and partly to an increase in carboxylase activity. Similarly, we found an increase in carboxylase activity (measured by peptide carboxylation) in lung microsomes from Warfarin-treated or vitamin K deficient rats. Presumably, the increased protein carboxylation observed in lung is also due to an increase in substrates for carboxylation.

Lung and spleen (8) have been added to liver, kidney and placenta, as mammalian tissues in which vitamin K dependent carboxylation has been observed. In addition this activity has been detected in embryonic chick bone and chorioallantoic membrane (16). In liver the formation of Gla residues in precursor proteins allows them to bind calcium and phospholipid which is necessary for conversion to the active clotting proteins. Carboxylation in bone, kidney and the chick membrane produces Gla containing proteins which may be important in the calcium binding abilities of these tissues. It is not clear what the function of vitamin K dependent carboxylation in lung, spleen and placenta could be.

Vitamin K dependent carboxylation in the various tissues appears very similar to that occurring in liver (TABLE 6). The biggest difference is that the liver appears to have much higher activity than lung, kidney or spleen (TABLE 7). Fried-

TABLE 6 Vitamin K_1 Dependent Carboxylation in Microsomes

	Rat Liver	Rat Lung	Rat Spleen	Rat Kidney	Chick Bone	Human Placenta	Chick Embryo Membrane
Requires NADH or DTE	+	+	+	+	?	?	?
Increased activity with K_1H_2	+	+	+	+	?	?	?
Increased activity with MK-3	+	+	?	?	+	+	+
Inhibited by TCP	+	+	+	+	?	?	?
Peptide carboxylation	+	+	+	+	+	+	−
Vitamin K-epoxide cycle	+	+	+	+	?	+	?

TABLE 7. Vitamin K dependent protein carboxylation in liver and extra-hepatic tissues

Microsomes from:	^{14}C protein produced cpm/mg of microsomal protein[a]
Lung	1,050
Kidney	90
Spleen	54
Liver	49,600

[a]See Materials and Methods. Microsomes were prepared from Warfarin-treated rats. Protein carboxylation in spleen, kidney and liver is taken from Buchthal and Bell (8).

man et al. (17) and Tuan (16) have reported that microsomes from human placenta and chick embryonic membrane also have lower activity than liver microsomes. However, the characteristics of the carboxylating systems are similar in many respects (TABLE 6). Most appear to require a reducing agent to convert vitamin K_1 to the hydroquinone and show increased activity with menaquinone-3. Most are inhibited by tetrachloropyridinol. All can carboxylate a peptide substrate except for chick membrane. The vitamin K-epoxide cycle, which appears to be necessary for carboxylation in liver (7), has been detected in all the mammalian tissues. This cycle involves the epoxidation of vitamin K to vitamin K epoxide and the reduction of the epoxide back to the vitamin by a coumarin-sensitive reductase.

ACKNOWLEDGEMENTS

This work was partially supported by Grant HL-14847 from the

National Institutes of Health. I thank Ms. Roxanne Johnson and Marilyn Panzica for excellent technical assistance.

REFERENCES

1. Hauschka, P.V., Lian, J.B. and Gallop, P.M. (1975) Proc. Natl. Acad. Sci. USA 72, 3925-3929.
2. Price, P.A., Otsuka, A.S., Poser, J.W., Kirstaponis, J. and Raman, N. (1976) Proc. Natl. Acad. Sci. USA 73, 1447-1451.
3. Hauschka, P.V., Friedman, P.A., Traverso, H.P. and Gallop, P.M. (1976) Biochem. Biophys. Res. Commun. 71, 1207-1213.
4. Lian, J.B., Skinner, M., Glimcher, M.J. and Gallop, P. (1976) Biochem. Biophys. Res. Commun. 73, 349-355.
5. Lian, J.B. and Friedman, P.A. (1978) J. Biol. Chem. 253, 6623-6626.
6. Matschiner, J.T. (1970) Fat Soluble Vitamins, pp. 377-397, Univ. of Wisconsin Press, Madison, Wisconsin.
7. Bell, R.G. (1978) Fed. Proc. 37, 2599-2604.
8. Buchthal, S. and Bell, R.G., This volume.
9. Esmon, C.T. and Suttie, J.W. (1976) J. Biol.Chem. 251, 6238-6243.
10. Suttie, J.W., Hageman, J.M., Lehrman, S.R. and Rich, D.H. (1976) J. Biol. Chem. 251, 5827-5830.
11. Hauschka, P.V. (1977) Anal. Biochem. 80, 212-223.
12. Sadowski, J.A., Esmon, C.T. and Suttie, J.W. (1976) J. Biol. Chem. 251, 2770-2776.
13. Friedman, P.A. and Shia, M. (1976) Biochem. Biophys. Res. Commun. 70, 647-654.
14. Marshall, F.N. (1972) Proc. Soc. Exp. Biol. Med. 139, 806-810.
15. Shah, D.V. and Suttie, J.W. (1978) Arch. Biochem. Biophys. 191, 571-577.
16. Tuan, R.S. (1979) J. Biol. Chem. 254, 1356-1364.
17. Friedman, P.A., Hauschka, P.V., Shia, M.A. and Wallace, J.K. (1979) Biochim. Biophys. Acta 583, 261-265.

REQUIREMENT OF EGG SHELL FOR EXPRESSION OF VITAMIN K-DEPENDENT CALCIUM-BINDING PROTEIN IN THE CHICK EMBRYONIC CHORIOALLANTOIC MEMBRANE

ROCKY S. TUAN

Developmental Biology Laboratory
Massachusetts General Hospital and Harvard Medical School
Boston, MA 02114

INTRODUCTION

During embryonic development of the chick, the chorioallantoic membrane (CAM) mobilizes a large amount of egg shell calcium into the embryonic circulation for the requirements of skeletal formation (1). Calcium accumulation by the embryo (2) and calcium transport by the CAM (3) are both development-dependent processes which begin around the 12-14th day of incubation. Concomitant with the onset of these functions, a calcium-binding activity is expressed in the CAM (4). A high-molecular-weight calcium-binding protein (CaBP) has been identified with this activity (5). Immunohistochemical studies using specific anti-CaBP antibodies demonstrate that the CaBP is associated exclusively with the calcium-transporting ectodermal cells of the CAM (6). The CaBP binds calcium with high affinity and specificity and, interestingly, contains several residues of γ-carboxyglutamic acid (γ-CGlu) (5). The vitamin K dependence of the CAM CaBP is demonstrated by subsequent studies which showed that vitamin K stimulates expression of the CaBP by organ-cultured explants of the CAM in a dose-dependent and warfarin-inhibitable fashion (7), and that a vitamin K-dependent γ-glutamyl carboxylase activity is present in CAM microsomes (8).

The present study proposes to investigate whether the availability of egg shell calcium itself may influence the expression of the CaBP in the CAM. It has been observed that, shortly prior to the onset of calcium transport, the CAM attaches to the shell membrane/egg shell and the ectoderm then undergoes extensive cytodifferentiation (1). This study compares normal chick embryos and embryos which have been maintained in long-term culture without the shell; and presents evidence strongly indicating that egg shell calcium is required for the expression of calcium transport function and CaBP in the CAM.

EXPERIMENTAL PROCEDURES

Chick embryos were maintained in shell-less cultures as described elsewhere (9). Calcium transport (3), calcium-binding (4), and vitamin K-dependent carboxylase (8) activities were assayed as described. Immunoreactive CaBP was quantified by single radial immunodiffusion against anti-CaBP antibodies (6,9). Immunoprecipitation of CaBP was carried out by the S. aureus method (10). Cross-immunoelectrophoresis (11) and SDS polyacrylamide gel electrophoresis (5) were performed as described.

RESULTS

Development of Shell-less Embryos and Their CAM

Around 4-5 days of incubation (total time), the allantois appears, gradually enlarging and fusing with the chorion to form the CAM. By about the 8-10th day, the CAM has enlarged considerably to face the air phase and cover the entire embryo. Compared to embryos incubated in ovo, the shell-less embryos develop normally until days 10-12, after which development appears retarded (e.g. Day 16: in ovo, Hamburger-Hamilton Stage 42, dry weight = 2.05 g; shell-less, Stage 38, 0.61 g). In addition, shell-less embryos are highly calcium deficient (e.g. Day 16: in ovo, 27 g calcium/embryo; shell-less, 4 g). Drastic anomalies in skeletal calcification were also observed in the shell-less embryos (Fig. 1).

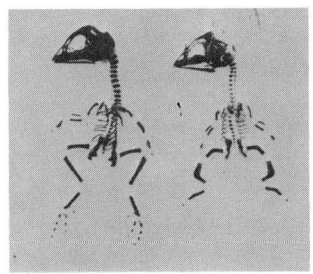
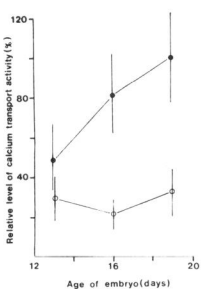

Fig. 1. Skeletal mineralization in normal (left) and shell-less (right) 15-day-old chick embryos. Alizarin stained.

Fig. 2. Age profiles of CAM calcium transport activity in normal (●) and shell-less (o) chick embryos.

CAM Calcium Transport and Calcium-Binding Activities

Figure 2 compares CAM calcium transport activities in normal and shell-less embryos during their development. Normal embryos exhibited the development-dependent onset of calcium transport in the CAM after incubation days 12-14 as previously reported (3), but shell-less embryos did not. The biochemical basis of the lack of calcium transport activity in shell-less embryos was next investigated. Figure 3 demonstrates that a

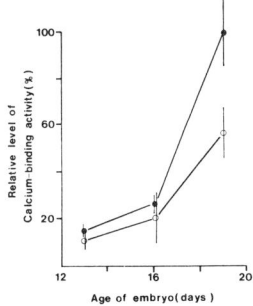
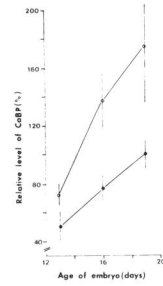

Fig. 3. Age profiles of calcium-binding specific activity in extracts of CAM from normal (●) and shell-less (o) embryos.

Fig. 4. Age profiles of immunoreactive CaBP level in the CAM extract of normal (●) and shell-less (o) embryos.

significant decrease in calcium-binding activity of the CAM resulted during ex ovo culture of the embryos. Specifically, the age-dependent, rapid rise in calcium-binding activity subsequent to incubation days 12-14 was considerably suppressed in the CAM of shell-less embryos. On the other hand, CAM carbonic anhydrase activity, previously shown to also increase in a development-specific manner (3), was expressed similarly in the shell-less embryos (9).

Expression and Biosynthesis of CaBP in the CAM

Since over 90% of the calcium-binding activity in the CAM is accountable by the CaBP (4), it is of interest to ascertain whether the lowered level of binding activity in the CAM of shell-less embryos during development reflects a parallel decrease in the concentration of CaBP. For this purpose, specific anti-CaBP antibodies were used to quantify the level of immunoreactive CaBP. Surprisingly, as shown in Figure 4, the results indicate that the level of CaBP was instead significantly elevated in the CAM of shell-less embryos. It thus appears that an immunoreactive but biochemically inactive (or less active) form of the CaBP is elicited in the CAM of shell-less embryos. Based on the data in Figures 3 & 4, the specific activity of CaBP in shell-less embryos is approximately 1/6 of that in normal embryos. This higher level of immunoreactive (biochemically inactive) CaBP in the shell-less embryos during late development appears to be a result of increased CaBP biosynthesis as demonstrated by the results in Figure 5. In particular, the rate of CaBP biosynthesis in the CAM on incubation day 16 was significantly higher in shell-less embryos. The accumulation of increasing amounts of the inactive CaBP may thus account for the subsequent depression of calcium-binding specific activity observed on day 19 (Fig. 3).

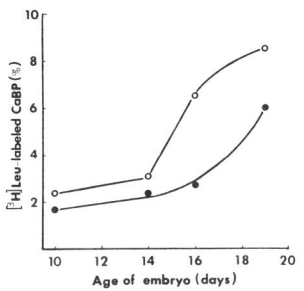

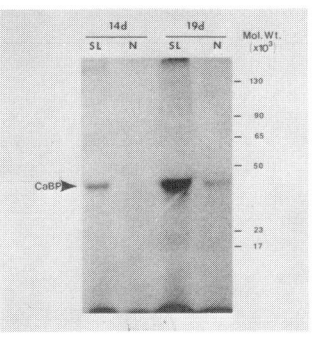

Fig. 5. Age profiles of CaBP biosynthesis rates in normal (●) and shell-less (o) embryos. The rates are the percentages of total proteinaceous radioactivity immunoprecipitated with anti-CaBP antibodies in extracts of CAM explants after 40 h organ culture with [^{3}H]leucine.

Fig. 6. SDS polyacrylamide gel electrophoretogram of [^{3}H]leucine-labelled CaBP after immunoprecipitation analyzed by fluorography. The ages (days) of normal (N) and shell-less (SL) embryos are as indicated.

The two respective forms of CaBP synthesized in the CAMs of shell-less and normal embryos appeared to be of similar molecular weight as determined by SDS gel electrophoresis (Fig. 6), suggesting that they may not differ in primary sequence but, perhaps, in other properties. One such difference was detected by means of cross-immunoelectrophoresis in the presence or absence of Ca^{2+} (Fig. 7). Although the two forms of CaBP behaved similarly in the absence of Ca^{2+} (10 mM EDTA), they migrated with different mobilities in the presence of Ca^{2+}. Calcium binding thus

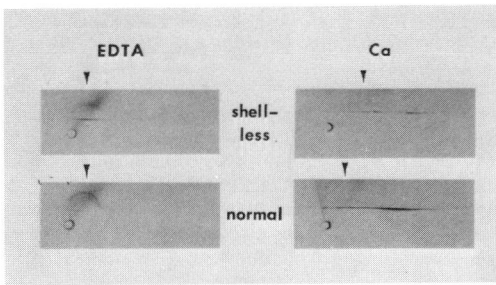

altered the ionic property of the active CaBP of normal embryos and reduced its electrophoretic mobility as compared to the inactive CaBP of shell-less embryos.

Fig. 7. Cross-immunoelectrophoresis analysis of CaBP in the CAM of normal and shell-less embryos.

Vitamin K-Dependent Carboxylase Activity in the CAM

The above observations, taken together with the known vitamin K dependence of the CaBP (7), suggest that the calcium-deficient, shell-less state of the embryo may also affect the vitamin K-dependent carboxylase activity of the CAM (8). The results in Table 1 clearly indicate that the level of endogenous vitamin K-dependent carboxylation in CAM microsomes was significantly depressed in the shell-less embryos.

TABLE 1. Activity of endogenous vitamin K-dependent carboxylase in CAM microsomes of normal and shell-less chick embryos.

Development	Assay Medium	^{14}C-radioactivity (CPM/mg dry wt)		
		Total	Vitamin K-dependent Carboxylation	%
Normal	vitamin K	555	401	100
	warfarin	154		
Shell-less	vitamin K	356	224	55
	warfarin	132		

DISCUSSION

The results presented here demonstrate that the presence of egg shell is absolutely required for the onset of calcium transport activity, and the expression of active CaBP and functional vitamin K-dependent γ-glutamyl carboxylation in the CAM of the developing chick embryo. In addition, these results are consistent with previous suggestions that the CaBP and vitamin K are integrally involved in the calcium transport system of the CAM (4-9).

The major and certainly primary physiological perturbation in the shell-less embryos is the lack of calcium, which is manifested explicitly in skeletal malformations. The limited yolk calcium resource (∼20 mg) is utilized for early ossification events of the embryo which, during normal development, needs to acquire over 100 mg of calcium from the shell. The present results indicate that calcium deficiency due to lack of egg shell (6 g of 95% $CaCO_3$) incapacitates the transport function of the CAM. Interestingly, two recent studies (12,13) have shown that the cytology of the CAM is unaltered in the shell-less embryos compared to normal embryos. Specifically, the CAM ectoderm of these embryos undergoes similar age-specific differentiation into capillary-covering and villus-cavity cells. The biochemical studies presented here therefore strongly suggest that the defect of these CAMs may be instead the inability to produce active

CaBP. On the other hand, the developmental expression of carbonic anhydrase, which is probably involved in localized acidification for eggshell dissolution and/or HCO_3^- scavenging (3), is not affected by the absence of the shell.

Although the exact cause of CaBP inactivation under calcium deficiency is not known, these data suggest that it may result from a defective vitamin K-dependent carboxylation system of the CAM. It needs to be pointed out that, since only endogenous carboxylation of CAM microsomes was measured here, the lowered activity may reflect either less availability of endogenous substrate and/or decreased carboxylase activity. Because immunoreactive CaBP is clearly detectable (in fact, in increasing amount) in the CAM of shell-less embryos, the possibility of decreased carboxylase enzyme activity in these embryos seems likely.

ACKNOWLEDGMENT

The author is grateful to Dr. Jerome Gross for generous support, encouragement, and laboratory facilities. This work was supported in part by grants from the Jane Coffin Childs Memorial Fund for Medical Research and the NIH (AM 3564). The author is a Fellow of the Jane Coffin Childs Fund. This is Publication No. 782 of the Robert W. Lovett Memorial Group for the Study of Diseases Causing Deformities.

REFERENCES

1. Terepka, A., Coleman, J., Armbrecht, H., and Gunther, T. (1976) Symp. Soc. Expt. Biol. 30, 117-140.
2. Romanoff, A. (1967) Biochemistry of the Avian Embryo. Wiley-Interscience, New York. p.39
3. Tuan, R. and Zrike, J. (1978) Biochem. J. 176, 67-74.
4. Tuan, R. and Scott, W. (1977) Proc. Natl. Acad. Sci. U.S.A. 74, 1946-1949.
5. Tuan, R., Scott, W., and Cohn, Z. (1978) J. Biol. Chem. 253, 1011-1016.
6. Tuan, R., Scott, W., and Cohn, Z. (1978) J. Cell Biol. 77, 743-751.
7. Tuan, R., Scott, W., and Cohn, Z. (1978) J. Cell Biol. 77, 752-761.
8. Tuan, R. (1979) J. Biol. Chem. 254, 1356-1364.
9. Tuan, R. (1979) Submitted to Develop. Biol.
10. Kessler, S. (1975) J. Immunol. 115, 1617-1624.
11. Ouchterlony, O. and Nilsson, L. (1973) In Handbook of Experimental Immunology. Vol. 1. Immunochemistry. D. Weir, Ed. Blackwell Scientific Publications, Oxford. Chapter 19.
12. Narbaitz, R. and Jande, S. (1978) J. Embryol. Expt. Morphol. 45, 1-12.
13. Dunn, B. and Fitzharris, T. (1979) Develop. Biol. In Press.

VITAMIN K DEPENDENT CARBOXYLATION IN SPLEEN AND KIDNEY

STEVEN D. BUCHTHAL and ROBERT G. BELL

Department of Biochemistry and Biophysics
University of Rhode Island,
Kingston, RI 02881

INTRODUCTION

Vitamin K-dependent carboxylation occurs in liver (1), kidney (2), placenta (3) and chick bone microsomes (4). Liver, kidney and bone have been shown to accumulate a high concentration of vitamin K and its metabolites when rats are fed tritiated vitamin K_1 over a period of days (5). The spleen had about the same concentration of ^3H as the liver. Therefore, we have examined spleen for vitamin K-dependent carboxylase activity. We also studied kidney in order to determine the characteristics of carboxylase activity in renal tissue and compare it to the liver.

MATERIALS AND METHODS

Peptide Carboxylation

Male Sprague-Dawley rats, 50-90 days old, were decapitated and the spleens and kidneys removed. A 25% homogenate in 0.25M sucrose, 0.025M imidazole, 0.1M KCl, 0.005M Mg Acetate, pH 7.2 was prepared from each tissue and centrifuged at 15,000 x g for 15 min. The supernatant was centrifuged at 105,000 x g for 65 min and the pellet was surface washed and resuspended in the above buffer.
Incubations contained 1 ml microsomes, 0.2% Triton, 1 mg peptide (phe-leu-glu-glu-leu from Vega Corp.), 1 mg NADH, 1 mg dithioerythritol (DTE), 0.5 mg pyridoxal phosphate, 1.3×10^7 cpm of $Na_2{}^{14}CO_3$ (Amersham) and 50 µg of vitamin K_1 hydroquinone (K_1H_2). Incubations were for 30 min at 27°. Incorporation of ^{14}C into the peptide was measured according to Suttie et al. (6).

Protein Carboxylation

Microsomes were prepared as above. Incubations contained 1 ml of microsomes, 0.2% Triton for spleen microsomes or 0.05% Triton for kidney microsomes, 1 mg NADH, 1 mg DTE, 5.2×10^7 cpm of $Na_2{}^{14}CO_3$ and 50 µg of vitamin K_1 or vitamin K_1 hydroquinone. Incubations were for 30 min at 27°. Incorporation of ^{14}C into microsomal protein was measured by chromatographing the incubation mixture on Sephadex G-25 and eluting with 0.025M imidazole buffer, pH 8.5. The fractions with protein were precipitated with TCA twice and the precipitate assayed for ^{14}C.

RESULTS

Vitamin K-Dependent Carboxylation in Kidney

In order to study the characteristics of vitamin K-dependent carboxylation in kidney microsomes, we tested their ability to catalyze the carboxylation of a pentapeptide containing adjacent Glu residues (TABLES 1 and 2). We found that vitamin K_1

TABLE 1. Vitamin K-dependent peptide carboxylation in spleen and kidney microsomes[a]

Microsomes from:	cpm in TCA supernatant		cpm/g of tissue
	No K added	K_1H_2 added	
Warfarin-treated spleen[b]	400 ± 30	2610 ± 280	12,600
Vitamin K-deficient spleen[c]	565 ± 95	5730 ± 475	31,680
Warfarin-treated kidney[d]	483 ± 102	2214 ± 409	4,130

[a]See Materials and Methods.
[b]Rats were treated with 1 mg/kg body wgt 16-18 hr prior to sacrificing the animals. The results are the average of 6 preparations of microsomes ± S.E.
[c]Rats were fed a vitamin K-deficient diet for at least 10 days. The results are the average of 3 preparations of microsomes ± S.E.
[d]Rats were treated as in b. The results are the averages of 5 preparations of microsomes ± S.E.

TABLE 2. Requirements for peptide carboxylation in spleen and kidney microsomes

	cpm in TCA supernatant % control[a]	
Variation	kidney	spleen
Omit peptide	2	0
Omit DTE and NADH	70	64
Omit pyridoxal phosphate	34	30
Add 0.2 mM tetrachloropyridinol	2	2
Add 1 mM Warfarin	86	56
Substitute vitamin K_1 for vitamin K_1 hydroquinone	3	21

[a]The control is the complete incubation mixture as described in Materials and Methods. The results are the averages of 2 or 3 preparations of microsomes from Warfarin-treated or vitamin K-deficient rats.

was inactive, but vitamin K_1 hydroquinone was able to stimulate peptide carboxylation in kidney microsomes isolated from Warfarin-treated rats. Optimal activity was obtained at 27° and with 0.2% Triton. The reducing agents, DTE and NADH, were required for optimal activity as was pyridoxal phosphate. Tetrachloropyridinol completely blocked carboxylation while Warfarin had little effect.

Vitamin K_1 did stimulate protein carboxylation, but the hydroquinone was more effective (TABLE 3). Protein carboxyla-

TABLE 3. Vitamin K-dependent protein carboxylation in kidney microsomes[a]

Microsomes from:	cpm in TCA precipitate			cpm/g of kidney	
	No K	K_1 added	K_1H_2 added	K_1	K_1H_2
Warfarin treated[b]	441 ± 58	1251 ± 269	1501 ± 343	654	1172
Vitamin K-deficient[c]	341 ± 86	1186 ± 624	2621 ± 701	766	1944

[a]See Materials and Methods.
[b]Rats were injected with 1 mg/kg body wgt 16-18 hr prior to sacrificing the animals. Results are the average of 4 preparations of microsomes ± S.E.
[c]Rats were fed a vitamin K-deficient diet for at least 10 days. Results are the average of 5 preparations of microsomes ± S.E.

tion in kidney microsomes was 3-5% of that observed in liver microsomes per gram of tissue.

Vitamin K-Dependent Carboxylation in Spleen

Vitamin K-dependent carboxylation of a peptide substrate was also demonstrated in spleen microsomes from Warfarin-treated and vitamin K-deficient rats (TABLES 1 and 2). The peptide carboxylase activity in spleen per gram of tissue was substantially higher than in kidney. The activity in spleen was about 3% of that found in liver microsomes. The characteristics of peptide carboxylation in spleen were similar to those of kidney.

Vitamin K_1 and vitamin K_1 hydroquinone were equally effective in stimulating protein carboxylation in spleen microsomes from Warfarin-treated rats (TABLE 4). In vitamin K-deficient rats, the hydroquinone was about twice as effective. The protein carboxylase activity in spleen per gram of tissue was 4-6% of that found in liver microsomes from Warfarin-treated and vitamin K-deficient rats.

TABLE 4. Vitamin K-dependent protein carboxylation in spleen microsomes[a]

Microsomes from:	cpm in TCA Precipitate			cpm/g Spleen	
	No K	K_1 added	K_1H_2 added	K_1	K_1H_2
Warfarin treated[b]	350 ± 58	614 ± 129	520 ± 114	766	757
Vitamin K-deficient[c]	419 ± 125	777 ± 299	1032 ± 357	768	1325

[a] See Materials and Methods.
[b] 1 mg/kg b.w. 16-18 hr prior to sacrificing the animals. Average of 4 microsomal preparations ± S.E.
[c] Rats were fed a vitamin K deficient diet for at least 10 days. Average of 3 preparations of microsomes ± S.E.

DISCUSSION

We have added spleen to the list of mammalian tissues which catalyze vitamin K-dependent carboxylation of endogenous protein(s) and synthetic peptide substrates. In addition, we have confirmed the presence of vitamin K-dependent carboxylation of kidney protein discovered by Hauschka et al. (2). The carboxylation is more easily detected if vitamin K_1 hydroquinone is used rather than vitamin K_1 or menaquinone-3. The kidney carboxylase will also catalyze the carboxylation of the peptide phe-leu-glu-glu-leu providing a convenient assay to determine the characteristics of the renal carboxylating system. The vitamin peptide carboxylating systems from liver, spleen, and kidney appear to be quite similar. They are readily inhibited by tetrachloropyridinol, but not by Warfarin, stimulated by pyridoxal phosphate and much more responsive to vitamin K_1 hydroquinone than the vitamin itself.

ACKNOWLEDGEMENTS

This work was partially supported by Grant HL-14847 from the National Institutes of Health. We thank Ms. Roxanne Johnson and Marilyn Panzica for excellent technical assistance.

REFERENCES

1. Esmon, C. T., Sadowski, J. A., Suttie, J. W. (1975) J. Biol. Chem. 250, 4744-4748.
2. Hauschka, P. V., Friedman, P. A., Traverso, H. P., Gallop, P. M. (1976) Biochem. Biophys. Res. Commun. 71, 1207-1213.
3. Friedman, P. A., Hauschka, P. V., Shia, M. A., Wallace, J. K. (1979) Biochim. Biophys. Acta 583, 261-265.
4. Lian, J. B., Friedman, P. A. (1978) J. Biol. Chem. 253, 6623-6626.
5. Matschiner, J. T. (1970) Fat Soluble Vitamins, pp. 377-397, Univ. Wisconsin Press, Madison, Wisconsin.
6. Suttie, J. W., Hageman, J. M., Lehrman, S. R., Rich, D. H., (1976) J. Biol. Chem. 251, 5827-5830.

ISOLATION OF A VITAMIN K-DEPENDENT PROTEIN CONTAINING γ-CARBOXYGLUTAMIC ACID FROM CHICKEN KIDNEY MICROSOMES

HECTOR P. TRAVERSO, PETER V. HAUSCHKA, and
PAUL M. GALLOP

Departments of Orthopaedic Surgery, Oral Biology and Biological Chemistry,
Harvard Schools of Medicine and Dental Medicine,
Children's Hospital Medical Center,
Boston, MA 02115

INTRODUCTION

Previous studies have identified γ-carboxyglutamic acid (Gla) as a constituent of one or more proteins synthesized by rat and chicken kidney microsomes in vitro in a vitamin K-dependent post-translational reaction (1). In most other sites of Gla-protein occurrence, Ca^{2+} metabolism and Ca^{2+}—protein interactions are important processes. Gla residues in proteins are essential not only for the binding of Ca^{2+} to the protein but for association of the protein with phospholipid in cells or plasma membrane fragments through Ca^{2+}-mediated salt bridges (2,3).

The kidney plays a central role in calcium homeostasis. This function is manifested through glomerular filtration and tubular re-absorption of both Ca^{2+} (about 10 grams/day in man) and phosphate. Control of mineral ion equilibria between bone and body fluids is achieved by Ca^{2+}-dependent fluctuation of parathyroid hormone, calcitonin levels, and renal regulation of vitamin D metabolites (4,5) and blood pH. Numerous pathological conditions attend the malfunction of any of these processes. Obviously there are mechanisms in the kidney for sensing Ca^{2+} levels and thereby regulating appropriate metabolic activities.

The synthesis of a Gla-protein by kidney (1) was of great interest to us because of its possible involvement in some aspect of renal Ca^{2+} metabolism. Since the kidney Gla protein has no known distinguishing feature other than its Gla content, specific radioactive labeling of the Gla residues was the logical approach for identifying this protein in subsequent purification and characterization studies. Vitamin K-dependent carboxylation with $^{14}CO_2$ by kidney microsomes in vitro (1) was patterned after the liver carboxylase system described by Suttie and his colleagues (6) and by Friedman and Shia (7). In the kidney system, about 90% of the non-dialyzable radioactivity is recovered in the γ-carboxyl carbon atom of peptidyl Gla residues (1). Preliminary characterization of the kidney Gla-protein is presented below.

MATERIALS AND METHODS

Day old male chicks (Buff - sex-linked) were raised for 3 to 6 weeks on Purina chow supplemented with 800 mg/kg of dicumarol (8). The chicks were deprived of food for 18 hours, before being killed by decapitation. The kidneys were quickly excised, placed in ice cold 0.9% NaCl, and adherent connective tissue was removed. Kidneys were then washed with cold 250 mM sucrose, 80 mM KCl, 25 mM imidazole-Hcl, pH 7.2 (buffered sucrose) and then homogenized for preparation of microsomes as previously described (1-9). The carboxylation reaction was performed by using a modified procedure of Friedman and Shia (7) described elsewhere (9). A scaled up reaction volume of 150 ml was used to prepare ^{14}C-Gla labeled kidney protein. After acidification with acetic acid to pH 4 and bubbling with CO_2 gas the mixture was dialyzed exhaustively against 50 mM NH_4HCO_3, using Spectrapor 3 membrane tubing and finally lyophilized. The yield was approximately 4200 cpm per gram of wet kidney tissue.

Radioactively labeled microsomal pellets were dissolved and dialyzed against 0.01M sodium phosphate, pH 7.2, 1% SDS, 1 mM DTT, before applying to a hydroxyapatite column (Clarkson Chemical Co.; 0.9 cm x 50 cm) equilibrated with the same buffer. A 200 ml linear gradient of 0.01M to 1 M sodium phosphate, pH 7.2, 1% SDS, 1 mM DTT at 9 ml/hr was effective in eluting all applied radioactivity. Agarose gel A5 (Bio Rad; 200-400 mesh) was packed in a 2.5 cm x 160 cm column and equilibrated with 0.05M NH_4HCO_3 buffer, pH 7.2, 0.5% SDS and eluted with the same buffer at a flow rate of 10 ml/hr. Removal of SDS from protein solutions was achieved by the Dowex-1 method of Weber and Kuter (10). After removal of the SDS, the labeled protein would neither precipitate nor aggregate during dialysis against water, in contrast to the SDS-solubilized crude microsomal protein.

RESULTS

Labelled kidney Gla-protein preparations were solubilized by exposure to detergents. Several detergents were examined (see Table 1), including cetylpyridinium chloride (CPC), Triton X-100, deoxycholate (DOC) and sodium dodecyl sulfate (SDS). Solubilization was defined as the fraction of non-dialyzable counts remaining in the supernatant after centrifugation at 10^5 x g for 60 min. SDS was chosen for use in further chromatography studies because it solubilized approximately 75% of the labeled protein. Non-detergent conditions such as high pH, low and high ionic strength, EDTA, 6M urea, 6M guanidine-HCl, were tested for their ability to solubilize the protein, but with little success.

TABLE 1. Solubilization of [^{14}C]-Gla protein from kidney microsomes.

Detergent	Concentration	% Soluble CPM
SDS	1%	73
CPC	1%	43
Triton X-100	1%	40
Deoxycholate	1%	27
Control	0	11

Dialyzed labeled kidney microsomal protein (2 mg) was suspended in 1 ml 0.02M Tris buffer, pH 7.2, after which detergents were added. After 30 min. at 30°C the mixture was centrifuged at 10^5 x g for 60 min. Aliquots of the supernatant were counted and the values are the average of duplicate samples.

Chromatography of the SDS-solubilized labeled kidney microsomal protein on hydroxyapatite shows two radioactive peaks eluting at 0.01M and 0.68M on the linear phosphate gradient (Fig. 1). Although the total concentration of SDS remains constant, the equilibrium monomer concentration of SDS drops as the ionic strength of the gradient increased. Apparently the labeled protein is strongly bound to the column and requires a rather high concentration of salt to desorb. The first peak (I) contains about 35% of the total protein, and about 10% of the total applied radioactivity; the volatility of this label suggests that it is residual, free

$^{14}CO_2$. The second peak (II) contains 65% of the total applied radioactivity, and from protein measurements its specific activity (CPM/mg protein) is 2- to 3-fold greater than the starting material. In order to identify the position of the [^{14}C] label in the protein, a sample from peak II was freed of SDS (see Methods), alkaline hydrolyzed, and applied to a Beckman 121M amino acid analyzer coupled to a flow scintillation counter (1). [^{14}C]γ-carboxyglutamic acid was present as the only labeled compound.

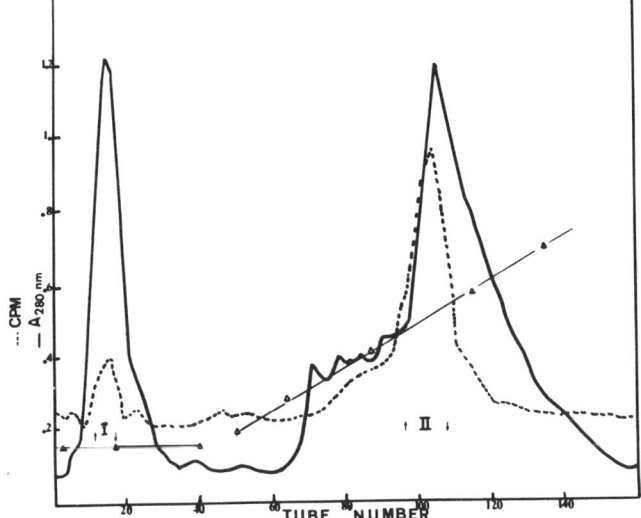

FIGURE 1. Hydroxyapatite chromatography of [^{14}C] labeled chicken kidney microsomal proteins solubilized in 1% SDS. A_{280} (solid line; CPM (broken line); phosphate gradient (-Δ-Δ).

Pooled peak II material from hydroxyapatite was next subjected to gel filtration on Agarose (Fig. 2), resulting in an additional purification of 3- to 4-fold.

DISCUSSION

Whole chicken kidney contains about 0.12 residues of Gla/1000 total amino acid residues (1). By comparison with amino acid compositions of several pure Gla-proteins [prothrombin = 17 res Gla/1000 res; chicken osteocalcin = 70 res Gla/ 1000 res (11)] one can estimate that the kidney Gla-protein comprises some 0.2% to 0.7% of the total kidney protein. Thus, purification to homogeneity will ultimately involve approximately 150-

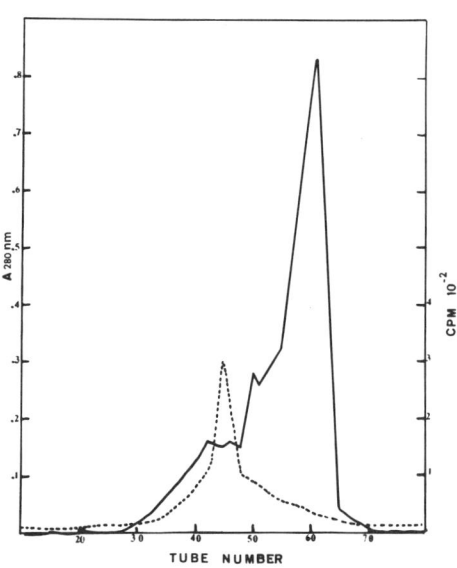

to 500-fold purification. The modest initial results in this study have achieved approximately 10-fold purification through the two column steps in 1% SDS. The ^{14}C-labeled kidney Gla-protein is intimately associated with the particulate microsomal fraction. Solubilization of this protein by detergents indicates that it has properties common to other membrane proteins and that it may be concentrated in the tubular membranes.

ACKNOWLEDGEMENTS

This work was supported by the National Foundation-March of Dimes and the National Institutes of Health (Grants AG 00376 and HL 20764).

REFERENCES

1. Hauschka, P.V., Friedman, P.A., Gallop, P.M. and Traverso, H.P. (1976) Biochem. Biophys. Res. Commun. 71, 1207-1213.
2. Esmon, C.T., Suttie, J.W., and Jackson, C.M. (1975) J. Biol. Chem. 250, 4095-4099.
3. Nelsestuen, G.L., and Lim, T.K. (1977) Biochemistry 16, 4164-4171.
4. DeLuca, H.F. (1975) Am. J. Med. 58, 39-47.
5. Russell, J.E., and Avioli, L.V. (1975) In Vitamin D and Problems to Uremic Bone Disease, Eds. Norman, A.W., Shaefer, K., Grigoleit, H.G., von Herrath, D., and Ritz, E., pp. 119-132, Walter de Gruyter and Co., Berlin.
6. Esmon, C.T., Sadowski, G.A., and Suttie, J.W. (1975) J. Biol. Chem. 250, 4744-4748.
7. Friedman, P.A., and Shia, M. (1976) Biochem. Biophys. Res. Commun. 72, 647-654.
8. Hauschka, P.V., and Reid, M.R. (1978) J. Biol. Chem. 253, 9063-9068.
9. Traverso, H.P., Hauschka, P.V. and Gallop, P.M. (1979) Eighth Steenbock Symposium, Madison, Wisconsin.
10. Weber, K., and Kuter, D.J. (1971) J. Biol. Chem. 246, 4504-4509.
11. Hauschka, P.V. (1977) Anal. Biochem. 80, 212-223.

PURIFICATION OF A PROTEIN CONTAINING
γ-CARBOXYGLUTAMIC ACID FROM BOVINE KIDNEY

ANNE E. GRIEP and PAUL A. FRIEDMAN

Department of Pharmacology,
Harvard Medical School and Center for Blood Research,
Boston, MA 02115

INTRODUCTION

In addition to coagulation factors II, VII, IX and X proteins containing γ-carboxyglutamic acid (γ-CGlu) have been identified in bone, kidney, spleen, placenta, chick chorioallantoic membrane, and possibly in ribosomes. Vitamin K-dependent carboxylation has been demonstrated in microsomes derived not only from liver, but also from kidney, bone, spleen, placenta, lung and chorioallantoic membrane. Except for the vitamin K-dependent coagulation factors, the functions of these proteins are not understood. As an initial attempt to define functions for these proteins, we have purified one protein rich in γ-CGlu from kidney.

MATERIALS AND METHODS

All steps in the purification scheme were carried out at 4°. Alkaline hydrolysis and amino acid analysis were performed as has been described (1) using a Beckman 121M column. Protein solutions were subjected to disc gel electrophoresis at pH 9.5 using a standard 10% analytical system (2). Agarose slab gel electrophoresis was done as described by Johansson (3). Protein concentration was determined by the method of Kalckar (4).

RESULTS

Calf kidneys, obtained at an abattoir within 15 to 30 minutes of exsanguination, were minced and immediately placed in cold 0.05 M Tris-HCl, pH 7.4, containing .002 M benzamidine and 0.015 M potassium oxalate (Buffer A). The minced kidneys were blotted, weighed (1.6 kg), and homogenized in 2 volumes Buffer A in an Omni-Mixer at top speed for 1 minute. The homogenate was centrifuged for 40 minutes at 10,000 x g. The resulting supernatant (3.25 L) which contained 60% and 80% of the γ-CGlu of the homogenate, was filtered through several layers of gauze to remove as much fat as possible. Barium sulfate (25 mg/ml) was added to the filtered supernatant and the suspension was stirred for 30 minutes. The BaSO$_4$ was then allowed to settle for 60 minutes, the supernatant poured off, and the remaining slurry centrifuged for 10 minutes at 2,500 x g. The BaSO$_4$ pellet was washed once with water and then resuspended into 180 ml of 0.2 M sodium citrate and stirred for 30 minutes. After centrifugation the eluate, which contains about 60-70% of the γ-CGlu of the original low speed supernatant, was frozen and stored at -70°. These steps were repeated twice on 2 consecutive days after which the BaSO$_4$ eluates were pooled (450 ml), diluted to 2.5 L with H$_2$O and applied to a QAE Sephadex A-25 column (300 ml bed volume), equilibrated with 0.01 M Tris-HCl, pH 7.2, 0.002 M benzamidine (Buffer B) containing 0.1 M KCl. The column was washed with 100 ml of Buffer B containing 0.1 M KCl and then developed with a KCl gradient - 0.1 to 1 M in Buffer B, 750 ml in each reservoir (Fig. 1A). Protein concentrations in the fractions were determined, and, based on these concentrations, fractions were combined arbitrarily into pools. The γ-CGlu content of the pools was determined; pool 3 contained the most γ-CGlu and possessed the highest specific activity (Table 1); it was purified further on a Sephadex G-50 column equilibrated with 0.1 M NH$_4$HCO$_3$ (600 ml bed volume) (Fig. 1B). Fractions

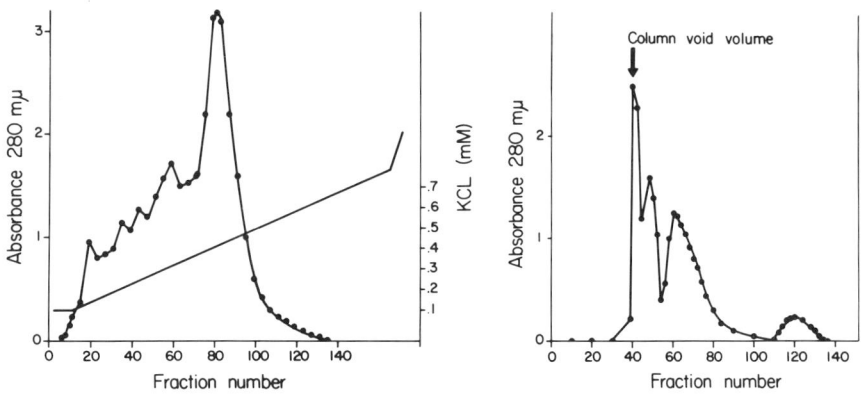

FIGURE 1A. Absorbance at 280 mμ of fractions (10 ml) was determined; fractions were pooled as follows: Pool 1 = unadsorbed material plus the wash; Pool 2 = fractions 11 to 68; Pool 3 = fractions 69 to 85; Pool 4 = fractions 86 to 105; Pool 5 = fractions 106 to 130. See text for details.
FIGURE 1B. Pool 3 (119 mg of protein) from the Sephadex QAE column was concentrated to 10 ml and applied to the Sephadex G-50 column. Absorbance at 280 mμ of fractions (5.4 ml) was determined and fractions were pooled as follows: Pool 1 = fractions 38 to 44; Pool 2 = fractions 45 to 55; Pool 3 = fractions 56 to 80; Pool 4 = fractions 81 to 110; Pool 5 = fractions 111 to 135. See text for details.

TABLE 1. Purification Scheme

Step	Volume (ml)	Protein (mg)	γ-CGlu (mμmoles)	Specific Activity (mμmoles γ-CGlu/mg protein)	Recovery of γ-CGlu[a]
Pooled BaSO$_4$ Eluates	500	1688	6703	3.97	100
Sephadex QAE					
Pool 1	2500	805	588	0.73	8.8
Pool 2	550	272	2050	7.54	30.6
Pool 3	400	119	2400	20.2	35.8
Pool 4	500	79	270	3.4	4.0
Pool 5	500	76	55.7	0.73	0.8
Sephadex G-50 Gel Filtration of QAE Pool 3					
Pool 1	38	32.5	34.5	1.06	0.5
Pool 2	54	17.5	37.5	2.14	0.5
Pool 3	135	12	926	77.2	13.8
Pool 4	162	12	58.8	4.9	0.9
Pool 5	81	8.7	9.1	1.05	0.1

[a] The γ-CGlu present in the BaSO$_4$ is taken as 100%.

containing protein were pooled, and γ-CGlu determinations again were done. Only pool 3 contained γ-CGlu. Repeat chromatography of pool 3 on Sephadex G-50 revealed a single symmetrical protein peak. This material has only one staining band of protein after either polyacrylamide disc gel or agarose slab gel electrophoresis (Fig. 2). A summary of the purification

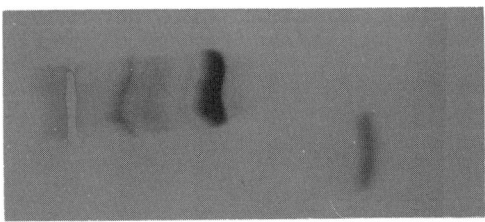

FIGURE 2. Agarose slab gel electrophoresis. Top - human serum; bottom - purified kidney protein containing γ-CGlu.

scheme is shown in Table 1. The molecular weight of the protein is about 8,000 daltons; its amino acid analysis (Table 2) shows a very high proportion of acidic residues, reflecting its pI of about 3.2.

TABLE 2. Amino Acid Composition[a] of the Purified Protein

Amino Acids	Residues/1000 amino acids	Amino Acids	Residues/1000 amino acids
Asp	175	Val	31
Thr[b]	21	Ile	13
Ser[b]	56	Leu	41
Glu[c]	231	Tyr	13
γ-CGlu[d]	26	Phe	17
Pro	38	Lys	45
Gly	165	His	15
Ala	61	Arg	32
Half Cys	19		

[a]Amino acid content determined by 6 N HCl hydrolysis except for γ-CGlu.
[b]Includes o-phosphoserine and o-phosphothreonine.
[c]Glu content corrected by subtraction of γ-CGlu.
[d]Determined by alkaline hydrolysis.

DISCUSSION

One protein containing γ-CGlu has been purified from bovine kidney. Its molecular weight as well as amino acid composition differs from those of the bone protein osteocalcin (5) as well as from those of several proteins containing γ-CGlu which are associated with renal stones (6). At present, neither the cell of origin, the function of the protein, nor whether this protein is the γ-CGlu-containing proteolysis product of a larger protein is known.

ACKNOWLEDGEMENTS

This research was supported by the U.S. Public Health Service Grant HL 11414. P.A.F. is a recipient of an RCDA HD 00023 grant.

REFERENCES

1. Hauschka, P., Lian, J., and Gallop, P. (1975) Proc. Natl. Acad. Sci. USA 72, 3925-3929.
2. (1965) Chemical Formulation for Disc Electrophoresis, Canal Industrial Corporation, Rockville, Maryland.
3. Johansson, B. (1972) Scand. J. Lab. Invest. 29(Suppl 124), 7-19.
4. Kalckar, H. M. (1947) J. Biol. Chem. 167, 461-475.
5. Price, P., Poser, J., and Raman, N. (1976) Proc. Natl. Acad. Sci. USA 73, 3374-3375.
6. Lian, J., Prien, E., Glimcher, M., and Gallop, P. (1977) J. Clin. Invest. 59, 1151-1157.

VITAMIN K-DEPENDENT CARBOXYLATION IN MICROSOMAL PREPARATIONS DERIVED FROM CULTURED KIDNEY CELLS, CHICK EMBRYO FIBROBLASTS, AND PANCREAS

HECTOR P. TRAVERSO, PETER V. HAUSCHKA, and
PAUL M. GALLOP

Departments of Orthopaedic Surgery,
Oral Biology, and Biological Chemistry,
Harvard Schools of Medicine and Dental Medicine,
Children's Hospital Medical Center,
Boston, MA 02115

INTRODUCTION

Vitamin K-dependent proteins contain γ-carboxyglutamic acid (Gla). Biosynthesis of Gla involves vitamin K-dependent carboxylation of specific glutamic acid residues in proteins (1). Most of the studies involving characterization of γ-carboxyglutamic acid-containing proteins have focused on the vitamin K-dependent plasma proteins such as prothrombin (2). Other Gla-proteins include osteocalcin from bone (3,4) and proteins of kidney (5), the matrix of Ca^{2+}-containing renal stones (6), calcified atherosclerotic plaque and other sites of pathological ectopic calcification (7), urine (8), placenta (9), chick chorioallantoic membrane (10), lung (11), and spleen (Friedman and Hauschka, unpublished).

Distribution of vitamin K-dependent carboxylase activity presumably parallels the occurrence of Gla-proteins in various tissues. The carboxylases of liver (1), cultured hepatocytes (12), bone (13), placenta (9), and kidney (5), have been characterized to various extents. The synthesis of a Gla-protein by kidney microsomes (5) was of great interest because of its possible involvement in some aspects of renal Ca^{2+} metabolism. This paper presents evidence that vitamin K-dependent protein carboxylation occurs in a cultured kidney cell line. Additionally, cultured chick embryo fibroblasts and chicken pancreas were found to synthesize Gla-proteins.

MATERIALS AND METHODS

The RAG cell line was originally derived from a transplantable renal adenocarcinoma in the BALB/cd strain of mice and shows an epithelioid morphology (14). Chicken embryo fibroblasts (CEF) were obtained from D. Giard at the Massachusetts Institute of Technology. Cells were grown in 499 cm^2 plastic roller bottles in Dulbecco's modified Eagle's medium supplemented with 5% fetal calf serum. Two days before harvesting, 10^{-4}M warfarin was added to the culture medium. Cells were harvested in late log phase by scraping and centrifuging in isotonic saline at 4°C. The yield was typically 0.6 ml packed cells per roller bottle. Pancreas was dissected from 6 week male chicks (buff sex-linked) fed a diet containing 800 mg dicumarol per kg of chow. Washed, packed cells or minced pancreas fragments were suspended in an equal volume of buffered sucrose (250 mM sucrose, 80 mM KCl, 25 mM imidazole, pH 7.2) and homogenized with a motor driven teflon-glass homogenizer (5).

Microsomes were prepared as described (5) and suspended in buffered sucrose to 60% of the volume of the original cell homogenate before addition to the carboxylation assay system. Protein carboxylation was performed using a modified procedure of Friedman and Shia (15). Incubation was at 37°C for 30 minutes in a capped vial. Each milliliter of reaction mixture contained 0.7 ml of suspended microsomes (5 to 10 mg protein) in 250 mM sucrose, 80 mM KCl, 25 mM imidazole, pH 7.2 buffer, 2.5 μmol magnesium acetate, 1 μmol ATP, 2 μmol NADH, 1 μmol phosphocreatine, 50 μg creatine phosphokinase, 2.5 μmol dithiothreitol (DDT), 47 μg cycloheximide, 47.5 μg 2-methyl 3-farnesyl 1-4 naphthoquinone (MK_3) in 10 μl ethanol, and 40 μCi [^{14}C]$NaHCO_3$ (specific activity 50 mCi/mmol). The reaction

311

was stopped by chilling on ice and adding, under the hood, 100 µl 100% TCA. The precipitate was collected by centrifugation, mixed with 300 µl 1M NaHCO$_3$, and then washed twice with 10 ml cold 10% TCA, and finally washed with acetone and diethyl ether. For preparation of [^{14}C]-labeled Gla-proteins, the above reaction was scaled up to 10 ml.

For [^{14}C]-Gla determination, alkaline hydrolyzed samples were applied to a Beckman 121M amino acid analyzer coupled to a flow scintillation counter as previously described (5,16). [^{14}C]NaHCO$_3$ (50 mCi/mmol) was purchased from New England Nuclear (Boston, MA). Sodium warfarin was generously provided by Endo Laboratories Inc. (Garden City, NY).

RESULTS

Assay of vitamin K-dependent protein carboxylation in vitro requires a suitable uncarboxylated peptide substrate which may be either endogenous to the microsomes or provided exogenously as a synthetic peptide. Since anticoagulant treatment in various in vivo situations generally decreases the Gla content of vitamin K-dependent proteins (17), it was anticipated that some accumulation of endogenous substrate for carboxylation might also be possible in this system. Two days previous to harvesting the RAG and CEF cells, 10^{-4} M sodium warfarin was incorporated into the growth medium. This level of sodium warfarin was chosen as the highest concentration at which cell growth appeared uninhibited. Microsomal fractions from RAG and CEF cells, normal and warfarin-treated, were examined for vitamin K-dependent carboxylation of endogenous protein. Vitamin MK$_3$ stimulates carboxylation by 1.5 to 4-fold, except that there is apparently no stimulation in the warfarin-treated RAG cells. This lack of stimulation may result from inhibition by residual warfarin in the assay mixture and is partially reversed by adding higher levels of MK$_3$.

For analysis of the position of [^{14}C] isotope incorporation, alkaline hydrolyzed smaples (5,16) were applied to a Beckman 121M amino acid analyzer coupled to a flow scintillation counter. In Figure 1a the chromatographic profile shows [^{14}C]-Gla to contain about 90% of the total radioactivity in the RAG microsome hydrolyzate. For proof of the putative [γ-carboxyl-^{14}C]-Gla structure, an aliquot of the alkaline hydrolyzed sample was acid hydrolyzed (6N HCl, 6 hr, 100°C) under conditions which are known to cause complete decarboxylation of Gla to glutamic acid (16).

TABLE 1

VITAMIN K-DEPENDENT INCORPORATION OF [^{14}C]NaHCO$_3$ IN VITRO

Microsome Preparation	[^{14}C] CPM	
	-MK$_3$	+MK$_3$
RAG cells (+ warfarin)	1494	1532
RAG cells (- warfarin)	260	975
CEF cells (+ warfarin)	1358	4520
CEF cells (- warfarin)	1119	3078
Chick pancreas (normal diet)	187	330
Chick pancreas (dicumarol diet)	642	967

Reaction volumes were 1 ml. Vitamin MK$_3$ was used at 47.5 µg/ml. Values are the average of duplicate incubations.

Because the two γ-carboxyl groups of Gla are equivalent, but only one carried the [^{14}C] isotopic label, it is expected that random decarboxylation will yield [^{14}C]-glutamic acid with only 50% of the original specific radioactivity (1,5,16). After acid hydrolysis and flash evaporation, the radioactive profile showed that 50% of the label was lost as volatile $^{14}CO_2$ and 50% remained as [^{14}C]-glutamic acid (Fig. 1b). Similar studies showed that >85% of incorporated [^{14}C] is associated with Gla in the pancreas and CEF systems as well. In all three tissues, the fraction of radioactivity lost by decarboxylation is approximately 50% (Table 2), thus confirming the presence of [^{14}C-γ-carboxyl]-Gla as the predominant labeled compound.

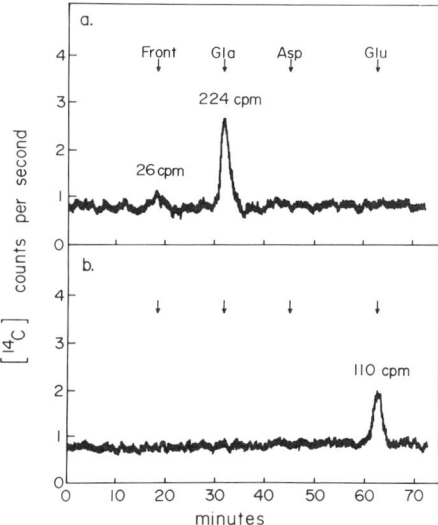

Figure 1. Ion-exchange chromatography of alkaline hydrolyzed RAG cell microsomes after [^{14}C]NaHCO$_3$ incubation. Total CPM in each peak is shown before (a) and after (b) hydrolysis in 6M HCl, 6 hr, 110°.

TABLE 2

DECARBOXYLATION OF [^{14}C]-Gla IN MICROSOMAL PREPARATIONS

Source of ^{14}C-labeled microsomal protein	Total ^{14}C CPM after 6M HCl treatment*		% loss of radioactivity
	unheated	heated	
RAG cells	1143	529	54%
	1142	542	53%
CEF cells	522	273	48%
Chicken pancreas	648	367	43%

* Alkaline hydrolyzed microsomal preparations were mixed with an equal volume of 12.2M HCl in duplicate tubes. One tube of each pair was heated 6 hours at 100°C while the other was stored at 0°C. All samples were then flash evaporated to dryness at 50° and washed twice with water.

DISCUSSION

Demonstration that vitamin K-dependent protein carboxylation occurs in a cultured kidney and fibroblast cell lines raises new possibilities for the study of this reaction. Just as RAG cells have been explored as a model for the kidney carboxylation system, the liver system has been studied in cultured hepatic cells (12). RAG cells show common features with renal tubular cells which are of primary importance in Ca^{2+}-reabsorption. Since Gla-proteins bind Ca^{2+} and exhibit Ca^{2+}-mediated adsorption to phospholipids (18, 19) it is possible that a Gla-protein is involved at the tubular level in the renal handling of Ca^{2+}. Thus the formation of a Gla-protein by RAG cells may be an expression of a specific Ca^{2+}-related renal tubular function *in vitro*. On the other hand, since a variety of other tissues also express Gla-proteins as a normal component, the RAG cell Gla-protein may not necessarily relate directly to the specific physiological Ca^{2+}-transport function of kidney.

ACKNOWLEDGEMENTS

E. Henson of these laboratories kindly synthesized the vitamin K analog MK_3. This work was supported by the National Foundation-March of Dimes and the National Institutes of Health (Grants AG 00376 and HL 20764).

REFERENCES

1. Esmon, C. T., Sadowski, J. A., Suttie, J. W. (1975) J. Biol. Chem. 250, 4744-4748.
2. Stenflo, J., and Suttie, J. W. (1977) Ann. Rev. Biochem. 46, 157-172.
3. Hauschka, P. V., Lian, J. B., Gallop, P. M. (1975) Proc. Natl. Acad. Sci. USA 72, 3925-3929.
4. Price, P. A., Otsuka, A. S., Poser, G. W., Kristaponis, J., Raman, N. (1976) Proc. Natl. Acad. Sci. USA 73, 1447-1451.
5. Hauschka, P. V., Friedman, P. A., Gallop, P. M., Traverso, H. P. (1976) Biochem. Biophys. Res. Commun. 71, 1207-1213.
6. Lian, J. B., Prien, E. L., Glimcher, M. J., Gallop, P. M. (1977) J. Clin. Invest. 59, 1151-1157.
7. Lian, J. B., Skinner, M. S., Glimcher, M. J., Gallop, P. M. (1976) Biochem. Biophys. Res. Commun. 73, 349-355.
8. Fernlund, P. (1976) Clin. Chim. Acta 72, 147-155.
9. Friedman, P. A., Hauschka, P. V., Shia, M. and Wallace, J. K. (1979) Biochim. Biophys. Acta 583, 261-283.
10. Tuan, R. S. (1979) J. Biol. Chem. 254, 1356-1364.
11. Bell, R. G. (1979) Fed. Proc. 38, 875.
12. Munns, T. W., Johnston, M. F. M., Liszewsky, M. K., Olson, R. E. (1976) Proc. Natl. Acad. Sci. USA 73, 2803-2807.
13. Lian, J. B., Friedman, P. A. (1978) J. Biol. Chem. 253, 6623-6626.
14. Klebe, R. J., Tchaw-Ren Chen, Ruddle, F. H. (1970) J. Cell Biol. 45, 74-82.
15. Friedman, P. A., Shia, M. (1976) Biochem. Biophys. Res. Commun. 72, 647-654.
16. Hauschka, P. V. (1977) Anal. Biochem. 80, 212-223.
17. Hauschka, P. V., Reid, M. R. (1978) J. Biol. Chem. 253, 9063-9068.
18. Esmon, C. T., Suttie, J. W., Jackson, C. M. (1975) J. Biol. Chem. 250, 4095-4099.
19. Nelsestuen, G. L., Lim, T. K. (1977) Biochemistry 16, 4164-4171.

MAMMALIAN VITAMIN K METABOLISM AND ANTICOAGULANT ACTION

NUTRITIONAL ASPECTS OF VITAMIN K IN THE HUMAN

M. J. SHEARER, V. ALLAN, Y. HAROON and P. BARKHAN

Guy's Hospital,
London, United Kingdom

INTRODUCTION

Despite recent advances in the understanding of the biochemical function of vitamin K, knowledge of the physiology of vitamin K in the human is incomplete. Information about dietary sources, requirements and turn-over of vitamin K is generally much less precise than for other fat-soluble vitamins. Even the fundamental question of the relative importance of the diet or intestinal micro-flora in providing man's requirements for vitamin K still remains to be answered.

In medicine, perhaps the most important nutritional problem concerning vitamin K, and certainly the most vexed (1) is the extent to which a deficiency of vitamin K contributes towards the incidence of bleeding in the newborn. In adults quantitative information about the sources of vitamin K is also relevant to medical practice because of the widespread use of oral anticoagulant drugs in the management of thrombo-embolic disease.

Undoubtedly a major reason for our ignorance in these nutritional areas is the difficulty in measuring the small amounts of vitamin K which are biologically effective. To date most nutritional data has derived from the chick bioassay which, although fairly sensitive, is cumbersome, and does not distinguish between molecular forms of vitamin K. Current methods for the chemical isolation and characterization of K vitamins from biological material mostly employ multi-stage chromatographic procedures requiring large amounts of starting material.

In the last few years the technique of high performance liquid chromatography (HPLC) has found increasing use in many areas. HPLC is of particular value in problems of trace analysis where its chief advantages are those of high chromatographic resolution, sensitive in line detection, speed of analysis, wide choice of separation principles, and adaptability to preparative or analytical requirements. These qualities suggested that HPLC would be well suited to the measurement of K vitamins in biological samples on a smaller scale than previously possible so that the technique could be used for routine analyses. In this report we describe the development of an HPLC assay procedure which was designed to study certain nutritional aspects of vitamin K in adults and the newborn. Some preliminary results are presented in which the technique has been used to assay vitamin K_1 in different biological materials, mostly foodstuffs.

MATERIALS AND METHODS

Lipid Extraction of Samples

To extract vitamin K_1 from vegetables, 10-50 g (fresh weight) was extracted with acetone as described by Lichtenthaler (2). Milk and commercial milk formulas were extracted with chloroform-methanol (2:1) by the method of Folch. Generally 10-20 ml of cows' milk, human milk and liquid forms of commercial milk formulas were extracted. For dried forms of milk formulas 1-10 g were reconstituted in water before extraction.

Gravity Column Chromatography

Lipid extracts were chromatographed on columns of Kieselgel 60, particle size 0.2-0.5 mm (E. Merck A.G., Darmstadt, Germany). After first eluting with hexane to remove hydrocarbons, a fraction containing K vitamins was obtained by elution with hexane-diethyl ether (97:3, v/v).

Adsorption HPLC

Adsorption HPLC was performed on columns packed with micro-particulate silica having an average particle size of 5 or 10 μm diameter (Partisil 5 or 10 from Whatman Lab Sales, Maidstone, UK). The mobile phase was hexane-dichloromethane (8:2, v/v) in which the dichloromethane component was 50% water-saturated. For the preparative purification of some milk samples, a cyano-bonded silica packing material was used (Partisil 10 PAC from Whatman) with the same mobile phase as for the normal columns above.

Reversed-Phase HPLC

The stationary phase was Zorbax ODS (DuPont, Hitchin, UK). For the assay of vitamin K_1, isocratic elution was employed with either methanol-dichloromethane (8:2, v/v) or acetonitrile-dichloromethane (7:3, v/v). To resolve menaquinones a solvent gradient was employed in which the concentration of dichloromethane in methanol was increased linearly at a rate of 5% min from an initial concentration of 20% to a final concentration of 50%. In all HPLC systems K vitamins were detected photometrically, usually at 250 or 270 nm.

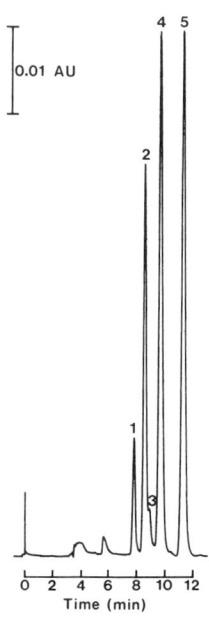

FIGURE 1. Silica adsorption HPLC of K vitamins on Partisil 5. Peaks 1. cis K_1, 2. trans K_1, 3. impurity, 4. MK-10, 5. MK-4. Detection 250 nm.

RESULTS AND DISCUSSION

HPLC of Vitamin K Standards

To explore the potential use of HPLC for the analysis of K vitamins in biological samples, the resolution of vitamin K standards by both adsorption and reversed-phase modes of HPLC was examined.

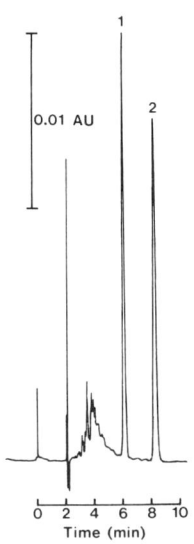 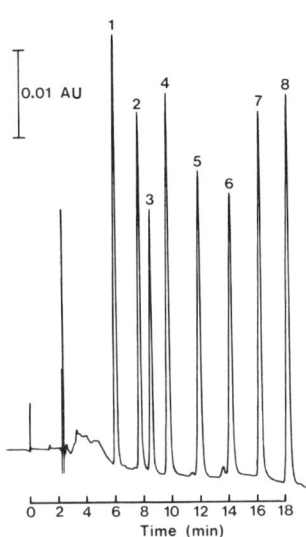

(Left) FIGURE 2. Resolution of K_1 epoxide (peak 1) and K_1 (peak 2) by reversed-phase HPLC on Zorbax ODS with methanol-dichloromethane (8:2) as mobile phase. Detection 250 nm.

(Right) FIGURE 3. Reversed-phase HPLC of K vitamins on Zorbax ODS using gradient elution (see Methods). Peaks 1, MK-4, 2. MK-5, 3. K_1, 4. to 8. MK-6 to MK-10. Detection 270 nm.

A typical separation of K vitamins by adsorption HPLC on columns of microparticulate silica is shown in Figure 1. Using hexane as the nonpolar component of the mobile phase, K vitamins could be eluted and partially resolved by the addition of a more polar modifier such as dichloromethane. Although adsorption HPLC could separate both cis and trans isomers of K_1 from menaquinones we were unable to resolve completely the individual members of the menaquinone series from each other.

The potential usefulness of the reversed-phase mode of HPLC in the separation of fat-soluble vitamins including vitamin K was shown some years ago (3). More recently the resolution of K_1 and K_1 epoxide has been reported using ODS bonded packing materials (octadecyl hydrocarbon groups chemically bonded either as a pellicular layer to inert beads or to porous silica particles) and aqueous-methanol mixtures as the mobile phase (4, 5). For our assay we chose a highly retentive ODS bonded phase (Zorbax ODS) based on porous microspheres of 6 μm diameter. To elute K vitamins it was necessary to combine a very polar solvent (e.g. methanol or acetonitrile) with a less polar solvent (e.g. dichloromethane). This type of chromatography has been termed non-aqueous reversed-phase HPLC (6). The separation of K_1 and K_1 epoxide on Zorbax ODS is shown in Figure 2. The high column efficiency of this separation enabled an on column detection of K_1 of about 1 ng.

Figure 3 shows that an efficient resolution of K_1 and menaquinones could also be achieved on Zorbax ODS by employing a methanol-dichloromethane mobile phase and gradient elution (see Methods).

Sample Purification Procedure

The purification and measurement of K_1 in biological material was usually carried out by the sequence of steps shown in Figure 4.

Owing to the low concentration of vitamin K in most biological samples it was not possible to determine K_1 by direct HPLC of crude lipid extracts either by adsorption or reversed-phase modes.

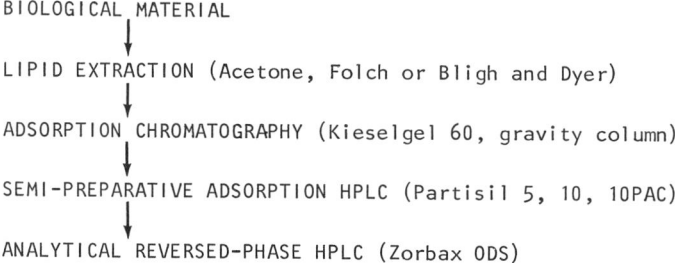

BIOLOGICAL MATERIAL
↓
LIPID EXTRACTION (Acetone, Folch or Bligh and Dyer)
↓
ADSORPTION CHROMATOGRAPHY (Kieselgel 60, gravity column)
↓
SEMI-PREPARATIVE ADSORPTION HPLC (Partisil 5, 10, 10PAC)
↓
ANALYTICAL REVERSED-PHASE HPLC (Zorbax ODS)

FIGURE 4 Flow Diagram of HPLC assay for vitamin K_1

Conventional gravity chromatography on an adsorption silica column was a very effective and simple initial purification step which exploits the low polarity of K vitamins compared with most other lipids present in biological samples. A major advantage of this column step was that it gave a fraction in which the remaining impurities had a similar polarity to K vitamins. This facilitated the subsequent adsorption HPLC stage by preventing both the accumulation of more polar compounds on top of the column (resulting in decreased column efficiencies) and their slow elution (resulting in interference with detection). The strategy by which we have been able to measure K_1 in this fraction was to employ two stages of HPLC. In the first stage we employed semi-preparative HPLC on silica columns (Partisil 5 or 10) or a cyano-bonded phase (Partisil 10 PAC). The K_1 present in the fraction collected from this stage was then measured by reversed-phase HPLC on Zorbax ODS.

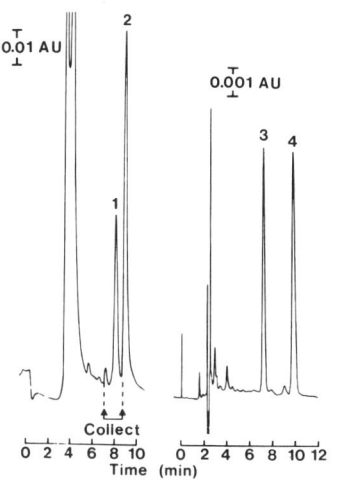

FIGURE 5. (Left) adsorption and (right) reversed-phase HPLC in assay of K_1 in dwarf beans. (Peaks) 1. K_1 plus K_1 epoxide, 2. P.Q., 3. K_1 epoxide, 4. K_1.

The general applicability of these HPLC steps to the analysis of biological material is illustrated in Figure 5 which shows the chromatograms obtained for the determination of K_1 in a vegetable (dwarf green beans). In this example the semi-preparative (adsorption) HPLC stage gave a clean K fraction which mostly contained K_1 and the internal standard K_1 epoxide. Not all biological samples gave such clean chromatograms. For example the final chromatograms obtained after the analysis of cows' milk, human milk and a commercial milk formula are shown in Figures 6 and 7. Despite the greater complexity of these chromatograms, the K_1 and K_1 epoxide peaks were generally resolved from interfering peaks. Although the 3-step chromatographic procedure has been successfully applied to a wide variety of biological samples, some commercial milk formulas containing non-milk

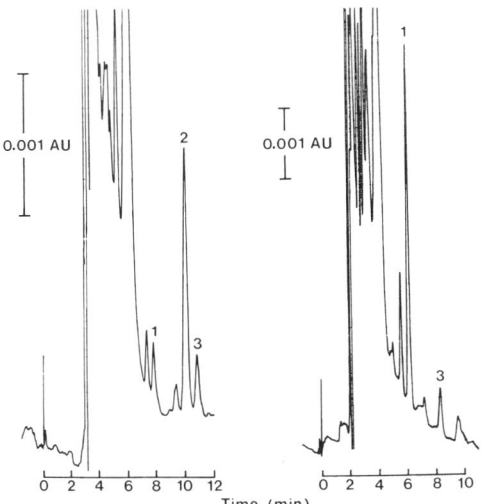
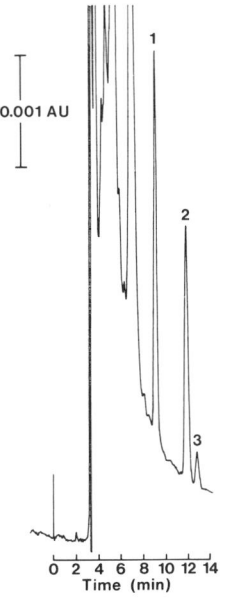

FIGURE 6. Chromatograms of reversed-phase HPLC stage on Zorbax ODS. (Left) infant formula product (Ostermilk Two) with acetonitrile-dichloromethane (8:2) as mobile phase. (Right) cows' milk with methanol-dichloromethane (8:2) as mobile phase. Peaks 1. K_1 epoxide (internal standard), 2. chloro-K_1 (added as marker for adsorption HPLC stage), 3. K_1. Detection (left) 270 nm, (right) 250 nm.

FIGURE 7.
Chromatogram of reversed-phase HPLC stage for human milk with acetonitrile-dichloromethane (7:3) as mobile phase. Peaks as Figure 6. Detection 270 nm.

oils gave contaminating peaks which interfered with those of K_1 or K_1 epoxide. Further modification of the assay is therefore required for such materials.

Quantitation and Internal Standardisation

Because of the multiple steps involved, the use of an internal standard had considerable attractions, both from the point of view of precision and the ease of manipulation and calculation. Because the assay contained two HPLC stages with different modes of chromatography, a prerequisite for an internal standard was that it should elute with the same or very similar retention volume on silica adsorption HPLC but a different retention volume on reversed-phase HPLC. So far the only suitable compound found to meet these requirements is vitamin K_1 epoxide and this compound has therefore been employed as an internal standard for the assay of K_1 in foodstuffs and certain other biological samples. The potential disadvantage that K_1 epoxide is a naturally occurring metabolite does not generally apply except when the metabolite accumulates in the presence of oral anticoagulants. A search for vitamin K_1 epoxide in biological material showed evidence that small amounts of K_1

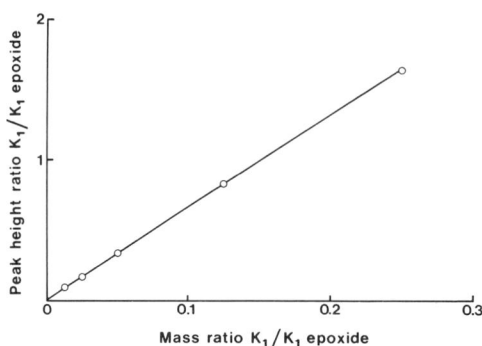

FIGURE 8. Calibration curve for HPLC assay of K_1 on a Zorbax ODS column with methanol-dichloromethane (8:2) as mobile phase.

epoxide are present in plants. At the wavelength of detection the peak height of endogenous K_1 epoxide was about 2% of the K_1 peak. Provided that the final peak height of the K_1 epoxide added as an internal standard was of a similar order to the K_1 peak this did not significantly affect the accuracy of the assay.

The chloro analog of K_1 (2-chloro-3-phytyl 1,4-naphthoquinone) was also examined as a potential internal standard but had the disadvantage that it eluted slightly before phylloquinone on adsorption HPLC. For this reason <u>cis</u> chloro-K_1 was useful as a marker compound for samples where the concentration of K_1 was too low to be detected as a peak during the semi-preparative adsorption HPLC step. The addition of chloro-K_1 provided a more accurate indication than retention times of the elution of the K_1 fraction. Since the collection of the K_1 fraction was started after most of the chloro-K_1 had been eluted only a small proportion of the marker was included in the K_1 fraction and was resolved from K_1 during the final analytical stage on Zorbax ODS (Figures 6 and 7).

To quantitate K_1 in a biological sample, a known quantity of K_1 epoxide was initially added to the lipid extract and the peak height ratio of K_1 to K_1 epoxide determined by the assay technique. Since peak height ratios of standard solutions were related linearly to mass ratios (Fig. 8), the amount of K_1 in the sample could be calculated by reference to the appropriate standard and the amount of K_1 epoxide added.

To check any possible difference in the chemical stability of K_1 and K_1 epoxide during the assay procedure (which might invalidate the use of K_1 epoxide as an internal standard), standard solutions of K_1 and K_1 epoxide were processed in the same way as the biological samples. Identical peak height ratios before and after the assay procedure showed that there was no differential loss of either K_1 or K_1 epoxide.

The accuracy of the assay was assessed by adding known quantities of K_1 to water or biological samples of previously determined K_1 content. There was good agreement between the calculated and added values of K_1.

Purity of Chromatographic Peaks

For any chromatographic assay solution it is important to establish that the peaks measured contain only the pure compounds of interest.

One method of checking the purity of peaks from UV photometers is to examine their ultraviolet absorption spectra. For K vitamins the UV absorption spectrum is a distinctive signature of their 2,3-disubstituted 1,4-naphthoquinone structure, and for some biological samples it was feasible to check the identity of the K_1 peak resolved by HPLC by directly recording the UV absorption spectra of compounds as they eluted

TABLE 1. Precision of HPLC assay for K_1 in different biological material

Biological material	n	Mean ($\mu g\ K_1/100\ g$)	SD (±)		CV (%)	
			Within run	Between run	Within run	Between run
Kale	20	729	34	42	4.7	5.8
Green beans	10	46.0	2.4	3.1	5.2	6.7
Infant formula	8	26.2	1.8	2.8	6.9	10.6
Infant formula	6	2.48	0.06	0.14	2.5	5.4

from the column. This required linking a specially designed double beam scanning spectrophotometer to the column outlet. To obtain an acceptable spectra of K_1 with this instrument a peak height of about 0.05 AU or greater was required.

When it is not possible to obtain a whole UV absorption spectrum, a good indication of peak purity may be obtained by comparing the absorbance ratios of peaks at two or more specific wavelength settings with those given by a pure standard of the suspected compound. Depending on the available instrumentation this ratioing technique can be applied in various ways. We have modified one of the techniques described by Yost et al. (7) and determined the peak height ratio of K_1 to K_1 epoxide for separate injections of the sample at different wavelengths. The ratio of the peak height ratios of K_1 to K_1 epoxide at the selected wavelengths was then compared with that given by a standard mixture of K_1 and K_1 epoxide.

Precision of HPLC Assay

An estimate of the precision of the HPLC assay was determined for different biological materials containing varying amounts of K_1 (Table 1). Since all analyses were performed in duplicate, the data from several duplicate determinations of the same sample performed over a period of time enabled both the within- and between-run precisions to be calculated from the same set of data. Table 1 shows that within-run precision was between 3 and 7% whilst between-run precision was between 5 and 11%. Although the results in Table 1 suggested that there was no apparent difference in the overall precision between samples with high and low K_1 content, other data (not shown in Table 1) suggested that a large part of the variation in the determinations of K_1 in vegetable tissues with a relatively high concentration of K_1 was due to the non-uniformity of tissue samples or to differences in extracting K_1. Thus when two separate lipid extracts of kale were sub-divided into four equal aliquots and analysed separately, the precision of the subsequent analytical steps for each set of quadruplicates was improved with coefficients of variation of 2.2% and 1.1% respectively.

Vitamin K_1 Content of Vegetables

Although there is some data of the K_1 content of plants determined by chemical assay (2, 8) these studies had a botanical rather than a nutritional bias. The chick bioassay has been applied to the determination of K_1 in certain vegetables and Olson (9) has collated the existing nutritional data. Table 2 shows some results obtained using the HPLC

TABLE 2. Vitamin K_1 content of some common vegetables determined by HPLC assay

Vegetable	µg/100 g fresh wt	
Potato	< 1	(3)
Parsnip	< 1	
White turnip	< 1	
Mushrooms	< 1	
Red pepper	2	
Celery	5	
Carrot	5	
Tomato	6	(5)
Green pepper	6	
Leek	10	
Cucumber	15	
Red cabbage	19	
Cauliflower	27	
Peas	39	(19)
Dwarf beans	46	(14)
Cress	88	
Lettuce		
(round variety)	120	(129)
(Webb's variety)	128	
White cabbage		
(outer leaves)	137	
(inner leaves)	83	
Winter cabbage		
(outer leaves)	189	
(inner leaves)	52	
Broccoli	147	(200)
Brussels sprouts		
(sprouts)	177	
(top leaves)	400	
Spinach	415	(89)
Spring cabbage	472	
Kale	724	

[a]Data in brackets are the results of bioassays taken from Olson et al. (9).

assay to determine the K_1 content of some common vegetables. As expected the HPLC assay gave values which were generally higher than those given by the chick bioassay.

Vitamin K_1 Content of Milk and Infant Formula Products

As part of investigations into the nutritional status of vitamin K in the newborn we are presently using the HPLC assay to measure dietary sources of vitamin K such as infant formula foods, human breast milk, and cows' milk. A comparison of two infant formula products marketed in the UK is shown in Table 3. One of these (Ostermilk) was based on cows' milk and had a K_1 concentration (4 µg/litre) which was similar to that found for fresh cows' milk (Table 4). Although another product (Gold Cap SMA) had been supplemented with K_1 at a level of 58 µg/litre, a consistently lower value (about 35 µg/litre) was obtained by HPLC assay (Table 4). Even so the concentration of K_1 in the formula supplemented with K_1 was much greater than the levels found naturally in either human or cows' milk (Table 4). Of the natural and artificial milk samples so far assayed for K_1, human milk (obtained from individual mothers after breast-feeding had been well-established) had the lowest levels of K_1, ranging from 1-2 µg K_1/litre. The K_1 content of human milk was 2-4 times lower than that found in homogenized milk from Friesian cows. An increased concentration of K_1 was found in milk from 'Channel Island' cows.

The only previous report of the chemical measurement of vitamin K in the foods of infants was a study in which the K_1 content of different infant formula foods marketed in the USA was assayed by reflectance densitometry after separation by conventional column and thin-layer chromatography (10). Using this method the K_1 levels in formulas without added K_1 ranged from 19 to 118 µg/litre. The same investigators also briefly reported that cows' milk analysed at different times of the year had average K_1 levels of 10, 47 and 85 µg/litre (10).

TABLE 3. Vitamin K_1 content of infant formula products by HPLC assay

PRODUCT	MANUFACTURER	ADDED K_1	K_1 CONTENT	
			powder (μg/100g)	reconstituted (μg/litre)
Ostermilk	Glaxo group	-	2.9 ± 0.2	4.5
Ostermilk Two	Glaxo group	-	2.5 ± 0.1	3.8
*Gold Cap SMA	Wyeth Labs	+	26.2 ± 1.0	33.2
*Gold Cap SMA	Wyeth Labs	+	28.9 ± 0.1	36.7
†Gold Cap SMA	Wyeth Labs	+	-	34.9 ± 0.3

Values are the mean (±SEM) of duplicate analyses
*Different batches of same product
†Marketed in liquid form

TABLE 4. Vitamin K_1 content of human milk and cows' milk by HPLC assay

HUMAN MILK			COWS' MILK		
Subject	month	K_1 (μg/litre)	Milk type	month	K_1 (μg/litre)
1	Nov	2.2 ± 0.1	Homogenized	Aug	8.9 ± 0.2
2	Feb	1.4 ± 0.2	" †	Aug	5.6 ± 0.1
3 (a)	Feb	1.9 ± 0.1	"	Apr	4.4 ± 0.3
(b)	Feb	1.3 ± 0.2	"	May	7.4*
4	Feb	1.4 ± 0.1	Channel Is.	Oct	17.8 ± 0.2
5	March	2.0 ± 0.1	"	Jan	12.3*
6	March	1.7 ± 0.2			

Except for single values* the values are the mean (±SEM) of duplicate analyses. Cows' milk was pasteurized except for one sterilized sample†.

Shortly after his discovery of vitamin K, Dam used the chick bioassay to determine the vitamin K content of human and cows' milk (11). For cows' milk analysed during the months from December to March the vitamin K activities of individual samples varied widely from 0 to 4000 Dam-Glavind units/litre with an average of 2000 units/litre. In the curative chick bioassay used in these studies an activity of 1000 units is equivalent to 30 μg menadione (12). Since menadione is not a nutritional form of vitamin K it is more appropriate to express vitamin K activity in terms of a natural form such as vitamin K_1. In this respect the activities of K_1 and menaquinones in the chick bioassay were approximately equal and 1000 Dam-Glavind units was equivalent to about 80 μg K_1 (13). The average activities for cows' milk and human milk of 2000 and 500 units are then equivalent to concentrations of K_1 of 160 and 40 μg/litre respectively. These values are much higher than the values for K_1 concentrations measured by HPLC (Table 4). As with cows' milk the bioassay of individual human milk samples showed a wide variation with a high proportion of samples showing no activity whilst the upper limit of 2000 units was equivalent to 160 μg K_1/litre. It is possible that this wide variation reflects the lack of sensitivity and precision of early chick bioassays. Although the levels of K_1 measured by HPLC were about one twentieth the average activity found by bioassay, all samples so far analysed by HPLC had a detectable level of K_1 and the range of values was much narrower (Table 4). In a preparative experiment designed to detect menaquinones in human milk by HPLC we could find no evidence that the much higher vitamin K activity recorded by bioassay reflected an increased proportion of menaquinones. If the relative proportions of individual forms of K vitamins reflect those found in human liver (14, 15) it might be expected that vitamin K_1 accounts for about half of the total vitamin K content of human milk.

Even though the concentrations of vitamin K determined by bioassay and HPLC assay were not in quantitative agreement a relative deficiency of human milk compared with cows' milk was found by both methods. The concentrations of K_1 in human milk found by HPLC assay (Table 4) suggest that the normal dietary intake of healthy breast-fed infants may be less than 1 μg vitamin K_1/day. Although the factors which may lead to a deficiency of vitamin K in the newborn are not known there is evidence that hypoprothrombinaemia in neonates is associated with breast-feeding and that feeding cows' milk protects against the development of a vitamin K deficiency (16, 17). In view of the relatively low levels of K_1 found in human milk fed to healthy infants, it is interesting to speculate that even lower levels in the milk of some mothers may be an important factor in the pathogenesis of the haemorrhagic disease of the newborn.

Assay of Vitamin K_1 in Plasma by HPLC

To study the absorption and metabolism of vitamin K in humans it would be useful to be able to measure blood levels of the vitamin directly, thus avoiding the use of isotopically labelled vitamin K. Figure 9 shows the time course of K_1 in the plasma determined by HPLC assay after a subject had been injected with 1 mg of K_1 (Konakion). The clearance of K_1 was very rapid and was very similar to that found in isotopic experiments in which the disappearance curve could be approximately described by two major exponential functions (18). The plasma levels of K_1 in the fasting state have not yet been accurately measured but appear to be less than 1 ng/ml plasma. To measure the range of K_1 levels shown in Figure 9 it was necessary to process 1-8 ml of plasma. Although the very low physiological levels of vitamin K in the circulation limit the use of this direct assay, the

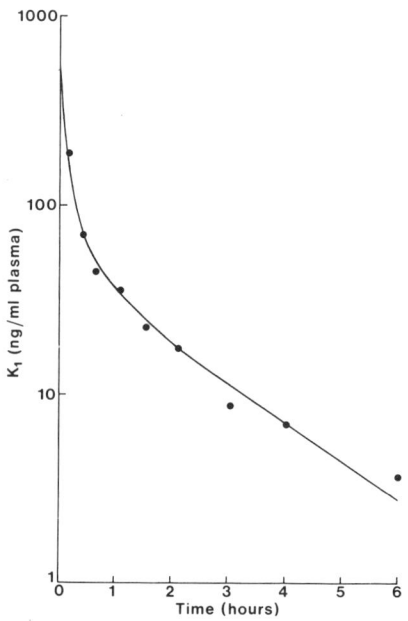

FIGURE 9. Plasma levels of vitamin K_1 determined by HPLC after i.v. injection of 1 mg vitamin K_1.

study showed the feasibility of measuring plasma levels in experimental situations to follow the time course of administered doses of vitamin K_1.

ACKNOWLEDGMENTS

We would like to thank all those who participated in the collection and donation of breast milk for these studies. Chloro-K_1 was kindly supplied by Dr R.G. Bell and Dr M.G. Townsend. The work was supported by a grant (G977/827) from the Medical Research Council, UK.

REFERENCES

1. Editorial (1978) Lancet 1, 755-757.
2. Lichtenthaler, H.K. (1962) Planta 57, 731-753.
3. Williams, R.C., Schmit, J.A., and Henry, R.A. (1972) J. Chromatogr. Sci. 10, 494-501.
4. Elliott, G.R., Odam, E.M., and Townsend, M.G. (1976) Biochem. Soc. Trans. 4, 615-617.
5. Bjornsson, T.D., Swezey, S.E., Meffin, P.J., and Blaschke, T.F. (1978) Thromb. Haemostasis 39, 466-473.
6. Parris, N.A. (1978) J. Chromatogr. 157, 161-170.
7. Yost, R., Stoveken, J., and MacLean, W. (1977) J. Chromatogr. 134, 73-82.
8. Egger, K. (1965) Planta 64, 41-61.
9. Olson, R.E. (1973) Modern Nutrition in Health and Disease Ed by Goodhart, R.S., and Shils, M.E. pp 166-174, Lea and Febiger, Philadelphia.
10. Schneider, D.L., Fluckiger, H.B., and Manes, J.D. (1974) Pediatrics 53, 273-275.
11. Dam, H., Glavind, J., Larsen, E.H., and Plum, P. (1942) Acta Med. Scand. 112, 210-216.
12. Dam, H., Dyggve, H., Larsen, H., and Plum, P. (1952) Adv. Pediatr. 5, 129-153.
13. Glavind, J., Larsen, E.H., and Plum, P. (1942) Acta Med. Scand. 112, 198-209.
14. Rietz, P., Gloor, U., and Wiss, O. (1970) Int. Z. Vitaminforsch. 40, 351-362.
15. Duello, T.J., and Matschiner, J.T. (1972) J. Nutr. 102, 331-335.
16. Sutherland, J.M., Glueck, H.I., and Gleser, G. (1967) Am. J. Dis. Child. 113, 524-533.
17. Keenan, W.J., Jewett, T., and Glueck, H.I. (1971) Am. J. Dis. Child. 121, 271-277.
18. Shearer, M.J., McBurney, A., and Barkhan, P. (1974) Vitamins and Hormones 32, 513-542.

DISPOSITION AND TURNOVER OF VITAMIN K_1 IN MAN

THORIR D. BJORNSSON*, PETER J. MEFFIN,
SARAH E. SWEZEY, and TERRENCE F. BLASCHKE

Divisions of Clinical Pharmacology and Cardiology,
Department of Medicine,
Stanford University Medical Center,
Stanford, CA 94305, and
Division of Clinical Pharmacology*,
Duke University Medical Center
Durham, NC 27710

INTRODUCTION

Although the interrelationships between vitamin K_1, vitamin K_1 epoxide, and vitamin K antagonist drugs, such as warfarin, have been under intense scrutiny for the past decade (1,2,3), few studies are available on the disposition of vitamin K_1 in man (4,5,6,7,8). Our knowledge in this area is therefore limited, and this includes information on the amount of vitamin K_1 in the body, the turnover of the vitamin in the body, its metabolism, the minimum and average daily intake of vitamin K_1, and concentrations of the vitamin in plasma. Research in this area is most significantly hampered by the nonavailability of an analytical method for determining vitamin K_1 in biological fluids, and studies to date are therefore based on radiolabelled vitamin K_1.

In a recent study (9), four healthy subjects received intravenous injections of tritiated vitamin K_1 as part of a detailed clinical study on the interaction between the drugs warfarin and clofibrate. This study showed that clofibrate caused a significantly enhanced anticoagulant effect of warfarin, and that this effect was not due to changes in the pharmacokinetics of warfarin. In this report we will focus on the analysis of the vitamin K_1 data in this study and arrive at some estimates of disposition and turnover parameters of vitamin K_1 in man.

METHODS

Four healthy male volunteers received specifically labelled vitamin K_1(2-methyl-3-phytyl-1,2-^{3}H-1,4-naphthoquinone, specific activity 87.5 mCi/mM, a gift from Hoffmann LaRoche, Basel, Switzerland) as an intravenous injection of 60 µCi on four different occasions. The first dose of tritiated vitamin K_1 was in the absence of drug administration, the second dose was after daily administration of warfarin for two weeks that yielded anticoagulant effect corresponding to prothrombin time 1½ times the control value, the third dose was after administration of clofibrate 2 g daily for two weeks, and the fourth dose was after concurrent administration of both drugs in same doses as before for two weeks. Following each dose of tritiated vitamin K_1, which corresponded to 300 µg of vitamin K_1, blood samples were collected from an antecubital vein into heparinized Vacutainer tubes at 10,20,30, and 45 minutes and at 1,1.5,2,3,4,5,6,7,8, and 10 hours.

Plasma radiolabelled vitamin K_1 and vitamin K_1 epoxide were quantitated by a high pressure liquid chromatographic method (10). The method involves the determination of total ether extractable radioactivity, which consists of the sum of the radioactivity due to vitamin K_1 and vitamin K_1 epoxide, and a chromatographic separation to determine the relative quantities of radiolabelled vitamin K_1 and vitamin K_1 epoxide. The method is reproducible and accurate over a wide range of relative amounts of the two compounds, and has a coefficient of variation of approximately

5%.

A non-linear least-squares regression analysis program, MLAB (11), was used to obtain the best fit of the radioactive vitamin K_1 concentration versus time data to a biexponential equation. Individual data points were weighted by the reciprocal of the squared concentration to prevent large numbers from predominating in the least-squares criteria. The area under the plasma radioactivity versus time curve up to 600 minutes was calculated using the trapezoidal rule, and the terminal area beyond the last data point was calculated by dividing the radioactive vitamin K_1 concentration at the time of the last data point by the best fit slope of the second exponential component. The apparent volume of distribution at steady-state (Vd_{ss}) was calculated by standard pharmacokinetic methods (12) based on the coefficients and exponents of the best fit biexponential equation to the data. The plasma clearance (Cl) was calculated by dividing the dose (in dpm) by the total area under the plasma radioactivity versus time curve. The turnover time (t_t) was calculated from the expression:

$$t_t = \frac{Vd_{ss}}{Cl}$$

and the fractional turnover rate (k) was calculated as the reciprocal of the turnover time (13):

$$k = \frac{1}{t_t}$$

Results are expressed as mean ± S.D.

RESULTS

When tritiated vitamin K_1 was administered in the absence of drug administration, it had an average initial half-life ($t_{\frac{1}{2}\alpha}$, corresponding to the first exponential decline) of 26.0±8.0 min, and an average terminal half-life ($t_{\frac{1}{2}\beta}$, corresponding to the second exponential decline) of 165.8 ±9.5 min. These values were similar when tritiated vitamin K_1 was administered in the presence of warfarin and/or clofibrate administration.

Table 1 lists the average computed parameters of vitamin K_1 dispo-

TABLE I. Disposition and turnover parameters of tritiated vitamin K_1 in man.

Study condition (presence of drugs)	Vd_{ss} (liters)	Cl (ml/min)	t_t (min)	k (hr^{-1})
No drugs	17.6±3.9	115±26	153±12	0.393±0.030
Warfarin	19.5±7.6	111±27	175±45	0.361±0.099
Clofibrate	17.9±2.6	120±24	151±14	0.399±0.037
Warfarin & Clofibrate	19.8±10.8	128±33	152±57	0.442±0.170

Symbols as defined in Methods

No statistically significant differences in disposition and turnover parameters between any study conditions ($P > 0.05$).

sition (Vd_{ss}, Cl, t_t, and k) when tritiated vitamin K_1 was administered in the absence of drug administration, and after chronic administration of warfarin or clofibrate, and after concurrent chronic administration of both drugs. No statistically significant differences were observed in these disposition parameters between any of the different study conditions.

In the absence of drug administration, essentially no radiolabelled vitamin K_1 epoxide was detected in plasma. After anticoagulant doses of warfarin substantial concentrations of tritiated vitamin K_1 epoxide appeared in plasma, although there were no apparent changes in the plasma disappearance curve of radiolabelled vitamin K_1. When the same doses of warfarin were administered with clofibrate, however, both the plasma disappearance curve of radiolabelled vitamin K_1 and the accumulation curve of radiolabelled vitamin K_1 epoxide fell below those observed after warfarin alone.

DISCUSSION

Radiolabelled vitamin K_1 has been administered to man by other investigators in studies on the metabolism of vitamin K_1 or the mechanism of action of warfarin (4,5,6,7,8), but complete pharmacokinetic analysis of its plasma disposition has not been carried out. The kinetic parameters reported have been an initial half-life of 20-24 min and a terminal half-life of 121-150 min (4); in another study these values averaged about 12 min and 200 min, respectively (8). These values are in general agreement with the values obtained in the present study. Several interesting aspects, however, of the disposition of vitamin K_1 from plasma and its turnover characteristics can be ascertained from its plasma radioactivity versus time profiles. This is based on pharmacokinetic analysis of the data, assuming the dose of the vitamin is physiological (i.e., dose of 300 µg), and this does not necessitate the determination of concentrations of unlabelled vitamin K_1 in plasma. One value which can be calculated from the data is the turnover time (t_t). The turnover time of a compound represents the average life time expectancy of each molecule in the body or the time required for the total body pool of a compound to "turn over", that is, to be replaced by new molecules (13). The fractional turnover rate (k) is the inverse of the turnover time, and represents the fraction of the total body pool which is replaced per time unit. Of note is the short turnover time (153 min) and rapid fractional turnover rate (0.393 hr^{-1}) of vitamin K_1. This indicates that the total body pool of vitamin K_1 is replaced approximately every 2½ hours. It is also interesting to note that the disposition parameters of vitamin K_1 did not change in the presence of warfarin when there is substantial accumulation of vitamin K_1 epoxide since this metabolite now constitutes a substantial portion of the administered dose of radiolabelled vitamin K_1.

The body pool size of vitamin K_1, however, cannot be calculated for these subjects, since both the plasma concentrations of unlabelled vitamin K_1 in plasma and the daily intake of vitamin K_1 are unknown. The minimum daily intake requirement of vitamin K_1 in man is not accurately known, but is thought to be lower than 1.5 µg/kg/day (14), and probably in the range of 0.5 - 1.0 µg/kg/day (3). Since the body pool size can be calculated as the product of rate of intake and turnover time, the pool size in an average weight subject ingesting that small amount would be expected to be less than 10 µg. The average daily intake is difficult to estimate because of synthesis of vitamins K by the intestinal flora, but is thought to be less than 1 mg (15). Intake of that magnitude would be expected to yield a body pool size of about 100 µg in an average subject. This estimate is of interest since the liver pool size of vitamin K_1 in man has been calculated to be about 100 μg based on experimental data (16), and since a substantial portion (>50%) of vitamin K_1 in animals appears to be stored in the liver (17,18). This suggests that our estimates of the disposition and turnover parameters of vitamin K_1 in man are physiologically realistic, though the precise characterization of vitamin K_1 disposition and turnover has to await the development of methodology for determining vitamin K_1 concentrations in plasma and other biological fluids. The average concentrations of vitamin K_1 in plasma are very low and no method is presently available. They may be estimated, however, from our data as rate of intake divided by total clearance which suggests a few ng/ml.

In spite of the short turnover time and small body pool size for vitamin K_1, the acute development of vitamin K deficiency is apparently avoided by the presence of higher molecular weight storage forms of the vitamin in man (17,19). These observations do have relevance to the dosing interval of exogenously administered vitamin K, which is used in the therapy of patients with excessive anticoagulation due to coumarins (20, 21), or in patients receiving parenteral nutrition and oral antibiotics (22).

ACKNOWLEDGEMENTS

Supported by Grant No. GM22209 and Training Grant GM 07065 from the National Institutes of Health, and Merck, Sharp & Dohme International Fellowship in Clinical Pharmacology (T.D.B.) and Pharmaceutical Manufacturers Association Foundation Faculty Development Award in Clinical Pharmacology (T.F.B.).

REFERENCES

1. Jackson, C.M., and Suttie, J.W. (1977) Progress in Hematol. 10:333-359.
2. Stenflo, J., and Suttie, J.W. (1977) Ann.Rev. Biochem. 46:157-172.
3. Suttie, J.W. (1978) The Fat-Soluble Vitamins. Ed. DeLuca, H.F., Handbook of Lipid Research Vol.2, Plenum Press, New York and London, pp. 211-277.
4. Shearer, M.J., Mallinson, C.N., Webster, G.R., and Barkham, P.(1972) Brit. J. Haematol. 22:579-588.
5. Shearer, M.J., McBurney, A., and Barkhan, P.(1973) Brit. J. Haematol 24:471-479.
6. Shearer, M.J., McBurney, A., and Barkhan, P. (1974) Vit. Horm. 32: 513-542.
7. Shearer, M.J., McBurney, A., Breckenridge, A.M., and Barkhan, P. (1977) Clin. Sci. Mol. Med. 52:621-630.
8. Shepherd, A.M.M., Wilson, N.M., and Stevenson, I.H. (1977) Clin. Pharmacol. Ther. 21:117.
9. Bjornsson, T.D., Meffin, P.J., Swezey, S.E., and Blaschke, T.F. (1979) J. Pharmacol. Exp. Ther. In press.
10. Bjornsson, T.D., Swezey, S.E., Meffin, P.J., and Blaschke, T.F. (1978) Thrombos. Hemostas. 39:466-473.
11. Knott, G.D., and Reece, D.K. (1972) Proceedings of the ONLINE 1972 International Conference, vol. 1, Brunel University, England, pp. 497-526.
12. Gibaldi, M., and Perrier, D. (1975) Pharmacokinetics, Marcel Dekker, Inc., New York, pp. 177-184.
13. Riggs, D.S. (1963) The mathematical approach to physiologic problems

Williams and Wilkins, Baltimore (paperback edition, MIT Press, 1970) pp. 126-129.
14. Frick, P.G., Riedler, G., and Brogli, H. (1967) J. Appl. Physiol. 23:387-389.
15. van der Meer, J., Hemker, H.C., and Loeliger, E.A. (1968) Thrombos. Diathes.Hemmorh. Suppl. 29: 1-95.
16. Duello, T.J., and Matschiner, J.T. (1972) J. Nutr. 102: 331-335.
17. Wiss, O., and Gloor, H. (1966) Vit. Horm. 24: 575-586.
18. Konishi, T., Baba, S., and Sone, H. (1973) Chem. Pharm. Bull. 21: 220.
19. O'Reilly, R.A. (1976) Ann. Rev. Med. 27: 245-261.
20. O'Reilly, R.A. (1976) Medicine 55: 389-399.
21. Bjornsson, T.D., and Blaschke, T.F. (1978) Lancet 2:846-847.
22. Pineo, G.F., Gallus, A.S., and Hirsh, T. (1973) J. Canad. Med. Assn. 109: 880-883.

EFFECT OF THE CHLORO ANALOG OF VITAMIN K ON PHYLLOQUINONE METABOLISM IN LIVER MITOCHONDRIA

M. J. THIERRY-PALMER, M. S. STERN, C. A. KOST,
and J. C. MONTGOMERY

Department of Natural Sciences
University of Michigan-Dearborn
Dearborn, MI 48128

INTRODUCTION

Synthetic vitamin K contains a mixture of cis- and trans-phylloquinone. Cis-phylloquinone is far less active than trans-phylloquinone in stimulating prothrombin synthesis (1), phylloquinone epoxide synthesis (2), and protein carboxylation (3) in the rat and is unable to participate effectively in oxidative phosphorylation in M. phlei (4,5). Knauer and coworkers (2) have demonstrated a slight enrichment of cis-phylloquinone in liver mitochondria after injection of a mixture of the cis and trans isomers. Disappearance of cis-phylloquinone from all subcellular fractions of the liver was slower than that of the trans isomer.

Thierry and Suttie (6) have shown that administration of the chloro analog of phylloquinone, 2-chloro-3-phytyl-1,4-naphthoquinone (chloro-K), simultaneously with radioactive phylloquinone caused a 1.5 fold increase in the amount of radioactivity found in the liver. Most of this increased radioactivity was shown to be in the mitochondrial fraction of the liver. There was also some indication of slower turnover of phylloquinone in the liver when chloro-K was administered. The studies reported here were designed to determine whether chloro-K affects the relative distribution of cis- and trans-phylloquinone in rat liver mitochondria.

MATERIALS AND METHODS

Animals

Normal male Sprague-Dawley rats were used. Rats were injected intravenously with ^{3}H-phylloquinone or with ^{3}H-phylloquinone and chloro-K in 0.05 ml ethanol. They were killed by decapitation three hours after injection and their livers were quickly excised.

Tissue Preparation

Mitochondria were isolated from a 10% liver homogenate in 0.25 M sucrose by centrifugation at 9,600 g for 10 minutes at 4°C after an initial sedimentation of nuclei and debris at 800 g for 10 minutes. Microsomes were prepared from the postmitochondrial supernatant by centrifugation at 105,000 g for 60 minutes at 4°C. All pellets were washed twice by resuspension in sucrose and centrifugation.

In vitro Incubation

Mitochondria equivalent to 400 mg original liver were incubated in medium containing 3 mM ATP, 10 mM sodium succinate, 10 mM tris buffer (pH 7.4), 80 mM NaCL, 4 mM inorganic phosphate (pH 7.4) and 10 mM $MgCl_2$ (7). A mixture of 0.5 µg ^{3}H-phylloquinone and 9.5 µg unlabeled phylloquinone in 0.1 ml ethanol was added to the control tubes at zero time. Chloro-K (70 µg) was added to the experimental tubes simultaneously with the vitamin. Total volume was 3.0 ml. Samples were incubated for 30 minutes at 30°C. Mitochondria were pelleted from the samples immediately after the incubation.

Chromatography

Lipids were extracted from the subcellular fractions by the method of Bligh and Dyer (8). The chloroform extracts of the subcellular fractions were evaporated under nitrogen and analyzed for cis- and trans-phylloquinone by thin-layer chromatography (1,2).

Chemicals

Radioactive phylloquinone, labeled with tritium in the napthoquinone ring, and chloro-K were generous gifts of Dr. John W. Suttie, University of Wisconsin-Madison. The specific activity of the labeled phylloquinone was 2×10^4 dpm/µg. Unlabeled phylloquinone was purchased from Sigma Chemical Co., St. Louis, Missouri. Phylloquinone and chloro-K were purified by the method of Matschiner (9). Ultraviolet spectra obtained for cis- and trans-phylloquinone were identical to that of the commercial vitamin. All operations with the vitamin were performed in dim light.

RESULTS

When ^{3}H-phylloquinone with a trans/cis ratio of 4.2 was administered to rats and the rats killed three hours later, phylloquinone isolated from the mitochondria of these rats exhibited a trans/cis ratio equal to 1.8 (Table 1). This enrichment of cis-phylloquinone in mitochondria was observed when the dosage of vitamin K was 1.0 µg and when it was 10.0 µg. There was a slight enrichment of the trans isomer in the microsomal fraction, but the relative distribution of the cis and trans isomers in the postmitochondrial supernatant did not differ significantly from that of the injected phylloquinone. The postmitochondrial supernatant contains both the soluble fraction and the microsomal fraction. Enrichment of trans-phylloquinone in the microsomes of the postmitochondrial supernatant may have been obscured by the presence of the soluble fraction.

In the presence of 300 µg chloro-K the trans/cis ratio of phylloquinone isolated from the mitochondria was 3.1, as compared with 1.6 in its absence. This response to chloro-K seems dose-dependent since 30 µg chloro-K injected simultaneously with 1 µg vitamin K did not affect the distribution of the two isomers in the mitochondria. The relative distribution of the isomers in the postmitochondrial supernatant and in the microsomes was unaffected by administration of chloro-K.

TABLE 1. Effect of the chloro analog of vitamin K on the relative distribution of cis- and trans-phylloquinone in rat liver in vivo.

	Trans/cis ratio	
Treatment	Mitochondria	Postmitochondrial supernatant (PM) or microsomes (M)
1 µg Vitamin K and 30 µg chloro-K	2.3 ± 0.2	5.2 ± 0.4(M)
1 µg Vitamin K	1.8 ± 0.1	5.1 ± 0.4(M)
10 µg Vitamin K and 300 µg chloro-K	3.1 ± 0.3	4.3 ± 0.3(PM)
10 µg Vitamin K	1.6 ± 0.1	4.3 ± 0.7(PM)

Male rats (200-250 g) were given ^{3}H-phylloquinone and chloro-K by intravenous injection and killed 3 hours later. The injected vitamin was 81% trans-phylloquinone (trans/cis ratio = 4.2). Values are means ± S.E.M. for 4-7 rats per group.

Incubation of ^{3}H-phylloquinone with mitochondria in vitro did not affect the trans/cis ratio of the phylloquinone (Table II). Inclusion of 70 µg chloro-K in the incubation medium, however, caused an increase in the trans/cis ratio. More than 95% of the radioactivity in the incubation medium was taken-up by the mitochondria. Uptake of radioactivity was unaffected by chloro-K. In the presence of chloro-K there was, however, a decrease in the proportion of the radioactivity which was phylloquinone (80% compared with 95% when chloro-K was not in the medium). Since the phylloquinone sample added to the incubation medium was 96% pure little or no metabolism of phylloquinone occurred in the absence of chloro-K.

TABLE 2. Effect of the chloro analog of vitamin K on the relative distribution of cis- and trans-phylloquinone in liver mitochondria in vitro.

Radioactivity inside the mitochondria	Minus chloro-K	Plus chloro-K
% Uptake	95.3 ± 1.2	96.9 ± 0.8
% as Phylloquinone	95.2 ± 0.5	80.0 ± 5.1
trans/cis Ratio of phylloquinone	1.8 ± 0.1	3.3 ± 0.4

Incubation conditions and assay were as described in text. Phylloquinone with a trans/cis ratio of 1.8 was added to the medium. The values are means ± S.E.M. for 3 rats.

DISCUSSION

Knauer and coworkers (2) have described the enrichment of cis-phylloquinone in liver mitochondria of deficient rats in vivo and have suggested that cis-phylloquinone is retained preferentially by liver mitochondria. These data show that enrichment of cis-phylloquinone also occurs in liver mitochondria of normal rats. A slight enrichment of trans-phylloquinone was observed in liver microsomes three hours after injection. Knauer and coworkers (2) have also found trans/cis ratios in microsomes which were slightly higher than that injected. One explanation is that a greater proportion of trans-phylloquinone is retained by the microsomes, but a greater proportion of cis-phylloquinone is retained by the mitochondria. Enrichment of cis-phylloquinone in liver mitochondria could not be demonstrated in vitro. Perhaps the physiologically intact animal is necessary for this phenomenon to take place.

Thierry and Suttie (6) have shown increased uptake of radioactivity from injected phylloquinone by liver mitochondria when chloro-K was simultaneously administered. In the in vitro studies reported here, however, chloro-K did not affect mitochondrial uptake of radioactivity from an incubation medium containing ^{3}H-phylloquinone. We are unable to explain this difference at this time.

An increase in the trans/cis ratio of mitochondrial phylloquinone in the presence of chloro-K can be demonstrated both in vitro and in vivo. Our laboratory is currently conducting experiments with cis-phylloquinone and trans-phylloquinone to determine whether the cis isomer is preferentially metabolized in the presence of chloro-K. Separation and identification of the metabolites produced in the mitochondria in response to chloro-K should help to elucidate the role of chloro-K in liver mitochondria.

ACKNOWLEDGEMENTS

The authors are indebted to Dr. John W. Suttie, University of Wisconsin, Madison, Wisconsin for advice and encouragement. They also wish to thank Kathleen Groff, Craig Jaynes, and David Straight for technical assistance. This research was supported by grants from the Campus Grant Committee of University of Michigan-Dearborn and the Rackham Graduate School and the Michigan Memorial Phoenix Project of University of Michigan-Ann Arbor.

REFERENCES

1. Matschiner, J.T. and Bell, R.G. (1972) J. Nutr. 102, 625-630.
2. Knauer, T.E., Siegfried, C., Willingham, A.K. and Matschiner, J.T. (1975) J. Nutr. 105, 1519-1524.
3. Friedman, P.A. and Shia, M. (1976) Biochem. Biophys. Res. Commun. 70, 647-654.
4. DiMari, S.J. and Rapoport, H. (1968) Biochemistry 7, 2650-2652.
5. Gutnick, D.L., Dunphy, P.J., Sakamoto, H., Phillips, P.G. and Brodie, A.F. (1967) Science 158, 1469-1471.
6. Thierry, M.J. and Suttie, J.W. (1971) Arch. Biochem. Biophys. 147, 430-435.
7. Lehninger, A.L., Rossi, C.S., and Greenwalt, J.W. (1963) Biochem. Biophys. Res. Commun. 10, 444-448.
8. Bligh, E.G. and Dyer, W.J. (1959) Can. J. Biochem. Physiol. 37, 911-917.
9. Matschiner, J.T., Taggart, W.V., and Amelotti, J.M. (1967) Biochemistry 6, 1243-1247.

FETAL/MATERNAL VITAMIN K DEPENDENT REACTIONS: SOME HORMONAL EFFECTS.

D. W. JOLLY, R. MCBRIDE, S. SEIBERT, B. KADIS, and T. E. NELSON, JR.

Southern Illinois University School of Dental Medicine,
Edwardsville, IL 62026

INTRODUCTION

For the past several years, our laboratory has been interested in the action of androgens and estrogens on vitamin K metabolism and vitamin K dependent reactions. In order to correlate the vitamin K dependent reactions of epoxidation and protein carboxylation in divergent rat systems (fetal and maternal liver homogenates, subcellular fractions and fetal bone cells), experiments have been designed to assess hormonal effects upon these different systems in the rat. This report presents data obtained from studies using these diverse tissue preparations.

Female rats resist the anticoagulant effect of dietary vitamin K deficiency or coumarin drugs more effectively than male or castrate rats of both sexes (1,2). Previously we showed that sex steroid administration to castrate male and female rats can modify vitamin K absorption (3). Moreover, androgen and estrogen administration to vitamin K deficient castrate male rats appears to act on clotting factor synthesis rather than degradation, while the difference in vitamin K metabolism between sexes and intact versus castrate rats is also affected by the administration of these sex steroids (4). Using a postribosomal supernatant isolated according to the procedure of Willingham and Matschiner (5), we found that the addition of methyltestosterone (MT) or ethynylestradiol (EE) had no effect upon the amount of vitamin K_1-2,3-epoxide (K_1O) found when incubated in the presence of warfarin and radioactive vitamin K_1. Intraperitoneal (i.p.) injection of these steroids into rats, however, does alter the in vitro activity of vitamin K_1-epoxidase, (Table 1). MT at a dosage of 100 μg injected into male castrate rats (in sesame seed oil carrier) at 5 days and again 1 day before sacrifice increases the K_1O production to as much as 32 nanomoles.

Table 1. Effect of Sex Steroids on Vitamin K_1 Epoxide Synthesis
(O castrate K-deficient rats; 27,000 g supernatant)

μg of Drug	nM Epoxide ±sem Formed/4 gm Liver	
	Estrogen	Androgen
100	2 ± 2	32 ± 3
50	5 ± 2	18 ± 4
20	7 ± 3	13 ± 4
0	9 ± 4	9 ± 4

On the other hand when EE is used, the K_1O formed is decreased to 2 nanomoles. Control animals were injected with sesame seed oil, only, and appear as the zero quantity in Table 1. Epoxidation of K_1 is proposed to be related to vitamin K dependent protein carboxylation of preprothrombin (5). To assess this possibility, liver homogenates from vitamin K-deficient male rats were fractionated to determine if vitamin K_1-epoxidation and K_1-dependent carboxylation activities occur in parallel.

METHODS

Supernatants, were isolated with a Beckman/Spinco L3-50 ultracentrifuge (Tl 60 rotor) at 27,000 x g (27 K), 42 K, 58 K and 105 K using 0.25 M sucrose-25mM imidazole buffer, pH 7.4. The corresponding isolated pellets were resuspended and washed in twice their original volume and resedimented. The pellets were then resuspended in one-fourth their original volume of 25mM imidazole-200mM sucrose buffer, pH 7.4, for assay.

Bone cells were isolated from 19 day fetal rat calvaria using a two stage collagenase/trypsin digestion (6),* and the isolated cells washed with BGJ_b medium and allowed to recover in a CO_2 incubator (5% CO_2, 95% air) at 37°C and 100% humidity for 2 hours. Approximately 10^6 cells were used in each incubation mixture. The cells were biochemically characterized and found to be alkaline phosphatase positive, acid phosphatase negative indicative of blast-like cells. The cells also actively synthesize a collagenase digestable collagen from either ^{14}C-proline or ^{3}H-glycine and cholesterol from ^{14}C-acetate. They also incorporate ^{3}H-thymidine and ^{3}H-uracil and utilize O_2 indicating growth. Furthermore, parathyroid hormone elicits a response as measured by cAMP concentration. The cells also exhibit both vitamin K-dependent carboxylation and epoxidase activity.

5μCi $H^{14}CO_3^-$ (New England Nuclear) was used / incubation of 10^6 cells in 1 ml BGJ_b for 30 minutes in the CO_2 incubator. The incubation was stopped with 4 volumes of acetone and chilled until all of the protein was precipitated. Subsequent centrifugation led to a small pellet which was dissolved in 2% Na_2CO_3. This procedure was repeated for a total of 3 times to remove the unincorporated $H^{14}CO_3^-$. All reactions and radioactive measurements were carried out on the washed, precipitated protein.

RESULTS AND DISCUSSION

The 27 K, 42 K and 58 K supernatants epoxidate ^3H-K_1 but neither the 105 K supernatants nor the 42 K, 58 K or 105 K resuspended pellets showed significant epoxidase activity, (Table 2). However, resuspension of either the 42 K or 58 K pellets with the 105 K soluble fraction resulted in a marked increase in epoxidase activity.

TABLE 2. K_1 Epoxide Formed

K-deficient Castrate ♂ Liver Fractions (g x 10^{-3})	DPM x 10^{-3} ±sem/mg Protein	
	Supernatants	Pellets
27	46 ± 6	-----
42	25 ± 5	2 ± 2
58	13 ± 2	7 ± 5
105	3 ± 2	2 ± 2

*Full manuscript in preparation

On the other hand, vitamin K-dependent protein carboxylation ($H^{14}CO_3^-$ incorporation) was found in the 27 K, 42 K, 58 K and 105 K supernatants while carboxylase activity was high only in the 42 K pellet.

TABLE 3. $H^{14}CO_3^-$ Incorporated.

K-deficient Castrate ♂ Liver Fractions ($g \times 10^{-3}$)	DPM x 10^{-2} C^{14} ±sem/mg Protein	
	Supernatant	Pellet
27	14.2 ± 0.8	----------
42	8.2 ± 0.8	13.5 ± 2.8
58	4.3 ± 0.9	2.7 ± 0.5
105	3.2 ± 0.4	1.0 ± 0.8

If vitamin K-epoxidation and vitamin K-dependent protein carboxylation are related, these data would suggest they are loosely coupled and in separate cellular compartments.

To further investigate steroid effects upon these two reactions, fetal livers from 19 day fetuses and their corresponding maternal livers were examined for epoxidase and carboxylase activity. The 27 K supernatants were isolated and assayed as described previously. The data listed in Table 4 shows that epoxidase levels in fetal liver obtained from control dams were higher when compared with that in maternal rat liver; whereas the epoxidase activity measured in warfarin treated fetal and maternal liver was essentially the same.

TABLE 4. Epoxidase Activity

	DPM x 10^{-3} K_1O ±sem/mg Protein	
	Fetal	Maternal
Control	80 ± 5	40 ± 6
Warfarin	142 ± 4	158 ± 7

Similar results were obtained for the observed carboxylase activity wherein the fetal levels were much greater than the corresponding maternal levels (Table 5).

TABLE 5. Carboxylase Activity

	DPM x 10^{-3} $H^{14}CO_3^-$ ±sem/mg Protein	
	Fetal	Maternal
Control	5.0 ± 0.6	1.0 ± 0.8
Warfarin	11.8 ± 0.5	6.0 ± 0.6

In warfarin treated animals, a doubling of fetal carboxylation occurred with a large increase in the base levels in the maternal tissue.

The higher levels of vitamin K_1 epoxidation found in fetal liver compared to maternal liver, paralleled the higher levels of vitamin K dependent protein carboxylation. An explanation for the observed differences between the fetal and maternal systems is not immediately apparent.

Fetal bone cells exhibit significant levels of vitamin K_1 epoxidase activity and were found to be responsive to hormone administration as shown in Table 6. When the cells were cultured with either physiological or pharmacological doses of testosterone (T_1) or estradiol (E_2) and compared to control treated cells, physiological doses of estradiol (two nanomolar) resulted in nearly a three-fold stimulation of epoxidase activity whereas pharmacological doses (two micromolar) increased activity by only 35 percent.

TABLE 6. K_1O Epoxide Formed in Bone Cells*
(CPM x 10^{-2})

		Physiological		Pharmacological	
Control	3.8	E_2	9.1	E_2	5.2
		T_1	5.0	T_1	4.7

*10^6 cells/inc

Both physiological (6 nanomolar) and pharmacological (6 micromolar) treatment with testosterone resulted in a 20 to 25 percent increase in epoxidation.

The effect of sex steroid administration on vitamin K dependent protein carboxylation in these cells appears to be opposite to that observed for epoxidation. All treatments resulted in a decrease of $H^{14}CO_3^-$ incorporation when compared to controls (Table 7). Estradiol treatment at both levels resulted in a slight decrease of 11 to 14 percent, while testosterone treatment resulted in decreases of 40 to 50 percent with the physiological dosage being more effective.

TABLE 7. $H^{14}CO_3^-$ Incorporation into Bone Cell Protein*
(CPM x 10^{-2})

		Physiological		Pharmacological	
Control	27	E_2	23	E_2	24
		T_1	13	T_1	17

*10^6 cells/inc

In four separate experiments, the effect of vitamin K alone upon protein carboxylation was examined, (Table 8). In all cases vitamin K enhanced $H^{14}CO_3^-$ incorporation into protein. In one experiment the mother was treated with warfarin 24 hours before sacrifice. That glutamic acid was carboxylated was shown by alkaline hydrolysis of the radioactive protein and subsequent dansylation followed by TLC and location established by radiochromatogram scan (Packard Model #7201). Filtration of the radiolabelled protein through an Amicon #PM 10 filter (cut off 10,000 daltons) was also performed with recovery of 86-90% of the radioactivity suggesting that the protein is of low molecular weight and is osteocalcin-like.

TABLE 8. $H^{14}CO_3^-$ Incorporation into Bone Cell Protein*
(CPM x 10^{-2})

	Group I	Group II	Group III
Control	12	3.5	13
Vitamin K	28	16	27

Group IV - in a separate experiment, bone cells were isolated from warfarin treated dams and when incubated, they exhibited a four-fold increase in the amount of $H^{14}CO_3^-$ incorporated into bone protein

*10^6 cells/inc

In conclusion, our observations from divergent studies using several rat liver systems suggest that if vitamin K-epoxidation and vitamin K dependent protein carboxylation are interrelated, it may well be through divergent, loosely coupled cell systems.

Additionally, our preliminary results obtained with bone cells suggests that this is a viable system for the study of vitamin K dependent reactions which occur in bone. Further experiments to define the role of the gla containing protein(s) are under way.

ACKNOWLEDGEMENTS

We are grateful to Dr. John Suttie for contributing the radioactive vitamin K and gamma carboxyglutamic acid used in these experiments. These investigations were supported by a S.I.U.E. Research and Projects Grant and a School of Dental Medicine Pilot Project Grant.

REFERENCES

1. Mellette, S. J. (1961) Am. J. Clin. Nutr. 9, 109-116.
2. Rama Rao, P. B., Paolucci, A. M. and Johnson, B. C. (1963) Proc. Soc. Exp. Biol. Med. 112, 393-396.
3. Jolly, D. W., Craig, C., and Nelson, T. E., Jr. (1977) Am. J. Physiol. 232:1, H12-H17.
4. Jolly, D. W., Kadis, B. M., and Nelson, T. E., Jr. (1977) Biochem. Biophys. Res. Commun. 74:1, 41-49.
5. Willingham, A. K. and Matschiner, J. T. (1974) Biochem. J. 140, 435-441.
6. Kadis, B., and Goodson, J. M. (1977) J. Dent. Res. 56, A70.

CLINICAL RESPONSES TO VITAMIN K_1

R. G. MALIA, F. E. PRESTON and C. D. HOLDSWORTH

Departments of Haematology and Medicine,
University of Sheffield, United Kingdom

INTRODUCTION

Vitamin K completes the final step in the biosynthesis of the coagulation factors II, VII, IX and X by converting glutamic acid residues on a precursor molecule into γ-carboxyglutamic acid residues, thus producing functionally normal procoagulant factors (1). In the absence or antagonism of Vitamin K, precursor proteins, designated proteins induced by Vitamin K absence or antagonists (PIVKA) are produced and released into the circulation (Fig. 1). The aim of this study was 1) to test the value of the modified thrombotest as a PIVKA screening test and an index of Vitamin K deficiency; and 2) to assess the response to Vitamin K_1 in various types of liver disease.

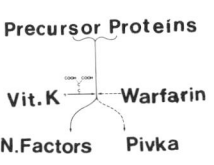

Figure 1

METHODS

Fourteen patients with liver disease aged between 35 and 75 years who required surgery or liver biopsy were included in the study. They were given 10 mgms (I.V.) Vitamin K_1 over a period of 10 minutes and venous blood samples were collected into hepes buffered sodium citrate (3.2%) at the following times: Pre (x2) then 30 minutes, 1 hour, 2 hours, 4 hours, 8 hours and 24 hours post infusion. Laboratory tests: 1) Modified thrombotest (PIVKA Screen) (Fig. 2), 2) Specific assays of factor II, VII, IX and X, 3) Antibody neutralization, and 4) One and two dimensional immunoelectrophoresis using an antibody to human factor II (Laurell). Calcium lactate 2.5mM was present in the first dimension of the 2D run when it was necessary to separate proteins in the presence of calcium.

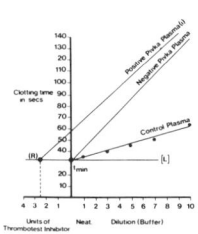

Figure 2

RESULTS

Value of the Modified Thrombotest (PIVKA screen)

The results of the modified thrombotest are shown in Table 1.

Table 1. Estimation of PIVKA units per ml in liver disease patients

Patients Group One	PIVKA (Units.Ml)	Patients Group Two	PIVKA (Units/Ml)
1. M.F.	0.0	8. J.D.	1.0
2. P.B.	0.1	9. E.T.	0.9
3. H.K.	0.1	10. M.C.	7.0
4. B.F.	0.1	11. S.W.	2.9
5. A.A.	0.0	12. M.T.	6.0
6. F.B.	0.1	13. M.M.	2.4
7. S.M.	0.0	14. S.L.	2.0

PIVKA Units/ml in normal patients ranged from 0.0-0.4 (mean 0.07) and in warfarin anticoagulated patients (19) ranged from 1.2-7.0 (mean 3.15).

On the levels of PIVKA (u/ml) detected it was possible to divide the patients into Group One: PIVKA negative: Mean 0.05 Units/ml and Group Two: PIVKA positive: Mean 3.17 and both groups were given 10 mgm (I.V.) Vitamin K_1.

Response to 10 mgm Vitamin K_1

The results of the response to Vitamin K1 are shown in Figures 3 and 4. They show that whilst Group One (PIVKA negative) patients did not respond to the Vitamin K_1, those in Group Two (PIVKA positive) did. Thus the modified thrombotest was of value as an index of Vitamin K deficiency.

Group One

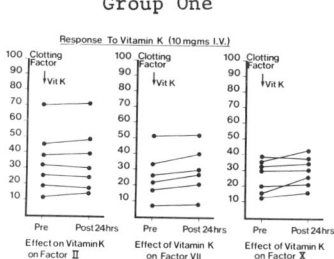

Figure 3

Group Two

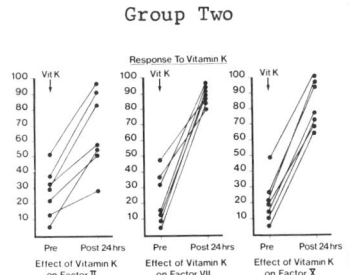

Figure 4

Effect of Vitamin K_1 on Circulating PIVKA Levels

Intravenous Vitamin K has an immediate effect on circulating levels of PIVKA (Figure 5). Normal levels of PIVKA are found within five hours of intravenous therapy.

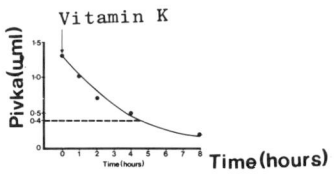

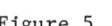

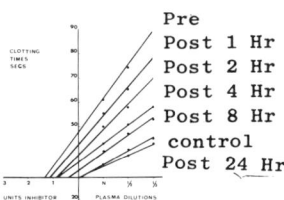

Figure 5   Figure 6

As well as changes in inhibitor values the plot of the clotting times alters during therapy (Figure 6). The slope of the lines expressed as the co-tangent i.e. 1/TAN, can be obtained for both the control α_N and patient α_X. The ratio between α_X and α_N is thought to indicate the amount of factor X present in the unknown plasma (3) (see Table 2).

Table 2. The relationship between the ratio of the slope and factor X assay

Sample	Ratio Slope $\frac{\alpha X}{\alpha N}$	Equivalent Factor X %	Clotting F.X. Assay %
Pre	0.33	33	31
Post 1 Hr	0.44	44	40
Post 2 Hr	0.50	50	55
Post 4 Hr	0.72	72	57
Post 8 Hr	0.74	74	69
Post 24 Hr	1.14	114	110

The results indicate that the modified thrombotest is sensitive to the circulating plasma level of factor X, in particular the _form_ of the circulating factor X.

Response to Vitamin K_1 in Liver Disease

$T_{50\% \text{ MAX}}$ (time for attainment of 50% maximum response) to Vitamin K_1. The mean time taken to attain 50% Max was taken as an index on the uptake and utilization of Vitamin K_1 in the synthesis of factors II, VII, IX and X and the results are shown in Table 3. The values show that overall no single Vitamin K dependent clotting factor is selected preferentially for the Vitamin K_1 to act upon.

Table 3. $T_{50\% \, MAX}$ response to 10 mg Vitamin K_1 (I.V.)

$T_{50\% \, MAX}$ for	Mean	Std D
F.II	Mean 5.13 Hrs	Std D 3.84 Hrs
F.VII	Mean 7.34 Hrs	Std D 7.2 Hrs
F.IX	Mean 6.5 Hrs	Std D 4.56 Hrs
F.X	Mean 4.86 Hrs	Std D 2.54 Hrs

Furthermore during the 24 hours analysis the rates of synthesis appeared to be bi-phasic. In order to summarize and compare the bi-phasic data an attempt was made to describe the time course with a two-term exponential equation.

$$C = C_1(1 - e^{-\alpha_1 t}) + C_2(1 - e^{-\alpha_2 t})$$

To obtain C_1, C_2, 1 and 2 this equation was re-arranged in the form of:

$$(100 - C) = C_1 e^{-\alpha_1 t} + C_2 e^{-\alpha_2 t}$$

Hence a plot of (100-C) Vs t(time) was constructed and the two exponential terms isolated by the "method of residuals" (3). An exponential curve fitting programme for a Hewlett-Packard H6-95 calculator was used to obtain least squares estimates for each co-efficient and exponent term. Half-lives ($T_{\frac{1}{2}}$) for the fast and slow phases were obtained using the equation: $T_{\frac{1}{2}} = \frac{0.693}{\alpha}$ and the values obtained are shown in Table 4.

Table 4. ($T_{\frac{1}{2}}$) for the fast and slow phases of clotting factor synthesis

	Fast Phase (α_1)	Slow Phase (α_2)
Factor II	2.57 Hrs	23.4 Hrs
Factor VII	2.73 Hrs	58.7 Hrs
Factor IX	2.10 Hrs	28.00 Hrs
Factor X	5.00 Hrs	22.4 Hrs

These results suggest that the factors possess the capacity for self-regulation of their reaction rate during Vitamin K therapy.

T_{LAG} (Time for significant response to Vitamin K)

The response of the clotting factors to Vitamin K_1 revealed a short T_{LAG} of one to two hours between uptake and utilization and further analysis was undertaken to determine whether this was due to 1) de novo synthesis of factors II, VII, IX and X, or 2) completion of the Vitamin K dependent step in an existing intracellular protein pool. The results are shown in Figures 7 to 12 and they indicate that within one hour of the Vitamin K_1 infusion normal factor II was detected in the circulation (Fig. 9). Analysis of the peak geometry of the immunoprecipitate showed apparent mirror images between the decline of PIVKA II and the synthesis of factor II (Figure 12). These findings, together with the one-dimensional immunoelectrophoresis analysis (Figure 11) suggest the alteration in the ratio between PIVKA II/normal II takes place within a constant amount of antigen.

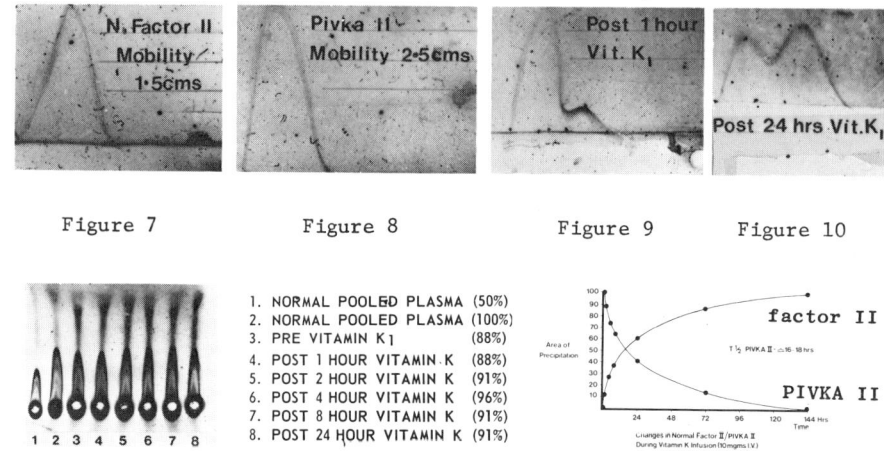

Figure 7 Figure 8 Figure 9 Figure 10

1. NORMAL POOLED PLASMA (50%)
2. NORMAL POOLED PLASMA (100%)
3. PRE VITAMIN K₁ (88%)
4. POST 1 HOUR VITAMIN K (88%)
5. POST 2 HOUR VITAMIN K (91%)
6. POST 4 HOUR VITAMIN K (96%)
7. POST 8 HOUR VITAMIN K (91%)
8. POST 24 HOUR VITAMIN K (91%)

Figure 11 Figure 12

DISCUSSION

In this study 14 patients with liver disease were investigated (without recourse to clinical information). Using the modified thrombotest it was possible to subdivide them into two groups: 1) PIVKA NEGATIVE and 2) PIVKA POSITIVE. The response to an infusion of 10 mgm (I.V.) Vitamin K_1 indicated that only the PIVKA POSITIVE group responded to the infusion. Further analysis (Figure 5 and Table 2) show that PIVKA levels alter during therapy and that the modified thrombotest is extremely sensitive to plasma levels of factor X. In particular the _form_ of circulating factor X is important since factor X has been shown to be rate limiting for the velocity of the reaction (3). From these studies it would appear that the modified thrombotest is of value as an index of Vitamin K deficieny. In order to assess the response to Vitamin K_1 50% MAX and LAG responses were analyzed. The 50% MAX values (Table 3) show that initially no single factor was selected preferentially for the Vitamin K_1 to act upon. It would appear that the precursor protein takes up the Vitamin K_1 and incorporates it into the Vitamin K dependent step simultaneously for all the individual factors. However, analysis using the method of residuals (2) showed that a bi-phasic synthesis of the Vitamin K factors occurred when Vitamin K_1 was infused (Table 4). Such a finding is consistent with the Vitamin K dependent factors functioning as part of a multi-enzyme system possessing the capacity for self regulation of their overall reaction rate i.e., regulatory or allosteric enzymes, during the response to Vitamin K_1. A short LAG following Vitamin K_1 infusion could have been due to 1) de novo synthesis, or 2) completion of a Vitamin K dependent step in an intracellular protein pool. Two-dimensional immunoelectrophoresis of factor II revealed that within one hour of the Vitamin K infusion two peaks were present (Figure 9) and the small peak with normal mobility was normal factor II. Prydz (4) found that intracellular protein synthesis took 240 minutes to complete, therefore this finding indicates that Vitamin K_1 completed existing precursor protein rather than institute de novo synthesis. As the one dimensional immunoelectrophoresis (Figure 11) showed the total amount of F.II antigen did not vary significantly, changes in the PIVKA II/ normal II ratio (Figures 7-12) must indicate allosteric enzyme function during the response to Vitamin K_1.

In conclusion these findings allow a tentative suggestion that the Vitamin K dependent clotting factors function as regulatory or allosteric heterophilic enzymes with a binding or catalytic site for substrates and a second site at which modulator molecules bind, e.g., phospholipids. In Vitamin K deficiency states this important second site for the modulator molecule to bind is incomplete and a reduced potential to form activated coagulation factors results, hence the biological importance of the Vitamin K dependent step.

REFERENCES

1. Brozovic, M. (1976) Brit. J. Haem., 32, 9.
2. Rescigno, A. and Segre, G. (1966) In: Drug and Tracer Kinetics. Blaisdell Publishing Co., p.20.
3. Hemker, H. C., Veltkamp, J. J. and Loeliger, E. A. (1968) Thromb. Diath. Haemorrh. 19, 349.
4. Prydz, H. (1973) Proc. IVth Int. Congress Thrmobosis and Haemostasis V, Vienna.

INVESTIGATION OF ANTICOAGULANTS AND VITAMIN K_1 IN THE RABBIT

B. K. PARK, J. B. LECK, A. WILSON and
A. M. BRECKENRIDGE

Department of Pharmacology,
University of Liverpool,
Liverpool, England

INTRODUCTION

Vitamin K_1 is essential for normal blood coagulation because it is a cofactor for the postribosomal synthesis of clotting factors II (prothrombin) VII, IX and X (1). The vitamin K_1 dependent step in clotting factor synthesis involves the γ-carboxylation of glutamic acid residues in clotting factor precursors (2). It has been suggested that cyclic interconversion of the vitamin to its biologically inactive epoxide and reduction back to the vitamin is necessary for continued clotting factor synthesis and that interruption of the vitamin K_1 cycle, by inhibition of either the epoxidase or the epoxide reductase will result in a reduction of clotting factor synthesis (3). Thus it has been shown that coumarin and indanedione anticoagulants inhibit the epoxide reductase whereas 2-chloro-3-phytylnaphthoquinone (Cl-K) and tetrachloropyridinol are thought to prevent clotting factor synthesis by inhibiting vitamin K_1 epoxidase (4). However, it is still not clear whether the γ-carboxylation and epoxidation reactions are chemically linked (5).

To date, most studies on the mechanism of anticoagulants which act by interfering with vitamin K_1 metabolism have been carried out in man or the rat. We have used the rabbit in order that the temporal relationship between changes in vitamin K_1 metabolism and clotting factor synthesis produced by anticoagulants, could be measured in the same individual animal. A further advantage is that there is no restriction on the dose of radioactivity or anticoagulant given. First we investigated the anticoagulants warfarin and Cl-K which have been studied in other species and then the action of acenocoumarol and the novel anticoagulants difenacoum and brodifacoum were studied. The effect of warfarin on the pharmacokinetics of $[^3H]$-vitamin K_1 was determined.

MATERIALS AND METHODS

$[1', 2'-{}^3H_2]$ vitamin K_1 was a gift from Hoffman La Roche, Basle. Sodium warfarin was obtained from Ward Blenkinsop, acenocoumarol from Geigy Pharmaceuticals and difenacoum, brodifacoum and 2-chloro-3-phytyl-naphthoquinone (Cl-K) were gifts from Sorex Laboratories, Widnes. For intravenous injections sodium warfarin and sodium acenocoumarol were dissolved in 0.9% saline while $[^3H]$-vitamin K_1 and Cl-K were dissolved in 5% Tween saline. For intramuscular injections difenacoum and brodifacoum were dissolved in dimethyl-sulphoxide.

The male New Zealand White rabbits (2.5 - 3.0kg) used in this study were caged individually and maintained on a diet of SGI pellets (Nutrients Ltd., Liverpool, U.K.) and water.

Plan of Study

Before each experiment the control prothrombin time for each animal was determined. Animals were dosed with anticoagulants either intravenously (warfarin, acenocoumarol, Cl-K) into the marginal ear vein or intramuscularly (difenacoum, brodifacoum) into the thigh. This injection was followed 1h later for animals dosed intravenously and 2h later in the case of animals dosed intramuscularly by an intravenous injection of [3H]-vitamin K_1. The metabolism of [3H]-vitamin K_1 was monitored by reversed-phase chromatographic (t.l.c. and h.p.l.c.) analysis of plasma (4ml) obtained from the marginal ear vein at 1,2,3,4,5 and 6h. For the more detailed pharmacokinetic study, additional plasma samples were obtained at 0.08, 0.17, 0.25, 0.5, 0.75 and 7h. Clotting factor activity was monitored by determining prothrombin complex activity (PCA) at four hourly intervals (6).

RESULTS

The pattern of [3H]-vitamin K_1 metabolites in rabbit plasma is similar to that observed in man (7). The effect of various anticoagulants on the metabolism of an intravenous dose of [3H]-vitamin K_1 (98 nmole), as indicated by the plasma ratio [3H]-vitamin K_1 epoxide: [3H]-vitamin K_1 at 3h, and on the rate of degradation of PCA and minimum PCA observed in the rabbit is shown in Table 1. There was no significant difference in the half-life of degradation of PCA between the groups and all anticoagulants produced significant ($P<0.01$) changes in the [3H]-vitamin K_1 epoxide: [3H]-vitamin K_1 plasma ratio compared to controls.

TABLE 1. Effect of anticoagulants on [3H]-vitamin K_1 metabolism and PCA in the rabbit.

Drug	Dose (mg/kg)	[3H]-epoxide: [3H]-K_1 (3h)	PCA $t_{\frac{1}{2}}$ (h)	PCA Min. (%)
None	–	0.23±0.04	–	100
Warfarin	2.5	0.62±0.08	6.13±0.53	16±6
Cl-K	10	0.06±0.01	6.05±0.93	<2
Warfarin / Cl-K	2.5 / 10	0.09±0.02	6.20±0.22	<2
Difenacoum	1	1.53±0.26	6.85±1.00	<2
Brodifacoum	1	2.50±0.59	7.20±0.38	<2
Acenocoumarol	10	0.92±0.15	6.33±0.46	17±8

Results are mean (n=4) ± S.D.

The effects of warfarin and Cl-K on the relationship between vitamin K_1 metabolism and prothrombin complex activity in the rabbit are shown in more detail in Figure 1.

The effect of warfarin on the pharmacokinetics of an intravenous dose of [^{3}H]-vitamin K_1 (4.76 nmole) is shown in Table 2. The animals received either warfarin (2.5mg/kg) or saline in a cross-over design. Warfarin did not significantly affect any of the [^{3}H]-vitamin K_1 parameters but did produce a significant increase in the area under the plasma concentration-time curve (AUC) of [^{3}H]-vitamin K_1 epoxide.

TABLE 2. The effect of warfarin on the pharmacokinetics of [^{3}H]-vitamin K_1 in the rabbit.

Pharmacokinetic parameter	Control	Warfarin
[^{3}H]-vitamin K_1 $t_{\frac{1}{2}}\alpha$ (h)	0.23 ± 0.11	0.21 ± 0.04
[^{3}H]-vitamin K_1 $t_{\frac{1}{2}}\beta$ (h)	1.88 ± 0.39	1.78 ± 0.21
[^{3}H]-vitamin K_1 V.D. (l)	3.00 ± 1.24	3.13 ± 1.22
[^{3}H]-vitamin K_1 A.U.C. (pmol.ml.$^{-1}$h)	4.40 ± 0.08	4.00 ± 0.37
[^{3}H]-vitamin K_1 epoxide A.U.C. (pmol.ml.$^{-1}$h)	0.41 ± 0.09	1.64 ± 0.18***

Results are mean (n=4) ± S.D.   *** $p < 0.001$

The effect of various doses of warfarin on the plasma [^{3}H]-vitamin K_1 epoxide: [^{3}H]-vitamin K_1 ratio, at 3h after a tracer dose of [^{3}H]-vitamin K_1 (4.76 nmole), and on rate of degradation of PCA is shown in Table 3. There was no significant difference in PCA at 6h indicating that the rate of onset of anticoagulation was the same in each group. The minimum PCA obtained was dose-dependent, reflecting the duration of inhibition of clotting factor synthesis.

TABLE 3. The effect of warfarin on [^{3}H]-vitamin K_1 metabolism and PCA in the rabbit.

Warfarin (mg/kg)	[^{3}H]-epoxide: [^{3}H]-K_1 (3h)	PCA $t_{\frac{1}{2}}$ (h)	PCA 6h (%)	PCA min. (%)
10	1.80±0.24	7.60±0.54	57±3	<5
2.5	1.24±0.23	6.78±0.25	66±4	11±4
0.63	0.71±0.33	7.35±0.33	61±5	19±2
0.16	0.48±0.14	10.75±3.16	64±5	24±10
0	0.20±0.02	-	100	100

Results are means (n=4) ± S.D.

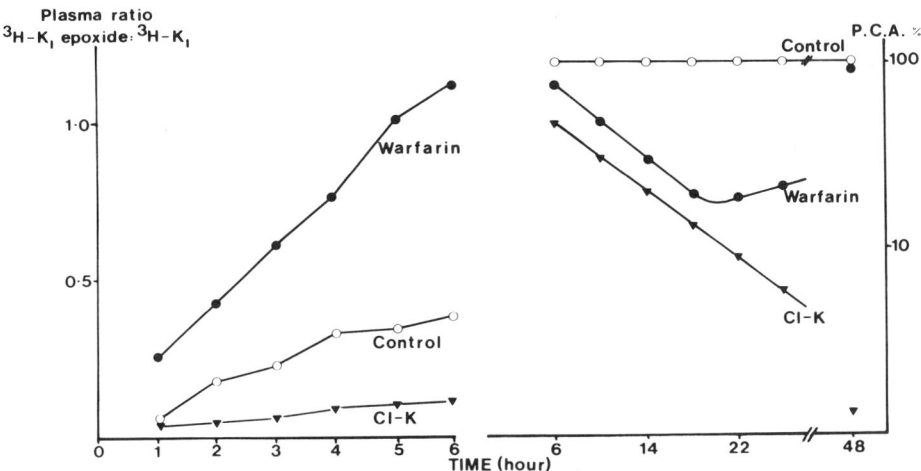

FIGURE 1. The effect of warfarin and Cl-K on the plasma [^{3}H]-vitamin K_1 epoxide: [^{3}H]-vitamin K_1 ratio and PCA in the rabbit.

DISCUSSION

The role of the vitamin K_1-epoxide cycle in the synthesis of clotting factors II, VII, IX and X has been studied previously in man (7) and the rat (3). Warfarin and Cl-K are thought to reduce clotting factor synthesis by inhibiting the vitamin K_1-epoxide cycle at the reductase and epoxidase steps respectively (8). In keeping with this hypothesis we found, in the rabbit, that Cl-K decreased the plasma [^{3}H]-vitamin K_1 epoxide: [^{3}H]-vitamin K_1 ratio whereas warfarin produced a significant increase in the ratio. When both anticoagulants were administered together Cl-K prevented the accumulation of [^{3}H]-vitamin K_1 epoxide that warfarin alone would have produced: consistent with the proposed relationship between the two enzymes.

The plasma concentration-time profile of [^{3}H]-vitamin K_1 in the rabbit is similar to that observed in man (7) and could be resolved into a fast and slow distribution phase. Administration of a dose of warfarin (2.5mg/kg) sufficient to inhibit completely clotting factor synthesis did not affect either the α or β elimination rate constants nor was there any significant change in the AUC of [^{3}H]-vitamin K_1 even though there was a significant increase in the AUC of [^{3}H]-vitamin K_1 epoxide. It would appear, therefore, that inhibition of [^{3}H]-vitamin K_1 regeneration does not significantly affect either the intrinsic hepatic clearance of [^{3}H]-vitamin K_1 or that hepatic clearance is blood flow dependent. This implies that if warfarin does act by simply reducing vitamin K_1 to ineffectual levels, its site of action must not be in equilibrium with plasma. Warfarin also produces an increase of radioactivity in plasma in man (7) but not in the rat (3, 9) indicating species difference in the disposition of [3H]-vitamin K_1 epoxide.

Using the rabbit, we studied acenocoumarol and two novel anticoagulants brodifacoum and difenacoum which, although possessing the same 4-hydroxycoumarin ring system as warfarin, are effective in warfarin-resistant rats (10). At the doses used, all three drugs produced the maximum rate of degradation of PCA and significantly increased the plasma [3H]-vitamin K_1 epoxide: [3H]-vitamin K_1 ratio, indicating that they act by inhibiting vitamin K_1 epoxide reductase. However, there was considerable inter-drug variation in plasma [3H]-vitamin K_1 epoxide concentrations despite the fact that each drug inhibited clotting factor synthesis for at least 20h (Table 1).

One possible explanation for the variation in the ratio is that the anticoagulants had different modes of action. We therefore investigated the effect of different doses of one anticoagulant, warfarin, on the relationship between [3H]-vitamin K_1 metabolism and clotting factor synthesis. From Table 3 it can be seen that 0.63, 2.5 and 10mg/kg of warfarin produced the same maximum rate of decay of PCA suggesting that 0.63mg/kg is sufficient to completely block clotting factor synthesis. The minimum PCA observed was dependent on dose but this reflects the duration, as well as the degree, of inhibition of clotting factor synthesis. Thus the dose of warfarin required to produce maximum decay of PCA does not necessarily produce the maximum [3H]-vitamin K_1 epoxide: [3H]-vitamin K_1 ratio. Similar results were obtained with brodifacoum indicating that the dose of anticoagulant required for maximum inhibition of clotting factor synthesis does not necessarily produce maximum perturbation of vitamin K_1 metabolism. This finding may explain why some workers have found a correlation between the [3H]-vitamin K_1 epoxide: [3H]-vitamin K_1 ratio and the anticoagulant effect (11), while others have not (12).

It is possible that only partial inhibition of the vitamin K_1- epoxide cycle is necessary for blocking the synthesis of complete clotting factors. An alternative explanation is that coumarin anticoagulants have more than one site of action in vivo, as indicated by in vitro experiments (13,14). We are currently testing the latter hypothesis by investigating the effect of synthetic vitamin K_1 analogues on the relationship between vitamin K_1 metabolism and clotting factor synthesis in the rabbit.

ACKNOWLEDGEMENTS

We would like to thank Dr. R. Long of Hoffman La Roche for a generous gift of tritiated vitamin K_1 and I.C.I. Central Toxicology Laboratory for financial support. We would also like to thank Mrs. B. Bath for typing the manuscript.

REFERENCES

1. Jackson, C.M., and Suttie, J.W. (1977) Progress in Haematology, Vol. 10, 333-359.
2. Stenflo, J., Fernlund, P., Egan, W., and Roepstorff, P. (1974) Proc. Natl. Acad. Sci., U.S.A. 71, 2730-33.
3. Bell, R.G. (1978) Fed. Proc. 37, 2599-2604.
4. Ren, P., Laliberte, R.E., and Bell, R.G. (1974) Mol. Pharmacol. 10, 373-380.
5. Suttie, J.W., Larson, A.E., Canfield, L.M., and Carlisle, T.L. (1978) Fed. Proc. 37, 2605-2609.
6. Quick, A.J. (1957) In: Haemorrhagic Diseases, (Quick, A.J. Ed) Lea and Febiger, Philadelphia, p. 379.
7. Shearer, M.J., McBurney, A., and Barkhan, P. (1973) Br. J. Haemat. 24, 471-479.
8. Willingham, A.K., Laliberte, R.E., Bell, R.G., and Matschiner, J.T. (1976) Biochem. Pharmac. 25, 1063-1066.
9. Leck, J.B. and Park, B.K.: unpublished.
10. Hadler, M.R. and Shadbolt, R.S. (1975) Nature (Lond.) 253, 275-276.
11. Ren, P., Stark, P.Y., Johnson, R.L., and Bell, R.G. (1977) J. Pharmacol. Exp. Ther. 201, 541-546.
12. Sadowski, J.A., and Suttie, J.W. (1974) Biochem. 13, 3696-3699.
13. Bell, R.G., and Stark, P. (1976) Biochim. Biophys. Acta 72, 619-625.
14. Wallin, R., Gebhardt, O., Prydz, H. (1977) Biochem. J. 169, 95-101.

STUDIES OF THE VITAMIN K EPOXIDE REDUCTASE SYSTEM

CHARLES M. SIEGFRIED

Department of Biochemistry,
University of Nebraska College of Medicine,
Omaha, NE 68105

INTRODUCTION

A major pathway of metabolism of vitamin K in the rat and man is conversion of vitamin K to vitamin K epoxide and reduction of the epoxide back to vitamin K (1-4). This interconversion of vitamin K and the epoxide occurs in liver microsomes and involves at least two membrane-bound enzymatic activities, vitamin K epoxide reductase (5) and vitamin K epoxidase (6). These enzymatic activities have also been found in several extrahepatic tissues (1). The enzymes involved in the interconversion of the vitamin are closely associated with and appear to be part of a membrane-bound enzyme complex which catalyzes the vitamin K-dependent carboxylation of peptide-bound glutamyl residues to form γ-carboxyglutamyl residues of proteins. Warfarin may exert its anticoagulant effect by inhibiting vitamin K epoxide reductase (5-9).

Our finding of an active vitamin K epoxide reductase in potassium cholate-treated microsomes (9) provided a suitable system to study simple kinetic parameters of the reduction of vitamin K epoxide to vitamin K and the relationship of vitamin K and vitamin K epoxide to vitamin K-dependent carboxylation. The results of these studies and of partial purification of a component from the cytosol which stimulates vitamin K epoxide reduction are the subject of this report.

MATERIALS AND METHODS

The materials and methods used in these studies were according to those described in or referred to by Siegfried (9) unless otherwise indicated. Briefly, potassium cholate-solubilized microsomes refer to the 105,000 x g supernatant obtained after resuspending microsomal pellets from vitamin K-deficient rats in homogenizing buffer (0.25 M sucrose, 0.025 M imidazole pH 7.8) and enough potassium cholate (20% w/v) to give a final concentration of 0.5%. The potassium cholate-solubilized microsomal preparations were diluted 1 to 8 with homogenizing buffer and stored at -70° until used. The standard incubation system contained 0.5 ml (equivalent to about 0.031 g of liver and about 0.5 mg of protein) of the diluted solubilized microsomes, 1 mm DTT, other additions in homogenizing buffer where indicated and homogenizing buffer to give a final volume of 1 ml. After preincubation for 1 min at 37°, the reactions were started by the addition of [^{3}H]vitamin K epoxide (4.7 x 10^5 dpm/nmole) or [^{3}H]vitamin K (2.4 x 10^5 dpm/nmole) in ethanol (0.05 ml) and conducted for 5 min unless otherwise indicated. When vitamin K-dependent protein carboxylation was measured, unlabeled vitamin and sodium [^{14}C]bicarbonate (20 µCi/incubation, 60 mCi/mmole) were included. Incubations and assays for vitamin K epoxide reductase, vitamin K epoxidase and vitamin K-dependent protein carboxylation were as described previously (9).

The 105,000 x g supernatant obtained in preparing the microsomal pellet was centrifuged at 105,000 x g 1 h and stored at -20° or -70°. This material (cytosol) was used to purify the vitamin K epoxide reductase stimulatory activity (ERSA) and was obtained from either vitamin K-deficient or normal rats. Aliquots (0.05 to 0.4 ml) of various fractions after chromatography of ERSA were assayed in the standard incubation system. Units of ERSA are defined as pmoles of vitamin K formed/min/ml of incubation minus the pmoles of vitamin K formed/min/ml of incubation containing solubilized microsomes without ERSA.

RESULTS

Purification of Vitamin K Epoxide Reductase Stimulatory Activity (ERSA) from Cytosol

Addition of cytosol to incubations stimulated the rate of reduction of vitamin K epoxide four to five fold (Table 1). The cytosol alone had essentially no epoxide reductase activity in the presence or absence of DTT and did not replace the requirement for DTT of the solubilized microsomal preparation. The activity of cytosol was heat-labile but stable when stored at -20° or -70°.

When the cytosol was purified by gel filtration or by ion exchange chromatography, two peaks of ERSA were observed. A typical elution profile after gel filtration of cytosol on a column of Sephacryl S-200 is shown in Figure 1. The major activity (Peak I) eluted first, partially separated from the unretarded protein and usually represented 80 to 85% of the activity recovered. A second peak of activity (Peak II) eluted later well separated from Peak I and represented from 15 to 20% of the activity recovered. The ERSA pooled from Peak I was purified further by chromatography on a column of DEAE Sephacel. The ERSA was slightly retarded and easily separated from the considerable bound protein. Pooled fractions of ERSA were then applied again to Sephacryl S-200. The results of a typical purification are shown in Table 2A.

TABLE 1. Effect of cytosol on the rate of vitamin K epoxide reduction[a]

Cytosol (mg protein added)	Vitamin K (pmoles/min)
0	39.8
0.28	61.8
0.55	106
1.10	132
2.20	151
4.40	172

[a]Incubations containing 0.35 ml of cytosol or dilutions of cytosol at the concentrations indicated were conducted for variable periods of time up to 10 min to determine initial rates. The results are the mean values from duplicate incubations.

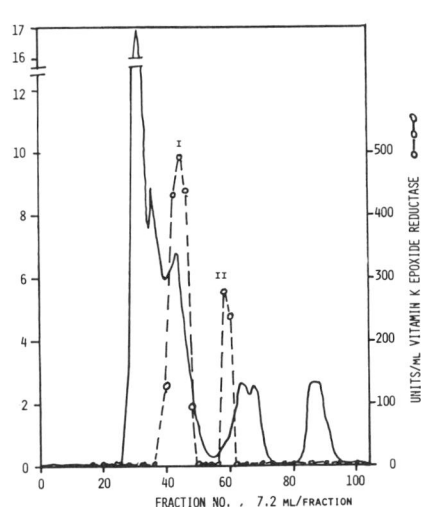

FIGURE 1. Cytosol (40 ml) was applied to Sephacryl S-200 (gel bed vol., 780 ml) and eluted with 0.1 M imidazole pH 7.8, flow rate 14 ml/h.

TABLE 2. Purification of vitamin K epoxide reductase stimulatory activity from cytosol

A Purification step	Protein (mg/ml)	ERSA (units/ml)	Total ERSA (units)	Specific Activity (units/mg)	Purification (fold)
Cytosol (40 ml)	12.6	718	28,700	57	1
Sephacryl S-200	2.50	316	21,500	126	2.2
DEAE Sephacel	0.010	89.4	9,120	8,940	160
Sephacryl S-200	0.0092	212	4,080	23,000	400
B					
Cytosol	6.60	280	140,000	42	1
DEAE Sephacel	0.250	287	170,000	1,100	27
[a]QAE Sephadex					
Peak I	(0.222)	(146)	(19,000)	(660)	(16)
Peak II	0.042	395	130,000	9,500	225
Sephacryl S-200	0.140	2,100	121,000	15,000	360

[a]ERSA from DEAE Sephacel from a similar preparation containing 160,000 units, 2890 units/mg and 55.1 mg of protein was combined with that above before chromatography on QAE Sephadex.

The scheme described above was not suitable for larger scale purification of ERSA. Because of the 70-fold purification achieved with DEAE Sephacel, this resin was used as the first purification step in subsequent procedures. A typical elution profile after chromatography of cytosol on a column of DEAE Sephacel is shown in Figure 2. Two peaks of ERSA were observed but the separation was poor. Although only about 50-60% of the ERSA applied was recovered, the purification was about 27-fold. No ERSA was detected after dialysis of aliquots and assay of material that eluted in the region associated with the salt gradient. A better separation of these activities on DEAE Sephacel could be achieved by substantially decreasing the flow rate. However, the two peaks of ERSA suggested from the results depicted in Figure 2 were readily separated when this activity was chromatographed on columns of QAE Sephadex A-50. ERSA pooled from appropriate fractions from DEAE Sephacel columns was concentrated by precipitation with ammonium sulfate, dissolved in and dialyzed against

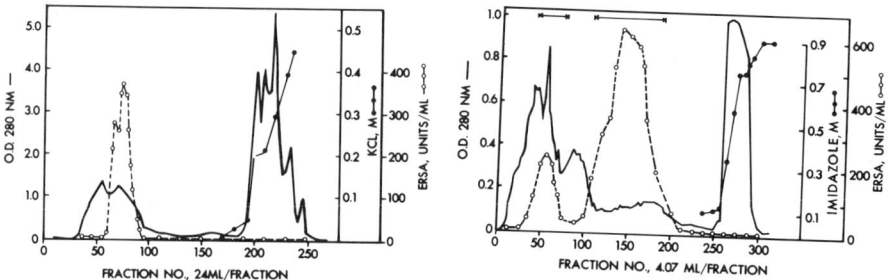

FIGURE 2. (Left) Cytosol was applied to DEAE Sephacel (gel bed vol., 1650 ml) and eluted with 0.1 M imidazole pH 7.8 and 0.1 M imidazole pH 7.8-KCl gradient as indicated; flow rate 93 ml/h.

FIGURE 3. (Right) Pooled fractions of ERSA from two preparations as in Figure 2 were applied to QAE Sephadex A-50 (gel bed vol., 190 ml) and eluted with 0.1 M imidazole pH 7.8; flow rate 23.4 ml/hr.

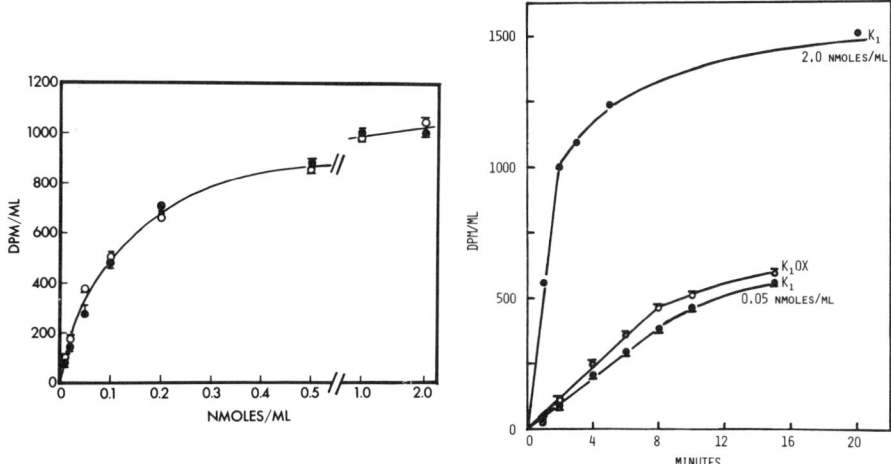

FIGURE 4. (Left) The effect of vitamin K (●) and vitamin K epoxide (O) on vitamin K-dependent carboxylation. The results are mean values ± SEM from triplicate incubations. A control value of 21 dpm/ml from incubations containing no vitamin has been subtracted.

FIGURE 5. (Right) Effect of time on vitamin K-dependent carboxylation in the presence of rate limiting amounts of vitamin K (K_1) and vitamin K epoxide (K_1OX) (0.05 nmoles/ml). Results are mean values from duplicate (upper curve) and mean values ± SEM from triplicate (lower curve) incubations.

elution buffer, and applied to a column containing QAE Sephadex A-50 (Fig. 3). Nearly complete separation of two peaks of ERSA was achieved. The recovered activity (about 13% in the first peak and 87% in the second peak) was distributed between the two peaks of activity in a manner similar to that observed after Sephacryl S-200 chromatography (Fig. 1), but the order of elution was reversed. The major peak of ERSA was concentrated by ultrafiltration and applied to a column of Sephacryl S-200. The results of a typical purification are shown in Table 2B. ERSA lost activity after ammonium sulphate precipitation and during the final stage of purification. ERSA was stable when stored at -20° in the elution buffer containing 10% sucrose. The material from the minor peak was similarly stored and has not been investigated further.

Vitamin K Epoxidase Reduction and Vitamin K-Dependent Carboxylation

Our previous studies showed that potassium cholate-solubilized microsomes retained an active vitamin K-dependent carboxylase (9). Both the vitamin K epoxide reductase and the vitamin K-dependent carboxylase activities required DTT and were inhibited by warfarin. NADH did not replace the requirement for DTT in these reactions. Furthermore, we observed that equivalent amounts of vitamin K and vitamin K epoxide resulted in nearly the same amount of vitamin K-dependent protein carboxylation.

Superficially, these data suggested that the conversion of vitamin K epoxide to vitamin K may not be required before the epoxide can be active in the carboxylation reaction. In order to examine this notion more carefully, kinetic studies were carried out on the relationship between vitamin K-dependent protein carboxylation and vitamin K epoxide reduction.

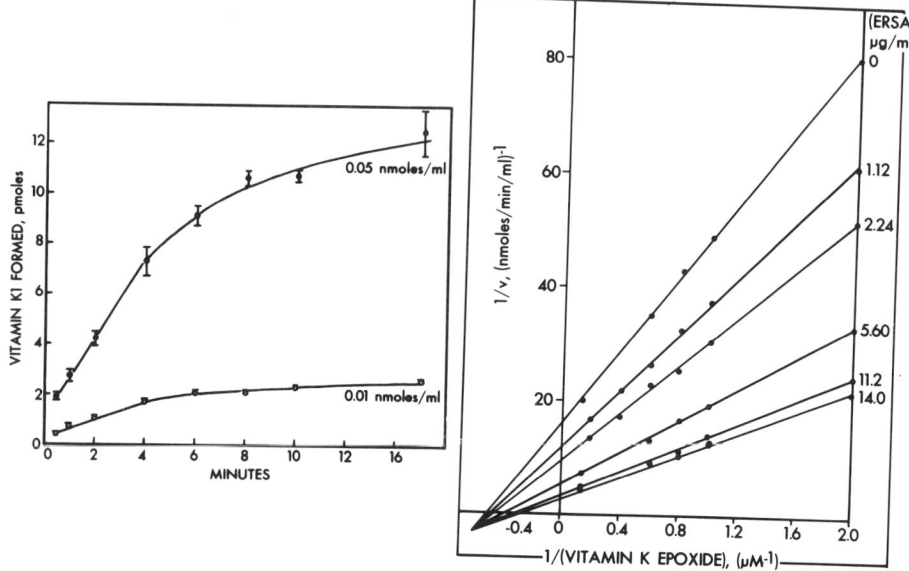

FIGURE 6. (Left) Rate of reduction of vitamin K epoxide at concentrations rate limiting with respect to vitamin K-dependent carboxylation. Standard incubations contained [^{3}H]vitamin K epoxide as indicated. Results are mean values ± SEM from triplicate incubations.

FIGURE 7. (Right) Effect of varying concentration of vitamin K epoxide on vitamin K epoxide reductase activity at different fixed concentrations of ERSA. The data are shown as a double reciprocal plot. Results are mean values from triplicate incubations.

The results (Fig. 4) show that either vitamin K or vitamin K epoxide served equally well as "effectors" for the carboxylation reaction at all concentrations tested. The effect of time on protein carboxylation was then examined at low concentrations (50 pmoles/incubation) of both vitamin K and vitamin K epoxide (Fig. 5). The rate of protein carboxylation was linear for at least 5 min, and both the rate and extent of carboxylation were about the same in the presence of either vitamin K or vitamin K epoxide (see Figure 8 also). The rate of formation of vitamin K from vitamin K epoxide was then studied at the same low concentration of vitamin K epoxide (0.05 nmoles/incubation) to determine whether the amount of vitamin K formed was sufficient to account for the amount of protein carboxylation observed (Fig. 6). Based on initial rates less than 10 pmoles of vitamin K were formed in 5 min, apparently not sufficient vitamin K to account for the amount of protein carboxylation observed (see Figures 4 and 5) when vitamin K epoxide was used to drive carboxylation if reduction of the epoxide to vitamin K is required for its action in carboxylation. These results are consistent with the view that vitamin K and vitamin K epoxide are converted to a common intermediate in their role in vitamin K-dependent carboxylation.

Stimulation by ERSA of Vitamin K Epoxide Reduction

The effect of ERSA on the stimulation of vitamin K epoxide reduction was studied with the preparation of ERSA partially purified as described in Table II (specific activity 15,000 units/mg). The rate of reduction of vitamin K epoxide was examined at variable concentrations of the epoxide

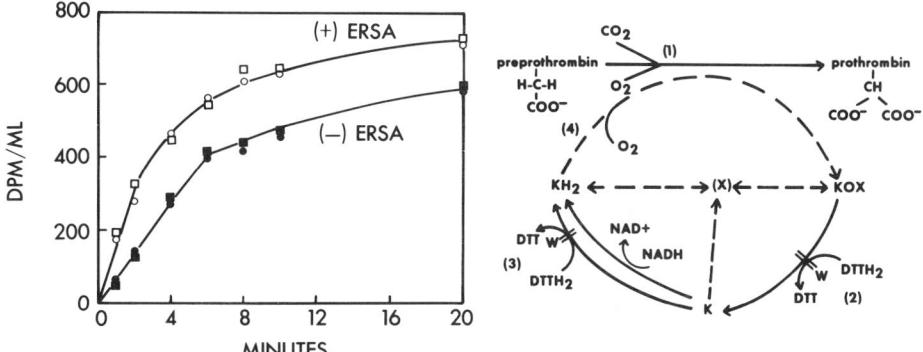

FIGURE 8. (Left) The effect of vitamin K (circles) and vitamin K epoxide (squares) on vitamin K-dependent carboxylation ± ERSA. Incubations contained vitamin K or vitamin K epoxide (0.05 nmoles) and ERSA (5.6 µg) as indicated. Control values from incubations with no vitamin were determined for each time point and subtracted. The results are mean values from duplicate incubations.

FIGURE 9. (Right) Model for vitamin K action. K = vitamin K_1, KOX = vitamin K_1 epoxide, KH_2 = vitamin K_1 hydroquinone, W = warfarin, X = hypothetical intermediate.

in the presence of different fixed concentrations of ERSA. The rate of reduction of vitamin K epoxide was stimulated four to five fold; very similar to the stimulation observed with cytosol. A double reciprical plot of the data obtained is shown in Figure 7. A replot of the 1/v intercepts versus [ERSA] or of the slopes of the lines versus [ERSA] gave hyperbolic functions. A replot of the reciprocal of (slope at variable [ERSA] minus slope at zero [ERSA]) gave a straight line. These data are consistent with intersecting hyperbolic non-competitive plots in the nomenclature of Cleland (10).

The rate of vitamin K-dependent protein carboxylation in the presence and absence of ERSA is shown in Figure 8. At the concentration of ERSA tested the rate of carboxylation was increased about two fold. Vitamin K and vitamin K epoxide at equal molar concentrations showed no difference in protein carboxylation with or without ERSA.

DISCUSSION

The mechanism of reduction of vitamin K epoxide to vitamin K is not understood. The source of physiological reducing equivalents is unclear, and other possible substrates involved in the reaction are not known. The role of ERSA is similarly vague. Consequently, to extrapolate the results of Figure 7 to a simple kinetic mechanism is not valid at this time. However, these results do indicate the usefulness of this solubilized system for examining other kinetic parameters.

Our results on the rate of reduction of vitamin K epoxide and the rate of carboxylation using vitamin K or vitamin K epoxide are consistent with the idea that vitamin K and vitamin K epoxide are converted to a common intermediate in their role as "effectors" for vitamin K-dependent carboxylation.

A model for the action of vitamin K, modified from that described by Whitlon et al. (8), incorporates this view. The intermediate (X) presumably is required to drive the carboxylation reaction. The potassium cholate-solubilized microsomal preparation retains an active DTT-sensitive vitamin K epoxide reductase but does not exhibit the NADH-supported vitamin K reductase (8, 11). Vitamin K epoxidase activity was not detected when vitamin K hydroquinone was incubated in the presence of sufficient warfarin to inhibit the epoxide reductase by greater than 90%. In this preparation vitamin K hydroquinone also serves as an effector for the carboxylation reaction and replaces the requirement for DTT. Where the primary site of warfarin action is and which reaction(s) is the most sensitive to warfarin are still unresolved.

The studies with ERSA are too preliminary to assign a clear role for it in the model. The primary action of ERSA may not be on reduction of the vitamin K epoxide but on a reaction subsequent to formation of the intermediate. Experiments are underway to clarify this question.

ACKNOWLEDGEMENTS

This work was supported by Grant HL 19322 from the National Heart and Lung Institute. The author thanks Chi-Chi Wood for excellent technical assistance and Theodore Mahowald for valuable discussions.

REFERENCES

1. Bell, R. G. (1978) Fed. Proc. 37, 2599-2604.
2. Matschiner, J. T., Bell, R. G., Amelotti, J. M., and Knauer, T. E. (1970) Biochem. Biophys. Acta 201, 309-315.
3. Caldwell, P. T., Ren, P., and Bell, R. G. (1974) Biochem. Pharmacol. 23, 3353-3362.
4. Shearer, M. J., McBurney, A., and Barkhan, P. (1973) Br. J. Haematol. 24, 471-479.
5. Zimmerman, A., and Matschiner, J. T. (1974) Biochem. Pharmacol. 23, 1033-1040.
6. Willingham, A. K., and Matschiner, J. T. (1974) Biochem. J. 140, 435-441.
7. Matschiner, J. T., Zimmerman, A., and Bell, R. G. (1974) Thromb. Diathes. Haemorrh., Suppl. 57, 45-52.
8. Whitlon, D. S., Sadowski, J. A., and Suttie, J. W. (1978) Biochemistry 17, 1371-1377.
9. Siegfried, C. M. (1978) Biochem. Biophys. Res. Commun. 83, 1488-1495.
10. Cleland, W. W. (1963) Biochem. Biophys. Acta 67, 173-187.
11. Wallin, R., Gebhardt, O., and Prydz, H. (1978) Biochem. J. 169, 95-101.

STUDIES ON THE *IN VITRO* REDUCTION OF VITAMIN K_1 EPOXIDE

MICHAEL G. TOWNSEND, EDWARD M. ODAM
and ALLAN K. NADIAN

Vertebrate Biochemistry Section,
Tolworth Laboratory,
Agricultural Science Service,
Ministry of Agriculture, Fisheries and Food,
Surbiton, Surrey KT6 7NF, England

INTRODUCTION

The isolation and identification of vitamin K_1 epoxide from the liver of warfarin-treated rats by Matschiner et al. (1) led to the discovery of the vitamin K_1 – vitamin K_1 epoxide cycle and the subsequent demonstration that the enzyme systems involved are located in the microsomal membranes of rat liver (2,3). Although the role that these reactions play in the vitamin K-dependent carboxylation reactions is currently being studied by several groups, it is not yet known whether epoxide formation is tightly coupled to carboxylation or merely a side reaction resulting from the production of activated oxygen (4,5,6).

Vitamin K_1 epoxide has a similar biological activity to vitamin K_1 in vitamin K-deficient rats, but it is ineffective in warfarin-treated animals (7). It was suggested that warfarin inhibited the in vivo production of the active form (vitamin K_1) from the epoxide and that this inhibition led to the observed increase in the tissue ratio of vitamin K_1 epoxide : vitamin K_1 and hypoprothrombinemia. Studies with a Sprague-Dawley derived warfarin-resistant rat strain showed that in the presence of warfarin these animals accummulated the epoxide to a smaller extent than susceptible ones (8). Subsequent in vitro studies using 6,7- ^3H - vitamin K_1 epoxide as substrate indicated that although the reductase system from resistant rats was less active, it was also less sensitive to warfarin inhibition (2,9). These findings would explain the increased dietary requirement for vitamin K_1 shown by resistant rats (10) and have formed the basis of a method for genotyping resistant rats (11).

Much less attention has been given to the in vitro studies of the system which regenerates vitamin K_1 from its epoxide. There is a need for a readily available assay for this reductase in order to determine the reaction mechanism, to study the site of action of warfarin and investigate the resistance shown by strains of rodents (12,13,14) as well as the effects of the rodenticidal compounds developed to control resistant populations (15). Recent work (16) showing that vitamin K_1 epoxide can replace the requirements of vitamin K_1 in the carboxylase reaction has cast doubt on the significance of the inhibition of the epoxide reductase activity, and this needs to be studied further. We have been assessing high performance liquid chromatography (HPLC) as a way of separating and measuring the products of the in vitro metabolism of vitamin K_1 epoxide (17,18) in order to study vitamin K_1 epoxide reductase.

MATERIALS AND METHODS

The enzyme assay used was based on that of Matschiner et al. (9) and has been published in detail elsewhere (18), but improvements have been made to the HPLC analysis. The best system was a 25 cm, 5µ Zorbax ODS column (DuPont Ltd) fitted with a 6 cm pre-column containing Co: Pell ODS (Whatman & Co. Ltd) and eluted with HPLC grade (Rathburn Ltd) acetonitrile-dichloromethane :: 825-175 (v/v) at a constant flow rate of

1 ml/min (Altex 110 metering pump). The extracts were applied with a 20 µl sample loop (Altex 905-23) and the solvent from the column was monitored at 248 nm (LC-UV detector, Pye Unicam Ltd). The 2-chloro-3-phytyl-1,4-naphthoquinone (Cl-K) was synthesised by the method of Lowenthal and Chowdhury (19). The cis- and trans-isomers of vitamin K_1 were separated from the commercially available material (Sigma Ltd) by column chromatography (20) and the epoxides produced by alkaline oxidation (21). N-acetyl cysteine was obtained from Boehringer Corporation (London) Ltd. and gifts of MK-6 (Hoffman-La Roche & Co. Ltd) and warfarin and difenacoum (Sorex (London) Ltd) were obtained.

RESULTS AND DISCUSSIONS

The liquid chromatographic method (18) has been used to investigate the epoxide reductase activity of several species and two resistant strains of rat (Table 1). The reductase activity of the three rat strains was

TABLE I

REDUCTASE ACTIVITIES FOR VARIOUS SPECIES AND STRAINS

Species or Strain	Activity *
Rat - Laboratory, Susceptible (TAS)	170
- Laboratory, Resistant (HS)	127
- Laboratory, Resistant (HW)	106
Mouse - Laboratory, Susceptible (LAC/GREY)	1270
Grey Squirrel - Wild, trapped	304 **
Red Squirrel - Wild, trapped	74
Japanese Quail - Laboratory strain	53

* The activities are expressed as nmoles vitamin K_1 produced per g. fresh wt. liver equivalent using the published method (18).
** Vitamin K_1 determined using the modified HPLC method described above.

inversely related to the quantity of vitamin K_1 required to restore 50% of the coagulant activity of vitamin K-deficient animals (22), and they therefore resemble the strains studied previously (2,9). The hamster has been shown to have a low epoxide reductase activity and to be more tolerant of warfarin than the rat (23) and a similar situation appears to occur with the Japanese quail where the LC_{50} of 400 ppm (equivalent to a dietary intake of 60 mg/kg/day) in a 14 day feeding study is associated with a low reductase activity (Table 1).

HPLC has been used to separate vitamin K_1 and MK-homologues and their epoxides (24,25,26) but in none of these studies has the amount of epoxide, which has the shorter elution time, exceeded the reduced form. When the epoxide reductase system is assayed in vitro the epoxide accounts for about 95% of the total and more when inhibitors are included in the enzyme incubation mixture. It is therefore essential to employ a chromatographic system which will separate these compounds as narrow bands. We have found that columns containing the newer 5µ particle packing materials give the best resolution of vitamin K_1 epoxide and vitamin K_1 coupled with an increased sensitivity. This greater resolution allows Cl-K which elutes between vitamin K_1 epoxide and vitamin K_1 (Figure 1), to be added as an internal standard. This analogue is preferable to MK-6 as it is chemically more stable and does

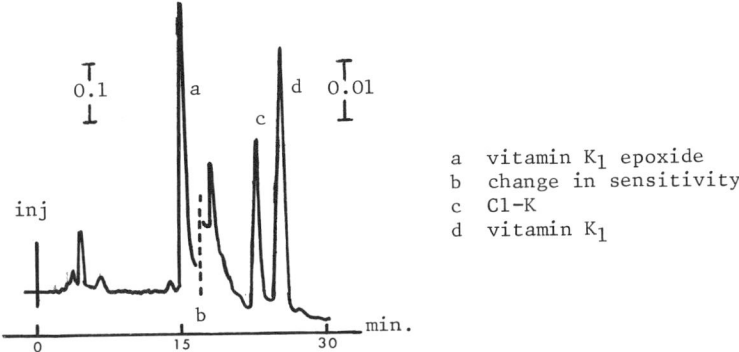

Figure 1. HPLC separation of an extract from an assay of vitamin K_1 epoxide reductase on a 25cm Zorbax ODS column by acetonitrile-dichloromethane (825-175) at 1.0 ml per minute.

a vitamin K_1 epoxide
b change in sensitivity
c Cl-K
d vitamin K_1

not prolong the analysis time. We have also found that although hexane and chloroform are better solvents for the final residues, when used with the small particle, higher resolution reverse phase column materials and the chromatographic solvent systems investigated, these solvents lead to anomalous changes in the elution profiles (Figure 2) analogous to

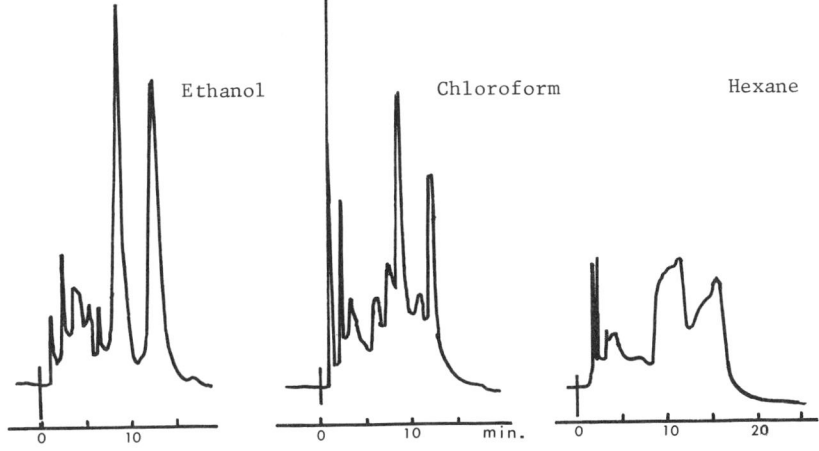

Figure 2. Solvent induced changes in the HPLC separation of 7μg vitamin K_1 epoxide and 2μg vitamin K_1 applied to a 30 cm Partisil ODS column and eluted with acetonitrile-methanol-water (40-40-20).

those reported for other compounds (27). Thus the solvent used to dissolve the final residues must be very similar to the eluting solvent. When acetonitrile-dichloromethane was the final solvent in the study with the grey squirrel (Table 1) it also provided a form of clean-up, as although all the extracted vitamin K_1 and epoxide were in solution after standing 4h at room temperature, much of the co-extracted lipid material remained undissolved. When it was found necessary to clean-up the concentrated extracts prepared from rat liver microsomal suspensions (4), a hexane solution of the material was added to a column of alumina, (activity IV) and eluted with hexane. The hexane was evaporated to dryness and the final residues treated as previously described. The introduction of a sample injector loop and pre-column did not appear to reduce the resolution and the presence of the guard column prevented contamination of the analytical column and consequent loss of resolution and changes in sensitivity.

As the endogenous reducing agent for vitamin K_1 epoxide reductase has not yet been identified most studies have employed dithiothreitol, although recently Bell (23) used dithioerythritol. It would appear that the cyclic conversions involve the hydroquinone form of vitamin K_1 (28) but it is not known whether the thiol compounds are responsible only for the reduction of the quinone or if they also play a role in the reduction of the epoxide.

We have found that the thiol protecting agent N-acetyl cysteine (10mM) cannot replace dithiothreitol, and it would seem that these sulphydryl compounds are not involved in stabilising the enzyme system. In a similar metabolic cycle found in the membranes of plant chloroplasts ascorbate was shown to act as the reducing agent with violaxanthin deepoxidase (29) although it has been shown to be inactive with vitamin K_1 epoxide reductase (30). Vitamin K_1 occurs naturally as the trans-isomer and this biologically active form is oxidised to a much greater extent than the cis-isomer (22). In the studies cited, vitamin K_1 epoxide has been prepared from a mixture of the cis- and trans-isomers of vitamin K_1, and we have now shown that when these isomers are separated by column chromatography (22) and each oxidised to the corresponding epoxide, they are equally effective as substrates for the rat liver system.

The epoxide reductase system is important to the practical aspects of rodent control as resistance in the rat appears to be accompanied by a reduced enzyme activity and the compounds based on 4-hydroxycoumarin which have been developed to control resistant rodents (17) are reported to inhibit this system (30,31). Further studies are being carried out to investigate this in vitro both in the rat and mouse.

REFERENCES

1. Matschiner, J.T., Bell, R.G., Amelotti, J.M., and Knauer, T.E. (1970) Biochim. Biophys. Acta. 201, 309-315.
2. Zimmerman, A., and Matschiner, J.T. (1974). Biochem. Pharmacol. 23, 1033-1040.
3. Willingham, A.K., and Matschiner, J.T. (1974). Biochem.J. 140, 435-441.
4. Esnouf, M.P., Green, M.R., Hill, H.A.O., Irvine, G.B., and Walter, S.J. (1978). Biochem. J. 174, 345-348.
5. Larson, A.E., and Suttie, J.W. (1978). Proc. Natl. Acad. Sci. USA 75, 5413-5416.
6. Wallin, R. (1979). Biochem. J. 178, 513-519.
7. Bell, R.G., and Matschiner, J.T. (1970) Arch. Biochem. Biophys. 141, 473-476.

8. Bell, R.G., and Caldwell, P.T. (1973) Biochemistry 12, 1759-1762.
9. Matschiner, J.T., Zimmerman, A., and Bell, R.G. (1974) Thromb. Diath Haemorrh. suppl. 57, 45-52.
10. Hermodson, M.A., Suttie, J.W., and Link, K.P. (1959). Amer. J. Physiol. 217, 1316-1319.
11. Martin, A.D., Steed, L.C., Redfern, R., Gill, J.E., and Huson, L.W. (1979). Larboratory Animals in press.
12. Greaves, J.H., and Ayres. P.B. (1967). Nature 215, 877-878.
13. Greaves, J.H., and Ayres, P.B. (1976). Genet. Res. 28, 231-239.
14. Wallace, M.E., and MacSwiney, F.J. (1976). J.Hyg., Camb.76, 173-181.
15. Hadler, M.R., and Shadbolt, R.S. (1975). Nature 253, 275-277.
16. Siegfried, C.M. (1978). Biochem. Biophys. Res. Commun. 83, 1488-1495.
17. Elliott, G.R., Odam, E.M., and Townsend, M.G. (1975). Biochem. Soc. Trans. 4, 615-617.
18. Elliott, G.R., Odam, E.M., and Townsend, M.G. (1979). Methods in Enzymology, Vol. 67 Part F in press, Academic Press, New York.
19. Lowenthal, J., and Chowdhury, M.N.R. (1970). Canad. J. Chem. 48, 3957-3958.
20. Knauer, T.E., Siegfried, C., Willingham, A.K., and Matschiner, J.T. (1975) J. Nutr. 105, 1519-1524.
21. Tishler, M., Fieser, L.F., and Wender, N.L. (1940) J. Amer. Chem. Soc. 62, 2866-2871.
22. Martin, A.D. (1973) Biochem. Soc. Trans. 1, 1206-1208.
23. Bell, R.G. (1978) Federation Proc. 37, 2599-2604.
24. Burt, V.T., Bee, E., and Pennock, J.F. (1977) Biochem.J. 162, 297-302.
25. Yamano, Y., Ikenoya, S., Tsuda, T., Ohmae, M., and Kawabe, K. (1977) Yakugaku Zasshi 97, 486-494.
26. Bjornsson, T.D., Swezey, S.E., Meffin, P.J., and Blaschke, T.F. (1978) Thrombos. Haemostas. (Stuttg). 39, 466-473.
27. Wu, C.-Y., and Wittick, J.J. (1975) Anal. Chim. Acta. 79, 308-312.
28. Wallin, R., Gebhardt, O., and Prydz, H. (1978). Biochem.J. 169, 95-101.
29. Siefermann, D., and Yamamoto, H.Y. (1975). Arch. Biochem. Biophy. 171, 70-77.
30. Whitlon, D.S., Sadowski, J.A. and Suttie, J.W. (1978) Biochemistry 17, 1371-1377.
31. Breckenridge, A.M., Leck, J.B., Park, B.K., Serlin, M.J., and Wilson, A. (1978) Brit. J. Pharmacol. 64, 399P.

R AND S WARFARIN AND METABOLITES AS PROBES OF VITAMIN K_1 EPOXIDE REDUCTASE

M. J. FASCO and L. S. KAMINSKY

New York State Department of Health,
Division of Laboratories and Research,
Empire State Plaza,
Albany, NY 12201

INTRODUCTION

The reduction of vitamin K_1 2,3 epoxide is catalyzed by vitamin K_1 2,3 epoxide reductase which is strongly inhibited by the coumarin and indanedione anticoagulant drugs. Current theory suggests that inhibition of this enzyme results in elevated levels of vitamin K_1 epoxide and diminished levels of vitamin K_1 insufficient to support protein synthesis (1).

S warfarin is considerably more active than R warfarin as an anticoagulant in both man and the rat (e.g. 2). Further, some, but not all, of the metabolites of warfarin are active as anticoagulants. The differential activities of the warfarin enantiomers and metabolites offer a means of determining physiologically relevant sites of warfarin action. We have, therefore, initially investigated the effects of these compounds on vitamin K_1 epoxide reductase.

MATERIALS AND METHODS

All chemicals were purchased from Sigma, St. Louis, Mo. Emulgen 911 was obtained from Kao Altas, Tokyo, Japan. The high performance liquid chromatograph (HPLC) was a Waters model 204 equipped with gradient former, WISP autoinjector, and Spectra-Physics 4000 recording integrator.

Hepatic microsomes from male, Wistar rats (250 g) were prepared and their protein concentration determined by methods described previously (3). Vitamin K_1 2,3 epoxide was prepared as described by Fieser et al. (4) and was separated from vitamin K_1 and other contaminants by HPLC on a µBondapak C_{18} preparative column (7.8 mm ID X 30 cm) using CH_3CN as the mobile phase at a flow rate of 3.0 ml/min. Vitamin K_1 was similarly purified. Emulgen 911 solutions (10% v/v) of vitamin K_1 and its 2,3 epoxide (10.0 mg/ml) were prepared as described by Lowenthal and Jaegar (5). R and S warfarin were resolved by the method of West et al.(6) to optical purities of 100 and 101% respectively. The warfarin metabolites were prepared as described previously (3). Solutions of these compounds were prepared by dissolving 2.0 mg of each in 1.0 ml CH_3CN, and further diluting first with an equal volume of 0.02M NaOH and then with water to the desired concentration.

In a final volume of 2.0 ml each reaction mixture contained: 8.0 mg microsomal protein, 1.0 mM dithiothreitol, 0.02 M tris buffer pH 7.4, and R or S warfarin or metabolites. Incubations were run at $25°C$ for 15 min with shaking. Reaction was terminated with 2.0 ml of isopropanol. Hexane (2.0 ml) was added, the mixture was vortexed for 30 sec and the phases were separated by centrifugation. An aliquot (1.5 ml) of the upper phase was evaporated to dryness in vacuo at $50°C$. The residue was redissolved in 0.2 ml of isopropanol and a portion (normally 50 µl) analyzed for vitamin K_1 content by HPLC utilizing a µBondapak C_{18} analytical column (3.9 mm ID X 30 cm). All experiments were performed in triplicate. The chromatographic conditions were: solvent A $H_2O/CH_3CN/MEOH$ (50:45:5), solvent B $CH_3CN/MEOH$ (9:1); the gradient (#7 Waters 660 solvent programmer) retaining the initial condition (75%B) for 1 min and then running to the final condition (100%B) in a near linear fashion over 4 min. The final condition was maintained for 20 min and the column reequilibrated for 5 min. Flow rate was 2.0 ml/min and detection was at 254 nm. Vitamin K_1 epoxide and vitamin K_1 were completely separated and eluted at approximately 610 sec and 740 sec respectively.

RESULTS

The rate of formation of vitamin K_1 from its 2,3 epoxide was essentially linear under the conditions employed. Rate of vitamin K_1 formation was independent of the type of atmosphere present (air or nitrogen), and increased linearly over an epoxide concentration range of 1.1-10.7 µM. Warfarin inhibition of vitamin K_1 formation was significantly less at low substrate epoxide concentrations than at high concentrations. A Dixon plot (Fig.1) has essentially parallel slopes and is consistent with a mixed type of inhibition where binding of the inhibitor to the enzyme promotes increased enzyme substrate binding. Rate of formation of vitamin K_1 was also inhibited to a greater extent by S warfarin than by R warfarin (Fig. 2). At fixed substrate and inhibitor concentrations inhibition of vitamin K_1 formation was 58±2% for R warfarin and 68±5% for S warfarin(insert). Similar differences in R and S warfarin inhibition of the reductase were obtained when enantiomer concentrations were varied over the range of 0.08-1.6 µM.

The effect of warfarin structural modification on reductase inhibition is presented in Figure 3. Hydroxylation of the aromatic portion of the coumarin nucleus diminished inhibition relative to warfarin with inhibition by 6-OH>7-OH>8-OH, the latter being totally inactive. In contrast, hydroxylation at the 4'-position of the side chain phenyl ring or reduction of the side chain ketone had relatively little effect, and these compounds retained considerable inhibitory activity. A hydroxyl substituent on the methylene carbon adjacent to the ketone group (10-hydroxywarfarin), did, however, produce a significant loss of reductase inhibitory activity. Removal of the carbonyl portion of the warfarin side chain (phenprocoumon) did not appreciably alter inhibitory activity. Restriction of the side chain in a configuration approximating a closed ring exo to the coumarin nucleus (cis-dehydrowarfarin) completely eliminated inhibition of vitamin K_1 formation.

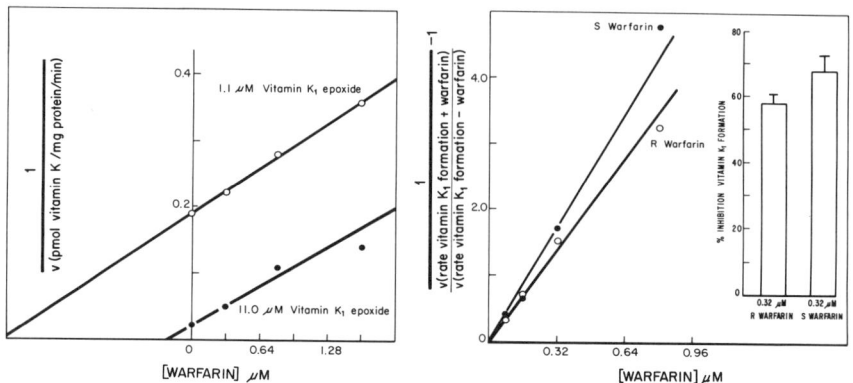

FIGURE 1 Dixon plot of warfarin inhibition of vitamin K formation values are the average of two independent experiments.

FIGURE 2 Inhibition of epoxide reductase by R and S warfarin. Epoxide concentration - 21 µM.

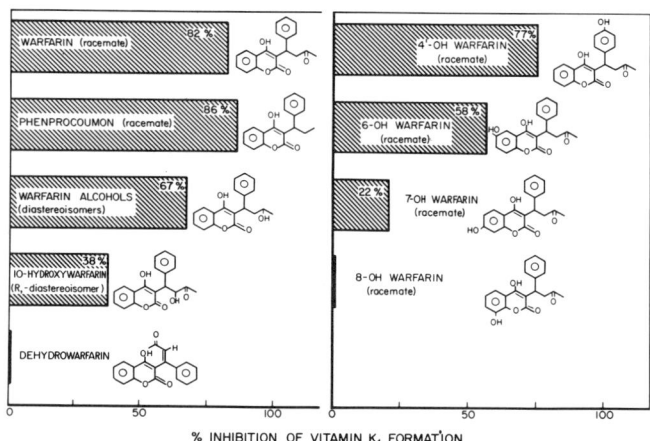

FIGURE 3 Effect of structural modification of warfarin on epoxide reductase inhibition. Warfarin or analog concentration 1.5 µM; epoxide concentration 21.4 µM.

DISCUSSION

Our in vitro results have demonstrated that for warfarin inhibition of vitamin K_1 2,3 epoxide reduction there is diminishing inhibition with decreasing epoxide substrate concentration. Extrapolation of these results to the in vivo situation suggests that warfarin would be a poor inhibitor of vitamin K_1 2,3 epoxide reductase at physiological concentrations of substrate, which are extremely low. This, coupled with a lack of pronounced stereoselectivity of inhibition of the reductase by R and S warfarin raises doubt about the validity of the hypotheses that inhibition of the enzyme is the primary mode of action of the coumarin and indanedione anticoagulant drugs.

The metabolites of warfarin exhibit varying ability to inhibit vitamin K_1 2,3 epoxide reductase. From the extent of inhibition produced by each metabolite we conclude that the functionally most important binding of warfarin to the enzyme is at the coumarin nucleus, most probably at the 4-hydroxy and lactone regions. Binding to both the acetonyl and phenyl regions also occurs, but to a lesser extent since the structural alterations at these regions (except for 10-hydroxy- and dehydrowarfarin) caused minimal losses in inhibitory activity. Results obtained with dehydrowarfarin and phenprocoumon strongly suggest that the ketonic function of warfarin is unnecessary for its activity and that the open chain form of warfarin or its metabolites is essential for inhibition of vitamin K_1 2,3 epoxide reductase.

ACKNOWLEDGEMENT

This research was supported by Grant R01 HL-19772 (M.J.F. and L.S.K.) from NIH, USPHS DHEW.

REFERENCES

1. Bell, R.G., (1978) Fed. Proc. 37, 2599-2604.
2. Breckenridge, A. and L.E. Orme, M. (1972) Life Sciences 11, 377-345.
3. Fasco, M.J., Dymerski, P.R., Wos, J.D. and Kaminsky, L.S. (1978) J. Med. Chem. 21, 1054-1059.
4. Fieser, L.F., Campbell, W.P., Fry, E.M., and Gates, M.D. Jr. (1939) J. Am. Chem. Soc. 61, 3216-3223.
5. Lowenthal J. and Jaeger, V. (1977) Biochem. Biophys. Res. Commum. 74, 25-32.
6. West, B.D., Preis, S., Schroeder, C.H. and Link, K.P. (1961) J. Am. Chem. Soc. 83, 2676-2679.

POSSIBLE PHENYLBUTAZONE POTENTIATION OF WARFARIN BY INHIBITION OF VITAMIN K DEPENDENT CARBOXYLATION

LINDA J. KELLY and ROBERT G. BELL

Department of Biochemistry and Biophysics
University of Rhode Island,
Kingston, RI 02881

INTRODUCTION

Many drugs interfere with anticoagulant therapy with coumarins. Inhibition of Warfarin activity was reported in patients receiving such sedatives as glutethimide or phenobarbital (1-5). Phenylbutazone, an anti-inflammatory agent, potentiated the response to Warfarin (6-8). The interaction of these drugs with Warfarin may be the result of altered availability or action of the anticoagulant. However, the effects may be due to drug interference with vitamin K action or availability. We have used the rat as a model to determine how these drugs alter the anticoagulant activity of Warfarin and to investigate the mechanism of drug interaction.

RESULTS

Rats were injected with a low dose of Warfarin (0.35 mg/kg body wgt) and the plasma prothrombin concentration was monitored over a 72 hr period (Fig 1). Prothrombin concentration

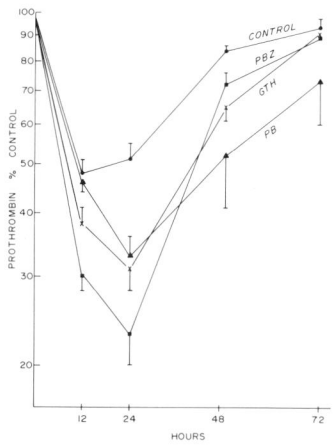

FIGURE 1. The effect of glutethimide, phenobarbital or phenylbutazone on Warfarin response. Female rats were injected intraperitoneally with glutethimide (20 mg/kg body wgt twice daily), phenobarbital (60 mg/kg twice daily or phenylbutazone (40 mg/kg every 4 hr for 12 hr and then every 12 hr throughout the test period). Warfarin (0.35 mg/kg) was in-

jected intraperitoneally at zero-time. The control group received Warfarin alone. Plasma prothrombin concentrations were determined at the times shown. The experimental results are the averages for 3-8 rats. The control results are the averages for 13 rats. The vertical bar represents the S.E. (glutethimide, GTH; phenobarbital, PB; phenylbutazone, PBZ).

decreased to 48% of normal at 12 hr and then slowly returned to its steady-state concentration. The effect of drugs on response to Warfarin was determined. When phenobarbital or glutethimide were administered to rats for 4 days prior to injection of Warfarin, the response to Warfarin was inhibited. However, if the sedatives were administered at the same time as Warfarin and twice daily throughout the 72 hr test period, they caused a potentiation of the effect of Warfarin (Fig 1). Similarly, when phenylbutazone was administered throughout the test period, it also caused potentiation of the response to Warfarin.

To determine if the drugs altered the metabolism of Warfarin, the effect of phenobarbital, glutethimide and phenylbutazone on the turnover of ^{14}C Warfarin in plasma was measured (Fig 2). Glutethimide or phenobarbital did not affect

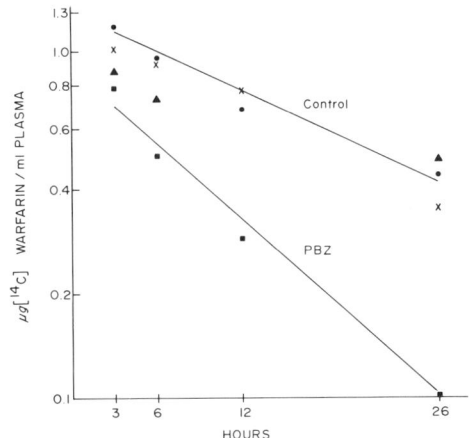

FIGURE 2. The effect of glutethimide, phenobarbital or phenylbutazone on ^{14}C Warfarin turnover in plasma. Female rats were administered drugs as in Fig 1. ^{14}C Warfarin (0.35 mg/kg, 0.15 µCi-0.19 µCi/mM) was injected intraperitoneally at zero-time. ^{14}C Warfarin was determined according to the procedure of Zimmermann and Matschiner (9). The experimental results are the averages for 4-7 rats. The control results are the averages for 12 rats. (glutethimide X; phenobarbital ▲; phenylbutazone ■ ; control ●).

the half-life of plasma Warfarin ($T\frac{1}{2}$ = 17 hr). However, phenylbutazone decreased the half-life to 8 hr.

To determine if the potentiation of Warfarin was due to an increase in the amount of anticoagulant in liver, rats were injected with ^{14}C Warfarin and hepatic ^{14}C Warfarin concentration was determined at 12 hr and 26 hr. Glutethimide or phenobarbital had little effect on the liver Warfarin concentration, suggesting that potentiation by these drugs is not due to altered Warfarin metabolism. Since phenylbutazone caused a rapid removal of plasma Warfarin, we expected to find more Warfarin in the livers of the phenylbutazone-treated rats. However, the hepatic ^{14}C Warfarin concentration in phenylbutazone-treated rats was similar to controls at 12 hr and slightly lower at 26 hr. Thus, phenylbutazone also does not appear to potentiate Warfarin response by increasing the liver concentration of the anticoagulant. To determine if phenylbutazone increased plasma Warfarin turnover by accelerating the excretion of the anticoagulant in the urine, the effect of phenylbutazone on ^{14}C Warfarin excretion was determined over the 72 hr test period. Phenylbutazone had little effect on the urinary excretion of Warfarin.

To determine if the drugs altered the metabolism of vitamin K, a tracer dose of ^3H vitamin K_1 was injected intracardially 15 min before Warfarin administration. Treatment with the drugs had little effect on the rapid decline of ^3H K_1 in the plasma. Similarly they had little effect on the amount of ^3H K_1 and its chief metabolite ^3H vitamin K_1 epoxide found in the liver 12 hr after the injection of Warfarin. This suggests that the drugs do not potentiate Warfarin response by interfering with vitamin K metabolism.

To determine if the drugs directly inhibited the synthesis of prothrombin, rats, treated with Warfarin 24 hr previously, were injected with vitamin K_1, which caused a rapid increase in plasma prothrombin. The administration of phenobarbital, glutethimide or phenylbutazone had little effect on the vitamin K stimulated synthesis of prothrombin. However, it would be difficult to detect a small inhibition of prothrombin synthesis using this method. A more sensitive method would be to measure the effects of drugs on vitamin K-dependent protein carboxylation in liver microsomes (TABLE 1). Phenylbutazone, at a concentration of 1 mM, had little effect on vitamin K-dependent carboxylation but 2.8 mM inhibited protein carboxylation by 33%. Thus, phenylbutazone may potentiate Warfarin action by inhibiting the carboxylation of precursor to active prothrombin. Glutethimide or phenobarbital did not inhibit vitamin K-dependent protein carboxylation. In fact, they stimulated carboxylation for unknown reasons. Thus, glutethimide and phenobarbital do not appear to potentiate Warfarin action by decreasing the availability or action of vitamin K.

DISCUSSION

It has been reported that glutethimide and phenobarbital inhibit the response to Warfarin (1-5). We found that glutethimide and phenobarbital inhibited the anticoagulant activity of Warfarin only if rats were pretreated with the drugs before Warfarin administration. If the sedatives were administered at the same time as Warfarin and throughout the 72 hr test

TABLE 1. The effect of glutethimide, phenobarbital or phenylbutazone on vitamin K-dependent protein carboxylation in liver microsomes[a]

	cpm in TCA precipitate		cpm/g liver	% of control
	No K_1	K_1 added		
Control	668	4537	13,747	
Phenylbutazone				
1 mM	668	4125	12,458	92 ± 16
2.8 mM	668	3623	10,978	67 ± 9
Glutethimide				
1.3 mM	668	6378	19,304	181 ± 24
Phenobarbital				
3.3 mM	668	5831	14,678	127 ± 22

[a]Liver microsomes were prepared from female rats treated with Warfarin (1 mg/kg body wgt) 16 hr previously. Vitamin K-dependent protein carboxylation was carried out as described by Esmon and Suttie (9). The results are the averages for 8 preparations of microsomes ± S.E.

period, they caused potentiation of Warfarin. Corn found that the inhibition of Warfarin action by glutethimide and phenobarbital in humans was accompanied by an increased turnover rate of plasma Warfarin (5). We confirmed this in rats if the drugs were administered for a few days before Warfarin injection. However, we found that the drugs had little effect on the Warfarin level in the plasma or liver if they were administered at the same time as the anticoagulant. Similarly, we found that the drugs had little effect on the turnover of vitamin K in plasma or its accumulation in liver. Glutethimide and phenobarbital also did not inhibit vitamin K-dependent prothrombin synthesis in vivo or vitamin K-dependent carboxylation in vitro. Thus, the mechanism of potentiation of Warfarin by glutethimide or phenobarbital is still unknown.

The potentiation of the anticoagulant activity of coumarins by phenylbutazone has been previously demonstrated. Phenylbutazone displaces Warfarin from plasma albumin (11) and increases its turnover rate (6,12). We also found that phenylbutazone reduced the plasma half-life of Warfarin by 53%. It has been suggested that the mechanism of phenylbutazone potentiation is by displacement of the anticoagulant into the liver where its increased concentration would inhibit clotting protein synthesis (13). However, phenylbutazone had little effect on hepatic Warfarin concentration. Phenylbutazone also did not affect the liver concentration of dicoumarol but potentiated its activity (14). We also found that phenylbutazone did not increase urinary excretion of Warfarin. Like the sedatives, phenylbutazone did not affect the metabolism of vitamin K but did inhibit vitamin K-dependent carboxylation in vitro. Although a relatively high concentration of drug was required for a 33% inhibition, this may be sufficient to account for the potentiation of Warfarin in vivo.

ACKNOWLEDGEMENTS

This work was partially supported by Grant HL-14847 from the National Institutes of Health. We thank Ms. Roxanne Johnson and Marilyn Panzica for excellent technical assistance.

REFERENCES

1. Udall, J.A. (1975) Amer. J. Cardiol. 35, 67-71.
2. MacDonald, M.G., Robinson, D.S., Sylvester, D. and Jaffe, J.J. (1969) Clin. Pharmacol. Therap. 10, 80-84.
3. MacDonald, M.G. and Robinson, D.S. (1968) J. Amer. Med. Assoc. 204, 95-98.
4. Robinson, D.S. and MacDonald, M.G. (1966) J. Pharmacol. Therap. 153, 250-253.
5. Corn, M. (1966) Thromb. et Diath. Haem. 16, 606-612.
6. Aggler, P.M., O'Reilly, R.A., Leong, L. and Kowitz, P.F. (1967) New Eng. J. Med. 276, 496-501.
7. Udall, J.A. (1970) Clin. Med. 40, 20-25.
8. Eisen, M.J. (1974) J. Amer. Med. Assoc. 189, 152-153.
9. Zimmermann, A. and Matschiner, J.T. (1974) Biochem. Pharmacol. 23, 1033-1040.
10. Esmon, C.T. and Suttie, J.W. (1976) J. Biol. Chem. 251, 6238-6243.
11. Solomon, H.M., Schrogie, J.J. and Williams, D. (1968) Biochem. Pharmacol. 17, 143-151.
12. Bachmann, K.A. and Burkman, A.M. (1975) J. Pharm. Pharmacol. 17, 832-836.
13. Brodie, B.B. (1965) Proc. Roy. Soc. Med. 58, 946-955.
14. Jahnchen, E., Wingard, L.B., Jr. and Levy, G. (1973) J. Pharmacol. Exper. Therap. 187, 176-184.

γ-CARBOXYGLUTAMATE EXCRETION AND VITAMIN K METABOLISM

ROBERT J. LEVY, JANE B. LIAN, CAREN GUNDBERG, and PAUL M. GALLOP

Departments of Cardiology and Orthopaedic Surgery
Children's Hospital Medical Center,
Boston, MA 02115

INTRODUCTION

Gammacarboxyglutamic acid (Gla) has been shown to be present in a number of Ca^{++} binding proteins including the vitamin K dependent clotting factor proteins (1), the bone protein, osteocalcin (2), and in proteins occurring in pathologic calcifications (3). Gla synthesis occurs as a post-translational vitamin K dependent enzymatic carboxylation in liver, bone and kidney (1,4,5). Furthermore, in the rat, Gla does not undergo metabolic degradation, but is excreted almost entirely as the free aminoacid (6). In humans as well, Gla is excreted primarily as the free amino acid (7). Therefore, urinary Gla excretion reflects turnover and metabolism of most Gla containing proteins, and may provide an informative index of the vitamin K coagulation system, normal and abnormal bone metabolism, and the progression of pathologic calcifications. The present study investigates these aspects of Gla and vitamin K metabolism.

METHODS

Clinical Aspects: The effects of warfarin anticoagulant therapy on urinary free Gla excretion were studied in 8 patients on stable warfarin anticoagulant therapy, who were receiving this treatment for prophylaxis of thromboembolic disease. These patients ranged in age from 7 to 42 years with 6 males and 2 females. In addition, one 16 year old boy was studied during the initiation of medically indicated warfarin anticoagulant therapy. An age and sex matched control population was also studied.
Urinary Gla excretion in patients with metabolic bone diseases and connective tissue disorders was studied in 23 patients ranging in age from 21 to 76. An additional patient with scleroderma and a subcutaneous skin calcification was also studied before, during and after a therapeutic trial of warfarin as a possible preventative for recurrence of the pathologic calcification. 15 normal adult volunteers (age range 20-54) were selected as a control population for this portion of the study.

Urine Gla Measurements and Clinical Chemical Analysis

24 hour urine collections were obtained from study participants. A blood specimen was obtained at the conclusion of the urine collection for measurement of the one stage prothrombin time by the clinical laboratory. A 5 ml aliquot of the urine was also sent to the clinical lab for measurement of creatinine concentration. 5 ml aliquots of each urine were combined with 1.6 nC of ^{14}C-Gla and chromatographed on columns of Dowex-1 followed by automated analysis of the ^{14}C Gla rich fractions on a Beckman Spinco 121-M aminoacid analyzer as previously published (8). Urinary Gla excretion was expressed either as micromoles per 24 hours, or nanomoles/mg creatinine (in groups where renal disease or muscle wasting was not present). Statistical analysis was performed with Student's t test, and % plasma prothrombin was calculated from Quick's equation (9).

RESULTS

<u>Anticoagulation Studies</u>: Patients on warfarin had decreased urinary Gla excretion (range 8.9 to 39.4 nm/mg Creatinine, mean 23.8) compared to normal (range 29.4 to 69.4, mean = 45.8), and these means differed significantly ($p = .001$). The percent plasma prothrombin concentration correlated with the urinary Gla excretion ($r = .79$) as shown in figure 1. The mean Gla/prothrombin time ratio differed significantly comparing anticoagulated patients to controls (1.17 vs. 3.55, $p = .001$) with overlap occurring with only one patient who was marginally anticoagulated (prothrombin time of 16.1 seconds). Finally, serial urine Gla measurements taken during the initial phases of anticoagulation (Figure 2) illustrate a marked drop from normal to subnormal levels in excretion with prolongation of the prothrombin time. There is also a notable time lag of several days in the drop in urine Gla compared to the prolongation of the prothrombin time.

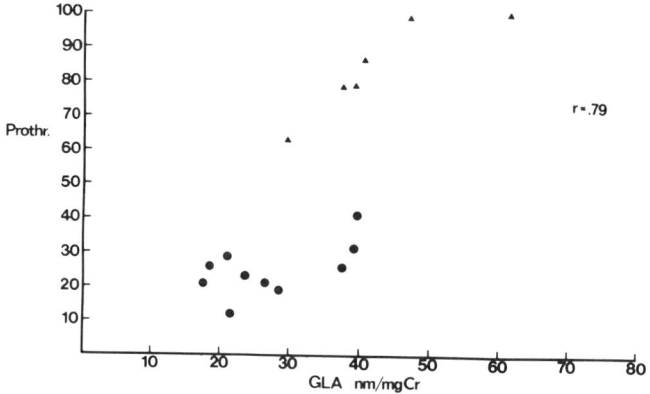

Figure 1. % Plasma Prothrombin vs. Urine Gla.
○ Anticoagulated; △ Normal.

<u>Bone Disorders and Connective Disease Studies</u>: Mean urinary Gla excretion was increased in the patients with osteoporosis, dermatomyositis, and scleroderma, but not in cases of Paget's Disease (Table I). For the Paget's patients, urine Gla levels were taken before their treatment with calcitonin and were not altered by therapy in the course of one year. A scleroderma patient, who underwent surgical resection of a recurrent, subcutaneous, skin calcification of her right knee was given a therapeutic trial of warfarin to inhibit the recurrence of the pathologic calcification during healing. After six months, complete healing was noted without calcification of the scar tissue (as determined by x-ray). The patient's urinary Gla excretion over the period of warfarin administration is illustrated in Figure 3. As can be seen, there was abnormally elevated urinary Gla excretion, which dropped with warfarin therapy to the normal range, with minimal prolongation of the prothrombin time. With cessation of warfarin, the urine Gla content returned to pretreatment levels. Studies are in progress to evaluate the status of any recurrence of calcification.

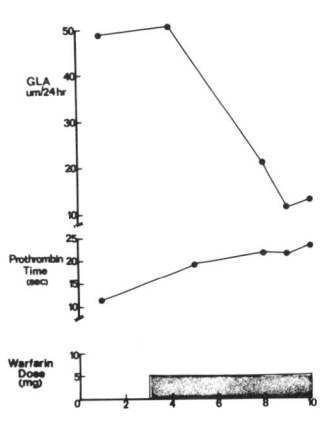
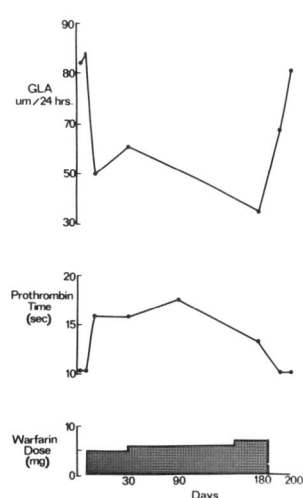

Figure 2. Serial Urine Gla During Warfarin Anticoagulation.

Figure 3. Serial Urine Gla During Warfarin Therapy in Scleroderma.

TABLE I

URINARY GLA EXCRETION IN BONE DISORDERS AND CONNECTIVE TISSUE DISEASE

Diagnosis	Number of Patients	Gla Excretion (nm/mg Creatinine) Range	Mean ($\pm$SEM)
Normal Adults	15	29-69	46.6 ($\pm$ 2.7)
Osteoporosis	7	56-105	69.4 ($\pm$ 6.9)
Paget's Disease	4	26-90	44.7 ($\pm$15.0)
Dermatomyositis	6	84-154	109.6 ($\pm$12.1)
Scleroderma	6	61-94	81.0 ($\pm$ 6.3)

DISCUSSION

Previous work from our laboratory (10) has established that there is decreased urinary Gla excretion in warfarinized patients. Lian has also previously shown increased urinary Gla excretion in several patients with collagen vascular diseases (5). It is of interest to note that our normal urinary Gla excretion values are higher than those published by Fernlund (11). This may reflect the fact that we were able to completely account for Gla recovery by an isotope dilution procedure (10).

Warfarin anticoagulant therapy clearly causes a decrease in urinary Gla excretion secondary to a decreased Gla synthesis occurring in the vitamin K dependent clotting factors (Figures 1 and 2), and in fact, urinary Gla levels correlated well with the plasma prothrombin activity. With stable anticoagulation (Figure 1) it can be seen that 10-20nm of Gla/mg creatinine are still excreted, and this probably represents the extrahepatic Gla-protein contribution, which may undergo a slower rate of metabolism, than the vitamin K dependent clotting factors. Serial Gla measurements during initial warfarin therapy (Figure 3) indicate that by day six of constant warfarin administration, urinary Gla excretion reaches a stable lowered value, and would therefore be useful from that time to monitor coagulation status. The fact that the drop in Gla excretion lags several days behind the prothrombin time probably reflects the rapid warfarin effect on Factor VII levels which would lower the prothrombin time after a single dose, while changing the urinary Gla level little (12).

Increased urinary Gla excretion in osteoporosis, probably reflects the increased rate of bone resorption whereas the normal to slightly elevated Gla excretion with Paget's disease, probably reflects the fact that bone deposition, rather than turnover is predominating. The high Gla excretion in the collagen vascular disease patients is difficult to interpret, but may be related in some way to the propensity of these patients to develop pathologic calcifications. The data on the patient with scleroderma receiving warfarin illustrate the fact that the increased urinary Gla excretion in her case may result from a rapid turnover of Gla containing proteins, apart from the vitamin K dependent coagulation system. It remains to be conclusively shown that inhibition of Gla synthesis in this disease process, will decrease pathologic calcium deposition (a problem which complicates about 20% of cases of scleroderma).

The clinical utility of urinary Gla measurements could be of broad value. It should be possible to check both coagulation status and drug compliance more accurately with urinary Gla levels than with the one stage prothrombin time (Figure 2). Also, Gla containing proteins are present in pathologic calcifications. Furthermore, the present study shows increased Gla levels in the urine of patients with collagen vascular diseases which are often associated with ectopic mineral deposits. Therefore, urine Gla measurements could be of value in this setting. Finally, urine Gla levels in bone disorders, such as osteoporosis could provide a convenient, noninvasive means of following disease activity. Once plasma assays become available for the various Gla containing proteins and their breakdown products, it should be feasible to identify their relative contribution to urinary Gla, and to therefore be cognizant of the major processes being monitored. It may be possible to separate vitamin K dependent clotting factor contribution to urinary Gla, from the contribution to the Gla level from bone metabolism as well as from ectopically calcified tissues. Changes in urinary Gla excretion could then be related most precisely to the relevant Gla protein system.

In summary, our study has demonstrated decreased urinary Gla excretion with warfarin therapy, and increased urinary Gla excretion with osteoporosis and several of the collagen vascular diseases. Monitoring urinary Gla in appropriate clinical situations might be valuable to examine in situations where acute vitamin K deficiency may result from 1) defective fat absorption, 2) diet, and 3) drugs and heritable factors. It may also be useful to monitor abnormal turnover of tissues which are rich in Gla proteins such as in bone. In the latter situation, the Gla proteins are already deposited in the bone mineral and the turnover of these proteins should contribute to the pool of urinary Gla essentially independently of the acute status of vitamin K level and the extent de novo Gla synthesis.

ACKNOWLEDGEMENTS

The authors would like to thank Ms. Kathleen Heroux for technical assistance, and Terry McCarthy and Margaret Wall for preparation of the manuscript. Thanks also to the following physicians for contributing patient urine collections: Dr. J. Barber, Santa Cruz, CA; Dr. L. Pachman, Chicago, IL; Dr. N. Partridge, Boston, MA; Dr. J. Steinberg, Boston, MA; and Dr. M. Whyte, St. Louis, MO. This work was supported by NIH grants: DE 04641, AG00376, and HL 05606.

REFERENCES

1. Stenflo, J., Fernlund, P., Egan, W., and Roepstorff, P. (1974) Proc. Natl. Acad. Sci. USA 71, 2730-2733.
2. Hauschka, P. V., Lian, J. B., and Gallop, P. M. (1975) Proc. Natl. Sci. USA 72, 3925-3929.
3. Lian, J. B., Skinner, M., Glimcher, M. J. and Gallop, P. M. (1976) Biochem. Biophys. Res. Comm. 71, 349-355.
4. Lian, J. B. and Friedman, P. (1978) J. Biol. Chem. 253, 6623-6625.
5. Hauschka, P. V., Friedman, P. A., Traverso, H. P. and Gallop, P. M. (1976) Biochem. Biophys. Res. Commun. 71, 1207-1213.
6. Shah, D. V., Tews, N. K., Harper, D. E. and Suttie, J. W. (1978) Biochim. Biophys. Acta. 539, 209-217.
7. Lian, J. B., Glimcher, M. J., and Gallop, P. M. (1977) in Wasserman, R. H. et al, editors, Calcium Binding Proteins and Calcium Function, pp. 379-381, Elsevier, North Holland.
8. Hauschka, P. V. (1977) Anal. Biochem. 80, 212-223.
9. Quick, A. J. (1939) Proc. Soc. Exper. Biol. and Med. 42, 788-797.
10. Levy, R. J. and Lian, J. B. (1979) Clin. Pharmacol. Ther. 25, 562-570.
11. Fernlund, P. (1976) Clin. Chim. Acta. 72, 147-155.
12. Hoag, M. S., Aggeler, P. M. and Fowell, A. H. (1960) J. Clin. Invest. 39, 554-563.

ANTITHROMBOTIC ACTIONS OF WARFARIN

SANFORD N. GITEL and STANFORD WESSLER

Department of Medicine
New York University School of Medicine
New York, NY 10016

INTRODUCTION

The stasis assay for thrombosis has been used to demonstrate the antithrombotic efficacy of small doses of heparin which can be correlated to an increase in Xa inhibitory activity (the ability of a plasma sample to inhibit activated Factor X) (1). Similarly, we have studied the antithrombotic actions of warfarin using the stasis assay. It was determined that at least two actions of warfarin: the depression of Factor VII activity and the increase in Xa inhibitory activity could account for the antithrombotic effect of warfarin in rabbits.

MATERIALS AND METHODS

Activated factor X (Xa) was prepared as described previously (2). Rabbit brain tissue thromboplastin (Simplastin) was a product of General Diagnostics, Morris Plains, NJ. Male New Zealand white rabbits, average weight 2 kg, were obtained from Camm Research Institute, Wayne, NJ. Normal rabbit plasma was a pool of plasma obtained from Pel-Freeze Biologicals, Inc., Rogers, AR. Rabbit blood was collected by venipuncture from the marginal ear vein and plasma harvested as described (3).

Factor X (4) and Factor II (5) activities were determined using published procedures. Factor VII activity was determined using a one stage assay and human Factor VII-deficient plasma obtained from George King Bio-Medical, Inc., Salem, NH. Xa inhibitory activity (3) and antithrombin III (6) were determined as described previously.

Assay for Thrombogenicity

Rabbits weighing 2 kg were injected intramuscularly with either saline (control) or one ml of a solution of 3 mg sodium warfarin (Lot #76-338, generously provided by Endo Laboratories) per ml in saline. The injections were administered daily between 9 and 10 AM except on the day on which the rabbit was subjected to the stasis assay. Plasma samples were obtained from each rabbit prior to initiation of the stasis assay. The stasis assay was performed as described previously (7) and the clots graded on a scale of zero (no clot) to 4 (complete cast of the isolated segment). An antithrombotic effect would be indicated by a decrease in the thrombotic scores of warfarin-treated rabbits compared to controls after injection of a standard dose of a thrombus initiator such as Xa or thrombin.

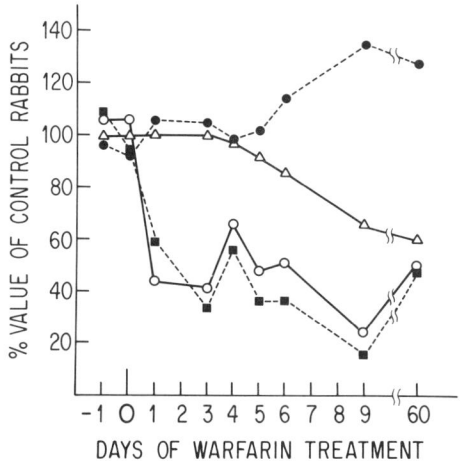

FIGURE 1. The effect of warfarin treatment in rabbits on Xa-induced thrombotic score (△), Xa inhibitory activity (●), Factor II activity (■), and Factor X activity (○). The data are expressed as % of the values obtained in an equivalent control group of rabbits. Factor II and X activities in warfarin treated rabbits were significantly different (p<0.01) from controls by day 1. Xa inhibitory activity was significantly increased (p<0.01) from day 6 of treatment. The thrombotic score of warfarin treated rabbits was significantly decreased compared to controls (p<0.05) from day 6 of treatment.

Statistical Analysis of Data

Data from the stasis assay were analyzed for statistical significance using the Wilcoxon rank sum test (8). Differences in mean clotting activities were analyzed for statistical significance using the Student's t test.

RESULTS

Effect of Warfarin on Factor II, Factor X, Factor VII, Antithrombin III and Xa Inhibitory Activity

Warfarin treatment resulted in a prompt, significant decrease in Factor II, VII, and X activities (Figs. 1 and 2). Xa inhibitory activity was unchanged for 5 days but was significantly increased by day 10 (Figs. 1 and 2), although the quantity of antithrombin III remained unchanged throughout the course of the experiments.

Effect of Warfarin Treatment on Xa-Induced Thrombosis

Figure 1 presents the effect of warfarin treatment on levels of Factors II and X, Xa inhibitory activity, and thrombotic response to Xa as a function of time. Factors II and X began to decrease within 24 hours of warfarin administration. Although these levels were maximally decreased within 3 days of the administration of warfarin, no significant change in Xa inhibitory activity or thrombotic response of the rabbits to Xa

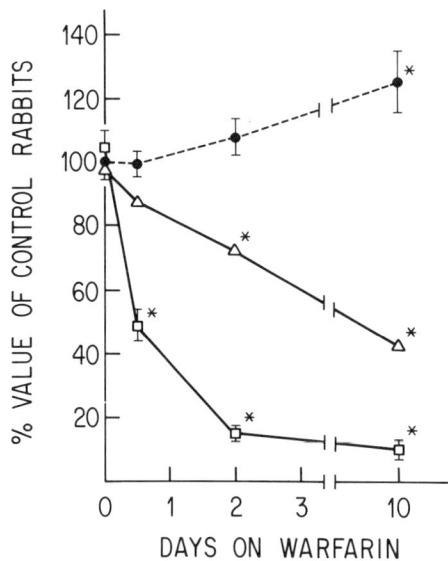

FIGURE 2. The effect of warfarin treatment in rabbits on tissue thromboplastin induced thrombotic score (△), Xa inhibitory activity (●), and Factor VII activity (□). The data are expressed as % of the values obtained in an equivalent control group of rabbits. The * indicates that the warfarin treated group differs significantly from control group ($p<0.05$).

appeared until the sixth day. The data indicate that the observed increase in Xa inhibitory activity occurred subsequent to the decrease in the activity of the vitamin K-dependent clotting proteins and that a decrease in the activity of these proteins was not a measure of the antithrombotic effect of warfarin, at least against Xa, as determined by the stasis assay. Figure 1 also demonstrates a temporal correlation between the warfarin-induced increase in Xa inhibitory activity and the decrease in stasis thrombosis.

Effect of Warfarin Treatment on Tissue Thromboplastin-Induced Thrombosis

Treatment of rabbits with warfarin resulted in a prompt depression of Factor VII activity (Fig. 2) as well as Factors II and X (data not shown), and, as before, Xa inhibitory activity was not significantly increased until the tenth day of treatment. In contrast to Xa-induced thrombosis, the antithrombotic effect against tissue thromboplastin appeared by the sixth hour after treatment, increased to significance on day 2, and was further significantly increased by day 10. These three stages of antithrombotic action correspond to the initial depletion of the vitamin K-dependent clotting factors, the maximum depletion of these proteins, and the increase in Xa inhibitory activity of rabbit plasma.

DISCUSSION

There are at least two independent actions of warfarin which contribute to its antithrombotic effect. The first action, which is specific for tissue thromboplastin-induced thrombosis, operates via the depression of Factor II, VII, and X activities. Although this antithrombotic action may be caused by the depression of any one or any combination of these factors, depression of Factor VII activity is the most likely contributor to this antithrombotic action. The second antithrombotic action of warfarin is more general and is dependent upon the ability of this drug to increase Xa inhibitory activity--an effect observed in man (2,9) as well as rabbits. This second action of warfarin is further substantiated by data which showed that thrombin-initiated thrombosis is inhibited once Xa inhibitory activity is elevated by warfarin use (2) and that there is a significant negative correlation ($p<0.05$) between Xa inhibitory activity and Xa-induced thrombotic score in warfarin-treated rabbits (2).

The data presented in this report indicate that the full antithrombotic effect of warfarin is expressed several days after the depression of the vitamin K-dependent clotting factors. Since there is no correlation between Xa inhibitory activity and prothrombin time (2), the latter assay, although required in order to determine hemorrhagic risk, may not be a measure of the antithrombotic efficacy of warfarin therapy in man.

ACKNOWLEDGEMENTS

This work was supported by a grant from the National Heart, Lung, and Blood Institute #HL-18333 and a grant from Endo Laboratories, Garden City, New York.

REVERENCES

1. Gitel, S.N., Stephenson, R.C., and Wessler, S. (1977) Proc. Natl. Acad. Sci. USA 74, 3028-3032.

2. Wessler, S., Gitel, S.N., Bank, H., Martinowitz, U., and Stephenson, R.C. (1978) Thrombos. Haemostas. 40, 486-498.

3. Gitel, S.N., Wessler, S., and Medina, V.M. (1977) Circ. Res. 41, 187-191.

4. Bachmann, F., Duckert, F., and Koller, F. (1958) Thrombos. Diathes. Haemorrh. 2, 24-38.

5. Hjort, P., Rappaport, S.L., and Owren, P.A. (1955) J. Lab. Clin. Med. 46, 89-97.

6. Gitel, S.N., and Wessler, S. (1975) Thrombos. Res. 7, 5-16.

7. Wessler, S., Reimer, S.M., and Sheps, M.C. (1959) J. Appl. Physiol. 14, 943-946.

8. Wilcoxon, F. (1947) Biometrics 3, 119-122.

9. Odegard, O.R., and Teien, A.N. (1976) Thrombos. Res. 8, 173-178.

CHROMOGENIC ASSAYS FOR THE DETERMINATION OF PROTHROMBIN RELATED MATERIAL IN RAT LIVER FRACTIONS

LINDA J. BEECROFT and J. H. SANDERSON

ICI, Central Toxicology Laboratory,
Alderley Park, Nr Macclesfield,
Cheshire, England

INTRODUCTION

Clotting assays are not applied easily to turbid solutions such as microsomal fractions and consequently results are expressed in a variety of units. With the development of chromogenic substrates the amidolytic activity of certain clotting factors can be assayed biochemically, allowing the expression of results in international units of activity.

Echis carinatus snake venom is known to activate both prothrombin and its precursor forms (ie. prothrombin related material). An assay system has been developed, using E.carinatus snake venom as activator, for the assay of prothrombin related material in plasma samples. This assay has been successfully applied to rat liver fractions, and the assay has been used to investigate the effect of warfarin on the distribution of prothrombin related material in these fractions.

MATERIALS AND METHODS

E.carinatus venom was obtained from Sigma Chemical Company (Poole, Dorset, England). Chromozym$^{(R)}$TH triethanolamine HCl and aprotinin were obtained from Boehringer Mannheim. Warfarin was obtained from Sorex (London) Ltd. All other chemicals were the finest grade available.

Warfarin administration

Male and female, Wistar derived rats were dosed orally with 0.05, 0.1, 0.2, 0.5, 1.0 and 2.0 mg warfarin/kg body weight for 1, 2 or 3 days, the last dose being twenty four hours prior to liver fraction preparation. Two animals from each group were bled by cardiac puncture.

Preparation of liver fractions

Liver fractions were prepared by the method of Sadowski et al.(1) except that the buffer pH was 7.5. The liver homogenate was centrifuged at 10,000 g for 10 minutes to yield supernatant 1. Supernatant 1 was further centrifuged at 105,000 g for 60 minutes to yield the microsomal pellet (resuspended in supernatant equivalent volume to give the microsomal fraction) and supernatant 2.

E.carinatus chromogenic assay

This is a modification of the method of Latallo et al (2) . 2.0 ml triethanolamine (TRA) - aprotinin buffer (0.1 M TRA, 0.2 M NaCl, 0.5 mg/L aprotinin, pH 8.4) was placed in a cuvette together with 0.1 ml of the suitably diluted sample (plasma or liver fraction). At zero time, 0.1 ml of E.carinatus snake venom (1 mg/ml) was added, and after thorough mixing the cuvette was placed in a Perkin Elmer 356 spectrophotometer at 37°C. The mixture was incubated for 3 minutes, after which time 0.25 ml Chromozym TH (1.5 mM) was added. The rate of change of absorbance at 395 nm was then recorded over the next 3 minutes, and from the slope of the line, enzyme activity was calculated. All results were corrected for the control assay in which sample was replaced by buffer.

Protein estimation

Protein was estimated by the Bio-Rad method.

RESULTS

The chromogenic assay was applied to plasma, microsomal fractions and supernatant 2 samples taken from rats dosed with warfarin for one, two or three days.

At dose levels where warfarin exerted an effect, the level of prothrombin related material (PRM) was found to decrease in plasma and supernatant 2 samples, but to increase in microsomal fractions. The changes were found to be more extreme with successive days of dosing (see Figure 1).

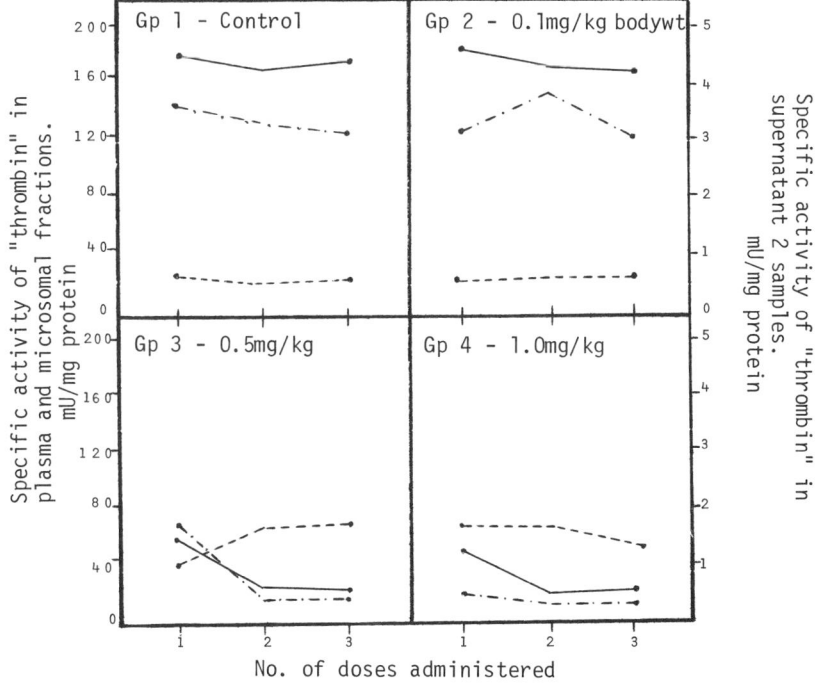

Figure 1 - Effect of various levels of warfarin on PRM in plasma (●——●), microsomal (●----●) and supernatant 2 (●-·-●) samples.

The relationship between warfarin dose, and effect in microsomal fraction and supernatant 2 samples was investigated further (see Figure 2).

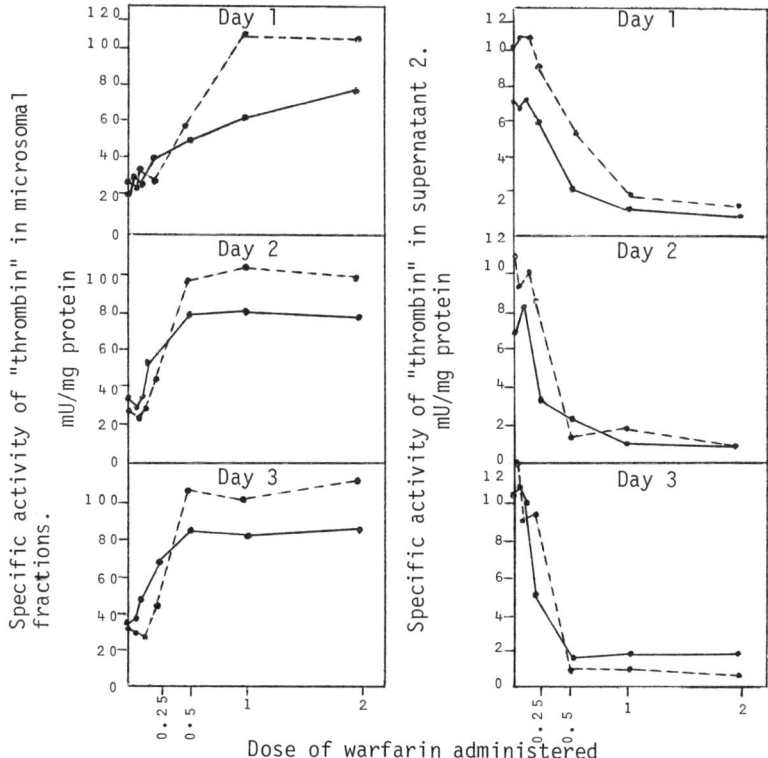

Figure 2 - Relationship between PRM in microsomal and supernatant 2 samples and warfarin dosage in male (•——•) and female (•---•) rats.

The results seem to indicate a sigmoidal relationship between dose and response. The lower doses of warfarin do not cause a measurable change in the levels of PRM in liver fractions. With increasing dose levels more and more PRM is found in the microsomal fraction and correspondingly less in the supernatant 2. At the highest dose levels, the PRM of the microsomal fraction seems to reach a plateau.

DISCUSSION

The chromogenic assay has been used to quantify the PRM in various liver fractions and to investigate the effect of warfarin administration on these levels.

Warfarin has been shown to cause a dramatic shift in PRM from supernatant 2 (presumably soluble forms) to microsomal fractions (microsome bound forms). These results are to be expected if warfarin inhibits vitamin K-dependent carboxylation and parallel the results of experiments using clotting assays to quantify PRM. The chromogenic assay demonstrates a clear relationship between dose level and response and indicates little sex difference. E.carinatus venom activates both prothrombin and precursor forms. Used in conjunction with an assay specific for more nearly completed PRM, eg. using Tiger snake venom as activator, it should be possible to investigate the relative proportions of precursor forms and their inter-conversion by vitamin K-dependent carboxylation.

ACKNOWLEDGEMENTS

The authors would like to thank Mrs C Shingles and Mrs J Jackson for technical assistance, and Mrs T Graham for typing of the manuscript.

REFERENCES

1. Sadowski, J. A., Esmon, C.T. and Suttie, J. W. (1976) J. Biol. Chem. 251, 2770-2775.

2. Latallo, Z. S. and Teisseyre, E. (1977) New methods for the analysis of coagulation using chromogenic substrates, pp. 181-192, Walter de Gruyter, Berlin, New York, Ed. I. Witt.

ISOLATION OF MULTIPLE FORMS OF DICOUMAROL-INDUCED PROTHROMBINS FROM BOVINE LIVER

JOYCE CASSEN and OM P. MALHOTRA

Veterans Administration Medical Center and the
Institute of Pathology, Case Western Reserve University,
Cleveland, OH 44106

INTRODUCTION

In 1972, isolation of three varieties of dicoumarol-induced atypical prothrombins from bovine plasma containing 17% or less normal activity were reported (1,2). However, at that time, some investigators questioned the existence of multiple forms of these atypical variants and even suggested that they quite possibly were artifacts. To prove or disprove this basic work, as well as to understand the mechanism of dicoumarol and vitamin K, we proceeded to isolate the prothrombins from liver, where the molecule is synthesized. Our results do confirm the existence of multiple forms of atypical protein. In this manuscript, we describe the isolation of one atypical form which is adsorbable onto barium citrate, another form adsorbable onto barium oxalate but not onto barium citrate, and the third form adsorbable onto alumina C-γ gel, but not onto the insoluble barium salts.

MATERIALS AND METHODS

Animal care and dicoumarol administration was the same as has been described previously (3). In general, livers from the dicoumarol-treated steers were procured when their plasma prothrombin activities (4) approximated 3 to 6% of normal. Before sacrifice, two or more liters of blood were drawn from each steer, and then the animals were anesthetized with pentobarbital. Immediately, the liver was removed and perfused with cold 0.154 $\underline{M}$ NaCl-0.14 $\underline{M}$ sodium citrate solution, pH 7.4, with 1 m$\underline{M}$ benzamidine-HCl, with the aid of a GE flow pump, type VW-1-101. For normal liver, perfusion was somewhat delayed (4 to 8 min), because of the time required for procuring the liver at a local slaughterhouse.

All purification steps were carried out at 4 to 6°C. The liver was suspended in cold homogenate buffer (0.05 $\underline{M}$ Tris-HCl containing 0.25 $\underline{M}$ sucrose, 0.014 $\underline{M}$ sodium citrate, and 6 m$\underline{M}$ benzamidine-HCl pH 7.4). After cutting the liver into small pieces and grinding it in a Straub meat mincer, the minced liver was homogenized in a tissue grinder (Houston Glass Co., 125 ml capacity) by using a drill press (Sears Rockwell, 1/2 horsepower, 1725 rpm). After removing mitochondria and nuclei by centrifugation, 12,800 x g for 10 min, the supernatant (of the homogenate) was then centrifuged at 105,000 x g for 1 h to obtain the heavy microsomal fraction. The resultant pellet was suspended in 0.028 $\underline{M}$ sodium barbital buffer (pH 7.4) containing 0.12 $\underline{M}$ NaCl, 0.014 $\underline{M}$ sodium citrate, and 6 m$\underline{M}$ benzamidine-HCl, and was homogenized again, as described above. Prothrombin was then extracted with 1% Triton X-100 in the same sodium barbital buffer by stirring the membrane of the heavy microsomal fraction for 30 min. The solubilized prothrombin was freed from cellular debris by centrifugation (105,000 x g for 1 h), and treated sequentially with barium citrate, barium oxalate and finally alumina C-γ gel (Bio-Rad), as described previously for the plasma prothrombins (1,2) to procure the normal and the three varieties of dicoumarol-induced prothrombins.

The adsorbed proteins from each of barium citrate, barium oxalate, and alumina C-γ gel, were eluted with 0.2 $\underline{M}$ sodium citrate in 0.154 $\underline{M}$ NaCl (pH 7.4) with 10 m$\underline{M}$ benzamidine-HCl, concentrated by ultrafiltration* (UM-10 filters, Amicon), and fractionated with solid ammonium sulfate (Schwarz-Mann, Ultrapure). The prothrombin fraction obtained between 22 to 67% saturation was dissolved in redistilled water and dialyzed against 0.03 $\underline{M}$ Tris-HCl buffer (pH 7.4) with 1 m$\underline{M}$ benzamidine-HCl. The clarified dialysate obtained after centrifugation was applied to DEAE-cellulose (Whatman) in columns of 2.5 x 20 to 50 cm (Pharmacia) equilibrated with the same buffer. Protein was eluted with a stepped increase of sodium chloride concentration from 0.0 to 0.3 $\underline{M}$ in 0.03 $\underline{M}$ Tris-HCl buffer (pH 7.4) containing 1 m$\underline{M}$ benzamidine-HCl. Presence of prothrombin molecules, normal and atypical, was monitored by antigen-antibody (antiprothrombin rabbit sera) precipitation reaction (immunodiffusion). After concentrating and dialyzing the prothrombin fraction in 0.03 M Tris-HCl buffer (pH 7.4) with 1 mM benzamidine-HCl, this sample was then subjected to heparin-agarose chromatography in a 1.5 x 50 cm column (Pharmacia), equilibrated with the same 0.03 $\underline{M}$ Tris-HCl buffer. Heparin was bound to cyanogen bromide-activated Sepharose 4B (Pharmacia), as described previously (5).

RESULTS

In normal liver, when each of the concentrated eluates from the adsorbents were tested for the presence of prothrombin-like molecules, only the barium citrate eluate from normal liver gave positive immunoprecipitation reactions. For dicoumarol-treated liver, on the other hand, each of the eluates from barium citrate, barium oxalate, and alumina C-γ gel, gave a positive reaction (Fig. 1). These results confirm our earlier observations with plasma (1,2), that multiple forms of atypical prothrombins are indeed produced during dicoumarol-regimen. Furthermore, as expected, the concentrated eluate from barium citrate used for normal, but not for dicoumarol-treated heavy microsomal fractions, revealed physiological activity - 176 U per kg liver. The bioactivity, however, was lost during subsequent purification steps, e.g., during ammonium sulfate fractionation.

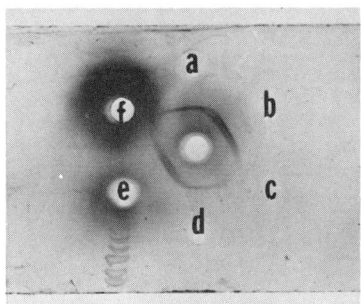

FIGURE 1. Ouchterlony double diffusion analysis of normal and dicoumarol-induced prothrombins. The central well contains rabbit antisera against normal bovine prothrombin. a) Normal hepatic citrate prothrombin, b) normal prothrombin, c) dicoumarol hepatic citrate, d) dicoumarol hepatic oxalate, e) dicoumarol hepatic alumina and f) normal hepatic oxalate.

---

*As our work progressed, the ammonium sulfate fractionation was performed without prior concentration of the eluates.

Each of the eluates containing antigenic (prothrombin) activity were processed for further purification by similar techniques, and the eluate from barium citrate, used for the normal microsomal fractions, is described in this paper. Upon ammonium sulfate fractionation, prothrombin was found to be present between 22 to 67% saturation. This fraction in 0.03 M Tris-HCl buffer (pH 7.4) containing 1 mM benzamidine-HCl, was subjected to DEAE-chromatography (Fig. 2a). Prothrombin fractions (135 to 176), after having been pooled, concentrated, and rechromatographed, were then subjected to heparin-agarose chromatography (Fig. 2b). Prothrombin was primarily present in fractions 45 to 73. The purified material, however, showed one minor component of low molecular weight and two major (adjacent) bands of equal intensity. One of the latter two bands was prothrombin, having a molecular weight of approximately 70,000, while the other band, representing extraneous protein, had a molecular mass of 75,000 daltons. The extraneous protein apparently consisted of two (or more) chains because its molecular weight decreased by 4,000 when the reduced sample was used for SDS-gel electrophoresis.

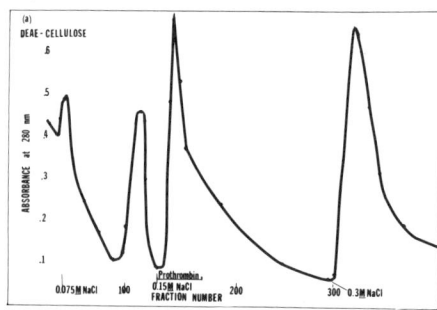 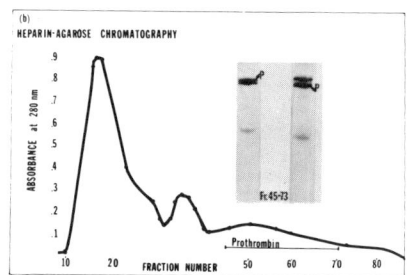

FIGURE 2. (a) DEAE-cellulose chromatography of normal hepatic prothrombin (column size 2.5 cm x 42 cm). Fractions of approximately 3 ml each were collected at a flow rate of 40 to 50 drops/min. Stepwise elution was begun at fraction 23, with 0.075 M NaCl in 0.03 M Tris-HCl (pH 7.4) with 1 mM benzamidine-HCl; 0.15 M NaCl in the same Tris buffer was begun at fraction 133, and 0.3 M NaCl at fraction 300. Prothrombin was noted primarily in the 0.15 M NaCl peak, which was rechromatographed; (b) Heparin-agarose chromatography in 0.03 M Tris-0.1 M NaCl (pH 7.4), column size 1.5 x 45 cm, and flow rate 10 to 15 drops/min. Fractions were 3 ml each. Prothrombin was primarily present in Fr. 45 to 73, which, however, by SDS-gel electrophoresis, showed prothrombin and an extraneous protein. Prothrombin (P) was about 70,000 daltons, shown without mercaptoethanol in the right gel. The extraneous protein consisted of two (or more) polypeptide chains in the presence of mercaptoethanol (left gel).

DISCUSSION

The first ten glutamyl residues, present in the amino portion of normal prothrombin, are carboxylated, γ-carboxyglutamic acid (Gla) (6-8). These extra carboxyl groups provide the calcium-binding ability to the normal molecule, which is essential for the generation of thrombin, physiologically. Dicoumarol interferes with the carboxylation mechanism; therefore, its administration results in the production of partially carboxylated (atypical) prothrombin molecules. From plasma studies, it has recently been reported that one of the atypical prothrombins adsorbs onto barium citrate as does normal prothrombin but contains 7-Gla's instead of 10. Another variant which adsorbs onto barium oxalate but not onto barium citrate contains 5-Gla's, and another variant adsorbable onto alumina gel (but not onto the insoluble barium salts) contains 2-Gla's. Other authors have been able to isolate a maximum of 2 forms only thus far (9,10). Our results with the hepatic prothrombins confirm not only the production of multiple forms of dicoumarol-induced prothrombins, but also differences in their adsorptive properties. Along the same lines, one is inclined to speculate that the Gla content of each of the hepatic atypical prothrombins, based upon their adsorbability, is similar to their plasma counterparts. Indeed, this remains to be investigated.

ACKNOWLEDGMENTS

This work was in part funded by a USPH Service Training Grant # 5 T01 GMO-1784-03 and in part by a grant from the Veterans Administration. Appreciation is expressed to Mrs. P. Mendelson for SDS gel electrophoresis and to Mr. P. Vano for help with biological prothrombin assays.

REFERENCES

1. Malhotra, O.P. (1972) Nature New Biology 239, 59-60.
2. Malhotra, O.P. (1972) Life Sci. 11 (Part II) 901-907.
3. Malhotra, O.P., and Carter, J.R. (1971) J. Biol. Chem. 246, 2665-2671.
4. Malhotra, O.P., and Carter, J.R. (1965) Fed. Proc. 24, 154.
5. Malhotra, O.P. (1979) Thromb. Res., in press.
6. Magnusson, S., Sottrup-Jensen, L., Peterson, T.E., Morris, H.R., and Dell, A. (1974) Fed. Europ. Biochem. Soc. Letters 44, 189-193.
7. Nelsestuen, G., Zytkovicz, T.H., and Howard, J.B. (1974) J. Biol. Chem. 249, 6347-6350.
8. Fernlund, P., Stenflo, J., Roepstorff, P., and Thomsen, J. (1975) J. Biol. Chem. 250, 6125-6133.
9. Esnouf, M.P., and Prowse, C.V. (1977) Biochem. Biophys. Acta 490, 471-476.
10. Friedman, P.A., Rosenberg, R.D., Hauschka, P.V., and Fitz-James, A. (1977) Biochem. Biophys. Acta 494, 271-276.

PRESENT DISTRIBUTION OF ANTICOAGULANT RESISTANCE IN THE UNITED STATES

WILLIAM B. JACKSON and A. D. ASHTON

Environmental Studies Center,
Bowling Green State University,
Bowling Green, OH 43403

INTRODUCTION

Although the discovery of anticoagulant-resistant Norway rats in North Carolina in 1971 was a unique event, the finding of resistant rats in American cities no longer is a rare occurrence. With the participation of federally-assisted urban rat control programs and other groups, collections of rats from nearly 100 sites have been examined by laboratories of the N.Y. State Health Department at Troy and Bowling Green State University. Previous reports have documented the initial analyses (1,2).

PROTOCOL

Anticoagulant resistance has been defined by the World Health Organization (3), and we have followed these criteria with only slight variations (4). A Norway rat surviving a 6-day, no-choice feeding test with bait (ground laboratory chow) containing 0.005% (50 ppm) warfarin is designated resistant. (For roof rats a 12-day, no-choice test with 0.025% bait is used.) We use a single lot of highly purified warfarin supplied by the Wisconsin Alumni Research Foundation to increase test uniformity. The rat must consume at least 12 mg/kg of warfarin during the test to qualify for inclusion. While the level of warfarin in the bait is one-fifth that found in commercial baits (0.025% or 250 ppm), the test is conducted under conditions that preclude feeding on alternate foods. Under normal conditions a rat feeding on a toxic bait also will feed on other available foods and thus ingest a smaller amount of toxic bait. Most rats surviving the 50 ppm bait in the laboratory also will survive with a 250 ppm bait, even under 6-day no-choice test conditions.

Rats resistant to warfarin (a coumarol compound) usually are resistant to the indandione anticoagulants (e.g., Pival, diphacinone, chlorophacine) as well. Thus warfarin-resistant rats properly have been referred to as anticoagulant-resistant rats. Initially in the test program rats were accepted from all sites and sources. More recently, participating cities have been required to submit randomly-trapped, 64-rat samples (4). Data from these latter collections permit estimates of resistance incidence with statistical limits.

RESULTS AND DISCUSSION

Data from these various tests conducted during this decade with Norway rats and roof rats are summarized in table 1 and figure 1. House mouse resistance apparently also is widespread, but comparable quantification is lacking. A low incidence of the resistance allele in populations is considered normal. When selection pressure from extended use of anticoagulants and persistence of poor environmental conditions occurs and the frequency of resistant animals in the sample exceeds 10%, management strategies that force concern for environmental conditions and utilize acute rodenticides (e.g., zinc phosphide) periodically (e.g., annually) should be implemented (5). The new, second generation anticoagulant rodenticides, Brodifacoum (Talon^{tm}) and Bromadiolone (Maki^{tm}), also are effective against rats resistant to the conventional anticoagulants but are available only under experimental registrations (EUP) at the present time.

ACKNOWLEDGEMENTS

These evaluations of anticoagulant resistant rat populations were made possible by support from the Urban Rat Control Program through the U.S. Public Health Service.

REFERENCES

1. Jackson, W. B., Joe E. Brooks, Alan M. Bowerman, and Dale E. Kaukeinen (1975) Pest Control 43, 12-16; 43, 14-24.
2. Jackson, W. B., and Dale E. Kaukeinen (1976) Proc. Third Intl. Biodegredation Symp. 303-308, Allied Sci. Pub., London.
3. WHO (U.N.) (1970) Tech. Rept. Ser. 443, 140-147.
4. Frantz, S. C. (1977) Procedures for collecting rats for anticoagulant resistance/urban rat control projects. U.S. Dept. H.E.W., Ctr. Disease Control, Atlanta, GA. 16 p.
5. Environmental Health Services Division/CDC, Environmental Studies Center/Bowling Green State University, Rodent Control Evaluation Laboratory/NY State Dept. Health (1978). Anticoagulant rodenticide rat resistance studies: policies and procedures manual. USDHEW, PHS, Center for Disease Control, Atlanta. 18 p.

TABLE 1. Summary of Norway rats (Rattus norvegicus) and Roof rats (R. rattus) subjected to WHO test for warfarin test for resistance. Animals come from federally assisted rat control projects, PCOs, local health departments, and others. Data combined from New York and Bowling Green laboratories as of March 31, 1979.

State and City	No. Rats Tested*	No. Surviving	% Resistant
Norway Rats			
Alabama			
Mobile	204	9	4.4
Alaska			
Kodiak	19	0	-
Arkansas			
Little Rock	69	4	5.8
Pine Bluff	38	1	2.6
West Memphis	19	0	-
California			
Fresno/Kerman	13	1	7.7
Los Angeles	78	1	1.3
Richmond	51	1	2.0
San Francisco	66	4	6.1
W. Oakland	68	5	7.4
Connecticut			
Hartford	140	17	12.1
District of Columbia	142	10	7.0
Florida			
Ft. Lauderdale	125	1	0.8
Miami	120	1	0.8
Tampa	36	1	2.8
Georgia			
Atlanta	89	8	9.0
Dekalb County	76	10	13.2
Illinois			
Chicago - Austin	62	44	71.0
- Englewood	69	30	43.5
- Garfield	11	8	72.7
- Lawndale	212	152	71.7
Indiana			
Ft. Wayne	70	2	2.9
Gary	56	5	8.9
Indianapolis	207	12	5.8
Iowa			
Sioux City	18	14	77.8
Kansas			
Kansas City	27	0	-
Kentucky			
Louisville	116	8	6.9
Lousiana			
New Orleans	58	0	-
Maryland			
Baltimore	167	18	10.7
Massachusetts			
Boston	175	20	11.4
Worcester	55	0	-

State and City	No. Rats Tested*	No. Surviving	% Resistant
Michigan			
Detroit	139	1	0.7
Minnesota			
Duluth	39	2	5.1
Missouri			
Kansas City	15	0	−
St. Louis	145	2	1.4
Nebraska			
Omaha	18	0	−
New Jersey			
Camden	190	5	2.7
E. Orange	13	2	15.4
Hoboken	91	2	2.2
Jersey City	216	15	6.9
Newark	88	3	3.4
Passaic	25	0	−
Paterson	117	8	6.8
Plainfield	116	1	0.9
Trenton	99	2	2.0
New Mexico			
Albuquerque	20	0	−
New York			
Binghamton	120	9	7.5
Buffalo	71	4	5.6
Cohoes	318	27	8.5
Dutchess Co./Poughkeepsie	345	116	33.6
Newburgh	52	1	1.9
New York City	641	16	2.5
Bushwick	79	1	1.3
Lower E. Side	51	1	2.0
Rochester	65	1	1.5
Syracuse	83	1	1.2
North Carolina			
Charlotte	19	5	26.3
Johnson Co.	160	81	50.6
Winston-Salem	19	0	−
Ohio			
Akron	52	5	9.6
Cincinnati	71	1	1.4
Cleveland	178	13	7.3
Columbus	121	11	9.1
Napoleon	20	0	−
Sandusky	27	3	11.1
Toledo	18	0	−
Oklahoma			
Tulsa	12	1	8.3
Pennsylvania			
Chester	108	11	10.2
Clairton	86	15	17.4
Harrisburg	27	0	−
N.E. Pennsylvania	46	0	−
Philadelphia	92	3	3.3
Pittsburgh	148	17	11.5
York	38	3	7.9

State and City	No. Rats Tested*	No. Surviving	% Resistant
Puerto Rico			
Mayaguez	18	1	5.6
San Juan	95	16	16.8
Tennessee			
Memphis	99	8	8.0
Nashville	60	2	3.3
Texas			
Houston	156	19	12.2
Virginia			
Chesapeake	78	6	7.7
Norfolk	149	13	8.7
Portsmouth	106	22	20.7
Washington			
Seattle	46	2	4.3
Wisconsin			
Milwaukee	61	2	3.3

Roof Rats

State and City	No. Rats Tested*	No. Surviving	% Resistant
Alabama			
Mobile	50	1	2.0
California			
Fresno	27	3	11.1
Los Angeles	23	8	34.8
Ontario	49	3	6.1
San Diego	22	1	4.5
Santa Ana	19	2	10.5
Florida			
Ft. Lauderdale	10	0	-
Tampa	167	4	2.3
Louisiana			
New Orleans	36	2	5.6
Puerto Rico			
San Juan	12	1	8.3
Texas			
Houston	20	4	20.0
Washington			
Seattle	14	1	7.1

* Only those cities or areas with collections of 10 or more rats are listed.

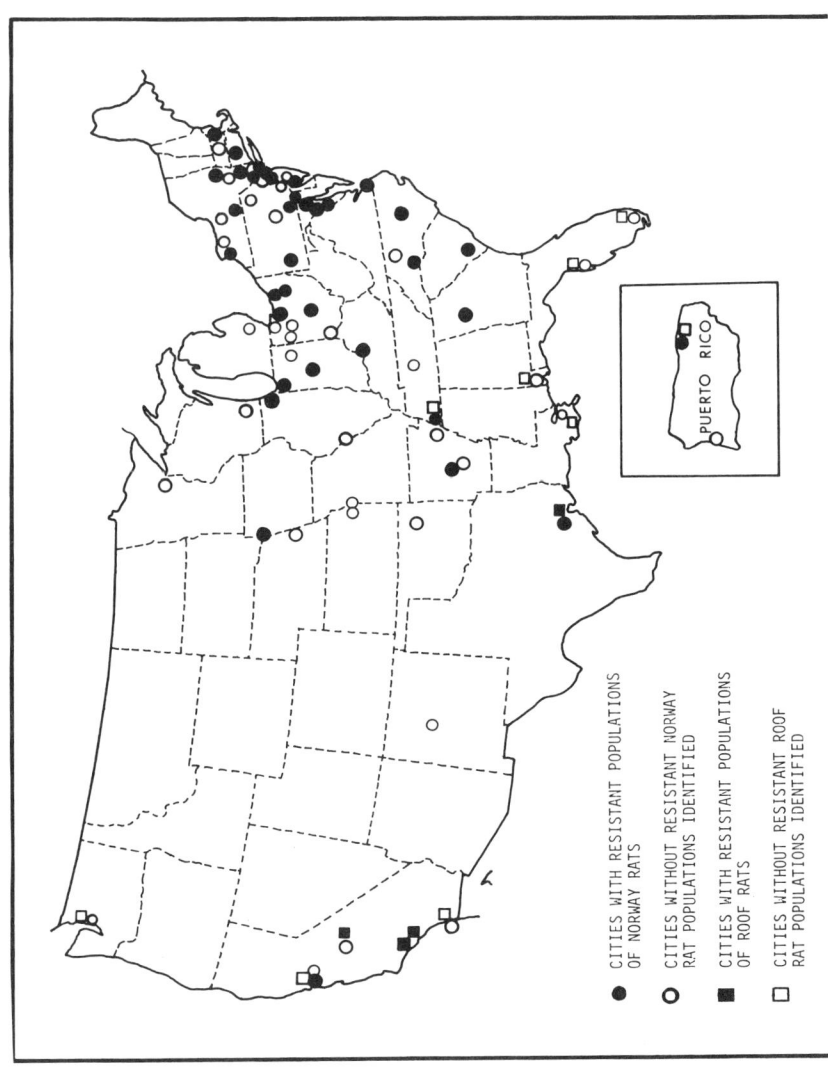

FIGURE 1. Collection sites of Norway and roof rats for WHO warfarin-resistance tests. Sites with samples (≥10 animals) having at least 5% (>3 animals) surviving are considered to have populations of resistant rats. Portions of the sample may have been collected at different times during the study period.

THE VITAMIN K-DEPENDENT CARBOXYLASE

DISSOCIATION OF VITAMIN K-DEPENDENT
γ-CARBON-HYDROGEN BOND CLEAVAGE FROM
CARBOXYLATION OF PEPTIDE-BOUND GLUTAMIC
ACID RESIDUES

PAUL A. FRIEDMAN

Department of Pharmacology,
Harvard Medical School and Center for Blood Research,
Boston, MA 02115

INTRODUCTION

Although the basic requirements of the vitamin K-dependent carboxylating enzyme system have been defined (1-5), the detailed mechanism by which the vitamin supports the post-translational conversion of specific glutamic acid (Glu) residues to γ-carboxyglutamic acid (γ-CGlu) in certain proteins remains unknown. Among several possible roles which have been proposed for the vitamin in the carboxylation event, two which would seem most reasonable are: 1) Vitamin K activates and/or is a carrier for CO_2; 2) The primary role of the vitamin is to facilitate γ-carbon-hydrogen bond cleavage. No experimental evidence to date supports one role to the exclusion of the other.

In recent experiments related to biotin-dependent carboxylations, Stubbe and Abeles (6) provide data strongly suggesting that proposals of concerted mechanisms of proton abstraction and carboxylation for biotin-dependent carboxylations are not feasible. They demonstrated that with β-fluoropropionyl coenzyme A as the substrate, the biotin-dependent enzyme propionyl-CoA carboxylase catalyzed the formation of ADP with the elimination of fluoride ion. In this study, the rate of fluoride release, indicative of the minimal rate of abstraction of the α proton, was six times that of ADP formation which is also equivalent to the rate of formation of biotin-CO_2. This indicated that hydrogen abstraction from the substrate could occur without concomitant CO_2 transfer from biotin to the substrate.

A similar approach also could be used with a vitamin K-dependent carboxylating enzyme system. Thus, the pentapeptide, Phe-Leu-Glu-Glu-Leu, tritiated at the γ carbon of both Glu residues has been synthesized. With the use of this peptide, a known substrate for the vitamin K-dependent carboxylating enzyme system (7), it has been possible to demonstrate that vitamin K-dependent enzymatic cleavage of the C-H bond in the gamma position of the glutamate residues can proceed in the absence of carboxylation (8).

MATERIALS AND METHODS

Preparation of Tritium-Labeled Pentapeptide

L-Glu (specific activity 50 Ci/mmole) tritiated at both the β and γ carbons (55% beta and 45% gamma as determined by tritium NMR analysis, with a random distribution between the R and S positions at each carbon) was obtained from New England Nuclear. The amino acid was benzyl-esterified specifically at the γ position (9); the γ-benzylglutamate was then treated with t-butoxycarbonyl (t-Boc) azide in triethylamine (10), and the resulting protected amino acid was used in the solid phase synthesis of the pentapeptide Phe-Leu-Glu-Glu-Leu. It was determined that 80% of the added tritiated Boc-L-Glu-γ-benzyl ester was coupled at each step. The finished peptide was cleaved from the resin by treatment with HBr in trifluoroacetic acid at room temperature for 90 min (11); after the resin was filtered and washed with trifluoroacetic acid, the combined filtrates were evaporated at reduced pressure. The pentapeptide was purified by gel filtration over a Bio-Gel P-2 column equilibrated with 1% acetic acid in water, on which the elution volume of unlabeled pentapeptide had been determined. The radioactive peak eluting in this volume was dried under reduced pressure. This peptide, which contained 10% of the original radioactivity in Glu, was 95% pure as judged by thin-layer chromatography (7). The amino acid composition was: Phe, 1.00; Leu, 2.08; Glu, 2.20. Tritium exchange with solvent was followed at each step in the preparation and was negligible. The specific activity of the peptide was 9,345 dpm/nmol.

For assay, peptide was dissolved in a minimal volume of 1 M KOH. This resulted in a solution of neutral pH which was then brought to the desired volume with H_2O; it was stored at 4°C and prior to assay was evaporated at reduced pressure to remove any traces of tritiated H_2O generated on storage.

Preparation of Vitamin K-Dependent Carboxylating System

A microsomal pellet, obtained from the livers of vitamin K-deficient rats (3), was extracted twice with a 40-fold excess (wt/vol) of cold acetone at 0°C in a Potter-Elvehjem homogenizer. After each extraction, the suspension was centrifuged at 7500 x g for 10 min at 4°C; the final pellet was dried under reduced pressure. The resulting powder was stored desiccated at 4°C; prior to assay, powder (50 mg/ml) was resuspended with a Potter-Elvehjem homogenizer in 0.25 M sucrose, 25 mM imidazole-HCl, pH 7.2, 2 mM dithiothreitol. The powder retains 70% of the carboxylating activity of the microsomal pellet, and the activity remains during storage (>75% after two weeks). A detailed study of the characteristics of this acetone powder vitamin K-dependent carboxylating system will be described elsewhere (12).

Conditions for Assay

The powder was incubated with the tritiated peptide in a total volume of 0.125 ml as described (3), with one modification. Pyridoxal-5'-phosphate (2 mM), reported by Suttie et al. (13) to stimulate carboxylation, has been included. After incubation, one aliquot of the deproteinized reaction mixture was desiccated at acid pH in a scintillation vial to remove remaining $NaH^{14}CO_3$ and then assayed for ^{14}C in a Searle Mark III liquid scintillation counter with a program that measured only 0.2% of the ^3H radioactivity present while retaining 70% efficiency for ^{14}C.

To measure ^3H release, an aliquot was placed in the side arm of a Thunberg vessel and frozen as the vessel was evacuated. The tube was placed in acetone/dry ice, and the ^3H in the water that lyophilized to the tube was counted at 40% efficiency.

Determination of CO_2 Content of Samples

The titration method described by Rose (14) was used with the following modifications. Incubation and titration were carried out in the sealed vial under N_2 that had been bubbled through KOH. $Ba(OH)_2$ was 10 mM; HCl was 10 mM. These modifications allowed detection of as little as 50 nmol of CO_2 with a reproducibility of ± 10%.

RESULTS

The tritiated pentapeptide could be carboxylated in the in vitro system as readily as commercially prepared unlabeled pentapeptide. Although ^3H should be released during these incubations from one or both Glu residues, it was possible that tritium would not be released in water and also that the tritium release would not be a vitamin K-dependent reaction. However, as shown in Table 1, 10 times more tritiated water was recovered from an incubation of the peptide with enzyme and vitamin K than was recovered when either the acetone powder or the vitamin was omitted, when the enzyme preparation was heated to 100°C, or when the complete system was assayed without incubation. The vitamin K-dependent tritium release,

TABLE 1. Vitamin K-Dependent ^3H Release

Condition	cpm
Complete system	1694
Omit acetone powder	94
Omit vitamin K	140
Boiled acetone powder	97
Complete system, no incubation	92

Incubations were for 30 min in room air at 27°C in a total volume of 130 µl. The reaction mixture contained 100 µl of resuspended acetone powder, 2 mM NADH, 2 mM pyridoxal 5'-phosphate, 1.6 mM tritiated pentapeptide (5 x 10^5 cpm), and either 5 µl of ethanol or 5 µg of vitamin menaquinone-3 (MK_3) in 5 µl of ethanol (penultimate addition). $NaHCO_3$ (0.5 µmol) was added last, and the tubes were capped during the incubation. Reactions were terminated by addition of 270 µl of 10% perchloric acid, and the mixtures were centrifuged to remove precipitated protein. An aliquot of the supernatant solution (200 µl) was assayed for tritiated water. Results are expressed as cpm for the entire 130 µl incubation mixture and are the average of triplicate determinations which differed by less than 15% (8).

which is a reflection of γC-H bond cleavage, could either precede or occur in concert with carboxylation. Although approximately 0.3% of the tritium on the peptide was recovered as water, the precise number of γC-H bonds cleaved during incubation cannot be determined without additional information: the isotope effect at the γ carbon is not known and, although it is quite unlikely, it is impossible to exclude the possibility that vitamin K-dependent tritium release occurs from both the β and the γ carbons. In addition, only a fraction of the tritium released may be recovered in water. This last possibility is unlikely since no tritium can be identified in molecules other than in the peptide and water after incubation. As shown in Fig. 1, time courses of tritium release from, and carboxylation of, the tritiated peptide paralleled each other throughout a 180-min incubation. If after 3 hr the acetone powder is centrifuged and resuspended with fresh reactants, no significant additional tritium release or carboxylation

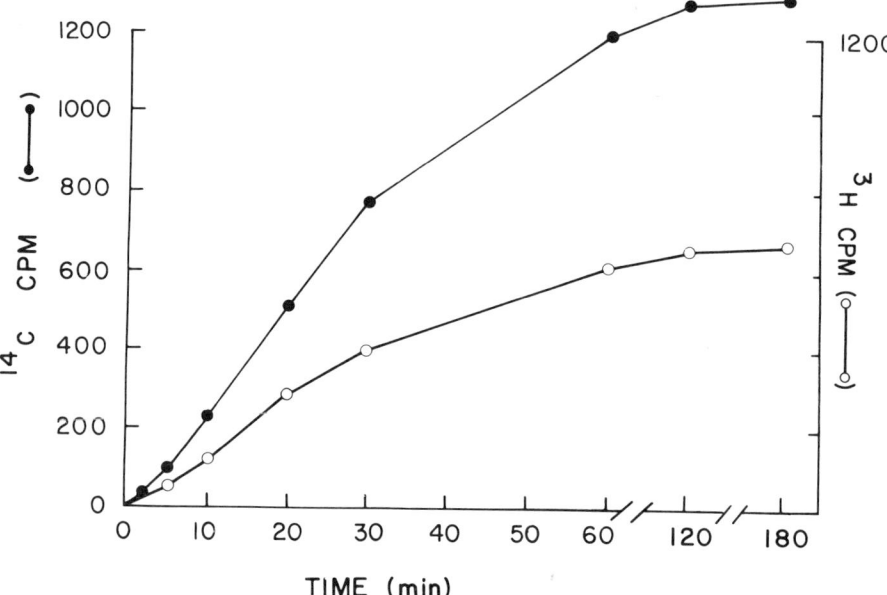

FIGURE 1. Time courses for carboxylation and tritium release. Incubations were for the times indicated; other conditions were as in Table 1. The last addition was 0.5 μmol of NaH^{14}CO$_3$ (specific activity 4000 cpm/nmol). One aliquot (100 μl) of the deproteinized reaction mixture was assayed for ^{14}C; a second (100 μl) was assayed for release of ^{3}H from the pentapeptide substrate (specific activity 3738 cpm/nmol). The results are the average of duplicate determinations from which controls incubated without vitamin K have been substracted and show the cpm measured in the respective aliquots (8).

occurs during further incubation. When we added known inhibitors of carboxylation to standard reaction mixtures or omitted compounds known to be required for carboxylation, we demonstrated a striking correlation between tritium release and carboxylation in every experiment (Table 2). In particular, tritium release and carboxylation required both the hydroquinone form of the vitamin and O$_2$. A recent study (15) suggests that a vitamin K hydroperoxide may be generated from the hydroquinone in the presence of O$_2$, and that this putative intermediate may support carboxylation. The data in Table 2 are compatible with the requirement for the formation of this intermediate to catalyze tritium release. Whether the stimulation by pyridoxal 5'-phosphate of ^{3}H release and carboxylation is an integral part in the carboxylation mechanism remains to be determined. As shown in Table 3, a detergent solubilized microsomal pellet, a better defined source for the vitamin K-dependent carboxylase, also catalyzes vitamin K-dependent ^{3}H release as water, as well as vitamin K-dependent fixing of ^{14}C. As has been reported (16), with this enzyme preparation vitamin K-dependent carboxylation is more efficient at lower temperatures; tritium release with this enzyme preparation also is more efficient at lower temperatures.

TABLE 2. Simultaneous Assay for Vitamin K-Dependent ^{14}C Fixation and ^3H Release Under Various Conditions

Condition	^{14}C fixed		[^3H]water recovered	
	cpm/incubation	%	cpm/incubation	%
Complete System	3756	100	1522	100
-NADH	404	11	134	9
-NADH, + vitamin K hydroquinone	3380	90	1354	89
-Dithiothreitol	3028	81	1332	88
-Pyridoxal 5'-phosphate	1728	46	684	45
-Pyridoxal 5'-phosphate, + pyridoxine	1368	36	536	35
-Oxygen	44	1	30	2
+Tetrachloropyridinol (50 μg/ml)	236	6	82	5
+2-Chloro-3-phytyl-1,4-naphthoquinone (50 μg/ml)	2176	58	926	61
+Warfarin (15 x μM)	3376	90	1358	89

Conditions were as described in Table 1. The last addition was 0.5 μmol of NaH^4CO_3 (4×10^6 cpm/μmol). The hydroquinone of vitamin MK_3, which was generated from the quinone with $NaBH_4$, was used immediately. Deproteinized reaction mixtures were assayed for ^{14}C and ^3H as described in Methods. Results are the average of triplicate determinations from which the appropriate control incubated without vitamin K has been subtracted (8).

TABLE 3. Simultaneous Assay for ^{14}C Fixation and ^3H Release Using a Triton X-100 Solubilized Microsomal Pellet as Enzyme Source

Condition	^{14}C fixed cpm/incubation	[^3H]water recovered cpm/incubation
17°; 45 min	7005	5091
17°; 90 min	8467	6883
8°;180 min	7200	6419

Conditions were as described in Table 2 except that the vitamin was phylloquinol (80 μg/ml). Temperature and time of incubation are indicated.

These data demonstrated correlation between tritium release and carboxylation, but they did not prove that a carboxylation must accompany each γC-H bond cleavage. By measuring the specific activities of $NaH^{14}CO_3$ in the reaction mixtures, the amounts of CO_2 fixed in incubations in which the bicarbonate concentrations are varied can be determined and compared with the recovery of tritiated water. When fixing of CO_2 and ^3H release are measured over a range of bicarbonate concentrations, there is essentially no change in the amounts of vitamin K-dependent ^3H released in experiments in which the amounts of CO_2 fixed varied by more than 10-fold (Table 4). If we assume that there is no ^3H released at the beta position, that all ^3H released is recovered as water and that the enzyme acts chirally as would be anticipated in these reactions, about 1950-2300 pmole of Glu undergo γC-H bond cleavage. This value, which is already 24-fold more than the amount of γ-CGlu formed at the lowest bicarbonate concentration, would be further increased if a significant isotope effect existed or if

TABLE 4. Dissociation of Vitamin K-Dependent Tritium Release from Carboxylation

HCO_3^- mM	CO_2 fixed pmol	[^{3}H]water recovered cpm	γC-H bonds cleaved[a] pmol
0.2	92	1669	1985
0.5	221	1869	2222
1	390	1816	2160
2	654	1922	2285
4	1028	1642	1952

Incubations were as described in Table 1 with the following exceptions: prior to the addition of bicarbonate, the test tubes were sealed with serum caps and the gas phase was made N_2/O_2 (80:20); reactions were initiated by injecting the indicated amounts of $NaHCO_3$ (containing 1.3×10^6 cpm of $NaH^{14}CO_3$) through the serum caps. Bicarbonate concentrations at zero time were determined by measuring total CO_2. For this, reaction mixtures identical to those that were incubated were made up in the sealed vials used for CO_2 determination. Extensive bubbling of reagent solutions with N_2 and multiple precipitations and resuspensions of the acetone powder in N_2-treated buffer reduced the total CO_2 concentration of reaction mixtures before addition of $NaH^{14}CO_3$ to less than 0.05 mM. No change in the specific activity of the bicarbonate occurred during incubations under these conditions. Results are the average of triplicate determinations from which controls without vitamin K have been subtracted.

[a]Calculations are based on the assumptions that no tritium is released from the β carbon, that all tritium is released in water, that a negligible isotope effect exists at the γ carbon, and that the enzyme is acting chirally. See text for details (8).

there were ^{3}H transfer to molecules other than water. Conversely, in the unlikely event that vitamin K were catalyzing the release of all the ^{3}H from Glu, γC-H bond cleavage of 490-575 pmol of Glu would have occurred. Since time courses (data not shown) of ^{3}H release at the bicarbonate concentrations used in Table 4 are parallel, the results cannot be explained by a prolongation of ^{3}H release at the lower bicarbonate concentrations. Rather, the experiment demonstrates that γC-H bond cleavage and carboxylation can be uncoupled.

DISCUSSION

The vitamin K-dependent carboxylating enzyme system will carboxylate appropriate endogenous protein substrates as well as certain added oligopeptides; the enzyme requires oxygen, CO_2 or bicarbonate, and the hydroquinone form of the vitamin; neither ATP nor biotin appears involved in the carboxylation (1-5,7). While the enzyme has been solubilized partially with nonionic detergents, it has not yet been extensively purified; hence, detailed mechanistic studies have been impossible. Conclusions concerned with reaction mechanism drawn from experiments conducted on enzyme systems as crude as those used here are fraught with hazard. Nonetheless, the data reported here are particularly compelling. It would seem that a concerted mechanism requiring an active form of the vitamin, enzyme, substrate, and CO_2 is not possible, and the data are equally incompatible with the concept that the vitamin functions solely to activate or transfer CO_2. Vitamin K is required for cleavage of the γC-H bond of appropriate glutamyl residues whether or not a carboxylation ensues. The data remain compatible with the possibility that, in addition, the vitamin is involved in the carboxylation event.

Finally, dissociation of γC-H bond cleavage from carboxylation raises the interesting possibility that vitamin K-dependent γC-H cleavage could precede the addition of reactants other than CO_2 to appropriate carbon atoms. Recently, both the vitamin K menaquinone-4 and its 2,3-epoxide have been identified in several invertebrate species (17) in which γCGlu has not yet been found.

ACKNOWLEDGEMENTS

This research was supported by U.S. Public Health Service Grant HL 11414. Dr. Friedman is the recipient of Research Career Development Award HD 00023.

REFERENCES

1. Jones, J. P., Gardner, E. J., Cooper, T. G., and Olsen, R.E. (1977) J. Biol. Chem. 252, 7738-7742.
2. Esmon, C. T., Sadowski, J. A., and Suttie, J. W. (1975) J. Biol. Chem. 250, 4744-4748.
3. Friedman, P. A., and Shia, M. A. (1976) Biochem. Biophys. Res. Commun. 72, 589-597.
4. Jones, J. P., Fausto, A., Houser, R. M., Gardner, E. J., and Olsen, R. (1976) Biochem. Biophys. Res. Commun. 72, 589-597.
5. Friedman, P. A., and Shia, M. A. (1977) Biochem. J. 163, 39-43.
6. Stubbe, J., and Abeles, R. H. (1977) J. Biol. Chem. 252, 8338-8340.
7. Suttie, J. W., Hageman, J. M., Lehrman, S. R., and Rich, D. H. (1976) J. Biol. Chem. 251, 5827-5830.
8. Friedman, P. A., Shia, M. A., Gallop, P. M., and Griep, A. E. (1979) Proc. Natl. Acad. Sci. USA, in press.
9. Stewart, J. M., Young, J. D., Benjamin, E., Shimizu, M., and Leung, C. Y. (1966) Biochemistry 5, 3396-3400.
10. Carpino, L. A. (1957) J. Am. Chem. Soc. 79, 4427-4431.
11. Stewart, J. M., and Young, J. D. (1969) Solid Phase Peptide Synthesis, pp. 40-41, Freeman, San Francisco.
12. Friedman, P. A., and Shia, M. A., unpublished data.
13. Suttie, J. W., Larson, A. E., Canfield, L. M., and Carlisle, T. L. (1978) Fed. Proc. Fed. Proc. Am. Soc. Exp. Biol. 37, 1605-2609.
14. Rose, J. G. (1976) Anal. Biochem. 76, 358-360.
15. Larson, A. E., and Suttie, J. W. (1978) Proc. Natl. Acad. Sci. USA 75, 5413-5416.
16. Suttie, J. W., Lehrman, S. R., Geweke, L. O., Hageman, J. M., and Rich, D. H. (1979) Biochem. Biophys. Res. Commun. 86, 500-507.
17. Burt, V. T., Bee, R., and Pennock, J. F. (1977) Biochem. J. 162, 297-302.

A RADICAL-RADICAL C-CARBOXYLATION REACTION AS A MODEL RELATED TO THE VITAMIN K-DEPENDENT CARBOXYLATION

PAUL M. GALLOP, PAUL A. FRIEDMAN*, and EDWARD HENSON

Departments of Orthopaedic Surgery,
Biological Chemistry, and Oral Biology,
Harvard Schools of Medicine and Dental Medicine,
Children's Hospital Medical Center;
and Center for Blood Research*;
Boston, MA 02115

INTRODUCTION

Recent work on the mechanism of the vitamin K-dependent protein carboxylation reaction has shown that both oxygen and the reduced form of the vitamin, vitamin K hydroquinone (KH_2) are required (1,2). Friedman et al., (3) were able to show that the glutamate substrate to be carboxylated was first oxidized as measured by tritium release and that this KH_2 and O_2 dependent oxidation could proceed without a concerted or concurrent CO_2 dependent carboxylation.

DISCUSSION OF POSSIBLE MODELS

Consideration of the basic outlines of various mechanisms consistent with the data suggested that the oxidation of KH_2 by oxygen was accompanied by either formation of a peptide substrate radical or a peptide substrate carbanion. Either generation of vitamin K hydroperoxide as an oxidant or a mixed function oxidative process could be involved. If a substrate carbanion was produced, it could then be carboxylated directly by carbon dioxide. However, if a substrate radical was produced, it could be carboxylated by a radical formed by reduction of carbon dioxide generated in the course of the overall oxidation of vitamin KH_2 to vitamin K epoxide. In Figure 1, these options are depicted to give reactions IA, IB or IIA and IIB as the possible mechanisms. Current evidence from Suttie's group (4) which suggests that a hydroperoxide may be the oxidant required by the peptide substrate would then favor route I, although it is too premature to rule out the MFO option depicted as route II.

In route A the substrate radical, S·, is further reduced by the K semi-quinone intermediate to generate a substrate carbanion which is carboxylated by CO_2. In the B route carbon dioxide is reduced by the vitamin K semiquinone intermediate, but not necessarily directly, to form a carbon dioxide radical species which condenses with the substrate radical leading to carboxylation. The B route which we currently favor by chemical intuition and not yet by any solid evidence can be tested by attempting to trap the carbon dioxide radical species by an appropriate one electron or hydrogen atom reduction which would lead to the formation of labelled formic acid. Such a detection reaction must be able to proceed specifically from the CO_2 radical to formate, but not from CO_2 to formate. It is also possible that CO_2 radical might, by a side reaction, couple to form oxalate or react with other species to form formate or other products and thereby reveal its transient existence.

In this paper we will discuss the Bernardi reaction (5) which has features which may relate to the B reaction route depicted in Fig. 1.

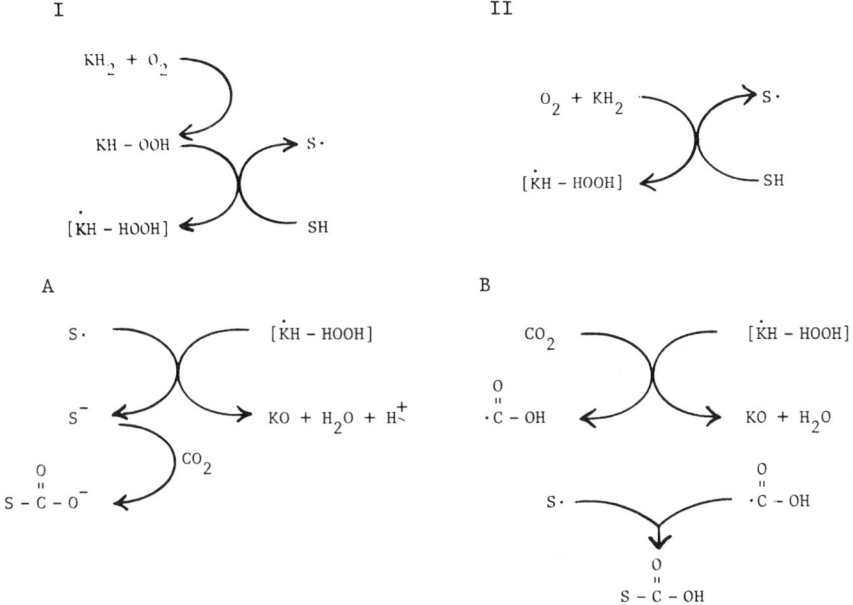

Figure 1

In the Bernardi reaction, one electron oxidation species are generated by ferrous ion and hydrogen peroxide. Oxidation of γ-ketoacid ethyl esters by the one electron oxidant generates ethoxycarbonyl radicals:

$$R - \overset{O}{\underset{\|}{C}} - \overset{O}{\underset{\|}{C}} - OEt + Fe^{++} + H_2O_2 \longrightarrow R - \overset{O}{\underset{\|}{C}} - OH + Fe^{+++} + OH^- + \cdot \overset{O}{\underset{\|}{C}} - OEt$$

In the presence of other appropriately generated radicals, carboxyethylation can occur:

$$R'H + Fe^{++} + H_2O_2 \longrightarrow R'\cdot + Fe^{+++} + OH^- + H_2O$$

$$R'\cdot + \cdot \overset{O}{\underset{\|}{C}}OEt \longrightarrow R' : \overset{O}{\underset{\|}{C}}OEt$$

A typical Bernardi reaction which proceeds about 80% yield is as follows:

[benzothiazole]-CH + CH$_3$ - $\overset{O}{\underset{\|}{C}}$ - $\overset{O}{\underset{\|}{C}}$OEt + 2Fe^{++} + 2H$_2O_2$ $\longrightarrow$

[benzothiazole]-C - $\overset{O}{\underset{\|}{C}}$OEt + 2Fe^{+++} + 2OH$^-$ + H$_2$O

Here the generation of the radical carboxylating species is by a one electron oxidation of a ketoacid ester.

In route B of the vitamin K dependent reaction described above, we are postulating a one electron or hydrogen atom reduction of CO_2 to the carboxylation radical by the vitamin K semiquinone or an intermediate (I) derived from it:

$$CO_2 + \dot{K}H \longrightarrow \cdot\overset{O}{\overset{\|}{C}}-OH + K$$

or

$$CO_2 + [\dot{K}H + HOOH] \longrightarrow \cdot\overset{O}{\overset{\|}{C}}-OH + KO + H_2O$$

or

$$\dot{K}H + I \longrightarrow I^{\frac{\cdot}{}} + K + H^+$$

and

$$I^{\frac{\cdot}{}} + CO_2 \longrightarrow I + \cdot\overset{O}{\overset{\|}{C}}-O^-$$

It is also noteworthy to remark that additional evidence exists for the production of carbon dioxide radical (6). In a system where CO_2 under pressure is in contact with water containing appropriate electron carriers, irradiation with light causes the formation of radical anions and cations:

$$2h\nu + 2A + 2B \longrightarrow 2A^{\frac{\cdot}{}} + 2B^{\overset{\cdot}{+}}$$

$$2A^{\frac{\cdot}{}} + 2CO_2 \longrightarrow 2\cdot\overset{O}{\overset{\|}{C}}-O^- + 2A$$

$$2\cdot\overset{O}{\overset{\|}{C}}-O^- \longrightarrow \begin{array}{c}\overset{O}{\overset{\|}{C}}-O^-\\ |\\ C-O^-\\ \overset{\|}{O}\end{array}$$

$$2B^{\overset{\cdot}{+}} + 2H_2O \longrightarrow 2B + HOOH + 2H^+$$

sum:

$$2h\nu + 2CO_2 + 2H_2O \longrightarrow \begin{array}{c}\overset{O}{\overset{\|}{C}}-OH\\ |\\ C-OH\\ \overset{\|}{O}\end{array} + HOOH$$

In such systems both oxalate, formate and hydrogen peroxide are produced with appropriate electron carriers present:

$$2h\nu + 2CO_2 + 2H_2O \xrightarrow{A,B} \begin{array}{c}\overset{O}{\overset{\|}{C}}-OH\\ |\\ C-OH\\ \overset{\|}{O}\end{array} + HOOH$$

$$h\nu + CO_2 + 2H_2O \xrightarrow{A,B} H-\overset{O}{\overset{\|}{C}}-OH + HOOH$$

In a system employed by the above authors (6; cited in Chem. Eng. News, April 9, 1979, p. 31), 70% aqueous acetonitrile with CO_2 at 70 psi was irradiated for 6 hours with a 300W high pressure mercury arc lamp. The solution contained dimethylaniline as an electron donor, terephthalonitrile as an electron acceptor, and pyrene as a sensitizer. A 3×10^{-5} M solution of formic acid was produced. When dithionite was added, 1.7×10^{-4} formic acid and 1.1×10^{-4} oxalic acid was produced. The authors suggest that light converts pyrene into a radical cation and terephthalonitrile to a radical anion. The radical anion reacts with CO_2 to form a carbon dioxide radical anion with regeneration of neutral terephthalonitrile. Two carbon dioxide radicals could condense to yield oxalate or the carbon dioxide could react with various hydrogen atom donors to form formic acid.

Hence, it is our current view that in the vitamin K-dependent formation of γ-carboxyglutamic acid a substrate radical anion is formed from the glutamic acid residue and this is coupled to the oxidation of the hydroquinone form of vitamin K (KH_2):

$$KH_2 \quad O_2 \quad \rightarrow \quad R - \dot{C}H - \overset{O}{\underset{\|}{C}} - O^-$$

$$[\dot{K}H - HOOH] \quad \leftarrow \quad R - CH_2 - \overset{O}{\underset{\|}{C}} - O^-$$

Next CO_2 is converted, in a process dependent on, but perhaps not directly coupled to, the semiquinone form of vitamin K:

$$[KH\cdot - HOOH] \quad \rightarrow \quad \dot{X}H \quad \rightarrow \quad \cdot \overset{O}{\underset{\|}{C}} - OH$$

$$KO + HOH \quad \leftarrow \quad X \quad \leftarrow \quad CO_2$$

Finally, the substrate radical anion and the CO_2 radical condense to form γ-carboxyglutamic acid:

$$R - \underset{\gamma}{\dot{C}H} - \overset{O}{\underset{\|}{C}} - O^- \quad + \quad \cdot \overset{O}{\underset{\|}{C}} - OH \quad \longrightarrow \quad R - \underset{\gamma}{CH} \overset{\displaystyle \overset{O}{\underset{\|}{C}} - O^-}{\underset{\displaystyle \underset{O}{\underset{\|}{C}} - OH}{}}$$

We are attempting to trap the hypothetical radical intermediates. It is noteworthy also that if labelled formate or labelled oxalate are found as side products in microsomal preparations given O_2, labelled CO_2, vitamin K + NADPH, or vitamin KH_2, and appropriate substrates, this observation would add strong corroborative evidence for a radical-radical carboxylation mechanism. Such a mechanism is proposed here with carbon dioxide radical as an important intermediate. This radical-radical mode of CO_2 fixation and formation of a carbon-carbon bond is a new type of biological reaction. All other known types of CO_2 fixation whether via CO_2 or via an activated bicarbonate intermediate appear to proceed from a nucleophilic carbanion attack on the electrophilic CO_2 or activated intermediate. One wonders if other biological systems exist in which CO_2 radical or CO_2 radical anion formed by a one-electron reduction of carbon dioxide is then employed to form other carboxylated compounds such as oxalate or to react with further reduction to form formate. One also wonders if vitamin KH_2 oxidations and the intermediates formed could be employed to promote one-electron reductions of compounds other than carbon dioxide; perhaps this is related to the presence of vitamin K in many microorganisms and plants.

REFERENCES

1. Olson, R. E. and Suttie, J. W. (1977) Vit. Horm. 35, 59-108.
2. Stenflo, J. and Suttie, J. W. (1977) Ann. Rev. Biochem. 46, 157-172.
3. Friedman, P. A., Shia, M. A., Gallop, P. M., and Griep, A. E. (1979) Proc. Natl. Acad. Sci. USA, in press.
4. Larson, A. E., and Suttie, J. W. (1978) Proc. Natl. Acad. Sci. USA 75, 5413-5416.
5. Bernardi, R., Caronna, T., Galli, R., Minisci, F., and Perchinunno, M. (1973) Tetrahedron Lett. 9, 645-648.
6. Tazuke, S., and Kitamura, N. (1978) Nature 275, 301-302.

INVESTIGATION OF THE ROLE OF OXYGEN IN THE VITAMIN K-DEPENDENT CARBOXYLASE REACTION

A. E. LARSON, J. J. MCTIGUE, and J. W. SUTTIE

Department of Biochemistry
College of Agricultural and Life Sciences
University of Wisconsin-Madison
Madison, WI 53706

INTRODUCTION

Early studies of the liver microsomal vitamin K-dependent carboxylase which converts peptide-bound glutamyl residues to γ-carboxyglutamyl (Gla) residues (1,2) established that the system required molecular oxygen. The reduced form of the vitamin, vitamin KH_2, has also been demonstrated (1,2,3) to substitute for [vitamin K + NAD(P)H] in the system and it appears to be the active form of the vitamin for the carboxylase reaction. One possible role for oxygen in this system would therefore be as a terminal electron acceptor for the reoxidation of the hydroquinone to the quinone form of vitamin K. The discovery (4) of an active vitamin K hydroquinone 2,3-epoxidase (5) in liver microsomal preparations and the possible involvement of this reaction in the carboxylation reaction (6) has raised the possibility of another function for oxygen. The largely indirect data which suggest that the formation of vitamin K 2,3-epoxide is in some manner coupled to the carboxylation reaction have recently been reviewed (7,8). If the epoxidation reaction is directly involved in the carboxylase system, the oxygen requirement of the carboxylase could be explained by the need to form this product. This report describes some recent experiments which relate to the possible role of vitamin K 2,3-epoxide in the carboxylation reaction and which attempt to define the mechanism by which microsomes form an oxygen derivative of the vitamin.

METHODS

Vitamin K-dependent carboxylase assays utilizing the peptide substrate, Phe-Leu-Glu-Glu-Leu, were carried out in Triton X-100-solubilized microsomes from vitamin K-deficient rats by methods previously described (9). Details of the experiments utilizing glutathione peroxidase as an inhibitor of the carboxylase and epoxidase reactions and those utilizing t-Butyl-OOH as an agonist of vitamin K have been described (10). Alterations in the standard incubation conditions required to assess the possible existence of various forms of activated oxygen are described in the appropriate figure legends and tables.

RESULTS

Evidence for a Vitamin K Hydroperoxide Intermediate

One way for the epoxidation of vitamin K to be coupled to the vitamin K-dependent carboxylation reaction would be for both reactions to use a common intermediate. The most logical intermediate in the conversion of

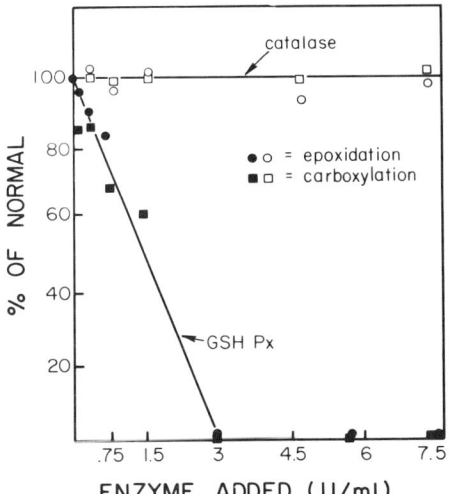

FIGURE 1. Effect of GSH-Px and catalase on vitamin K-dependent carboxylation and epoxidation. Incubations with GSH-Px contained purified enzyme, 2 mM glutathione, 2 U/ml glutathione reductase, 1 mM EDTA, 1 mg/ml NADPH, and 0.5 mM peptide. Vitamin KH_2 concentration was 10 μg/ml, and carboxylation and epoxidation were determined using aliquots of the same incubation. Catalase incubations had no GSH-Px, glutathione, EDTA, or glutathione reductase. Vitamin KH_2 concentration was 20 μg/ml for carboxylation and 4 μg/ml for epoxidation assays (10).

vitamin K to its 2,3-epoxide would be the 2- or 3-hydroperoxide of the vitamin. The enzyme glutathione-peroxidase (GSH-Px) will reduce a wide range of organic hydroperoxides to the corresponding alcohols; and, when increasing amounts of this enzyme were added to the standard incubation mixtures (Fig. 1), there was a corresponding inhibition of both vitamin K-dependent carboxylase activity and vitamin K-epoxidase activity. GSH-Px will also utilize H_2O_2 as a substrate, but the addition of catalase which would also act on H_2O_2 in the system had no influence on either reaction. These data strongly suggested that some type of vitamin K hydroperoxide might be an intermediate in the action of the vitamin K-dependent carboxylase, and suggested that other organic hydroperoxides might be agonists of the vitamin in this reaction. When the stable organic hydroperoxide, t-Butyl-OOH, was added to vitamin K-deficient rat liver microsomes in the absence of vitamin K (Table 1), a weak but significant carboxylation reaction was observed. When the carboxylated product was isolated, the relatively high blank was eliminated and the stimulation by t-Butyl-OOH was about ten-fold over background. Subsequent experiments demonstrated

TABLE 1. Stimulation of the carboxylation of Phe-Leu-Glu-Glu-Leu by t-Butyl-OOH.

Stage of Product Purification	dpm/ml		Stimulation % of Cont.
	− t-Butyl-OOH	+ t-Butyl-OOH	
Perchlorate supernatant	8000	13,300	166
Isolated product	450	4,410	980

The incubations contained 0.5 mM substrate, 1 mM NADPH, and when included, 20 μl/ml of t-Butyl-OOH in the standard triton X-100 solubilized microsomal preparation. The radioactivity in the isolated (15) carboxylated product was shown to be present as Gla by thin-layer chromatography of the acid and base hydrolysis product (10). The inclusion of t-Butyl-OOH in the incubation also stimulated the incorporation of $^{14}CO_2$ into endogenous microsomal proteins (10).

that this stimulation was inhibited by GSH-Px and that the requirement for O_2 was eliminated when t-Butyl-OOH, rather than vitamin KH_2, was utilized to drive the carboxylation reaction. Further evidence that the action of t-Butyl-OOH in stimulating the carboxylation is related to some normal function of the enzyme was gained by the demonstration that this compound acts as an apparent competitive inhibitor of both the carboxylation and epoxidation reactions (Fig. 2). The mechanism by which t-Butyl-OOH is able to function as an analog of vitamin K is not yet clear; it may be that it directly substitutes for a vitamin hydroperoxide to drive the carboxylation event or it may be activating some component of the system that normally interacts with an oxygenated form of vitamin K, and this component subsequently catalyzes the actual carboxylation event.

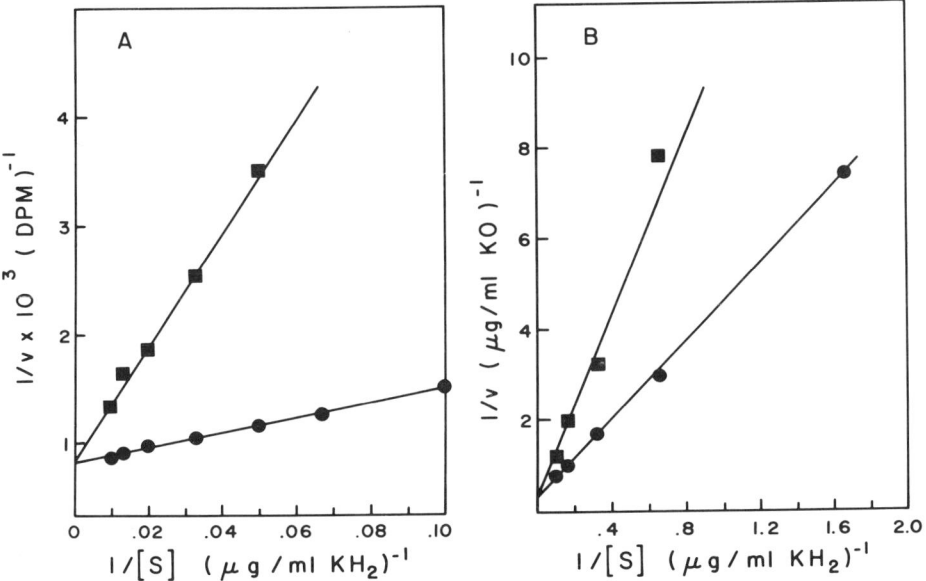

FIGURE 2. Double reciprocal plots of vitamin K-dependent peptide carboxylase (A) and vitamin K epoxidase (B) activity in the presence and absence of 10 mM t-Butyl-OOH. Apparent K_i's were 10 mM for epoxidation and 2.5 mM for carboxylation. —●— No t-butyl-OOH; —■— + t-Butyl-OOH.

Possible Role of a Vitamin Hydroperoxide

Possible roles suggested (7,11) for a vitamin K hydroperoxide in the carboxylase reaction have included the stabilization of a vitamin K hydroquinone carbonate ester or the formation of percarbonate at the 2- or 3-position of the vitamin. The available evidence (12,13) would suggest that the vitamin is not involved in CO_2 transfer, but rather that it functions by labilizing the hydrogen on the γ-position of the substrate glutamyl residue so that some form of CO_2 may attack. The data of Friedman et al. (14) on the vitamin K-dependent exchange of tritium from this position would strongly support this hypothesis.

It has been demonstrated (5) that the oxygen of the vitamin K epoxide ring arises from molecular oxygen, and it is possible that the epoxide may be generated from a vitamin hydroperoxide as part of a reaction where the hydroperoxide is acting to labilize a γ-hydrogen of the glutamic acid residues. Among the possible carboxylation mechanisms involving the hydroperoxide form of the vitamin is one which would require the incorporation of an oxygen atom from the hydroperoxide into the substrate. This pathway requires the vitamin to aid in the abstraction of the γ-hydrogen by forming a peroxyester with a glutamyl residue (Fig. 3). The strong electron attracting nature of the acyloxy group would increase the stability of a carbanion formed if the γ-hydrogen was removed as a proton and facilitate the attack of CO_2. Subsequent breakdown of the acyloxy group would leave one of the original oxygen atoms on the Glu residue.

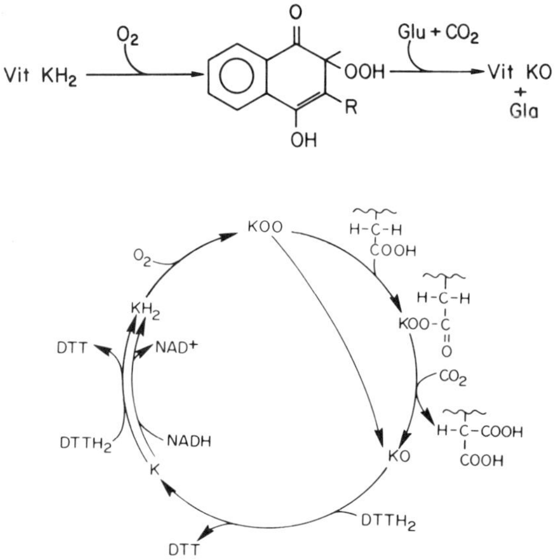

FIGURE 3. (Top) Generalized mechanism showing the formation of a hydroperoxide of the vitamin and the utilization of this species to drive the carboxylation and be converted to vitamin K epoxide (KO). (Bottom) A hypothetical scheme which would use a hydroperoxide or peroxyradical of the vitamin (KOO) to form a peroxyester of the glutamic acid residue and to promote the carboxylation. In in vitro systems KO is reduced by dithiothreitol (DTT), and the vitamin is reduced to the hydroquinone (KH_2) by DTT or by NADH.

To test for the possible existence of this pathway, rat liver microsomes were incubated with a simple low-molecular-weight substrate of the enzyme, t-BOC-Glu-α-benzyl-ester (15) in the presence of $^{14}CO_2$ and in an atmosphere of 15% $^{18}O_2$ and 85% N_2 for 4 h at 0° C. This incubation resulted in an overall enzyme catalyzed conversion of 0.01% of the substrate into the corresponding γ-carboxyglutamic acid derivative. The product was purified by DEAE-sephadex ion exchange chromatography and Bio-Gel P-2 exclusion chromatography with a recovery of 80%. To obtain a volatile derivative for mass spectral analysis, the Gla-containing product was reacted with diazomethane and the methyl esterified product (0.3 μmoles) was purified by silica gel chromatography on 1,000 micron plates (hexane-ethyl acetate 9:1 (v/v)). The mass fragmentation spectrum of the methylated Gla derivative did not exhibit a molecular ion peak because the benzyl group was lost during isolation of the product prior to methylation and because of instability of the t-Butyl-functional groups. The parent molecular ions in the spectrum would, therefore, be those of tri-methyl-t-BOC-γ-carboxyglutamic acid (mw 333). The mass fragmentation spectrum of the ^{18}O-incubated system (Fig. 4) was found to exhibit peaks characteristic of fragments derived from the expected γ-carboxyglutamic acid product at m/e 277 (M-56, loss of t-Butyl), 218 (277-59, loss of carboxymethyl), and 174 (218-44, loss of CO_2). These fragmentation peaks were identical to the peaks obtained for the ^{16}O-incubated system and indicated that the ^{18}O-isotope was not present. The small isotope labeling exhibited at major peaks + 2 m/e is due to the presence of the small amount of $NaH^{14}CO_3$ present in the incubation in order to follow the carboxylated product during the purification procedure. These data suggest that peroxyester formation with a glutamyl residue is not the mechanism by which a hydroperoxide participates in the carboxylation reaction.

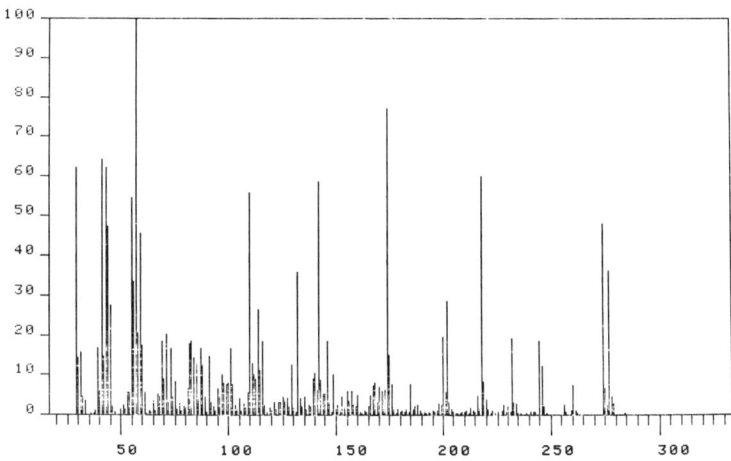

FIGURE 4. Mass fragmentation spectrum of tri-methyl-t-BOC-Gla isolated from an incubation containing $^{18}O_2$.

Vitamin K-O_2 Interaction

The available evidence suggests that the oxygenation of vitamin K, at least to a hydroperoxide, plays an important role in the carboxylation reaction. Ground state, or triplet oxygen, is a diradical; and, because of spin conservation principles, it cannot react directly with an organic molecule such as vitamin K which has no unpaired electrons to form singlet products. For all organic oxygenation reactions, there must be either free radical intermediates or an activation of oxygen, an activation of the substrate to a radical, or a metal oxygen complex in which the electrons are delocalized. Biologically active oxygen species which might conceivably be involved include superoxide ($\cdot O_2^-$), a hydroxyl radical ($\cdot OH$), and singlet oxygen ($^1O_2$). The possible role of these various species in the oxygenation of vitamin K and in the carboxylase reaction was therefore investigated through the use of specific scavengers of the active species and through the use of systems to generate these active forms of oxygen.

The $^1O_2$ scavengers, β-carotene and diphenylfuran, did not inhibit either the carboxylation or epoxidation reactions. Diphenylfuran forms cis-dibenzoylethylene when it reacts with $^1O_2$ in the standard detergent-solubilized microsome preparation as judged by this method (data not shown). Superoxide dismutase (SOD) which catalyzes the reaction ($2 \cdot O_2^- + 2H^+ \rightarrow H_2O_2 + O_2$) has been used as a scavenger to indicate the involvement of

TABLE 2. Effect of superoxide dismutase on vitamin K-dependent carboxylation and vitamin K epoxidation.

Superoxide Dismutase	Vitamin K-dependent Carboxylation % of Control	Vitamin K Epoxidation % of Control
0	100	100
2 µg/ml	96	–
8 µg/ml	90	–
20 µg/ml	90	–
40 µg/ml	87	100
40 µg/ml + 50 U/ml catalase	95	100

Incubations were done in 0.025 M imidazole, 0.125 M K_2SO_4, 0.25 M KCl, and 0.2% triton X-100 instead of the usual SIK-1.5% Triton system. Superoxide dismutase (3760 U/mg) was obtained from Sigma.

·O_2^- in various reactions (16). In solubilized microsomes, SOD at levels less than 2 µg/ml had no effect on either vitamin K-dependent carboxylation or epoxidation (Table 2). At higher levels, SOD slightly inhibited the system. This inhibition was partly relieved by catalase, suggesting that the slight inhibition seen was due to production of H_2O_2 by the SOD. In addition, Kellog and Fridovich (17) have shown that SOD acts as a peroxidase at concentrations greater than 10 µg/ml. The slight inhibition of the carboxylase observed in the presence of SOD might therefore be occurring by the same mechanism as the inhibition seen in the presence of GSH-Px. Generation of ·O_2^- by a xanthine/xanthine oxidase system or a KO_2/NaOH system did not stimulate either carboxylation or epoxidation, again making it unlikely that ·O_2^- is the active species of oxygen involved in these reactions.

The effect of various radical scavengers on the carboxylase system was also investigated. The data shown in Figure 5 indicate that these were effective inhibitors of the vitamin K-dependent systems. Para-nitrosodimethylaniline (PNDA) which was a good inhibitor of both carboxylation and epoxidation has been reported (18) to react with ·OH but not other oxyradicals. However, spectrophotometric analysis indicated that PNDA reacted with menadione semiquinone and would presumably also react with vitamin K

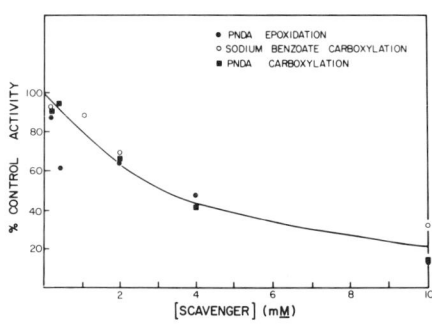

FIGURE 5. Effect of the addition of radical scavengers on the vitamin K-dependent carboxylation reaction and the vitamin K epoxidase reaction. All activities are expressed relative to the uninhibited control. PNDA = Para-nitrosodimethylaniline.

semiquinone. The possible involvement of ·OH was also investigated through the generation of ·OH with a Fenton system, and it was found that this system did not stimulate carboxylation in either the presence or absence of additional oxygen. These data would suggest that ·OH is not involved in the carboxylase or epoxidase reactions. However, hydroxyl radical is a very reactive species and may be so destructure to the system that no stimulation would be observed from its generation.

TABLE 3. Stimulation of carboxylation and epoxidation by UV irradiation with dithiothreitol.

Treatment	Carboxylase (dpm)		Epoxidase nMole KO/g Liver
	Bkg	+KH$_2$	+KH$_2$
No UV	111	665	1.4
10 sec UV	130	1328	2.1

1 mM DTT was added to triton-solubilized microsomes immediately before irradiation. Irradiation was with a short-wave mineral light, approximately 2 x 10^3 μwatt/cm^2. Peptide, vitamin KH$_2$, and H^{14}CO$_3$ were added immediately after irradiation.

An alternate mechanism to those considered above would be that dioxygen is not activated but rather that the first step in the oxygenation may be reaction of molecular O$_2$ with a vitamin K semiquinone to form a hydroperoxide or hydroperoxide radical. This hypothesis is supported by the data in Table 3 which show that irradiation of the standard microsomal preparation in the presence of dithiothreitol stimulates carboxylation approximately two fold and stimulates epoxidation somewhat less. Irradiation of DTT is known to form DTT radicals (19) which probably interact with vitamin K or vitamin K hydroquinone to form the semiquinone. The data in Figure 5 demonstrate that the addition of vitamin K semiquinone to the vitamin KH$_2$-driven carboxylation reaction significantly stimulates the initial rate of carboxylation above that observed with vitamin KH$_2$ alone. These observations also support a mechanism involving the vitamin K semiquinone.

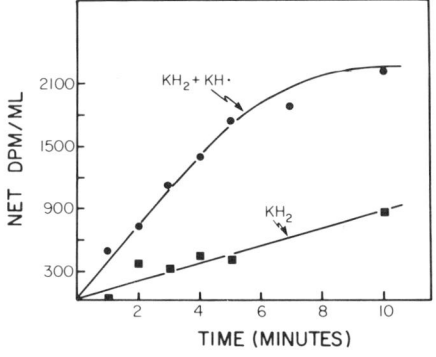

FIGURE 6. Time course of peptide carboxylation with vitamin K hydroquinone and vitamin K semiquinone. Vitamin K semiquinone was produced by irradiation of an anaerobic solution of vitamin K quinone. Vitamin KH$_2$ was 50 μg/ml and vitamin K semiquinone was 5 μg/ml. Incubations were done at 25° C and were warmed to temperature by a 30-sec preincubation prior to addition of the vitamin.

DISCUSSION AND CONCLUSION

These data strongly suggest that a hydroperoxide of vitamin K is the active oxygenated species involved in the carboxylation reaction and provide additional evidence that carboxylation is closely associated with the vitamin K epoxidation reaction. Whether t-Butyl-OOH is acting as an analog of the presumed hydroperoxide intermediate when it is used to stimulate carboxylation or if its role is more indirect cannot be ascertained at this time. However, any reaction mechanism proposed must be consistent with the observation that this organic hydroperoxide can be used to drive the carboxylation reaction that forms γ-carboxyglutamic acid.

There is no direct evidence available at the present time to indicate how a vitamin K hydroperoxide could be used to mediate the carboxylation event. There is little evidence to suggest that the vitamin is associated with CO_2 activation or transfer in this system, and it is more likely that it is used to labilize a hydrogen at the γ-position of the glutamyl residue. A vitamin K hydroperoxide could be directly involved in the removal of a proton or hydrogen radical from the γ-position, or it could be used to stabilize a radical formed by some other means or to increase the acidity of the γ-hydrogen. One possible mechanism of action would be through the formation of a peroxyacyl derivative of the glutamyl residue which would have much the same influence on the hydrogen α to this carboxyl group as would the formation of a thioester. The breakdown of such an intermediate should lead to the incorporation of $^{18}O_2$ into the carboxylated product. The experiments reported here indicate that no such incorporation could be detected, and this mechanism seems unlikely.

The data presented here also suggest that the presumed hydroperoxide or any other oxygenated form of the vitamin is not formed by the interaction of an activated oxygen species with the vitamin, but rather by an attack of the semiquinone form of the vitamin on oxygen. Although far from conclusions, the data obtained fail to provide any evidence that any of the activated oxygenated species investigated are involved in the carboxylation reaction. The stimulation of the carboxylase system by the direct generation of vitamin K semiquinone would support indirect evidence (3,20) of the involvement of this species in the reaction and again argue against the need for oxygen activation. It has been reported (21) that superoxide is an

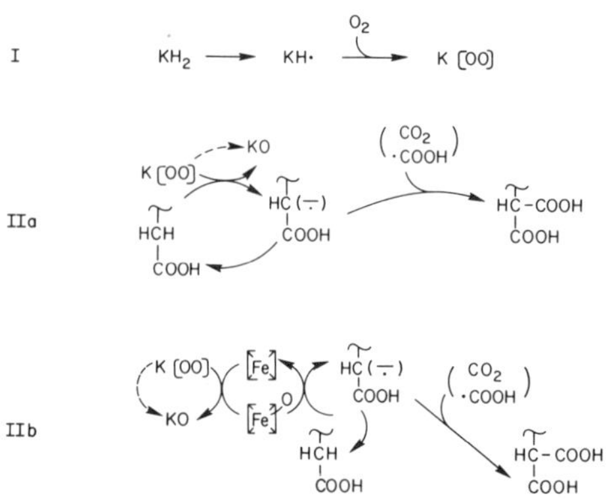

FIGURE 7. Possible molecular role of vitamin K. Current evidence would suggest (I) that the attacks of the semiquinone (KH·) on oxygen forms some oxygenated intermediate (hydroperoxide or peroxyradical). This intermediate may then be used (IIa) to drive the carboxylation event and generate the epoxide. Either a radical or carbanion on the γ-carbon of the glutamyl residue could be used, and the electronic nature of the attacking species is not known. It is also possible (IIb) that the vitamin intermediate is used to activate a heme or other reaction center which drives the carboxylation. In either case, it must be possible for the epoxide to form without the carboxylation reaction occurring. Other mechanisms of vitamin action are not ruled out by the available data.

important component of the reaction. The data presented here fail to support this observation, and it is likely that the large amounts of superoxide dismutase used in the previous experiments led to artifactual results. The data reported here have cleared up some of the questions associated with the involvement of oxygen in the vitamin K epoxidation--vitamin K-dependent carboxylation reaction, but have failed to provide any clear evidence of a unique molecular mechanism. The hypothetical reactions shown in Figure 7 are consistent with the available data and provide models which can be used to stimulate further investigation.

ACKNOWLEDGEMENTS

This research was supported by the College of Agricultural and Life Sciences, University of Wisconsin-Madison, and in part by grants AM-14881, DE-07031, and GM-07215 from the National Institutes of Health.

REFERENCES

1. Sadowski, J. A., Esmon, C. T., and Suttie, J. W. (1976) J. Biol. Chem. 251, 2770-2775.
2. Friedman, P. A., and Shia, M. (1976) Biochem. Biophys. Res. Commun. 70, 647-654.
3. Girardot, J.-M., Mack, D. O., Floyd, R. A., and Johnson, B. C. (1976) Biochem. Biophys. Res. Commun. 70, 655-662.
4. Matschiner, J. T., Bell, R. G., Amelotti, J. M., and Knauer, T. E. (1970) Biochim. Biophys. Acta. 201, 309-315.
5. Sadowski, J. A., Schnoes, H. K., and Suttie, J. W. (1977) Biochemistry 16, 3856-3863.
6. Willingham, A. K., and Matschiner, J. T. (1974) Biochem. J. 140, 435-441.
7. Suttie, J. W., Larson, A. E., Canfield, L. M., and Carlisle, T. L. (1978) Fed. Proc. 37, 2605-2609.
8. Bell, R. G. (1978) Fed. Proc. 37, 2599-2604.
9. Suttie, J. W., Hageman, J. M., Lehrman, S. R., and Rich, D. H. (1976) J. Biol. Chem. 251, 5827-5830.
10. Larson, A. E., and Suttie, J. W. (1978) Proc. Natl. Acad. Sci. USA 75, 5413-5416.
11. Olson, R. E., and Suttie, J. W. (1978) Vitamins and Hormones 35, 59-108.
12. Suttie, J. W., and Jackson, C. M. (1977) Physiol. Rev. 57, 1-70.
13. Suttie, J. W. (1978) In Handbook of Lipid Research 2, "The Fat-soluble Vitamins" (DeLuca, H. F., ed.) pp. 211-277, Plenum Press, NY.
14. Friedman, P. A., Shia, M. A., Gallop, P. M., and Griep, A. E. (1979) Proc. Natl. Acad. Sci. USA, in press.
15. Finnan, J. L., and Suttie, J. W. (1979) these proceedings.
16. Strobel, H. W., and Coon, M. S. (1971) J. Biol. Chem. 246, 7826-7829.
17. Kellog, E. W., and Fridovich, I. (1975) J. Biol. Chem. 250, 8812-8817.
18. Rigo, A., Stevanato, R., Finazzi-Agro, a., and Rotilio, G. (1977) FEBS Letters 80, 130-132.
19. Haugaard, N. (1968) Physiol. Rev. 48, 311-373.
20. Wallin, R. (1979) Biochem. J. 178, in press.
21. Esnouf, M. P., Green, M. R., Allen, H., Hill, O., Irvine, G., and Walter, S. J. (1978) Biochem. J. 174, 345-348.

THE ROLE OF SUPEROXIDE IN THE CARBOXYLATION OF GLUTAMYL RESIDUES

M. P. ESNOUF*, A. I. BURGESS, S. J. WALTER*, M. R. GREEN,
H. A. O. HILL and M. J. OKOLOW-ZUBKOWSKA

Nuffield Department of Clinical Biochemistry*,
The Radcliffe Infirmary and Inorganic Chemistry Laboratory,
South Parks Rd., Oxford, United Kingdom

INTRODUCTION

The present view of the vitamin K dependent carboxylation of glutamic acid residues has been well reviewed by Olson & Suttie (1) and Suttie et al., (2). The mechanism that is proposed is essentially that a hydroperoxide derivative of the vitamin is formed first, which either reacts with CO_2 and acts as a carbon carrier, or that the hydroperoxide activates the γ-position of the glutamic acid, prior to the attack by CO_2. In support of this, Larson & Suttie (3) show that glutathione peroxidase, which reduces both organic peroxides and hydrogen peroxide, is a potent inhibitor of the carboxylation reaction. They further show that in the presence of 100mM t-butyl hydroperoxide carboxylation can occur in the absence of vitamin K, albeit at a reduced level. In discussing the formation of vitamin K hydroperoxide Suttie et al., (2) suggest that it might arise from a reaction of the vitamin with superoxide. Esnouf et al., (4) have shown that in the presence of superoxide dismutase, the carboxylation of both protein and peptide substrates is substantially inhibited and it is suggested that superoxide reacts directly or indirectly with CO_2 to form an intermediate in the carboxylation reaction. We present here evidence to support this view.

MATERIALS & METHODS

Microsomes were prepared from the livers of 3-5 days old calves, normal and vitamin K deficient male Sprague-Dawley rats by the methods previously described (4). The microsomal suspensions were diluted differently so that carboxylase activity of the preparations from each source was approximately the same. In the case of the vitamin K deficient rats, 1ml of the suspension was obtained from 0.5g liver, while with normal rats the suspension was twice as concentrated. When calf liver was used, 1ml of the suspension was derived from 2g liver. The e.p.r. experiments were carried out using a more concentrated suspension, such that 1ml of microsomes was prepared from 5g rat liver. Where indicated the microsomal preparation was solubilized with triton X-100 (5).

The pentapeptide substrate PHE-LEU-GLU-GLU-VAL was synthesised by the active ester procedure (4). Superoxide production by rat liver microsomes was assayed by the method of Esnouf et al. (4).

Superoxide dismutase was a generous gift from Dr. J. V. Bannister; catalase, vitamin K, NADH and NADPH were obtained from Sigma and $NaH^{14}CO_3$ was from The Radiochemical Centre, Amersham.

5,5'dimethyl-Δ'-pyroline-N-oxide was prepared as described by Bonnet et al. (6) and further purified by the method of Buettner et al. (7). t-Butyl hydroperoxide was obtained from Aldrich Chemical Co. Ltd.

The copper and nickel complexes were prepared as follows:

Copper penacillamine ($[\text{D-penacillaminato}]_{2n}[\text{aqua}]_{2n}[\text{Copper(II)}]_n$) and copper aspirinate. (tetrakis-μ-acetyl salicylato-di-copper(II), (8). Copper tyrosine (bis[L-tyrosinato (O.N.)] copper(II)), (9). Nickel glycinate (Di-aquo-bis-glycinato nickel(II)), (10). Stock solutions (1-8mM) were made up in water and the metal content determined by atomic absorption spectroscopy. The superoxide activity of the complexes and the superoxide dismutase were assayed essentially by the photoreduction method (11).

Electron paramagnetic resonance spectra were recorded using a Varian E109 Spectrometer with 100 KHz field modulation in the first derivative mode. Samples of the incubation mixtures were drawn rapidly into a Varian flat quartz cell (0.2ml) by a simple syringe technique (12). To monitor the signal height continously the magnetic field sweep was set to zero and the magnetic field adjusted to the resonance field of the peak under study. Signal intensities were calibrated using the spin label, 4-hydroxy-2,2,6,6-tetramethyl piperidine-N-oxide (Aldrich Chemical Co. Ltd). The incubation mixtures contained 0.1ml of the microsomal suspension, 0.05ml of an aqueous solution containing Triton X-100 (20%), DMPO (100mM), diethylene triamine pentaacetic acid (DTPA) (1mM), and 0.02ml vitamin K hydroquinone (10mg/ml) in ethanol, which was added last. The volume was adjusted to 0.5ml with the same buffer in which the microsomes were suspended.

The coupled glutathione peroxidase: glutathione reductase system when added contained 2mM glutathione, 1mM NADPH, glutathione reductase (Sigma) 2 units/ml and glutathione peroxidase (13).

Potassium hydrogen peroxomonocarbonate ($KHCO_4$) and dipotassium peroxodicarbonate ($K_2C_2O_6$) were prepared by the method of Firsova et al. (14).

RESULTS

The carboxylation of the prothrombin precursor or a synthetic substrate based on residues 5-9 of bovine or rat prothrombin (15) requires molecular oxygen and vitamin K hydroquinone (16). Rat liver microsomes in addition to the carboxylase activity also possess an NADH dependent vitamin K reductase activity (17). Patel & Willson (18) have shown that reduced vitamin K reacts with molecular oxygen to form superoxide. Recently, Bartoli et al. (19) have found that rat liver microsomes generated superoxide by an NADPH dependent pathway and Esnouf et al. (4) have shown that the release of superoxide by normal rat liver microsomes can be stimulated by adding vitamin K. In these experiments the release of superoxide was assayed by the conversion of adrenalin to adrenochrome. This was inhibited by the addition of superoxide dismutase (10μg/ml).

In the experiment shown in Table 1, we have repeated that experiment and also included the result obtained with microsomes obtained from vitamin K deficient rats. In both cases there is a considerable increase in superoxide formation following the addition of vitamin K. In these experiments the microsomes were suspended in 0.15M KCl/50mM Tris/HCl buffer, pH 7.5 (buffered KCl), if 0.25M sucrose (buffered sucrose) was added the vitamin K stimulated release of superoxide was considerably reduced.

TABLE 1

Production of Superoxide by Normal and Vitamin K Deficient Rat Microsomes

		Superoxide produced (pmol/min/ml)
Normal Rat microsomes		0
	+ NADH	60
	+ NADH + vitamin K_1	230
	suspended in sucrose + NADH	79
	suspended in sucrose + NADH + vitamin K_1	117
Vitamin K deficient rat microsomes		0
	+ NADH	157
	+ NADH + vitamin K_1	545

Incubations contained 2ml of O_2-saturated 0.15M-KCl/50mM Tris/HCl buffer, pH 7.5; 0.1ml microsomes; 0.1ml of adrenaline (4mg/ml); 0.05ml NADH (10mg/ml) and 0.1ml vitamin K_1 (10mg/ml).

The techniques of 'spin trapping' whereby a short-lived or otherwise undetectable radical reacts with a 'spin-trap' to yield a relatively stable nitroxide radical (20,21), provides a more direct method of detecting radicals generated in biological processes (22,23). The electron paramagnetic resonance (e.p.r.) spectrum of the nitroxide is often characteristic of the radical trapped and indeed in favourable instances several radicals may be identified simultaneously. Figure 1a shows the e.p.r. spectra obtained when normal rat liver microsomes, suspended in buffered KCl, were incubated with liposomes or liposomes containing vitamin K (17). The spectrum is that expected from the product of the reaction of superoxide and the hydroxyl radical with DMPO (7,24). The signal due to the superoxide adduct was stimulated approximately 2.5 times by including vitamin K in the liposomes, and was not evident when superoxide dismutase (10 μg/ml) was added (Fig. 1b). If the microsomes were prepared in buffered sucrose, the superoxide was not detected, as is consistent with the results of the adrenochrome assay (Table 1).

A signal very similar to the superoxide adduct of DMPO in water was also evident during the reoxidation of vitamin K hydroquinone by dioxygen in an ethanol:water mixture (Fig. 2a). [A_N = 13.6G, A_H^β = 10.8G, A_H^γ = 1.5G, g = 2.009]. This is further evidence that vitamin K hydroquinone is capable of reducing oxygen to superoxide. If this reaction mixture was scanned about 15 min later, by which time the superoxide adduct had decayed, a new 'six-line' signal was more clearly seen (Fig. 2b) [A_N = 15.5G; A_H^β = 22.2G; g = 2.009]. A similar signal was also observed when rat liver microsomes suspended in sucrose were incubated with DMPO and vitamin K hydroquinone (Fig. 3) [A_N = 15.9G; A_H^β = 21.8G; g = 2.007]. A comparison of the parameters derived from these e.p.r. spectra with

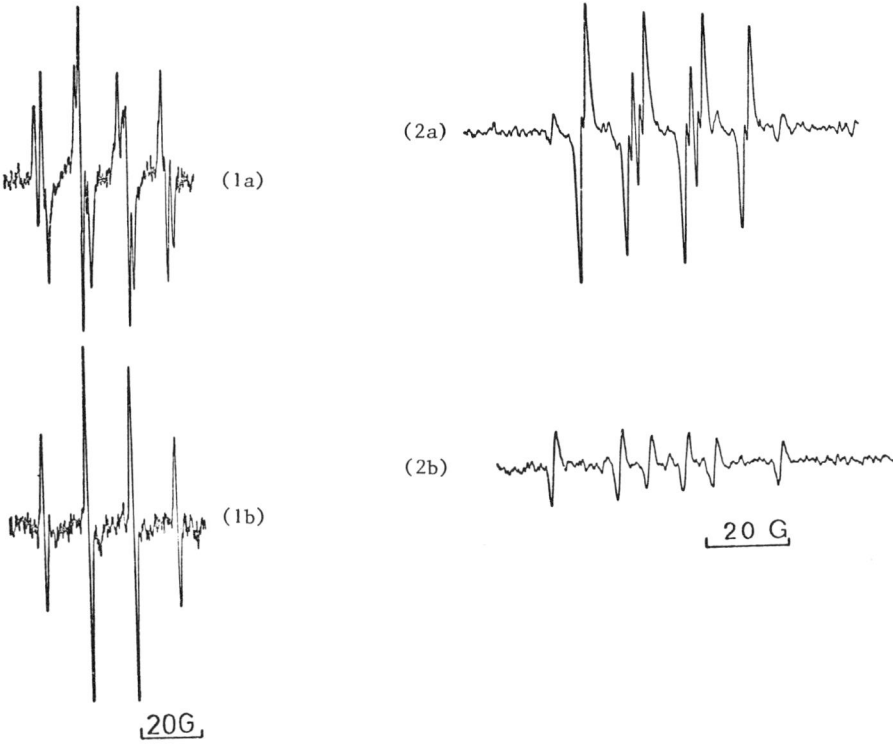

Figure 1

E.p.r. spectra obtained from incubating vitamin K replete rat liver microsomes suspended in buffered KCl (see text) with DMPO. 1a, microsomes (0.1ml), DMPO (100mM), NADH (200 g ml^{-1}), Triton X100 (2%), 0.250ml of liposomes containing vitamin K. The sample was made up to 0.5ml with buffered KCl. 1b with superoxide dismutase 10 μg/ml. Field 3385G, frequency 9.462GHz, power 30mW, modulation 1G, time constant 0.5s, scan rate 0.2Gs^{-1}, gain 1.25 x 10^5.

Figure 2

2a, e.p.r. spectrum obtained immediately after adding 0.1ml of vitamin K hydroquinone in ethanol to DMPO (100mM final concentration) in 0.4ml of 66% ethanol:water (v/v) mixture. The ethanol:water mixture had previously been gassed with CO_2 and O_2.

2b, spectrum observed after 10 minutes. Field 3385G, frequency 9.460GHz, power 30mW, modulation 1G, time constant 0.5s, scan rate 0.4Gs^{-1}, gain 5 x 10^4.

published data (25) suggests that this nitroxide may be formed by the reaction of DMPO with a carbon radical.

In a previous paper (4) we have shown that the carboxylation of both pentapeptide substrate and prothrombin precursors by rat liver microsomes are inhibited by 64% and 35%, respectively, by bovine superoxide dismutase

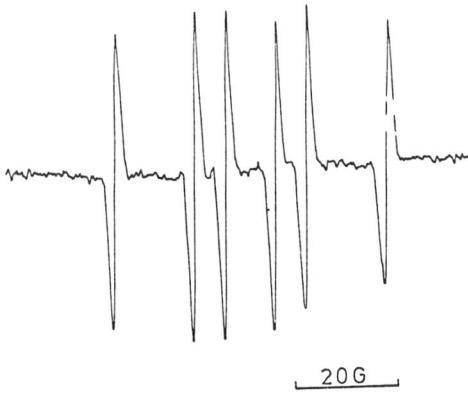

Figure 3

E.p.r. spectrum obtained from vitamin K replete rat liver microsomes suspended in buffered sucrose (see text). The sample contained microsomes (0.1ml), DMPO (100mM), DPTA (1mM), Triton X100 (2%), vitamin K hydroquinone (400 g ml^{-1}) made up to 0.5ml with buffered sucrose.

Field 3385G, frequency 9.500GHz, power 10mW, modulation 1G, time constant 0.5s, scan rate 0.2Gs^{-1}, gain 5 x 10^4.

(10mg/ml). We have now shown that the carboxylation of the pentapeptide substrate by calf liver microsomes is inhibited to the same extent by SOD at one tenth the concentration (Table 2). Catalase similarly was more effective in the calf system compared with the rats, the reason for the increased sensitivity of the calf system has not yet been explained. Esnouf et al. (4) suggested the relative insensitivity of the rat carboxylation reaction to superoxide dismutase might be explained by the inaccessibility of the superoxide generating site to the dismutase.

TABLE 2

Inhibition of Pentapeptide Carboxylation by Various Agents in Calf Liver Microsomes

	DPM ml mics	% Inhibition
Microsomes + vitamin K$_1$ quinol + 1mg bsa	3,234	0
+ 1mg SOD	1,305	60
+ 1mg CAT	1,788	45
+ K$_1$ + 0.65μmole Cu asprinate	120	96

Incubations contained 1ml microsomes, pentapeptide (2mM) NaH^{14}CO$_3$ (10 Ci) NADH (1.4mM), dithiothreitol (60 M), vitamin K$_1$ quinol (100 g) in a volume of 1.25ml.
bsa = bovine serum albumin (Sigma)
SOD = superoxide dismutase
CAT = catalase

A similar situation arises in the cytochrome P-450 dependent hydroxylation reactions, which are not inhibited by the dismutase if intact microsomes are used, but are when a reconstituted hydroxylation system is studied (26). However Richter et al. (27) have shown that hydroxylation reactions in intact microsomes can be inhibited by a copper-tyrosine complex. In the experiment shown in Table 3, we have tested the effect of three copper(II) complexes with known superoxide dismutase activity on the carboxylation of prothrombin precursor by vitamin K deficient rat liver microsomes. To show that the inhibition is related to the dismutase activity, we tested the effect of nickel(II) glycinate, which has no dismutase activity and, as can be seen from the results, did not inhibit the carboxylation reaction at a concentration of 830µM. In the experiment with calf liver microsomes (Table 2), the carboxylase activity was completely inhibited by 650µM copper asprinate.

TABLE 3

Comparison of Superoxide dismutase activity and inhibition of ^{14}C incorporation into prothrombin precursors by Metal (II) complexes, DMPO and SOD

	Carboxylation K_i (µM)	Superoxide generation K_i (nM)
Copper penicillamine	135	140
Copper tyrosine	100	145
Copper Asprinate	65	125
Nickel glycinate (No inhibition) at	830	8300
DMPO	155×10^3	30×10^6
SOD	- 500	1

Incubations contained 1ml microsomes, NADH (1.4mM), DTT (60µM), $NaH^{14}CO_3$ (10µCi), Vitamin K quinone (100µg) in a volume of 1.25 ml.

The 'spin-trap' DMPO has a K_i at least three orders of magnitude higher than the copper complexes, and in our hands is a relatively poor inhibitor of carboxylation. Girardot et al. (28) obtained 50% inhibition with 5mM DMPO, but their experimental conditions were considerably different from those used here.

The formation of the 'six-line' signal (Fig. 3) obtained when DMPO is incubated with rat liver microsomes is also inhibited by copper asprinate (200µM) (Fig. 4). This suggests that the carboxylation reaction and the generation of the radical trapped by DMPO in the microsomes may be linked.

Larson & Suttie (3) suggest that vitamin K hydroperoxide is formed as an intermediate in the carboxylation reaction, and they show that t-butyl hydroperoxide, in high concentrations, will support the carboxylation of both pentapeptide and protein in the absence of vitamin K. We have obtained essentially the same results (Table 4) as Larson & Suttie (3)

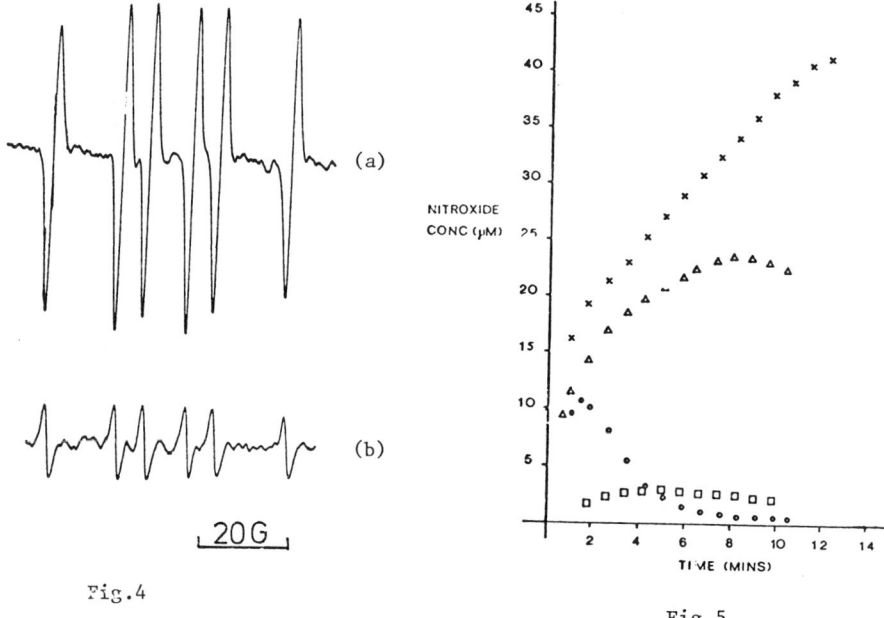

Fig.4

Fig.5

Figure 4

E.p.r. spectra obtained after incubating vitamin K deficient rat liver microsomes in buffered sucrose (see text) with DMPO. 4a, microsomes (0.1ml), DMPO (100mM), DTPA (1mM), NADH (200 g ml^{-1}), Triton X100 (2%), vitamin K (400 g ml^{-1}) and enough buffered sucrose to make the sample up to 0.5ml. 4b, as 4a + 200 g ml^{-1} copper asprinate. Both spectra were commenced 8 minutes after mixing the samples.

E.p.r. conditions as in figure 2.

Figure 5

Plots of nitroxide concentration (μM) against time (mins) of the e.p.r. spectrum obtained in figure 3 (see experimental) and the effect of the coupled glutathione peroxidase system. (a) □ , vitamin K replete rat liver microsomes in buffered sucrose (0.1ml) (see text) DMPO (100mM), DTPA (1mM), Triton X100 (2%) and enough buffered sucrose to make the volume up to 0.5ml. (b); x, As a, + NADPH (1mg ml^{-1}) and vitamin K hydroquinone (200 g ml^{-1}) (c); Δ, as (a), + vitamin K hydroquinone and the coupled glutathione system (glutathione peroxidase: 2 units ml^{-1}) d; O, as (c) except 5 units ml^{-1} glutathione peroxidase. The e.p.r. spectra used to prepare this figure were obtained under the following conditions; Field 3387.1G, frequency 9.498GHz, power 10mW modulation 1G, time constant 1s, gain 10^5.

in terms of the percentage change in C^{14} incorporated over the background (151% against 57%), but we consider the effect small when seen against an experiment where vitamin K has been added.

It is of interest to note that the addition of vitamin K to t-butyl hydroperoxide results in the rapid formation of vitamin K epoxide and this probably explains the low incorporation of C^{14} seen when the two are added together.

TABLE 4

Comparison of the Effect of t-butyl-OOH and Vitamin K_1 quinol on Carboxylation of Pentapeptide

	DPM ml/mics	% above background
Microsomes + Vitamin K_1 quinol + NADH	39,816	1,385
+ K_1 quinol + NADPH + t-butyl-OOH	5,430	185
+ t-butyl-OOH + NADPH	4,343	151
+ t-butyl-OOH + NADH	372	13

Incubations contained 1ml solubilised microsomes made from vitamin K deficient rats, NADH (1.4mM) or NADPH (1.4mM), Dithiothreitol (60μM), $NaH^{14}CO_3$ (20μCi), vitamin K_1 quinol (100μg), pentapeptide (2mM), t-butyl-OOH (0.1M) in a volume of 1.25ml.

The glutathione peroxidase: glutathione reductase system is a potent inhibitor of carboxylation as previously shown by Larson & Suttie (3). However, we find that glutathione reductase alone inhibits carboxylation by about 30%, and that our preparations of glutathione peroxidase cause about 20% inhibition in the absence of the other components. This inhibition probably due to small amounts of glutathione peroxidase and glutathione reductase present in the microsomal preparations. The coupled glutathione peroxidase system also inhibits the formation of the 'six-line' nitroxide adduct of DMPO in rat liver microsomes (Fig. 5). Glutathione peroxidase (2 units/ml) caused partial inhibition, while the signal was strongly suppressed at 5 units/ml.

In order to study the interaction with DMPO of some of the products of the reactions between reduced dioxygen ($O_2^{\cdot-}$ and H_2O_2) and CO_2 (29), we have examined the e.p.r. spectra formed on the decomposition of the potassium peroxocarbonates [$KHCO_4$ and $K_2C_2O_6$] in various media, in the presence of DMPO and the coupled glutathione peroxidase system (Figs. 6 & 7). In a 66% ethanol:water mixture (Figs. 6a/7a) the hydroxyl radical and the 'six-line' nitroxide adducts are observed. The splitting constants for the 'six-line' adduct are as follows [A_N = 15.4G; A_H^β = 22.8G; g = 2.009]. In the buffered sucrose solution used for preparing the microsomes, only the hydroxyl signal is seen (Fig. 7b). The 'six-line' adduct can be detected in a 32% glycerol:water mixture (Fig. 6b) [A_N = 15.8G; A_H^β = 23.0G; g = 2.007]; these parameters are very close to those observed for the 'six-line' signal in the experiemnts with the rat liver microsomes (Fig.3). The characteristic spectra due to both the hydroxyl and the 'six-line' nitroxide adducts with $KHCO_4$ in 32% glycerol (Fig. 6c) are not observed in the presence of the coupled glutathione peroxidase system (2 units/ml glutathione peroxidase).

DISCUSSION

Both the adrenochrome assay and e.p.r. measurements show that there is a marked vitamin K stimulated release of superoxide from rat liver microsomes suspended in buffered KCl, confirming the observations made

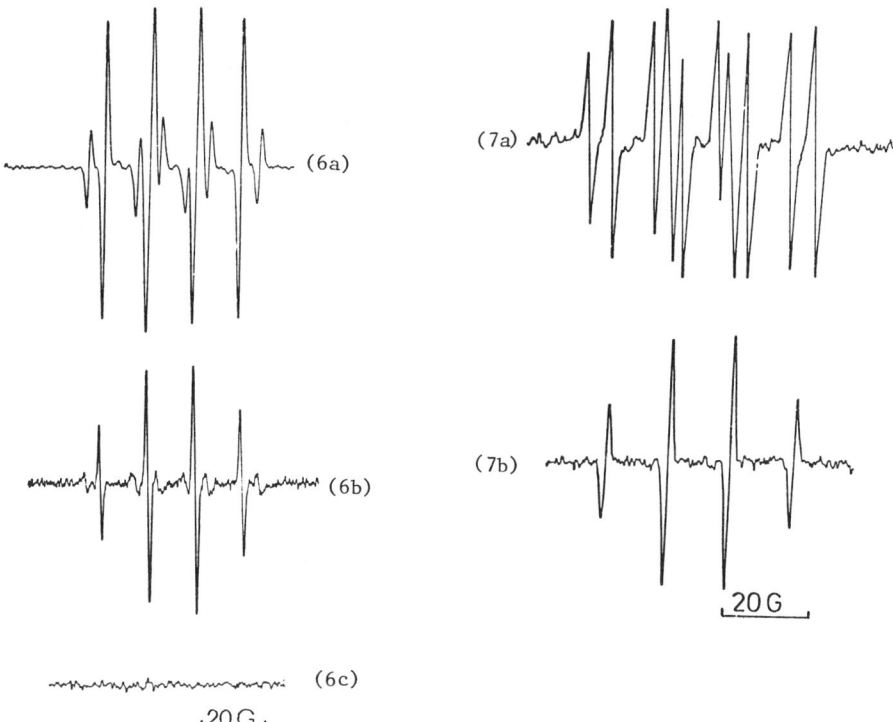

Figure 6

E.p.r. spectra obtained after adding c.a. 5mg of freshly prepared potassium peroxomonocarbonate (KCHO4) to 0.5ml of various media containing 100mM DMPO. The effect of the coupled glutathione peroxidase system was also investigated.

6a, 66% Ethanol:water (v/v)
6b, 32% Glycerol:buffered sucrose (2/v)
6c, 32% Glycerol (final concentration):buffered sucrose (w/v) + coupled glutathione system (glutathione peroxidase, 2 units ml^{-1}).
6a; field 3385G, frequency 9.460GHz, power 10mW, modulation 1G, time constant 0.5s, scan rate $0.4Gs^{-1}$, gain 1.6×10^4.
6b and 6c; field 3385G, frequency 9.500 GHz, power 10mW, modulation 1G, time constant 0.128s, scan rate $0.8Gs^{-1}$, gain 2×10^4.

Figure 7

E.p.r. spectra obtained after adding c.a. 5.5mg of potassium peroxodicarbonate ($K_2C_2O_6$) to 0.5ml of various media containing DMPO (100mM).

7a; 66% Ethanol:water (v/v) mixture
7b; Buffered sucrose (see text)
7a; Field 3385G, frequency 9.456GHz, power 10mW, modulation 1G, time constant 0.5s, scan rate $0.4Gs^{-1}$, gain 3.2×10^5.
7b; as e.p.r. conditions for 6b, 6c.

earlier (4). The release of superoxide seen in the absence of vitamin K probably arises from the microsomal NADPH dependent cytochrome c reductase (19) and the microsomal cytochrome P-450 (26). The increased rate of superoxide release seen when the microsomes are suspended in buffered KCl without sucrose may arise from the disruption of microsomal membrane and the enzyme complexes which produce superoxide. Strobel & Coon (26) have observed that hydroxylation reactions catalysed by cytochrome P-450 are influenced by the concentration of sodium chloride in the suspending medium.

The inhibition of both the carboxylase and the appearance of the 'six-line' e.p.r. spectrum by the copper(II) asprinate and the coupled glutathione peroxidase system, suggests that the radical generated in the rat liver microsomes and 'trapped' by DMPO may be involved in the vitamin K dependent carboxylation reaction. The splitting parameters of the 'six-line' signal, together with generation of a similar signal from the decomposition of the peroxomonocarbonate, provides a convincing arguement that the 'trapped' radical contains carbon. Further experiments are in progress to establish the identity of this radical.

If the 'trapped' radical arises from peroxocarbonates generated in the microsomes during carboxylation, it is possible that the peroxocarbonates are generated directly by a reaction between superoxide or peroxide and CO_2 (14, 30, 31). An alternative source could be the reaction of CO_2 with the hydroperoxide of vitamin K, the vitamin K hydroperoxide being formed by the reaction of superoxide with vitamin K quinone (32).

The inhibitory action of the copper(II) complexes is most likely to be due to their superoxide dismutase activity, although it is possible that they may act as general radical scavengers. In the case of the coupled glutathione peroxidase system, which is remarkably effective at low enzyme concentrations, the site of action may be either on vitamin K hydroperoxide as suggested by Larson & Suttie (3), or free hydrogen peroxide, or even peroxomonocarbonate which is itself a hydroperoxide. The peroxodicarbonate anion may break down in an aqueous environment to yield peroxocarbonic acid (H_2CO_4) or the peroxomonocarbonate anion (33).

The hydroxyl radical observed in Figs. 6 & 7 may arise from the cleavage of the O-O bond in potassium peroxomonocarbonate. This decomposition would generate the CO_3^- radical, which may possibly be the carbon radical or the precursor to the radical giving rise to the 'six-line' signal.

On the basis of the evidence present here it is reasonable to suggest that radicals are involved as intermediates in the vitamin K dependent carboxylation of glutamyl residues.

ACKNOWLEDGEMENTS

The authors thank Professor M. C. R. Symons for the use of his e.p.r. spectrometer to obtain the data in Fig. 5. M.R.G., M.J.O-Z., I.A.B. are supported by the SRC. S.J.W. is supported by the MRC. We thank the SRC, the MRC and the British Health Foundation for support. This is a contribution from the Oxford Enzyme Group of which two of us M.P.E. and H.A.O.H. are members.

REFERENCES

1. Olson, R.E. & Suttie, J.W. (1978) Vitamin & Hormones 35: 59-108
2. Suttie, J.W., Larson, A.E., Canfield, L.M. & Carlisle, T.L. (1978) Federation Proc. 37: 2605-2609
3. Larson, A.E. & Suttie, J.W. (1978) Proc. Natl Acad. Sci. U.S.A. 75: 5418-5416
4. Esnouf, M.P., Green, M.R., Hill, H.A.O., Irvine, G.B. & Walter, S.J. (1978) Biochem. J. 174: 345-348
5. Esmon, C.T. & Suttie, J.W. (1976) J. Biol. Chem 251: 6238-6243
6. Bonnet, R., Brown, R.F.C., Clark, W.M., Sutherland, I.O. & Todd, A. (1959) J. Chem. Soc. 2094-2102
7. Buetnner, G.R. & Oberley, L.W. (1978) Biochem. Biophys. Res. Commun. 83: 69-74
8. Sorenson, J.R.J. (1976) J. Medicinal Chemistry 19: 135-148
9. Brigelius, R., Hadman, H.J., Bors, W., Sara, M., Lengfelder, E. & Weser, U. (1975) Hoppe-Seyler's Z. Physiol. Chem. 356: 739-745
10. McAuliffe, C.A. & Perry, W.D. (1969) J. Chem. Soc (A) 634-636
11. Beauchamp, C. & Fridovich, I. (1971) Anal. Biochem. 44: 276-287
12. Miller, R.W. & Rapp, U. (1973) J. Biol. Chem. 248: 6084-6090
13. Nakamura, W., Hosoda, S. & Hayashi, K. (1974) Biochim. Biophys. Acta 358: 251-261
14. Firsova, T.P., Molodkina, A.N., Morozova, T.G. & Aksenova, I.V. (1964) Russ. J. Inorg. Chem. 9: 583-586
15. Suttie, J.W., Lehrman, S.R., Geweke, L.O., Hageman, J.M. & Rich, D.M. (1979) Biochem. Biophys. Res. Commun. 86: 500-507
16. Sadowski, J.A., Esmon, C.T. & Suttie, J.W. (1976) J. Biol. Chem. 251: 2770-2775
17. Martius, C., Ganser, R. & Viviani, A. (1975) FEBS Lett. 59: 13-14
18. Patel, K.B. & Willson, R.L. (1973) J. Chem. Soc. Faraday Trans. 69: 814-825
19. Bartoli, G.M., Galeotti, T., Palombini, G., Parisi, G. & Azzi, A. (1977) Arch. Biochem. Biophys. 184: 248-257
20. Janzen, E.G. (1971) Acc. Chem. Res. 4: 31-40
21. Lagercrantz, C. (1971) J. Chem. Phys. 75: 3466-3475
22. Harbour, J.R. & Bolton, J.R. (1975) Biochem. Biophys. Res. Commun. 64: 803-807
23. Saprin, A.N. & Piette, L.H. (1977) Arch. Biochem. Biophys. 180: 480-492
24. Harbour, J.R., Chow, V. & Bolton, J.R. (1974) Can. J. Chem. 52: 3549-3553
25. Janzen, E.G. & Lui, J.I.P. (1973) J. Mag. Res. 9: 510-512
26. Strobel, H.W. & Coon, M.J. (1971) J. Biol. Chem. 246: 7826-7829
27. Richter, C., Azzi, A., Weser, U. & Wendel, A. (1977) in Superoxide & Superoxide Dismutases 375-385 (Michelson, A.M., McCord, J.M. & Fridovich, I. eds) Academic Press, London.
28. Girardot, J.M., Mack, D.O., Floyd, R.A. & Connor-Johnson, B. (1976) Biochem. Biophys. Res. Comm. 70: 655-663
29. Hill, H.A.O. (1978) in 'New Trends in Bioinorganic Chemistry. (ed. Williams, R.J.P. and da Silva, J.J.R.F.) Academic Press, pp 173-208.
30. Mel'nikov, A.Kh. & Firsova, T.P. (1961) Russ. J. Inorg. Chem 6: 1137-1139
31. Spangler, G.E. & Collins, C.I. Analytical Chemistry 47: 393-402
32. Saito, I., Otsuki, T. & Mutsuura, T. (1979) Tet. Lett 19: 1693-1696
33. Mel'nikov, A.Kh. & Firsova, J.P. (1961) Russ. J. Inorg. Chem 6: 1251-1252.

VITAMIN K-DEPENDENT CARBOXYLASE FOR PEPTIDE-BOUND GLUTAMATE

ANNE L. HALL, PAUL M. TURNER, BARBARA F. DUNKLE,
DAVID A. WING and ROBERT E. OLSON

Edward A. Doisy Department of Biochemistry,
St. Louis University School of Medicine,
St. Louis, MO 63104

INTRODUCTION

The carboxylation of selected glutamate (GLU) residues in the N-terminal portion of prothrombin precursors and in selected glutamate-containing peptides is vitamin KH_2-dependent. The chemical mechanism by which vitamin K accomplishes this CO_2 fixation to form γ-carboxyglutamate (GLA) residues is still obscure. Our demonstration that CO_2 rather than bicarbonate is the active form of "CO_2" in this carboxylation reaction (1) and our failure to demonstrate γ-carboxyglutamate synthesis from chemically synthesized carbonates of menaquinone-2 hydroquinone (2), has led us to the belief that vitamin K is not a carbon dioxide carrier. The report by Larsen and Suttie (3) that t-butyl-OOH is able to stimulate carboxylation of a GLU-containing pentapeptide in the presence of NADPH, but in the absence of oxygen, led them to postulate a vitamin K-hydroperoxide as an intermediate in the carboxylation reaction. It seemed possible to us that organic peroxides of suitable structure might react with a final common metalloenzyme to generate an enzyme-peroxide derivative which, in turn could produce the base required to abstract a γ proton from peptide-bound glutamate (4). This view of the mechanism would make CO_2-fixation the last step in an ordered reaction within the relative anhydrous reticulum membrane.

In order to test this hypothesis, we carried out experiments to study the chromatographic behavior of proteins concerned with t-butyl-OOH activation and those concerned with the terminal carboxylation of the pentapeptide Phe-Leu-Glu-Glu-Ile. On heparin affinity columns the enzymes responsible for the incorporation of radioactivity into a TCA-soluble acid under the influence of t-butyl-OOH are entirely different from those required for the synthesis of γ-carboxyglutamic acid via the vitamin KH_2-dependent reaction. Our investigation leads us to believe that the product of the t-butyl-OOH driven carboxylation is not γ-carboxyglutamic acid, but some other acid that resembles it in some respects.

MATERIALS AND METHODS

Chemicals: NADPH, avidin, vitamin K_1 (2-methyl-3-phytl-1,4-napthoquinone), warfarin, sephadex G-25, heparin sodium salt, and cyanogen bromide activated sepharose 4B were purchased from Sigma Chemical Co. Sodium [^{14}C]-bicarbonate (>50 Ci/mmol) and aqueous counting scintillant (ACS) were obtained from Amersham Corp. Tert-butyl-hydroperoxide was obtained from Aldrich Chemical Co., Silica G-25 TLC plates were from Brinkman Instruments, and Bio-gel P-2 was purchased from Bio-Rad Laboratories. γ-Carboxyglutamic acid (GLA) and the pentapeptide Phe-Leu-Glu-Glu-Ile were also synthesized in this laboratory (5). Reduced vitamin K_1 was prepared by mixing 10 mg/ml of the vitamin in oxygen free ethanol with H_2 plus Pd (10% carbon 5 mg/ml) for 2-4 min at room temperature in airtight containers. The mixture was centrifuged to remove the catalyst and used immediately. All other chemicals were reagent grade or better.

Animals: Male 200-250 g ARS Sprague-Dawley strain rats were used throughout the study. Vitamin K deficiency was produced by feeding a vitamin K-deficient diet for 10-14 days to rats in raised bottom cages to minimize corprophagy. To insure prothrombin levels of less than 2% of normal, the overnight fasted rats were given 1.5 mg Warfarin, i.p. 12 hours before sacrifice.

Preparations of Microsomes: Liver from decapitated rats were removed, minced, and homogenized with two parts of ice cold buffer (w/v) containing 0.25 M sucrose, 25 mM imidazole, 0.5 M KCl, pH 7.2 using a glass homogenizer with three strokes of a teflon pestle at 250 rpm. The homogenate was centrifuged at 12,500 x g for 20 min. Microsomes were prepared from this first mitochondrial supernatant by centrifuging at 105,000 x g for 60 min in a Beckman model L-2 ultracentrifuge. The microsomal pellet was surface washed with the original homogenizing solution and resuspended with six strokes of a Dounce homogenizer in a volume of solubilizing buffer (original buffer plus 1.5% Triton X-100) equal to 0.7 ml/g rat liver. The membranous material was removed by centrifugation at 105,000 x g for 60 min. The supernatant solution was either removed immediately for studies of carboxylation or was frozen at -70°C for future use.

Incubations: The incubation consisted of 0.3 ml of solubilized microsomes, 0.1 ml of solubilizing buffer containing 1 mM peptide, NADPH, and other compounds as described in text. Tert-butyl-OOH was added directly to the incubation mixtures. Reduced vitamin K was added in ethanol. 20 μCi of $NaH^{14}CO_3$ (59-50 mCI/mmol. Amersham Searle) was added per 0.4 ml of reation mixture. The mixture was incubated in 8 x 95 mm screw top tubes in a Dubnoff metabolic shaking incubator at 18° for 45 min. Reactions were stopped by adding an equal volume of

10% TCA. The samples were allowed to stand at least 30 min before centrifugation to remove protein. The residual $^{14}CO_2$ was removed by gassing the supernatant with CO_2 for 5 min. Aliquots of the TCA-soluble extract (0.2 ml) were counted in 7 ml ACS fluid in a Beckman scintillation counter at 70% efficiency.

Preparation of Heparin Column: Cyanogen bromide activated sepharose 4B was washed with 300 mls of 1 mM HCl/g sepharose at room temperature through sintered glass filter under suction to remove stabilizer (dextrose, etc.). Five mg heparin, sodium salt 169 U5PK units/mg was dissolved in 1 ml 0.1 M sodium carbonate pH 9.0. The heparin solution was added with gentle stirring at 4°C to the activated sepharose at a concentration of 25 mg heparin/g sepharose. The solution was stirred very gently overnight at 4°C. A 2 x 60 cm column was prepared and washed with starting buffer 25 mM imidazole, 0.1 M KCl, 0.01% Triton, pH 7.2. The elution buffer was 0.5 M KCl, 0.01% Triton, 1 mM DTT, 25 mM imidazole, pH 7.2. Samples applied to heparin column were either extracted at 0.15 M KCL salt concentration or dialyzed overnight against 0.1 M KCL buffer before applying to column. They all contained 10^{-3} benzamidine HCl.

Amino Acid Analysis: Pooled degassed TCA soluble (2-3 ml) was applied to 2.5 x 60 cm Bio-gel P-2 column (mesh 200-400) in 0.05 M NH_4CO_3 buffer, pH 9.5 and the column developed with same buffer. The eluates were pooled, lyophilyzed, dissolved in either 6 M HCl or KOH and hydrolyzed for specific times (see text) in sealed vials. The hydrolyzed samples were neutralized and insoluble material removed. The solubilized material was evaporated to dryness (flash evaporator) and chromatographed on a AA-15 resin in a Beckman 120 amino acid analyzer. Samples were collected at 2 min intervals and 0.3 ml aliquots were removed for counting. Standards of GLA and GLU were run as controls.

Thin-layer Chromatography: Radioactive eluates from the A.A. analyzer were pooled, lyophilyzed, dissolved in appropriate buffer and chromatographed on G-25 TLC plates (silica gel 5x20 cm) in four different solvent systems. Standard GLA, GLU and citrate were also chromatographed in each system. The plates were scraped in 5 mm segments, placed in 10 ml ACS fluid and counted in a Beckman counter. The solvent systems used were: a) 95% EtOH 70, H_2O, 30; b) EtAC 80, HOAC 8, EtOH 16, H_2O 16; c) EtAC 2, HOAC 1, H_2O 1; and d) 95% EtOH 78, H_2O 9.5, 25% NH_4OH, 12.5.

RESULTS

The results of heparin affinity chromatography of a Triton X-100 extract of vitamin K-deficient rat liver microsomes are shown in Fig. 1. The biological activity associated with t-butyl-OOH driven carboxylation eluted with the void volume in fractions 20-42, whereas the biological activity associated with vitamin KH_2-dependent carboxylation eluted with increased salt and appeared in fractions 79-108. As shown in Table 1, no t-butyl-OOH activity appeared in the vitamin KH_2 active fraction, although small amounts of vitamin KH_2 activity were present in the void volume because of apparent overloading. The degree of purification of the KH_2-dependent enzyme was about 30-fold in this particular experiment and is of the magnitude as reported earlier (6).

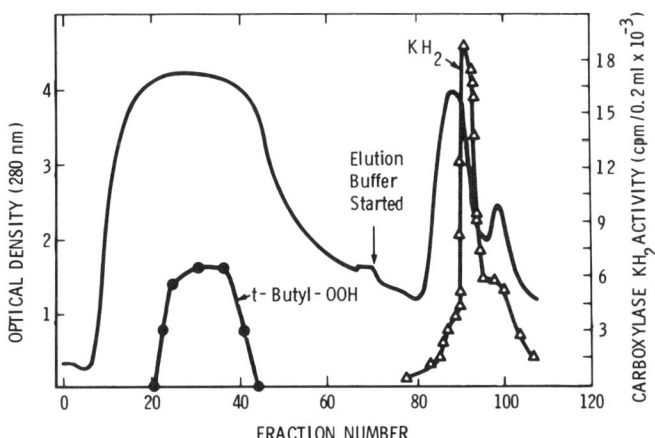

FIGURE 1. A Triton X-100 extract of vitamin K-deficient rat liver microsomes was prepared as in MATERIALS AND METHODS and loaded onto the column in the presence of 10^{-3}M benzamidine HCl. The column was washed with the same buffer minus Triton. The elution buffer, introduced at the arrow, was 0.5 M KCl in the same buffer plus 1 mM DTT and 0.01% Triton X-100.

TABLE 1. Heparin Affinity Chromatography of Carboxylase Activities (t-Butyl-OOH versus KH_2)

Sample	cpm/mg protein			
	t-butyl-OOH + NADPH (30 mg/ml)		Reduced Phylloquinone (100 µg/ml)	
	Absent	Present	Absent	Present
Initial extract	105	670	35	1,324
15-30	200	1,400	40	120
38-58	0	0	0	0
79-101	0	0	35	33,000

Carboxylase for Peptide-bound Glutamate 437

It might also be pointed out that Echis carinatus determinations were run on all fractions. The Echis units paralleled the KH_2 carboxylase activity almost exactly. This was consistent with our previous findings that a complex between carboxylase and precursor exists in the membrane. No such complex exists between the t-butyl-OOH activity and the prothrombin precursor. From previous studies we have found that microsomes prepared from vitamin K-supplemented rats gave the same t-butyl-OOH activity as those prepared from K-deficient rats, whereas KH_2-dependent carboxylase activities are highly augmented in K-deficient rats (7).

The hypothesis that there is a common final pathway for t-butyl-OOH driven and KH_2 driven carboxylation necessitates some complementarity between the major fractions from the heparin column. Experiments to test this interaction are shown in Fig. 2. When one-half fraction of the void volume containing t-butyl-OOH activity was mixed with one-half of the heparin eluate containing KH_2 activity, there was an augmentation of about 3-fold in the KH_2-dependent carboxylation of pentapeptide. On the other hand, when one-half the void volume plus one-half the heparin eluate was tested for activity with t-butyl-OOH there was no synergism. In fact, the total activities were less than that expected (50%) if there was no interaction between the fractions. This result was not consistent with the view that a final common enzyme was reacting with t-butyl-OOH and vitamin KH_2 peroxide.

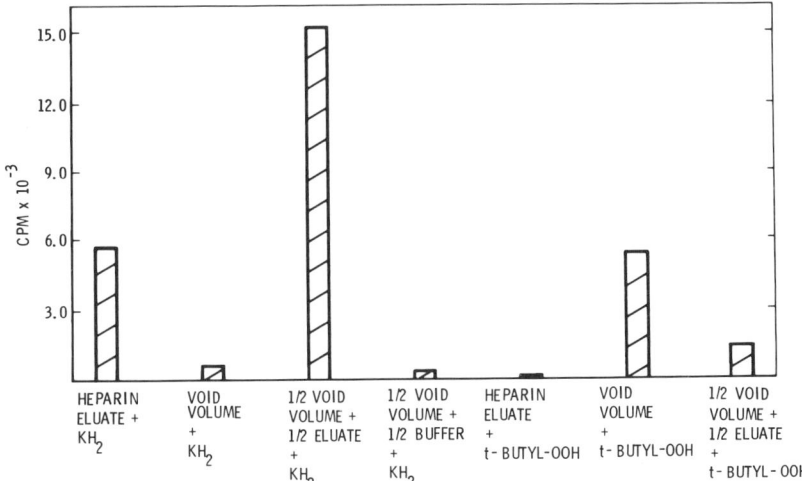

FIGURE 2. Complementarity of fractions from the heparin column with respect to KH_2-dependent and t-butyl-OOH dependent carboxylation activity. The first 4 samples were incubated with KH_2; the last 3 samples with t-butyl-OOH.

As shown in Table 2, dialysis of a microsomal extract against either water or imidazole buffer containing 0.5 M KCl pH 7.2, resulted in the loss of t-butyl-OOH activity, whereas no KH_2-dependent carboxylase activity was lost.

TABLE 2. Effect of Dialysis on Carboxylase Activity

	cpm/mg protein			
	t-Butyl-OOH (30 mg/ml)		Vitamin KH_2 (100 μg/ml)	
	Absent	Present	Absent	Present
Non-dialyzed extract	80	750	40	1,400
Dialyzed extract	20	20	20	1,400
Non-dialyzed void vol. (Heparin column)	80	1,400	40	120
Dialyzed void volume (Heparin column)	20	20	40	120
Boiled ext. supernatant	20	20	20	20
Dialyzed void volume + dialysate	20	1,350	--	--
Dialyzed void volume + boiled extract	20	1,450	--	--

Under more acid conditions, Larsen, Whitlon, and Suttie (8) report loss of KH_2-dependent activity upon dialysis against 5 mM EDTA. Although the KH_2-dependent enzyme may be metal dependent, the t-butyl-OOH activity is clearly metal-dependent and can be distinguished from the KH_2 activity by the ease of dissociation of its metal. Furthermore, 1 mM EDTA added to the reaction mixture totally inhibits t-butyl-OOH activity without affecting the KH_2 activity.

These findings led us to re-examine the product of the t-butyl-OOH reaction in more detail. The material resulting from alkaline hydrolysis of the radioactive carboxylation product of the t-butyl-OOH-dependent reaction was compared with that from the KH_2-dependent reaction. It was found that both hydrolysis products eluted identically on the AA-15 cation exchanger used in the Beckman amino acid analyzer. Standard GLA eluted at the same place. Upon acid hydrolysis, the t-butyl-OOH product was not converted to glutamic acid but eluted in the same spot as previously (Fig. 3). The KH_2 products did yield glutamic acid and very small amounts of residual GLA after 24 hours of acid hydrolysis. We also discovered that the t-butyl-OOH driven carboxylation occurred whether or not the pentapeptide was added (Fig. 3). This shows clearly that the t-butyl-OOH reaction is not related to the vitamin KH_2 driven carboxylation reaction.

Carboxylase for Peptide-bound Glutamate   439

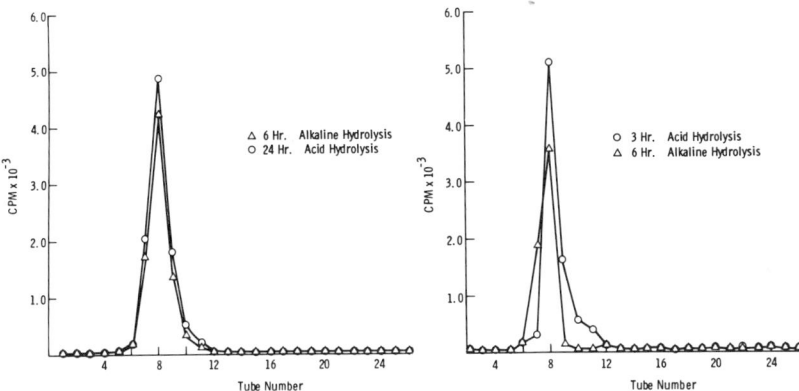

FIGURE 3. Chromatography on AA-15 resin of the carboxylation product of t-butyl-OOH after acid and alkaline hydrolysis. The left panel shows the results in the presence of peptide substrate, whereas the right panel shows the results in the absence of peptide substrate. Authentic GLA eluted in tubes 6-12 and standard GLU eluted in fractions 18-22.

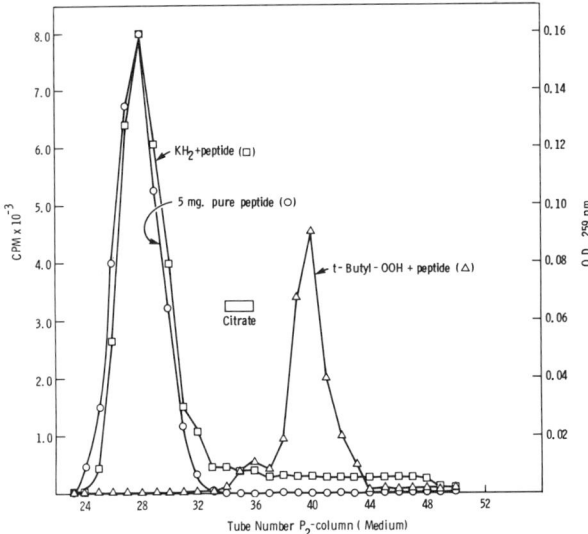

FIGURE 4. Chromatography of the peptide substrate, the KH_2-dependent carboxylation product and the t-butyl-OOH-dependent carboxylation product on a P-2 gel. The position of citric acid elution is shown by a box. Optical density at 259 nm (for the peptide) is at the right, radioactivity at the left.

Figure 4 shows the elution from a P-2 gel of the uncarboxylated peptide as measured by optical density, the product of KH_2 carboxylation, the product of t-butyl-OOH carboxylation, and citric acid. It is clear that the product of KH_2 carboxylation is not identical with the product of t-butyl-OOH carboxylation. The t-butyl-OOH product is not only acid stable, but of lower molecular weight. A number of di- and tricarboxylic acids have been tested to determine if any of them have the same properties as the t-butyl-OOH-dependent product, but as yet we have not identified this product. Table 3 shows that in four TLC systems there is no correspondence between migrations of γ-carboxyglutamic acid and the t-butyl-OOH carboxylation product.

TABLE 3. Thin Layer Chromatography (Rfs) of t-Butyl-OOH Carboxylation Product after Alkaline Hydrolysis and AA-15 Chromatography

Solvent System	GLU	GLA	CIT	Alkaline Hydrolysis Product
(a)	0.55	0.36	0.04	0.60
(b)	0.30	0.10	0.19	0.19
(c)	0.41	0.19	0.43	0.33
(d)	0.57	0.17	0.03	0.37

The acid hydrolysis products of the t-butyl-OOH carboxylation furthermore co-migrate with the alkaline hydrolysis products. In the absence of t-butyl-OOH, NADPH yields a carboxylation product of lesser radioactivity which does not appear to be identical with that found with t-butyl-OOH.

Larsen and Suttie (3) did not report the details of the chromatographic procedures by which they isolated the t-butyl-OOH carboxylation product except to say that after perchloric acid deproteinization and a sephadex G-25 sizing column, the product migrated with the carboxylation product of KH_2 on DEAE-sephadex A-25, and yielded GLA (as determined by TLC) after basic hydrolysis. Two products of t-butyl-OOH metabolism were not mentioned by them. It is possible that under the conditions of our study, the peptide carboxylation product of t-butyl-OOH action might be vanishingly small, although we are inclined to doubt that it would be undetectible.

In light of these findings, the points of evidence which remain to implicate a vitamin K hydroperoxide as an intermediate in the vitamin KH_2-dependent peptide-bound glutamate carboxylation are 1) the inhibitory effect of glutathione peroxidase, 2) the inhibitory effect of t-butyl-OOH (which is largely vitiated in the presence of NADPH), and 3) the formation of vitamin K epoxide as a byproduct of the reaction. Stronger, more direct evidence is needed. Since t-butyl-OOH imitates the structure of a hypothetical hydroperoxide derivative of vitamin K around carbon atom 2, we have synthesized structurally more closely related compounds such as t-butyrophenone-OOH (t-BP-OOH). t-BP-OOH has a potency of 10^3 times that of t-butyl-OOH in inhibiting the KH_2-dependent carboxylation and appears to be competitive. Isolation and characterization of intermediates in the vitamin K-dependent carboxylase reaction would provide even more convincing evidence.

CONCLUSIONS

The products of the t-butyl-OOH-dependent and vitamin KH_2-dependent carboxylation reactions in Triton X-100 solubilized hepatic microsomes from vitamin K-deficient rats are distinctly different under our conditions of incubation. Vitamin KH_2 clearly stimulated incorporation of $^{14}CO_2$ into the peptide substrate, Phe-Leu-Glu-Glu-Ile, to yield a GLA residue as has been previously reported (9,10). t-Butyl-OOH, on the other hand, yields a radioactive product distinct from the peptide which is not GLA, and which is produced in the absence of the peptide substrate. It is both alkali and acid stable, does not yield GLU on acid hydrolysis, and does not resemble GLA, GLU or citrate in four TLC systems. It is not identical with any of the Krebs tricarboxylic acid cycle intermediates.

t-Butyl-OOH does not appear to be an agonist for vitamin K in the vitamin KH_2-dependent carboxylation reaction. t-Butyl-OOH, however, is a competitive antagonist for this reaction. An even more potent inhibitor is t-butyrophenone-OOH which imitates the structure of vitamin K around carbon atom 2 more completely. More direct evidence is needed to establish vitamin KH_2-peroxide as an intermediate in GLA synthesis.

ACKNOWLEDGEMENTS

This investigation was supported by Grant AM-09992 from the National Institutes of Health, Bethesda, Maryland. We thank Dr. Robert K.Y. Zee-Cheng for the synthesis of GLA and t-butyrophenone-OOH, and Richard Pinkston for amino acid analysis.

REFERENCES

1. Jones, J.P., Gardner, E.J., Cooper, T.G., and Olson, R.E. (1977) J. Biol. Chem. 252, 7738-7742.

2. Olson, R.E. and Suttie, J.W. (1978) Vit. and Horm. 35, 59-108.

3. Larsen, A.E. and Suttie, J.W. (1978) Proc. Natl. Acad. Sci. USA 75, 5413-5416.

4. Dunkle, B.F., Turner, P.M., Hall, A.L., Wing, D.A., Houser, R.M., and Olson, R.E. (1979) Fed. Proc., 38, 723.

5. Zee-Cheng, R.K.Y. and Olson, R.E. (1979) Vitamin K, pp. (this proceedings), (J.W. Suttie, ed.).

6. Olson, R.E. and Houser, R.M. (1977) Circulation 56, Suppl. 3, 78.

7. Shah, D.V. and Suttie, J.W. (1978) Arch. Biochem. Biophys. 191, 571-577.

8. Larsen, A.E., Whitlon, D.S., and Suttie, J.W. (1979) Fed. Proc. 38, 876.

9. Suttie, J.W., Hageman, J.M., Lehrman, S.R., and Rich, D.H. (1976) J. Biol. Chem. 251, 5827-5830.

10. Houser, R.M., Carey, D.J., Dus, K.M., Marshall, G.R., and Olson, R.E. (1977) FEBS Lett. 75, 226-230.

SPECIES VARIATION, INDUCTION, AND SUBCELLULAR LOCALIZATION OF THE LIVER VITAMIN K-DEPENDENT CARBOXYLASE

T. L. CARLISLE, D. V. SHAH, and J. W. SUTTIE

Department of Biochemistry
College of Agricultural and Life Sciences
University of Wisconsin-Madison
Madison, WI 53706

INTRODUCTION

The vitamin K-dependent carboxylase of liver microsomes has been most extensively studied in crude microsomal preparations from vitamin K-deficient rat liver, and only limited information regarding carboxylase activity in other species is available. The available data (1,2) suggest that the activity of this enzyme is higher in the rough rather than the smooth microsomal fractions, but no careful study of the complete subcellular distribution of this enzyme or of the relative localization of this carboxylase and other vitamin K metabolizing enzymes in liver is available. This report summarizes recent studies in our laboratory of the carboxylase activity of various species, the induction of the activity during the development of a hypoprothrombinemic state, and the subcellular and membrane localization of various vitamin K-dependent activities of rat liver microsomes.

METHODS

Young male animals obtained from commercial suppliers were used to determine the carboxylase activity in the liver of various species. A plasma hypoprothrombinemia (two-stage prothrombin activity of less than 20% of normal) was developed by oral anticoagulant administration or by maintaining the animals on a vitamin K-deficient diet. All animals were starved for 18 h before they were killed by decapitation and the livers obtained. A Triton X-100 solubilized preparation of liver microsomes was used to determine the vitamin K-dependent incorporation of $H^{14}CO_3^-$ into the endogenous microsomal precursor protein (protein carboxylation) or into the substrate Phe-Leu-Glu-Glu-Leu (peptide carboxylation) as previously described (3). The alteration of carboxylase activity during the development of a hypoprothrombinemic state was assayed as previously described (4). For the determination of the subcellular distribution of vitamin K metabolizing enzymes in liver from vitamin K-deficient rats, rough and smooth microsomes were prepared as described by Dallner (5), and mitochondria as described by Sattocason et al. (6). Details of the separation procedure, proof of cleanliness of fractions, procedures for trypsin treatment of microsomes, and details of assays for vitamin K-dependent carboxylase, vitamin K epoxidase, and vitamin K epoxidase reductase are available (7).

RESULTS

The rat liver microsomal vitamin K-dependent carboxylase activity was originally shown (8) to be dependent on the level of prothrombin precursors in the microsomes and, therefore, on the degree of hypoprothrombinemia of the animals. The initial report (9) of the carboxylation of a peptide substrate indicated that this activity was also increased 2-3 fold in microsomes from hypoprothrombinemic rats, and suggested that not only the substrate for the carboxylase, but the enzyme itself, was increased by a vitamin K deficiency. The data in Figure 1 illustrated this response and demonstrated that liver microsomes from rats fed a vitamin K-deficient diet for 7 days or injected with Warfarin for 18 h have an increased capacity to carboxylate both endogenous precursors and a peptide substrate.

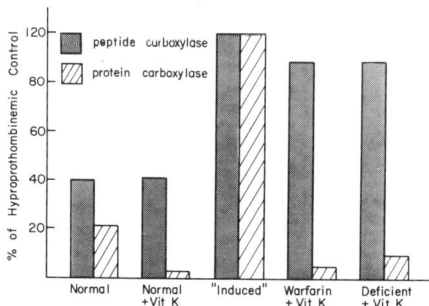

FIGURE 1. Effect of vitamin K status on vitamin K-dependent carboxylase activity. The fully "induced" animals represent 7-day vitamin K-deficient rats or rats given Warfarin 18 h before the assay. When administered, vitamin K was given 15 min before the rats were killed.

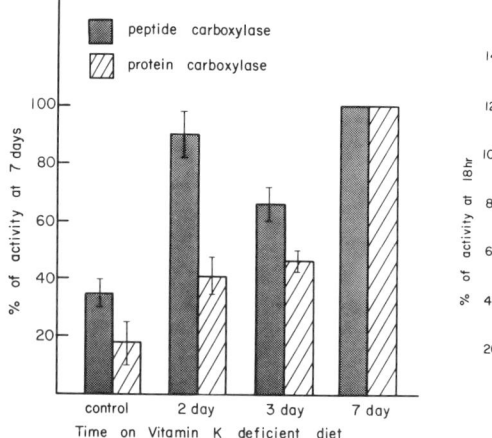
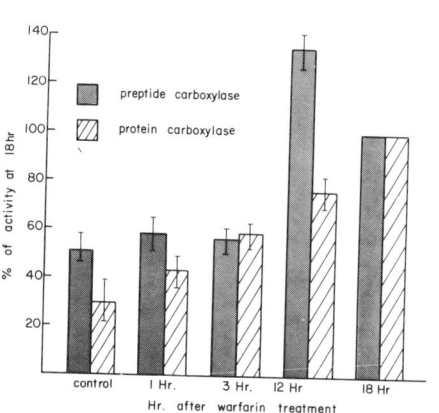

FIGURE 2. Vitamin K deficiency and Warfarin treatment on alterations in vitamin K-dependent carboxylase activity.

Pretreatment of the animals with vitamin K reduces the protein carboxylase activity as the precursor substrates have been converted to prothrombin, but has little influence on the high activity demonstrated toward the peptide substrate. The increase in carboxylase activity with time is shown in Figure 2, and the relative alteration in plasma prothrombin and liver prothrombin precursor in Figure 3. When these data are considered, it seems apparent that the extent of endogenous protein carboxylation is a reflection of the amount of precursor(s) available at any given time. The peptide carboxylase activity, which presumably is an indication of the actual amount of activity of the carboxylase enzyme, responds more rapidly to the development of hypoprothrombinemia and reaches its maximum level before the maximum level of liver precursor has been achieved.

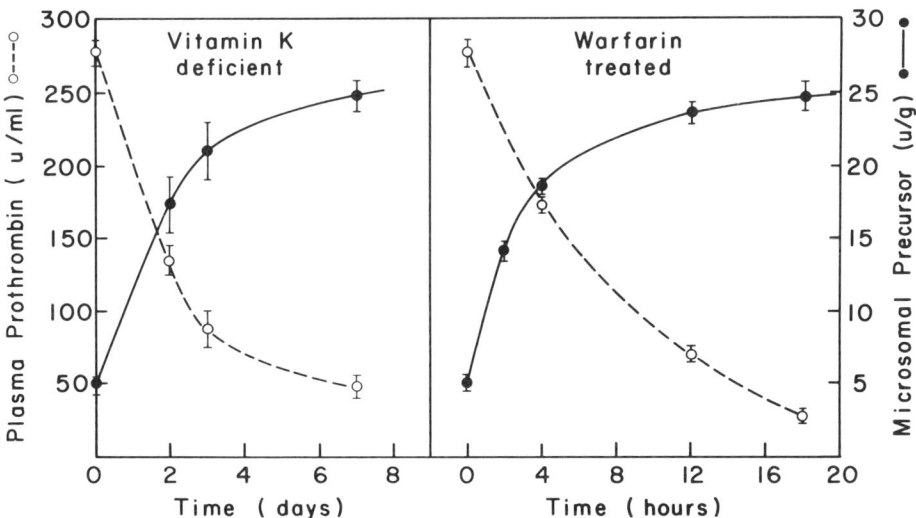

FIGURE 3. Effect of vitamin K deficiency and Warfarin treatment on plasma prothrombin and microsomal prothrombin precursor concentrations.

The vitamin K-dependent carboxylase activity of microsomes obtained from normal and hypoprothrombinemic animals of various species is shown in Figure 4. With the exception of the guinea pig, the activity was enhanced in hypoprothrombinemic animals. The degree to which the vitamin K deficiency enhanced the activity in other species was variable, but peptide carboxylation was usually increased 2-4 fold. It seems likely that this represents an increase in amount or activity of the enzyme. The increase in endogenous protein carboxylation is probably a better measure of the amount of precursor protein which built up in the microsomes of these animals when vitamin K action is blocked. The highest vitamin K-dependent carboxylase activity was found in hamsters and Warfarin-resistant rats. The activity in hypoprothrombinemic hamsters was 2-3-fold higher than in vitamin K-deficient rats and nearly 10 times higher than in normal rats. The carboxylase activity in the normal chick and calf was much lower than in other species, and peptide carboxylase activity remained relatively low even after anticoagulant treatment. The remainder of the species studied exhibited activity that was seen in the same general range as that observed for the rat.

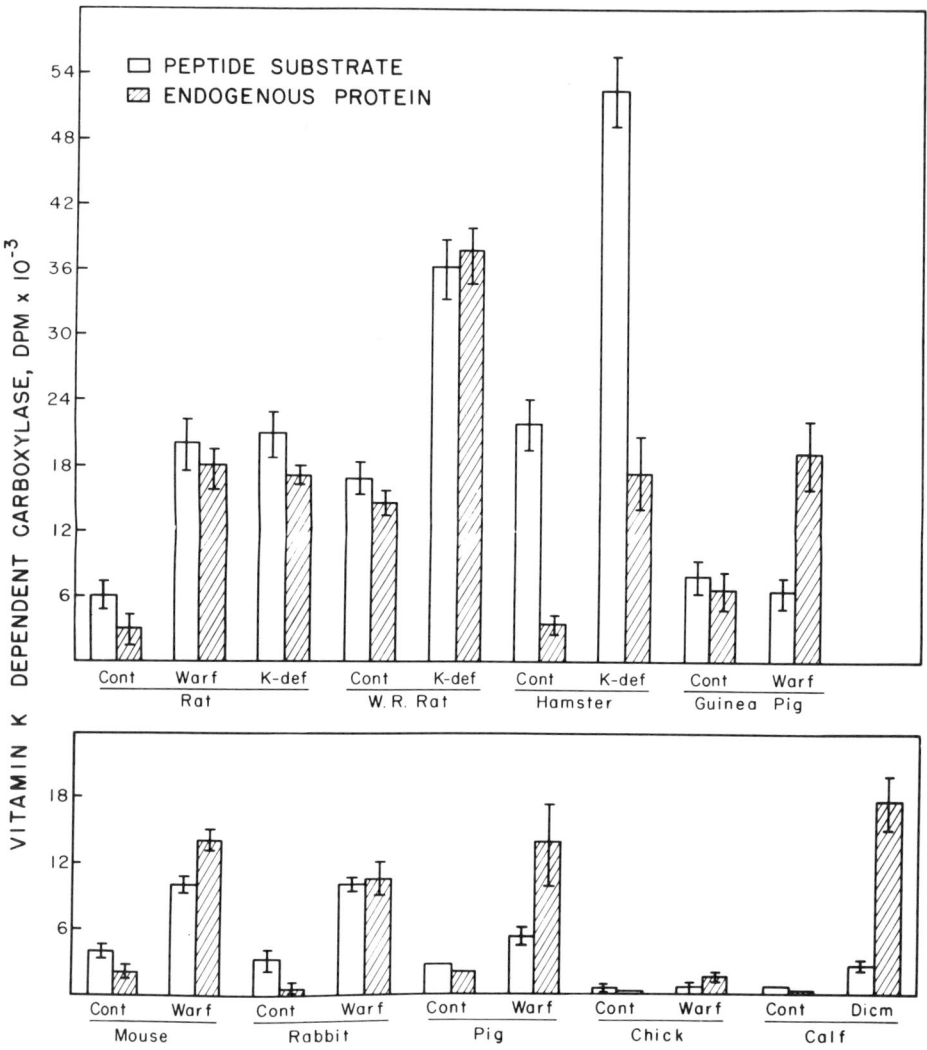

FIGURE 4. Vitamin K-dependent liver carboxylase activities in control, vitamin K-deficient, and anticoagulant-treated animals.

When the activity of various vitamin K-dependent enzymes in rat liver was assayed in subcellular fractions (Fig. 5), it was clear that for all enzymes measured, the highest activity was found in the rough microsomal fraction. When appropriate corrections are made for the contamination of the rough microsome fraction with smooth microsomes and the relative amounts of the two fractions are considered, it appears that 80-90% of the total enzyme activity as measured with a peptide substrate is present in the rough membrane fraction. The vitamin K epoxidase and epoxide reductase activities are also predominately present in the rough membrane fraction. In contrast to the other activities, the amount of the

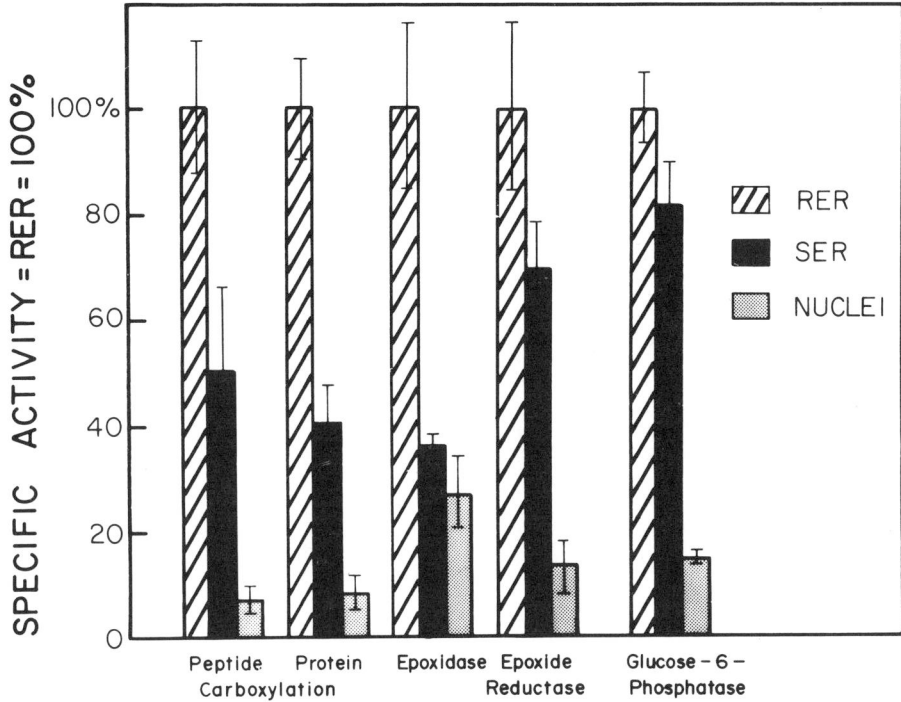

FIGURE 5. Relative activity of various vitamin K-related activities in rough endoplasmic reticulum (RER), smooth endoplasmic reticulum (SER), and nuclei. Glucose-6-phosphatase activity is included as a marker.

vitamin K epoxidase found in the nuclear fraction might be more than can be explained by contamination of this fraction with microsomal enzyme. Intact microsomes do not utilize low-molecular-weight peptides as substrates for the carboxylase, and this suggests that the enzyme is not located at the cytoplasmic surface of the membrane. Trypsin does not penetrate microsomal membranes, and treatment of this vesicular preparation with this proteolytic enzyme provides another approach to determining the orientation of the vitamin K-dependent enzyme within the membrane. The data in Figure 6 indicate that the vitamin K-dependent carboxylase and the vitamin K-epoxide reductase behave as typical intrinsic membrane proteins. They are not influenced by treatment with trypsin until the membrane integrity has been destroyed by treatment with the detergent Triton X-100. The partial inhibition of the vitamin K epoxidase activity treatment with trypsin suggests that this enzyme might have some component which is at least partially accessible to proteolysis; but, for the most part, it too is protected by the membrane.

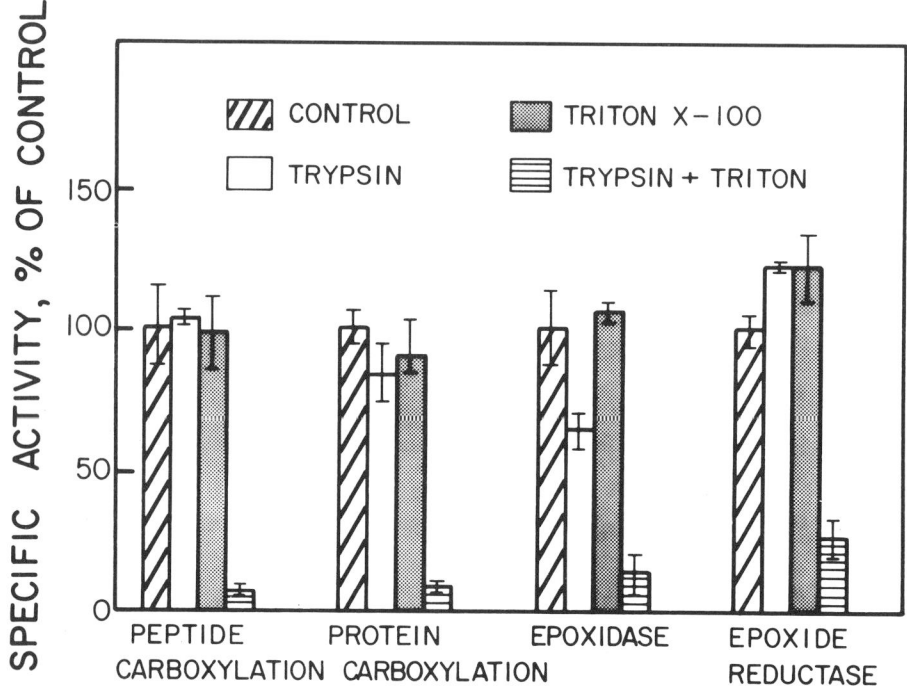

FIGURE 6. Effect of trypsin treatment on liver microsomal vitamin K-related activities. Microsomes were incubated in the presence or absence of 0.15 mg/ml trypsin and/or 0.2% Triton X-100 for 15 h at 4° C before being assayed under standard conditions.

DISCUSSION

These data indicate that the activity of the vitamin K-dependent carboxylase is increased during those periods when vitamin K action is blocked. Neither the basis for this increase nor the physiological signal responsible for it has been determined, but the available data (4) would be most consistent with a true increase in amount of enzyme. Although it seems logical to look upon this as a control function which would aid in the maintenance of the plasma levels of the vitamin K-dependent clotting factors, such a role is only supposition at the present time. The survey of various species for carboxylase activity has shown that most other species respond in the same fashion as the rat, and increase carboxylase activity when vitamin K activity is blocked. These data also indicate that the rat has been a reasonable choice in the study of this activity. With the exception of the hamster, it has as good an activity as any other readily obtainable species. The hamster shows the same Warfarin resistance (10) as does a strain of Warfarin-resistant rats, and both of these animals have a high carboxylase activity. They also have a high requirement for vitamin K, and this may represent an attempt to maintain adequate carboxylation in the face of an inadequate amount of the vitamin.

These data have expanded on the previous reports (1,2,11) that the vitamin K-dependent carboxylase is localized in the rough microsomal fractions, and have presented evidence that the enzymes responsible for vitamin K epoxidation and reduction of the epoxide are also located predominately in this subcellular fraction. The evidence that there is a close connection between the vitamin K epoxidase activity and the vitamin K-dependent carboxylase activity has been reviewed (12), and these data on the localization of the activities would also support some type of interrelationship of the two activities. The enrichment of the epoxidase activity in rough microsomes contrasts with the distribution of most mixed function oxidases which are predominately located in the smooth membrane fraction. The various activities measured also appear to be present predominately as intrinsic microsomal proteins and suggest a model in which the carboxylase active site is exposed on the cisternal side of the microsomal membrane. This would be consistent with the carboxylation of glutamyl residues of vitamin K-dependent precursor proteins being a very early event in a series of posttranslational modifications required for the complete synthesis of a complex plasma glycoprotein such as prothrombin. The similar location of the vitamin K epoxidase and epoxide reductase again points out the physiological importance of the cycling of the liver stores of vitamin K between these various forms.

ACKNOWLEDGEMENTS

These studies were supported by the College of Agricultural and Life Sciences, University of Wisconsin-Madison, and in part by grant AM-14881 from the National Institutes of Health.

REFERENCES

1. Helgeland, L. (1977) Biochim. Biophys. Acta 499, 181-193.
2. Wallin, R., and Prydz, H. (1979) Thrombos. Haemostas. (Stuttg.) in press.
3. Shah, D. V., and Suttie, J. W. (1979) Proc. Soc. Exp. Biol. Med., in press.
4. Shah, D. V., and Suttie, J. W. (1978) Arch. Biochem. Biophys. 191, 571-577.
5. Dallner, G. (1974) Meth. Enzymol. 31, 191-201.
6. Sottocasa, G. L., Kuylenstierna, B., Ernster, L., and Bergstrand, A. (1967) Meth. Enzymol. 10, 448.
7. Carlisle, T. L. (1978) Ph.D. Thesis, University of Wisconsin-Madison.
8. Esmon, C. T., Sadowski, J. A., and Suttie, J. W. (1975) J. Biol. Chem. 250, 4744-4748.
9. Suttie, J. W., Hageman, J. M., Lehrman, S. R., and Rich, D. H. (1976) J. Biol. Chem. 251, 5827-5830.
10. Shah, D. V., and Suttie, J. W. (1975) Proc. Soc. Exp. Biol. Med. 150, 126-128.
11. Carlisle, T. L., and Suttie, J. W. (1978) Fed. Proc. 37, 708 (abstr.).
12. Suttie, J. W., Larson, A. E., Canfield, L. M., and Carlisle, T. L. (1978) Fed. Proc. 37, 2605-2609.

EFFECT OF PYRIDOXAL PHOSPHATE ON THE VITAMIN K-DEPENDENT CARBOXYLASE

J. W. SUTTIE, L. O. GEWEKE, J. L. FINNAN, S. R. LEHRMAN, and D. H. RICH

Department of Biochemistry
College of Agricultural and Life Sciences and School of Pharmacy
University of Wisconsin-Madison
Madison, WI 53706

INTRODUCTION

The inhibition or stimulation of the vitamin K-dependent microsomal carboxylase which converts a peptide-bound glutamyl residue to γ-carboxyglutamyl residues by various compounds has recently been reviewed (1-3). The mechanism of action of most compounds which influence this system can be explained on the basis of their specific interaction with vitamin K or their general effect on this sulfhydryl-containing enzyme. The major carboxylase systems of green plants, the ribulose bisphosphate carboxydismutase enzyme, has been shown (4) to be inhibited by pyridoxal-phosphate (PLP). In this case, an essential amino group of the enzyme presumably formed a Schiff base with PLP, and its activity was effectively titrated by PLP. When the influence of PLP on the vitamin K-dependent carboxylase was determined, it was found (5) to stimulate rather than inhibit the reaction. This report describes a series of investigations which were carried out to determine the mechanism by which this coenzyme influences the activity of the vitamin K-dependent carboxylase.

METHODS

Vitamin K-dependent carboxylase assays utilized a triton X-100 solubilized rat liver microsomal preparation from vitamin K-deficient rats. The conditions of incubations were those previously described (5,6); and, unless otherwise indicated, incubations contained 100 μg/ml of vitamin KH_2, 1 mM pyridoxal-phosphate, and 0.5 mM Phe-Leu-Glu-Glu-Leu as a substrate. Samples were incubated for 30 min at 27° C, and $^{14}CO_2$ incorporation into the substrate was measured as previously described (5,6).

RESULTS

The data in Figure 1A indicate the maximum effect of PLP phosphate was seen at a concentration of 1 mM and that the addition of this coenzyme had no effect on the carboxylation of the endogenous microsomal proteins which were present in the preparation. At 27° C, the carboxylation of endogenous proteins is essentially complete within 5-10 min of incubation, and the effect of PLP on the rate of endogenous protein carboxylation would not be evident in the standard assay. Incubations were therefore carried out at 5° C where it is possible to observe the initial rate of endogenous protein carboxylation. The data in Figure 1B clearly show that the rate of this reaction is not influenced by the presence of PLP. The data in Figure 1A were from single time-point assays, and it was possible that PLP could have been influencing either the initial rate of peptide substrate

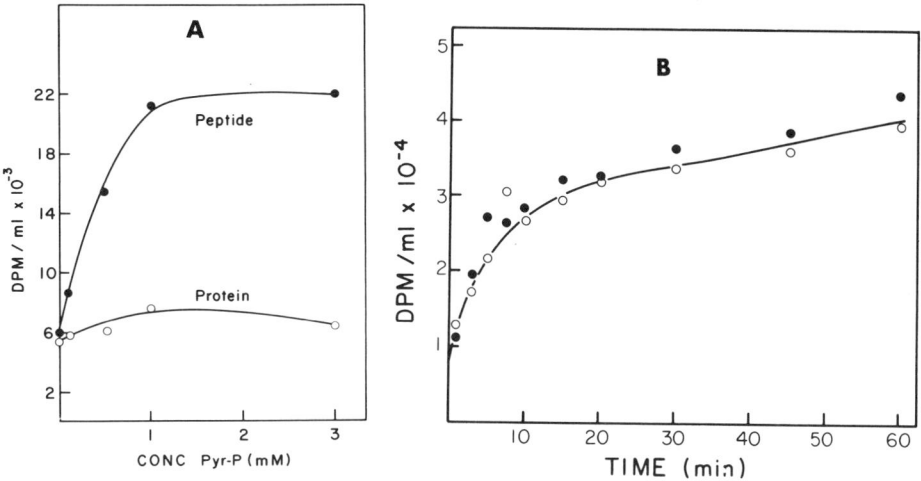

FIGURE 1. (A) Effect of pyridoxal phosphate on the vitamin K-dependent carboxylation of both a soluble peptide substrate and endogenous microsomal proteins. (B) Rate of carboxylation of endogenous microsomal proteins in the presence (●—●) and absence (○—○) of pyridoxal phosphate.

carboxylation, or that it could have extended the period of linearity of the reaction. The data in Figure 2A clearly show that the initial rate of the reaction is increased and that the addition of PLP at various times after the start of the reaction allows the reaction to proceed at a more rapid rate. A number of other pyridoxine derivatives or structurally unrelated aldehydes were assayed in an attempt to determine the specificity of this response. The effect of the addition of formaldehyde, pyridoxal·HCL,

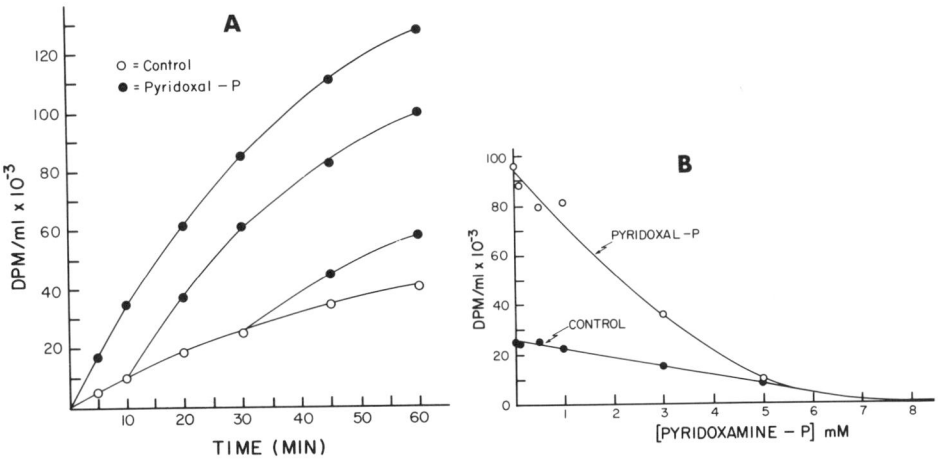

FIGURE 2. (A) Effect of pyridoxal-phosphate on the rate of soluble peptide substrate carboxylation. (B) Effect of pyridoxamine phosphate on the vitamin K-dependent carboxylase activity.

Na pyrophosphate, 2,3-diphosphoglycerate, 4-deoxypyridoxine, pyridoxamine-phosphate, and pyridoxic acid on the carboxylase system was determined. None of these compounds stimulated the carboxylase; and pyridoxal HCl, pyridoxic acid, and pyridoxamine-phosphate showed significant inhibition of the reaction at a concentration of 3 mM. The inhibition of the system by pyridoxamine-phosphate was considered in more detail (Fig. 2B), and it was found that addition of this compound overcame the effect of pyridoxal-phosphate, and at high concentration it inhibited the control reaction.

Although these data clearly demonstrated the effect of PLP on the vitamin K-dependent carboxylation reaction, they offered no evidence for its mechanism of action. The carboxylation of peptide substrates is much more sensitive to the vitamin K concentration of the incubation than is the carboxylation of endogenous protein (5), and it was possible that PLP was influencing the efficiency of vitamin K utilization. The data in Figure 3A indicate that this was not the case. At all vitamin K concentrations the effect of PLP was similar. The most logical explanation for the effect of PLP would appear to be that it might form a Schiff base with the free amino group of the substrate, Phe-Leu-Glu-Glu-Leu, and that the formation of this adduct might influence the efficiency of binding of the substrate. A number of lines of evidence argue against this explanation. The apparent K_m for this substrate is not influenced by the presence or absence of PLP (Fig. 3B). An effect of PLP on substrate binding would have been expected to lower the K_m for the substrate, but it apparently did not

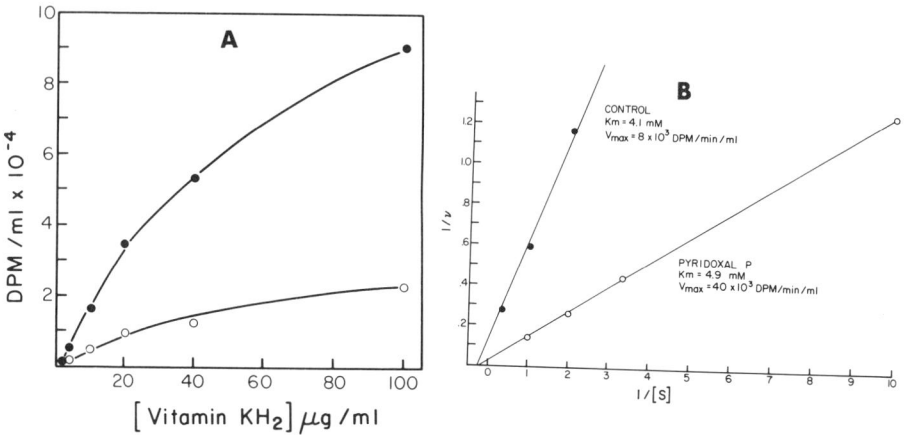

FIGURE 3. (A) Vitamin K-dependent carboxylase activity in the presence (●—●) and absence (o—o) of pyridoxal phosphate at varying vitamin K concentrations. (B) Double reciprocal plot of vitamin K-dependent carboxylase activity in the presence and absence of pyridoxal phosphate.

as the observed values were essentially identical. The postulated Schiff base adduct of the peptide and PLP can be formed. When a 1.5 molar excess of PLP was reacted with Phe-Leu-Glu-Glu-Leu in methanol, a bright yellow compound was formed. This adduct was reduced with $NaBH_4$ and the covalently bound product isolated by chromatography on Sephadex G-25 and DEAE Sephadex. This compound, which should have substrate binding properties very similar to the Schiff base formed between PLP and the pentapeptide substrate, was not as good a substrate for the enzyme as the unmodified peptide (Table 1).

It does not have a free amino group, yet its activity was stimulated by PLP. The activity of four other substrates which do not have a free amino group and could not enter into Schiff base formation was also stimulated by PLP. These included a simple modified glutamic acid derivative, t-BOC-Glu-α-benzyl-ester, which is carboxylated (7) by this system. These data (Fig. 3B and Table 1) make it unlikely that the effect of PLP on the system is mediated through Schiff base formation with the exogenous substrates.

TABLE 1. Effect of pyridoxal phosphate on various carboxylase substrates.

Substrate	Activity Relative to Phe-Leu-Glu-Glu-Leu	% Stimulation by Pyridoxal-phosphate
Phe-Leu-Glu-Glu-Leu	100	316
Acetyl-Phe-Leu-Glu-Glu-Leu	42	274
Propionyl-Phe-Leu-Glu-Glu-Leu	153	120
Pyridoxal-Phe-Leu-Glu-Glu-Leu	26	170
BOC-Leu-Glu-Glu-Leu	54	160
BOC-Glu-Bz	5	129

All substrates were assayed at 1 mM in the presence or absence of 1 mM pyridoxal-phosphate.

The lack of effect of PLP in the carboxylation of endogenous substrates suggests that the participation of PLP in this reaction is not of any physiological significance. The vitamin K-dependent carboxylase activity of PLP-deficient rats was not significantly influenced. Rats which were fed a vitamin B_6-deficient diet for a sufficient length of time show a drop in the activity of other PLP-dependent enzymes did not show a significantly decreased vitamin K-dependent carboxylase activity.

DISCUSSION

These data have expanded on our initial observation that PLP stimulated the activity of the liver microsomal vitamin K-dependent carboxylase, but have failed to provide an unambiguous explanation to response. The lack of effect on endogenous substrate carboxylation suggests that PLP has nothing to do with the basic reaction mechanism of this enzyme. It should be realized, however, that in most respects the carboxylation of a peptide substrate is more sensitive to inhibition or stimulation than the endogenous microsomal protein substrates (5). It is possible that PLP is interacting with the enzyme at a site near the binding of these exogenous substrates and is in some manner increasing their rate of carboxylation. The rate of endogenous protein carboxylation is much faster than the rate of peptide substrate carboxylation, and it may be that in this case the PLP responsive step is not rate limiting. What this step in the reaction is was not apparent from these studies and will depend on further studies of this system.

ACKNOWLEDGEMENTS

These studies were supported by the College of Agricultural and Life Sciences, University of Wisconsin-Madison, and in part by grants AM-14881, AM-21472, DE-07031, and HL-05649 from the National Institutes of Health.

REFERENCES

1. Suttie, J. W. (1978) Handbook of Lipid Research 2, "The Fat-soluble Vitamins" (DeLuca, H. F., ed.) pp. 211-277, Plenum Press, New York.

2. Olson, R. E., and Suttie, J. W. (1978) Vitamins and Hormones 35, 59-108.

3. Stenflo, J. (1978) Adv. in Enzymol. 46, 1-31.

4. Paech, C., Ryan, F. J., and Tolbert, N. E. (1977) Arch. Biochem. Biophys. 179, 279-288.

5. Suttie, J. W., Lehrman, S. R., Geweke, L. O., Hageman, and Rich, D. H. (1979) Biochem. Biophys. Res. Commun. 86, 500-507.

6. Suttie, J. W., Hageman, J. M., Lehrman, S. R., and Rich, D. H. (1976) J. Biol. Chem. 251, 5827-5830.

7. Finnan, J. L., Goodman, H. L., and Suttie, J. W. (1979) these proceedings.

VITAMIN K ANALOGS IN THE STUDY OF VITAMIN K-DEPENDENT CARBOXYLATION

B. C. JOHNSON, D. O. MACK, R. DELANEY,
M. R. WOLFENSBERGER, C. ESMON, J. A. PRICE, E. SUEN,
and J. -M. GIRARDOT

Oklahoma Medical Research Foundation, and
University of Oklahoma Health Sciences Center,
Oklahoma City, OK 73104

INTRODUCTION

As one way of studying vitamin K-dependent carboxylation in solubilized liver microsomes from vitamin K-deficient rats, we have examined many compounds for inhibitory activity and sought to determine the structural requirements of naphthoquinones for activity in the system.

This work led to the discovery of a number of compounds (many of them vitamin K analogs) which inhibit vitamin K-dependent carboxylation. This, in turn, led to the study of other specific inhibitors, compounds which vary from those closely related in structure to vitamin K, to those unrelated to the naphthoquinones, but which block the reaction similarly.

In studying the structural requirements for activity or inhibition of vitamin K-dependent carboxylation, two different criteria can be used to evaluate the effectiveness of any compound studied. The most usual is to carry out the reaction at a standard temperature for a standard time and compare the plateau values for obtainable carboxylation with the compound being tested. A more valid procedure for evaluating the relative effects of various compounds is to compare the relative rates ("initial rates") of carboxylation (the slope, prior to plateau). This latter method involves comparing rates at a constant temperature and at various concentrations of the compound.

Most of the values reported here will be based on plateau amounts of carboxylation obtained at 20 or 25°.

MATERIALS AND METHODS

Materials

The compounds used were purchased, when available, and those not available were synthesized by modifications of published methods. Purity was checked by UV spectra, thin-layer and gas-liquid chromatography. Identification of synthetic compounds was by GLC-Mass Spectrometry (2).

Methods

The methods of producing vitamin K-deficient rats, preparing liver microsomes, and from them a "solubilized" microsomal system, which we have used to study the incorporation of $[^{14}C]CO_2$ into endogenous protein precursor or into synthetic pentapeptide (PheLeuGluGluLeu) (3), are given in recent publications (1,2) and will not be repeated here. Any modifications of these methods will be given in the Tables and Figures.

The use of particulate microsome carboxylation system (4) will not be considered here and we will restrict this discussion to the solubilized microsome system. The nutritionally vitamin K-deficient rat is the usual source of liver microsomes.

RESULTS

Since the solubilized microsomal carboxylation system carries out the carboxylation reaction with the addition of vitamin K_1 quinone plus NADH, or with the addition of vitamin K_1 hydroquinone, most of the data reported here will be on the carboxylation reaction as defined by its dependence on the hydroquinone. In this way, those compounds which are required for the vitamin K reduction step, will be eliminated from consideration.

The very rapid rate of endogenous precursor protein carboxylation at 20°, when carboxylation is initiated by vitamin K hydroquinone is shown in Figure 1. The figure shows that at 37°, optimum carboxylation is not obtained. This is apparently because the enzyme system is so rapidly inactivated at 37°. At 0°, the reaction will proceed at a straight-line rate for at least 120 min, eventually almost reaching the same carboxylation reached at 20°.

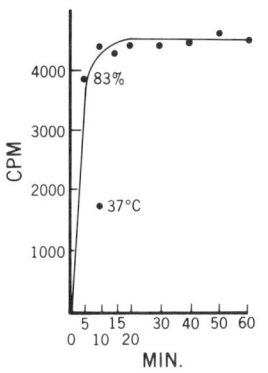
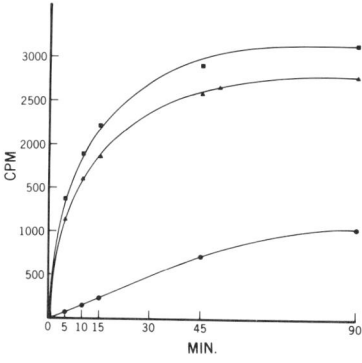

FIGURE 1. Rate of endogenous protein carboxylation at 20°. Vitamin K_1 hydroquinone, 0.55 mM. The point at 37° for 10 min shows the optimum carboxylation with the same vitamin K-deficient hepatic microsomal Triton X-100 solubilized system and the same level of vitamin K_1 hydroquinone and $[^{14}C]CO_2$.
FIGURE 2. Comparison of rate of carboxylation of endogenous protein, endogenous protein plus pentapeptide and pentapeptide. Vitamin K_1 hydroquinone, 0.55 mM. ■——■ , carboxylation of endogenous protein in the presence of 4 mM pentapeptide in pellet; ▲——▲ , carboxylation of endogenous protein in pellet; ●——● , carboxylation of added pentapeptide in supernatant.

The relative rates of endogenous carboxylation and pentapeptide carboxylation are shown in Figure 2. Pentapeptide (PheLeuGluGluLeu) carboxylation has proven to be very useful in studying the reaction. Perhaps, because it has a much slower carboxylation rate and is thus much more sensitive to changes in reactants than is endogenous protein carboxylation.

Before presenting the vitamin K analog data on carboxylation, I would like to give one table on the vitamin K quinone plus NADH solubilized microsome carboxylation system, since reducing capacity (vitamin K hydroquinone and/or sulfhydryl) is so important in the carboxylation system. The results given in Table 1 are for a large number of compounds, which were studied for their ability to replace the NADH requirement in carboxylation initiated by vitamin K quinone.

TABLE 1 The ability of various reducing compounds to replace NADH in carboxylation initiated by vitamin K quinone.

Compound	Concentration	Relative Carboxylation Activity (%)
NADH	2 mM	71
Dithiothreitol	2 mM	77
Dithioerythritol	2 mM	80
NADH + dithiothreitol	2 mM + 4 mM	100^{a}
Reduced glutathione	4 mM	9
β-mercaptoethanol	4 mM	10
Sodium bisulfite	4 mM	0
Sodium dithionite	10 mM	0
Vitamin K hydroquinone (replacing vitamin K quinone)	0.11 mM	190
Coenzyme A -SH	30 mM	0
Sodium borohydride	1.5 mM	46
Ascorbic Acid	4 mM	0

^{a}4,000 cpm.

The results will be presented in three sections:

1. Compounds which were expected to be inhibitory, and which proved to have little or no activity, hence, eliminating some potential reaction sequences.

2. Analogs of vitamin K which were functional in place of vitamin K_1.

3. Compounds including a number of analogs of vitamin K, which strongly inhibited the carboxylation reaction.

---

1. Compounds, some of which were expected to be inhibitory to the carboxylation reaction

The results given in Table 2 were obtained with a large number of potential inhibitors of the vitamin K hydroquinone-initiated reaction. There were a number of surprises as this work progressed. None of the cytochrome p450 inhibitors had any effect, even though the reaction, requiring as it does both reduced vitamin K and oxygen, could be similar to or include a mixed-function oxygenase. This soluble system is relatively insensitive to cyanide and warfarin, although high enough levels of either compound will cause some inihibition. The lack of effect of azide appears to rule out catalase as a part of the reaction, as the lack of an effect of H_2O_2 appears to rule out this compound as an intermediate in the reaction. The almost two-fold stimulation by perchlorate is interpreted as destruction of an inhibitor.

TABLE 2 Metabolic inhibitors which proved inactive in significantly inhibiting vitamin K hydroquinone-initiated endogenous carboxylation

Compound	Concentration	Carboxylation^a
SKL-525A	0.2 mM	100%
Aminoglutethimide (Elipten)	0.1 mM	100%
7,8-benzoflavone	0.1 mM	100%
Carbon monoxide	--^{b}	100%
Metyrapone	0.1 mM	100%
Atabrine (quinacrine)	10 mM	100%
Potassium cyanide	1 mM	100%
Potassium cyanide	10 mM	52%
Sodium azide	2-20 mM	100%
Avidin	250 units/ml	100%
EDTA	10 mM	100%
Phytol	0.2 mM	100%
Warfarin	0.1 mM	100%
Sodium perchlorate	0.5 %	190%
Hydrogen peroxide	0.1 mM	100%
H_2O_2 + NaN_2	0.1 mM	100%
Glutamic acid	50 mM	92%
ATPase (3.6.1.3)	10 units/ml	100%
Formate	50 mM	100%
Nitrite	50 mM	100%

^{a}5,000 cpm

^{b}3 min CO, followed by 3 min O_2.

2. Vitamin K analogs which were functional in place of vitamin K in the carboxylation reaction

Fieser et al (5), in 1941 reported the in vivo activity of a very large number of vitamin K analogs in preventing hypoprothrombinemia in vitamin K-deficient chicks. Is in vitro activity similarly dependent? In Table 3, the relative activities (height of plateau of carboxylation reached) for a large number of quinones and hydroquinones are given.

The experiments which produced the data shown in the various sections of this table gave us some surprises and some disappointments over the years. Probably the first, both surprise and disappointment, was the finding in 1974, that neither the chromanol, nor the chromanol phosphate were active. They were tried on the basis of numerous publications (e.g., 6-9), which postulated the role of the chromanols in bacterial oxidative-phosphorylation. These compounds were very generously synthesized for us by Dr. Patchett and co-workers at Merck, Sharp, and Dohme Research Laboratories. The inactivity of the β-γ dihydrate [and of the cis β-γ unsaturation (10)] seemed to support this early finding. It was also surprising that the epoxide of vitamin K was without activity in the solubilized microsomal system, since it functions essentially as well as vitamin K quinone when intact microsomes are used. Apparently, some conversion factor to a functional form is lost in the solubilization.

What was perhaps most surprising in this early work (Table 3-A) was the inactivity of menadione and menadiol, since in the 1941 feeding experiments, these had been the most active vitamin K compounds on a weight basis, and equal in activity to the natural forms of vitamin K on a molar basis.

Some of these surprises are cleared up by section B of Table 3. From this set of results, it can be seen that a polyprenoid side chain at position 3 of 2-methyl-1,4-naphthoquinone (menadione) is not necessary, but that this position does need to be filled by an uncharged, relatively hydrophobic group.

TABLE 3 Analogs of vitamin K which were tested for activity in the vitamin K carboxylation reaction.

Compound[b]	Plateau Activity (%)[a]
A. Specificity of vitamin K structure for carboxylation activity in the solubilized microsomal system.	
Vitamin K quinone	100[c]
Vitamin K hydroquinone	190
Vitamin K epoxide	0
Vitamin K chromanol	0
Vitamin K chromanol phosphate	0
Menadione	0
Menadiol (+ NADH + dithiothreitol)	0
Vitamin K_1 dihydride	0
B. Thioethers of menadione	
2-methyl-3-thiomethyl-NPQ[d]	92
2-methyl-3-thioethyl-NPQ	38
2-methyl-3-thiobutyl-NPQ	64
2-methyl-3-thio-1,2-propandiol-NPQ	64
2-methyl-3-thioethanol-NPQ	56
2-methyl-3-(dithiothreitol)-NPQ	150
2-methyl-3-(dithioerythritol)-NPQ	200
2-methyl-3-(1,4-thiobutane)-NPQ	150
2-methyl-3-thiophenol-NPQ	15
2-methyl-3-thiobenzyl-NPQ	48
2-methyl-3-(3-thiopropionic acid)-NPQ [Vitamin K-S(II)]	0
2-methyl-3-(3-thiopropionyl ethyl ester)-NPQ	32
2-methyl-3-(3-thioacetyl ethyl ester)-NPQ	25
3-methyl-3-(cysteine)-NPQ	0
2-methyl-3-(thioaminoethane)-NPQ	0
2-methyl-3-(thioaminobutane)-NPQ	0
2-methyl-3-(thio)-diethylaminoethane-NPQ	0
2-methyl-3-(glutathionyl)-NPQ	0
2-methyl-3-(coenzyme A)-NPQ	0
2-methyl-3-thiol-NPQ	0
C. Thioether hydroquinones	
2-methyl-3-thioethyl-1,4-naphthohydroquinone	100
2-methyl-3-(2-amino ethyl)-1,4-naphthohydroquinone	0
2-methyl-3-(thiopropionic acid)-1,4-naphthohydroquinone	0

[a] Since this is a summation of many experiments, various times and temperatures have been used. For this reason, the various plateau values reported are only approximately comparable. The level of vitamin K analog used was 0.11 mM in all cases.
[b] Plus 2 mM NADH, except when hydroquinone replaced quinone, and plus dithiothreitol (10 mM), except where a quinone with an open 3-position is used.
[c] The 100% value varies in different experiments (all assembled in one table here). It normally varies within 3000-6000 cpm per assay tube, with a blank (no added vitamin K compound) which normally varies between 30 and 60 cpm.
[d] NPQ is used here for 1,4-naphthoquinone.

As can be seen when studying the thioethers, some are highly active (particularly in the presence of excess dithiol compound, e.g. dithiothreitol, dithioerythritol, or dithiobutane), but all activity is lost if the 3-side chain carries a positive or negative charge, or both. It is not lost, however, in the case of the relatively hydrophilic, but neutral thio-ethanol and thio-1,2-propandiol derivatives.

Table 3-C shows the high activity of one of the neutral 3-thioethers as the hydroquinone and the complete inactivity of two of the 3-thioethers with charged side-chains, even used as the hydroquinones.

As can be seen from Figure 3 (2), the rate of carboxylation initiated by 2-methyl-3-thiomethyl-1,4-naphthoquinone plus NADH is similar to that with vitamin K_1 plus NADH (Figure 1).

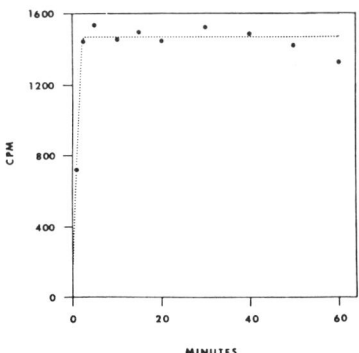

FIGURE 3 Rate of response of carboxylation to 0.25 mM, 2-methyl-3-thiomethyl-1,4-naphthoquinone.

Table 4-A shows the relative plateau activities of some 3-O-ethers as the quinones, while 4-B shows the activity of one derivative of menadiol with a long chain alkyl at the three position. These data also show the non-specificity of the 3-position side chain.

TABLE 4 Activities of other vitamin K derivatives

Compound	As Hydroquinone
A. Activity of phthiocol and its alkyl ethers as hydroquinones compared to vitamin K_1[a].	
Vitamin K_1	100%
Phthiocol	15%
2-methyl-3-methoxy-1,4-naphthoquinone	20%
2-methyl-3-ethoxy-1,4-naphthoquinone	60%
2-methyl-3-n-propoxy-1,4-naphthoquinone	32%
B. Activity of hydroquinones of various structures compared to vitamin K_1 (at 0° for 10 min)[b]	
Vitamin K_1	190%
Durohydroquinone	0
2-methyl-3-pentadecyl-1,4-naphthoquinone	37%
2-ethoxy-3-(3-methyl-2-butenyl)-1,4-napthoquinone (lapachol)	2%

[a]These carboxylations were carried out at 0° for 10 min. The hydroquinones were used at 1.0 mM.

[b]All analogs added at 1.5 mM, except vitamin K_1, which was used at 0.55 mM.

3. Compounds including vitamin K analogs which inhibit carboxylation

Figure 4 illustrates the wide range of inhibition activities shown by different quinones. Duroquinone was the most inhibitory of the compounds studied in these experiments. In regard to the naphthoquinones, those with a hydroxyl or methoxyl in the 2-position were all much more inhibitory than the dicoumarol compound to which they were compared. This probably reflects the ability of these quinones to rapidly oxidize vitamin K hydroquinone.

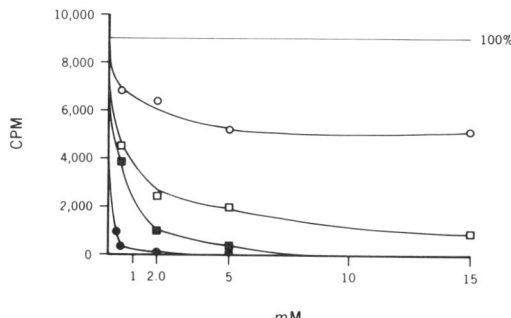

FIGURE 4 Concentration dependency of quinone and 7-ethoxycoumarin inhibition of vitamin K_1 hydroquinone-initiated carboxylation. ☐──☐, lapachol quinone [2-hydroxy-3-(3-methyl-2-butenyl)-1,4-naphthoquinone]; ■──■, phthiocol quinone [2-methyl-3-hydroxy-1,4-naphthoquinone] (2-methoxy-1,4-naphthoquinone gave the same inhibition); ●──●, duroquinone; ○──○, 7-ethoxycoumarin. Vitamin K_1 hydroquinone at 0.55 mM. Carboxylation at 20° for 10 min.

As can be seen from Table 5, the most active non-analog inhibitors of endogenous carboxylation in the soluble system are tetrachloropyridinol, parahydroxymercuribenzoate (pHMB), and Cu^{2+}. In all three cases, this inhibition was totally reversible by sulfhydryl reagents such as dithiothreitol. In all these cases also, pentapeptide carboxylation was considerably more sensitive to the inhibitor, than was endogenous protein carboxylation, indicating that the essential sulfhydryl is not on the carboxyl acceptor molecule.

TABLE 5 Some inhibitors of endogenous carboxylation by the soluble system when carboxylation is initiated by vitamin K_1 hydroquinone

Compound	Concentration[a]	% Carboxylation Activity Remaining
NAD	30 mM	0
Sodium dithionite	500 mM	1.5
Dicoumarol	1 mM	53
Warfarin	20 mM	50
7-ethoxycoumarin	1 mM	100
Tetra-chloropyridinol	0.2 mM	6
Potassium ferricyanide[b]	10 mM	0
para-hydroxymercuribenzoate[b,c] (pHMB)	1 mM	0
phenyl-N-tert·-butyl-nitrone[d]	100 mM	6
Cu^{2+}[b]	1.5 mM	2
Chloro-vitamin K_1[e]	1.1 mM	50
Sodium Arsenite[f]	50 mM	0
Zinc acetate	50 mM	5
Pyridoxal-5'-phosphate	25 mM	34
Pyridoxine	2.5 mM	88
$FeCl_3$	2.5 M	100
EDTA	10 mM	100

[a]Minimum level used to obtain this inhibition
[b]All these inhibitions were reversible by dithiothreitol.
[c]Pentapeptide carboxylation blocked at 0.25 mM pHMB.
[d]A spin-trapping agent
[e]Not reversible by dithiothreitol (10 mM). Chloro-K inhibits pentapeptide carboxylation about 30% at this level.
[f]Inhibition prevented by prior addition of dithiothreitol.

The results shown in Figure 4 are expanded to include many more vitamin K analog inhibitors in Table 6. This table continues the theme proposed earlier that there appear to be two general classes of antagonists: 1) those which react with a sulfhydryl group, thereby blocking the reaction (Table 6-A) and; 2) those which are, in general, considerably less inhibitory, and appear to inhibit by oxidation of vitamin K hydroquinone back to the quinone (Table 6-B).

TABLE 6 Analogs of vitamin K quinone which are inactive in replacing it and are inhibitors of the reaction. Endogenous protein carboxylation initiated by vitamin K_1 hydroquinone[a]

Compound	Minimal Level for this Inhibition	Activity Remaining (%)
A. All these inihibitions are totally reversible by 10 mM dithiothreitol, except the inhibition by 2-methyl-5-hydroxy-1,4-naphthoquinone.		
None		100
1,4-naphthoquinone	0.3 mM	2
Menadione	0.3 mM	6
Vitamin K-S(II)	0.2 mM	5
2,3-dichloro-1,4-naphthoquinone	0.3 mM	0
2-methyl-3-thioethylamine-1,4-napththoquinone	0.3 mM	6
2-methyl-3-(cysteine)-1,4-naphthoquinone	0.3 mM	45
2-methyl-5-hydroxyl-1,4-naphthoquinone (Plumbagin)	0.3 mM	0
3-methyl-5-ethoxy-1,4-naphthoquinone	0.3 mM	3.5
B. Inhibitory compounds not reversed by dithiothreitol.		
Duroquinone	2.0 mM	1
2-hydroxy-1,4-naphthoquinone	0.3 mM	69
2-methoxy-1,4-naphthoquinone	0.5 mM	5
2-methoxy-1,4-naphthoquinone epoxide	3.0 mM	78
2-methyl-3-hydroxy-1,4-naphthoquinone (phthiocol)	0.5 mM	55
2-hydroxyl-3-chloro-1,4-naphthoquinone	0.3 mM	79
2-hydroxy-3-(3-methyl-2-butenyl)-1,4-naphthoquinone (lapachol)	15 mM	5
C. Compounds inactive, but not inhibitors		
Coenzyme Q (Ubiquinone 10)		

[a]Vitamin K_1 hydroquinone at the level of 0.11 mM, no NADH or dithiothreitol added.

The compound, 2-methyl-5-hydroxy-1,4-naphthoquinone (plumbagin) (Table 6-A), is a highly active inhibitor which is not reversed by dithiothreitol. Its inhibitory activity resides in the 5-hydroxy group, since the 5-ethoxy analog is readily reversed by dithiothreitol. As can be seen from Table 6-C, ubiquinone (CoQ_{10}) is without activity either as an inhibitor or a carboxylation co-factor.

Since there were a number of analogs which were highly inhibitory as the quinone, a number of examples of each class of inhibitor were studied as the hydroquinone (Table 7). As can be seen, the inhibitory activity was slight as compared to sulfhydryl-inhibiting quinones and the only compounds with significant inhibitory activity as the hydroquinones, were those compounds which contained a 2-hydroxyl or methoxyl replacing the required 2-methyl of vitamin K.

TABLE 7 Vitamin K analogs used as their hydroquinones to inhibit endogenous protein, soluble system, carboxylation. Carboxylation initiated by vitamin K_1 hydroquinone (0.55 mM)[a]

Compound	Residual Carboxylation
1,4-naphthohydroquinone	78%
2-methyl-1,4-naphthohydroquinone[b]	117%
2-methyl-5-hydroxy-1,4-naphthohydroquinone[c]	87%
2-methyl-5-ethoxy-1,4-naphthohydroquinone	133%
2-hydroxy-1,4-naphthohydroquinone	62%
2-methoxy-1,4-naphthohydroquinone	66%
2-hydroxy-3-(3-methyl-2-butenyl)-1,4-naphthohydroquinone[d]	52%
No inhibitor	100%[e]

[a]The different 1,4-naphthohydroquinones were added at 1.1 mM and vitamin K_1 hydroquinone at 0.55 mM. Their addition to the soluble system was carried out simultaneously.
[b]Menadiol
[c]Plumbagin hydroquinone
[d]Lapachol hydroquinone
[e]5,000 cpm

These results led us to further examine the sulfhydryl requirement of vitamin K_1 hydroquinone-initiated carboxylation. In Table 8 and Figure 5, it is shown that the three sulfhydryl reagents, N-ethyl maleimide, iodoacetamide, and iodoacetic acid are much less active inhibitors of carboxylation than is pHMB (Figure 6).

TABLE 8 Carboxylating activity of the soluble system after preincubation with sulfhydryl-blocking compounds[a,b]

Preincubation at 0° C for 60 min in the dark with the compounds below	Activity remaining when Vitamin K_1 was used to initiate carboxylation
N-ethyl malemide (10 mM)	49%
Iodoacetamide[c] (20 mM)	100%

[a]Vitamin K_1 hydroquinone was at 0.55 mM. Carboxylation was for 10 min at 0° C.
[b]100% - 5000 cpm
[c]Iodoacetic acid gave similar results.

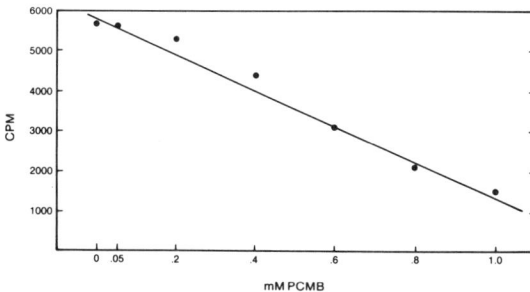

FIGURE 5 Inhibition of carboxylation initiated by vitamin K_1 hydroquinone by parahydroxymercuribenzoate. Vitamin K_1 hydroquinone at 0.11 mM. Carboxylation for 10 min at 0°, immediately after all additions.

In Table 9, the almost complete block in carboxylation, previously shown by menadione (Table 6) is shown to be reversible by dithiothreitol, even in the presence of N-ethylmaleimide or acetamide. This appears to indicate that the essential sulfhydryl(s) is more accessible to menadione and pHMB than to the other reagents. However, Figure 6 does show that with time, even iodoacetamide can markedly inhibit carboxylation.

TABLE 9 Effects of menadione and dithiothreitol on carboxylation after incubation with sulfhydryl blocking agents[a,b]

Preincubation for 60 min at 0° C with the compounds below	Menadione	Menadione plus Dithiothreitol
N-ethylmaleimide (10 mM)	3%	45%
Iodoacetamide (20 mM)	6%	80%

[a]Vitamin K_1 hydroquinone was 0.55 mM; menadione was 0.3 mM; dithiothreitol was 2.0 mM.

[b]100% - 5000 cpm

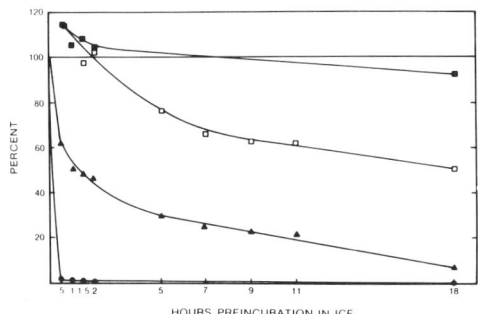

FIGURE 6 Relative time course of inhibition of vitamin K_1 hydroquinone-initiated carboxylation with four different sulfhydryl blocking agents. The times given are hours preincubation at 0°. Carboxylations were carried out for 10 min at 0°. Vitamin K_1 hydroquinone at 0.55 mM. ●——●, parahydroxymercuribenzoate (2.0 mM); ▲——▲, 5,5'-dithiobis (2-nitrobenzoate) (10.0 mM); □——□, iodoacetamide (10.0 mM); ■——■, iodoacetic acid (10.0 mM); ————, no blocking agent added, served as control and set at 100% for each time.

From Figure 7, it is clear that, as with other agents, pentapeptide carboxylation is more sensitive to sulfhydryl blocking agents than is endogenous protein substrate carboxylation. This is particularly noticeable for N-ethylmaleimide and iodoacetamide.

It has been shown that pyridoxal phosphate markedly stimulates pentapeptide carboxylation (11), but that the activation effect of the pyridoxal phosphate appears to be on the carboxylation system, rather than on the pentapeptide (3). Therefore, it was necessary to determine whether pyridoxal phosphate-stimulated carboxylation was equally sensitive to sulfhydryl reagents. The data in Figure 8 show that the stimulated carboxylation is equally sensitive to pHMB.

Vitamin K Analogs   465

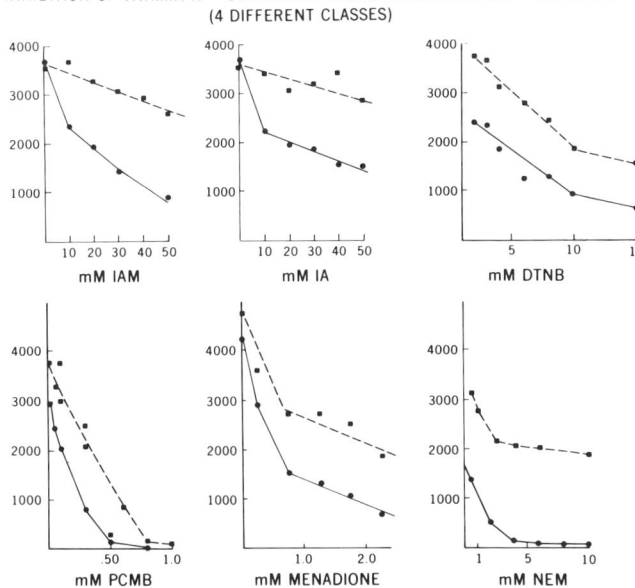

FIGURE 7   Inhibition of carboxylation of endogenous protein and of added exogenous pentapeptide (PheLeuGluGluLeu) substrates by SH blocking agents. Vitamin K_1 hydroquinone at 0.55 mM. ■----■ , endogenous protein carboxylation; ●——● , pentapeptide carboxylation.

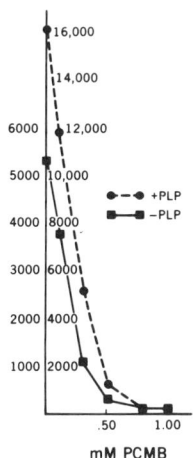

FIGURE 8   Effect of pyridoxal phosphate on inhibition of carboxylation by paracholoromercuribenzoate (pCMB).   Conditions as in Figure 7.   ●----● , plus pyridoxal phosphate (+PLP); ■——■ , minus pyridoxal phosphate (-PLP).

CONCLUSION

1. Most inhibition of vitamin K hydroquinone-induced carboxylation, by vitamin K analogs, as well as other reagents, is reversible by dithiothreitol (and dithioerythritol). It appears that the carboxylation system contains an essential sulfhydryl.

2. Pentapeptide carboxylation is more sensitive to inhibition or stimulation than is endogenous protein carboxylation.

3. The "initial rate" of endogenous protein carboxylation is several orders of magnitude faster than pentapeptide carboxylation.

4. No hydroquinone analog appears to be a highly active inhibitor of vitamin K hydroquinone-initiated carboxylation. This may indicate little or no competition for a binding site.

5. The hydroquinones, which do inhibit carboxylation, all lack the 2-methyl group, supporting the essentiality of that group for the reaction.

ACKNOWLEDGEMENTS

This work was supported in part by NIH grant No. HL17619.

We wish to acknowledge the technical assistance of Ms. Vicki Bartels, Mr. Tom Curtis, and Ms. Julie Miller. We also wish to thank Ms. Patricia Ownbey for her help in the preparation of this manuscript.

REFERENCES

1. Mack, D.O., Wolfensberger, M., Girardot, J.M., Miller, J.A. and Johnson, B.C. (1979) J. Biol. Chem. 254, 2656-2664.
2. Mack, D.O., Suen, E.T., Girardot, J.M., Miller, J.A., Delaney, R. and Johnson, B.C. (1976) J. Biol. Chem. 251, 3269-3276.
3. Dubin, A., Suen, E.T., Delaney, R., Chiu, A. and Johnson, B.C. (1979) Biochem. Biophys. Res. Commun. (In Press).
4. Esmon, C.T., Sadowski, J.A. and Suttie, J.W. (1975) J. Biol. Chem. 250, 4744-4748.
5. Fieser, L.F., Tishler, M. and Sampson, W.L. (1941) J. Biol. Chem. 137, 659-692.
6. Chmielewska, I. and Ciesak, J. (1958) Tetrahedron 4, 135-146.
7. Vilkas, M. and Lederer, E. (1962) Experientia 18, 546-549.
8. Wagner, A.F., Wittreich, P.E., Arison, B., Trenner, N.R., and Folkers, K. (1963) J. Am. Chem. Soc. 85, 1178-1181.
9. Watanabe, T. and Brodie, A.F. (1966) Proc. Nat. Acad. Sci. 56, 940.
10. Friedman, P.A. and Shia, M. (1976) Biochem. Biophys. Res. Commun. 70, 647-654.
11. Suttie, J.W., Lehrman, S.R., Geweke, L.D., Hageman, J.M. and Rich, D.H. (1979) Biochem. Biophys. Res. Commun. 86, 500-507.

STIMULATION OF VITAMIN K_1 PROTEIN CARBOXYLATION BY SEVERAL 1,4-NAPHTHOQUINONES

D. O. MACK, T. A. CURTIS and B. C. JOHNSON

Oklahoma Medical Research Foundation and
University of Oklahoma Health Sciences Center
Oklahoma City, OK 73104

INTRODUCTION

A 2% Triton X-100 extract of liver microsomes from nutritionally vitamin K-deficient rats carries out the carboxylation of specific glutamic acid residues on protein substrates to yield γ-carboxyglutamate (1). In this system, the minimum requirements for promoting vitamin K-dependent carboxylation are CO_2, O_2 and vitamin K_1 hydroquinone (1-3). The vitamin K_1 hydroquinone can be replaced by vitamin K_1 plus NADH. The vitamin K carboxylation system is inhibited by menadione (4). The menadione inhibition is prevented and/or reversed by dithiothreitol through the formation of an active menadione-dithiothreitol adduct (4). This behavior of menadione in the vitamin K-dependent carboxylation system led us to investigate the effect of other 1,4-naphthoquinones on the vitamin K-dependent carboxylation. Several of these 1,4-naphthoquinones, which were found to stimulate vitamin K_1-dependent protein carboxylation initiated by vitamin K quinone plus NADH, are the subject of this paper.

MATERIALS AND METHODS

The preparation of liver microsomes from vitamin K-deficient rats, the Triton X-100 solubilized carboxylation system, and the carboxylation assay were carried out as previously described (4).

Lapachol, 2-methoxy-1,4-naphthoquinone, 2-hydroxy-1,4-naphthoquinone, and 2,3-dichloro-1,4-naphthoquinone were obtained from Aldrich Chemical Co. Technical grade 1,4-naphthoquinone was obtained from Eastman Kodak Co. and purified by recrystallization from ethanol. The 2-hydroxy-3-chloro-1,4-naphthoquinone was prepared by sodium hydroxide hydrolysis of 2,3-dichloro-1,4-naphthoquinone, and the 2-amino-1,4-naphthoquinone was synthesized from 1,4-naphthoquinone by reaction with sodium azide (5).

RESULTS AND DISCUSSION

In the course of investigating the effects of various 1,4-naphthoquinones on the vitamin K protein carboxylation system, a few of the compounds investigated were observed to stimulate carboxylation when carboxylation was initiated by vitamin K quinone plus NADH, although not when it was initiated by vitamin K_1 hydroquinone (Table I). This phenomenon was not given by the benzoquinones, duroquinone, or coenzyme Q_{10} and, thus, is presumably a property of the naphthoquinone nucleus, as well as the substituents. These compounds, which stimulate carboxylation, are ineffective in promoting carboxylation when added to the vitamin K-dependent carboxylation system either as the quinone form plus NADH or as the hydroquinone form.

TABLE 1. Effect of several 1,4-naphthoquinones on vitamin K carboxylation.

Addition	Carboxylation initiated with	
	K_1 + NADH	K_1 hydroquinone
None	100%	100%
2-methoxy-1,4-naphthoquinone	362%	75%
2-hydroxy-1,4-naphthoquinone	214%	70%
Lapachol	250%	80%
Phthiocol	180%	65%
2-hydroxy-3-chloro-1,4-naphthoquinone	189%	75%
2-amino-1,4-naphthoquinone	291%	100%

Figure 1 shows that the stimulation by these naphthoquinones is concentration-dependent. The maximum effect is observed at 0.1 mM, which is the concentration of the vitamin K_1.

The experiments in Table 1 and Figure 1 were carried out at a temperature of 37° for a 20 min incubation period. Thus, the values obtained are maximum plateau levels for 37°, not rates of carboxylation. The observed stimulation of carboxylation could, therefore, be due to any one of

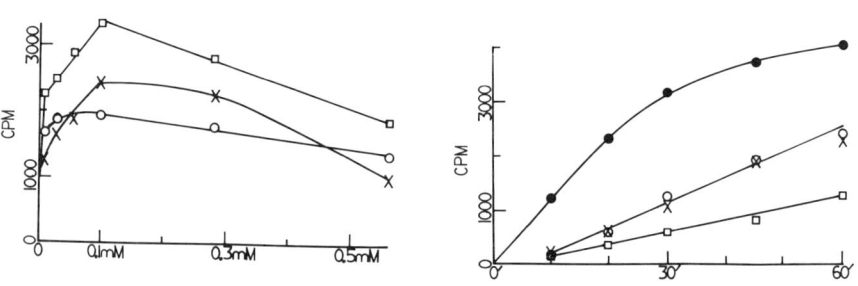

FIGURE 1. (Left) Concentration Dependence. Carboxylation was initiated with 0.1 mM vitamin K_1 and 2 mM NADH at 37° for 20 min. □ , 2-methoxy-1,4-naphthoquinone; X, Lapachol; and ○ , 2-hydroxy-1,4-naphthoquinone.

FIGURE 2. (Right) Rate of Vitamin K_1 Carboxylation. Effect of 2-methoxy-1,4-naphthoquinone, 2-hydroxy-1,4-naphthoquinone and Lapachol. Carboxylation was initiated with 0.1 mM vitamin K_1 and 2 mM NADH at 0° for the indicated times. Addition to the carboxylation assay: □ , no addition; X, 0.1 mM Lapachol; , 0.1 mM 2-hydroxy-1,4-naphthoquinone; and ● , 0.1 mM 2-methoxy-1,4-naphthoquinone.

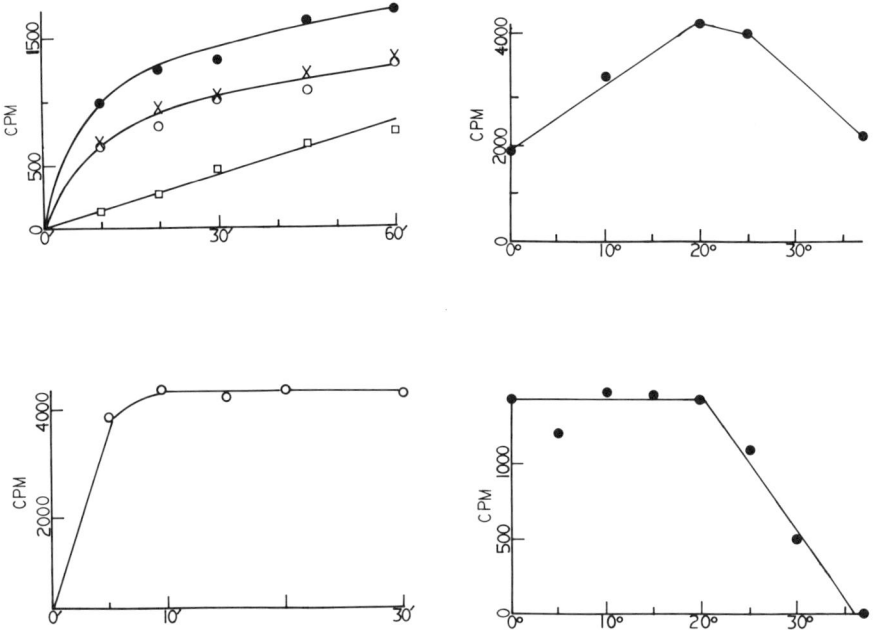

FIGURE 3. (Upper Left) Rate of Carboxylation: Comparison of 2-methoxy-1,4-naphthoquinone Added to Vitamin K_1 plus NADH with Vitamin K_1 Hydroquinone. Carboxylation was carried out at 0° for the indicated times. Carboxylation was initiated with: □, 0.1 mM vitamin K_1 and 2 mM NADH; ○, 0.1 mM vitamin K_1 and 2 mM NADH with 0.1 mM 2-methoxy-1,4-naphthoquinone; X, 0.1 mM vitamin K_1 hydroquinone with 2 mM NADH; and ●, 0.1 mM vitamin K_1 hydroquinone.

FIGURE 4. (Upper Right) Effect of Incubation Temperature on Plateau Level Carboxylation. Carboxylation was initiated with 0.1 mM vitamin K_1 hydroquinone. The incubation time was 2 h for 0° and 10°, and 30 min for 20° and higher.

FIGURE 5. (Lower Left) Rate of Carboxylation at 20° for the Indicated Time.

FIGURE 6. (Lower Right) Effect of Preincubation. The assay tube without vitamin K_1 hydroquinone or $[^{14}C]CO_2$ was incubated for 30 min at the indicated times, then cooled to 0°. The $[^{14}C]CO_2$ was added with carboxylation initiated by 0.1 mM vitamin K_1 hydroquinone and allowed to proceed 2 h at 0°.

several possibilities leading to an increased plateau level of carboxylation. The first variable studied was, hence, the initial rate of carboxylation. Since the rate of carboxylation proceeds too rapidly at 37° to determine the initial rate, the investigation of the initial rates of carboxylation was carried out at 0° (Figure 2). Lapachol and 2-hydroxy-1,4-naphthoquinone increased the initial rate three-fold, while

2-methoxy-1,4-naphthoquinone gave a five-fold stimulation. Thus, the stimulation observed in Table 1 is principally due to an increase in the initial rate of carboxylation.

The initial rate given by 2-methoxy-1,4-naphthoquinone added to vitamin K quinone plus NADH appeared to give about the same rate of carboxylation as was previously observed for vitamin K_1 hydroquinone at 0° (6). This possibility is investigated in Figure 3. The rate of vitamin K_1 hydroquinone was greater than the 2-methoxy-1,4-naphthoquinone-stimulated vitamin K_1 plus NADH rate. However, the addition of NADH to vitamin K_1 hydroquinone lowered the initial rate to essentially the 2-methoxy-1,4-naphthoquinone-stimulated rate. Therefore, the effect of the 2-methoxy-1,4-naphthoquinone is to remove the reduction of vitamin K_1 as the rate-limiting step.

The carboxylation reaction, if allowed to reach a plateau, proceeds to a similar amount of $[^{14}C]CO_2$ incorporated into protein at 0° and at 37°. This prompted an inquiry into what effect other temperatures would have on the plateau carboxylation (Figure 4). Increasing the temperature from 0° to 20° resulted in an increase in carboxylation, with a decrease observed at 37°. The plateau level of carboxylation at 20° is achieved within 10 min (Figure 5). The previously known instability of the soluble system to 37° (7) might account for the lower amount of carboxylation at 37°, as compared to 20°. The soluble system was preincubated at selected temperatures for 30 min, then cooled to 0° prior to adding $[^{14}C]CO_2$ and vitamin K_1 hydroquinone, with the carboxylation assay done at 0° (Figure 6). Preincubation of the soluble system at a temperature of 25° or higher gave a decreased amount of carboxylation. Thus, the decrease in carboxylation at 37° appears to be due to instability of the carboxylation system at that temperature.

ACKNOWLEDGEMENTS

This work was supported in part by NIH grant No. HL17619.

We would like to thank Ms. Patricia Ownbey for aid in the preparation of this manuscript.

REFERENCES

1. Mack, D.O., Suen, E.T., Girardot, J.M., Miller, J.A., Delaney, R. and Johnson, B.C. (1976) J. Biol. Chem. 251, 3269-3276.
2. Girardot, J.M., Mack, D.O., Floyd, R.A. and Johnson, B.C. (1976) Biochem. Biophys. Res. Commun. 70, 655-662.
3. Johnson, B.C., Girardot, J.M., Suen, E.T., Mack, D.O. Floyd, R.A. and Delaney, R. (1978) World Review of Nutrition and Diet 31, 202-209.
4. Mack, D.O., Wolfensberger, M., Girardot, J.M., Miller, J.A. and Johnson, B.C. (1979) J. Biol. Chem. 254, 2656-2664.
5. Fieser, L.F. and Hartwell, J.L. (1935) J. Am. Chem. Soc. 57, 1482-1484.
6. Girardot, J.M. (1977) Dissertation, University of Oklahoma.
7. Mack, D.O., Miller, J.A. and Delaney, R. (1977) Fed. Proc. 35, 305.

RAT LIVER VITAMIN K-DEPENDENT CARBOXYLASE: SUBSTRATE SPECIFICITY

DANIEL H. RICH, S. RUSS LEHRMAN, MEGUMI KAWAI,
H. L. GOODMAN and J. W. SUTTIE

School of Pharmacy and Department of Biochemistry,
College of Agricultural and Life Sciences
University of Wisconsin-Madison
Madison, WI 53706

INTRODUCTION

Vitamin K functions in the post ribosomal modification of liver microsomal precursors to form biologically-active prothrombin and the other K-dependent clotting factors (1,2). This modification involves a carboxylation of specific glutamyl residues in these proteins to form γ-carboxyglutamic acid (Gla) residues. Although many posttranslational modifications of amino acid residues in proteins have been identified in nature (3) carboxylation of glutamic acid is the only postribosomal modification in which a carbon-carbon bond is formed. Extensive studies have shown that the basic requirements for the enzyme catalyzing this unique transformation are reduced vitamin, oxygen, carbon dioxide and substrate peptide (4-17).

We have reported that the pentapeptide, Phe-Leu-Glu-Glu-Val, will serve as a substrate for the carboxylase (17) and other substrate peptides have subsequently been identified (12, 16, 18). Because improved substrates and substrate-related inhibitors of the carboxylase could facilitate mechanistic studies, we have carried out experiments to define the substrate specificity of rat liver vitamin K-dependent carboxylase. Our approach has been to systematically alter the structure of known pentapeptide substrates by chemical synthesis and determine the extent each analog is carboxylated.

RESULTS AND DISCUSSION

The structures and activities of a series of synthetic peptides containing glutamic acid residues are shown in Table I. Some of these (1, 2, 10-12) were prepared using solid phase methods (19, 20) as previously described (17). More recently we have prepared the peptides, 3-8 using solution synthesis. The solution procedure will be described separately. Each peptide was assayed by established methods (17,18) and the biological activity is expressed as a percentage relative to pentapeptide 1 which will be referred to as the standard pentapeptide.

The data in Table I indicate that several properties of the molecule determine its susceptibility to the carboxylase. For example compounds 2 and 3 indicate that increasing the hydrophobic properties of the molecule can lead to improved substrates. Protection of the N-terminal and C-terminal residues of 2 by preparing the Boc-methylester derivative 3 neutralizes two charges on the molecule and also adds the hydrophobic tert-butyl group to the molecule. Peptide 3 is carboxylated about 9-fold more than tetrapeptide 2. Similarly, neutralization of charges on the N- and C-termini of pentapeptide 1 by forming the N-propyl peptide methyl ester 4 leads to an improved substrate. Neither result is unexpected since the corresponding sequence of amino acids 5-9 in prothrombin precursor is part of a larger peptide and is not ionized at residues 5 and 9.

TABLE I. Activity of Various Peptides as Substrates for Vitamin K-K-Dependent Carboxylase.[a]

		Relative Activity (%)
1	H-Phe-Leu-Glu-Glu-Leu-OH	100
2	H-Leu-Glu-Glu-Leu-OH	8.4
3	Boc-Leu-Glu-Glu-Leu-OMe	77
4	CH_3CH_2CO-Phe-Leu-Glu-Glu-Leu-OMe	149
5	Boc-Phe-Leu-Glu-Glu-Leu-OMe	24
6	C_6H_5CO-Phe-Leu-Glu-Glu-Leu-OMe	27
7	Boc-Glu-Glu-Leu-OMe	107
8	Boc-Glu-Leu-OMe	<1
9	Boc-Glu-$OCH_2C_6H_5$	5
10	H-Phe-Glu-Leu-Glu-Leu-OH	<1
11	H-Phe-Leu-Glu-Leu-OH	<1
12	H-Phe-Glu-Ala-Leu-Glu-Ser-Leu-OH	5.5

[a] All peptides were incubated at a concentration of 1 mM with [vitamin K + NADH] as the source of vitamin. The activity is expressed as the % of the incorporation observed into peptide 1 utilizing the same microsomal preparation. Incubations were carried out on different days and the values are means of duplicate incubations which differed by less than 10%.

There may be a limit to the size of the group that can be placed on the N-terminus of 1 without lowering substrate activity. As the size of the N-acyl substituent is increased by addition of a Boc- or a benzoyl group as in 5 and 6, the analogs formed are not carboxylated as readily by the enzyme. This pattern could be caused by altered substrate conformation or by the bulkier groups encountering steric hinderance to binding to the enzyme. In prothrombin precursor, residue 4 is occupied by glycine, a residue that is isosteric with the propionyl group.

It has been reported that carboxylation of pentapeptide 1 is stimulated by addition of pyridoxal phosphate (18,21). Stimulation might be caused by Schiff base formation between the aldehyde of the vitamin and the free amino group in 1. To test this idea we synthesized the N-benzoyl derivative 6. The benzoyl group is approximately isosteric with the aromatic ring of pyridoxal. However we found that carboxylation of both N-protected peptides 5 and 6 was stimulated 1.5 fold by pyridoxal phosphate. Since neither 5 nor 6 could form the Schiff base with the vitamin, pyridoxal phosphate stimulation of carboxylation must be caused by some other mechanism.

One unexpected finding in Table I is that the tripeptide 7 is a very good substrate for the carboxylase and is carboxylated to about the same extent as pentapeptide 1. Tripeptide 7 may be more useful than pentapeptide 1 because the Boc group is easily removed by acid and the site of carboxylation can be determined after only one Edman degradation.

In contrast to substrates Boc-Glu-Glu-Leu-OMe (7) and Boc-Glu-OCH$_2$C$_6$H$_5$ (9), the structurally related dipeptide Boc-Glu-Leu-OMe (8) was not carboxylated to a measurable extent. Compound 9 establishes that adjacent glutamic acid residues are not an absolute requirement for carboxylation (22).

Peptides 10, 11 correspond to other permutations of the sequences found in substrates 1 and 2, and these peptides are not carboxylated. Compound 12 which corresponds to sequence 29-35 in prothrombin precursor is carboxylated. The relatively small carboxylation observed is comparable to that observed in other peptides lacking adjacent glutamic acid residues.

The specificity of the carboxylase for the side chain of glutamic acid residues was studied (Table II) using tripeptide 7 as the standard. We obtained evidence that residues with longer (Homo glutamic acid) or shorter (Asp) side chains are not carboxylated. The glutamic acid containing peptides 14, 15 have not been sequenced but it is assumed the carboxyl group added by the enzyme was added to the glutamic acid residue and not the aspartic acid residue.

TABLE II. Activity of Analogs of Tripeptide Substrate as Substrates for Vitamin K-Dependent Carboxylase.[a]

		Biol. Act. (%)
7	Boc-Glu-Glu-Leu-OMe	107
13	Boc-Asp-Asp-Leu-OMe	<1
14	Boc-Glu-Asp-Leu-OMe	11
15	Boc-Asp-Glu-Leu-OMe	11
16	Boc-Gln-Gln-Leu-OMe	<1
17	Boc-D,L-HGlu-D,L-HGlu-Leu-OMe	<1

[a]Incubation conditions are described under Table I. All values are means of duplicate workups differing by less than 10%.

The effect of optical configuration or chirality of the glutamic acid residues in substrates 5 and 7 also was studied (Table III). It appears that substrates with D-Glutamic acid residues are not carboxylated. At a lower substrate concentration peptide 20 appeared to have been carboxylated but at higher substrate concentration no carboxylation was detected.

Substitution of a D-amino acid for an L-amino acid in protease substrates often leads to protease inhibitors. With this in mind we tested to see if any of our non-substrate peptides especially those with D-Glu residues inhibited the carboxylase (Table IV). Some of the peptides have been tested at concentrations 4 to 8 times that of substrate but we have not observed inhibition of pentapeptide carboxylation.

TABLE III. Effect of Optical Configuration of Glutamic Acid on Activity of Various Peptides as Substrates for Vitamin K-Dependent Carboxylase.[a]

		% at 0.25 mM	% at 1.0 mM
5	Boc-Phe-Leu-L-Glu-L-Glu-Leu-OMe		24
18	Boc-Phe-Leu-D-Glu-D-Glu-Leu-OMe	1.8	0.6
19	Boc-Phe-Leu-L-Glu-D-Glu-Leu-OMe	<1	<1
20	Boc-Phe-Leu-D-Glu-L-Glu-Leu-OMe	4.5	<1
7	Boc-L-Glu-L-Glu-Leu-OMe	112	113
21	Boc-D-Glu-D-Glu-Leu-OMe	<1	<1
22	Boc-D-Glu-L-Glu-Leu-OMe	<1	<1
23	Boc-L-Glu-D-Glu-Leu-OMe	<1	<1

[a] Assay conditions are described under Table I. Peptide 1 was used as standard and assigned a value of 100%. All values are means of duplicate runs.

We conclude from the data in Tables I-IV that vitamin K-dependent carboxylase is able to select specific L-glutamic acid residues for carboxylation. The available evidence indicate the carboxylase carboxylates only L-glutamic acid residues and does not carboxylate D-glutamic acid, aspartic acid or homoglutamic acid residues. It is possible that substrates with adjacent glutamic acid residues (or two glutamic acid residues that approach each other in space) may be better substrates for the enzyme than substrates with isolated, non-interacting glutamyl residues. However the single amino acid derivative Boc-L-Glu-OBzl (9) shows that adjacent glutamyl residues are not an absolute requirement for carboxylation to occur.

Possible Factors Affecting the Recognition Process

Specificity has been observed in post-ribosomal modification of amino acids in proteins. Because many of these modifications occur before extensive tertiary structure is formed, the recognition processes seem to depend largely on the primary sequence of the substrate (3). However, because the K-dependent carboxylase carboxylates prothrombin precursor which has a defined tertiary structure, it is likely that substrate conformation will be much more important for successful carboxylation of either prothrombin precursor or low molecular weight substrates than it is in other posttranslational modifications. The glutamic acid residues in the F-1 segment of prothrombin precursor are found in peptide segments with different primary sequences. These sequences all are carboxylated when present in prothrombin precursor (1,2) but not all of the glutamic acid residues are carboxylated in the low molecular weight peptides (23). Furthermore the rate of carboxylation of individual glutamic acid residues in the small peptides varies considerably depending on the primary

TABLE IV. Effect of a Poor Carboxylase Substrate on Protein and Peptide Carboxylation[a]

Peptide	Concentration	Relative activity	
		Peptide	Protein
Phe-Leu-Glu-Leu (1)	0.5 mM	100	100
Phe-Gly-Glu-Glu-Leu (25)	0.5 mM	3.7 ± 0.3	110 ± 5.6
Phe-Gly-Glu-Glu-Leu (25)	1.0 mM	6.5 ± 1.2	92 ± 4.4
1 + 25	0.5 mM + 0.5 mM	109 ± 8.3	107 ± 5.5
1 + 25	0.5 mM + 1.0 mM	106 ± 7.0	104 ± 3.7
Phe-Glu-Ala-Leu-Glu-Ser-Leu (12)	0.5 mM	5	78
Phe-Glu-Ala-Leu-Glu-Ser-Leu (12)	1.0 mM	10	92
1 + 12	0.5 mM + 0.5 mM	112	99
1 + 12	0.5 mM + 1.0 mM	106	86
1 + Boc-Glu-Leu-OMe (7)	0.25 mM + 1.0 mM	100	not determined
1 + Boc-Phe-Leu-D-Glu-Glu-Leu-OMe (20)	0.25 mM + 1.0 mM	100	not determined
1 + Boc-D,L-HGlu-D,L-HGlu-Leu-OMe (17)	0.25 mM + 1.0 mM	100	not determined

[a]Carboxylase activity is expressed as a % of the incorporation observed into peptide 1 utilizing the same microsomal preparation. Values for incubations utilizing peptide 25 are means s.e.m. for four separate incubations, and values for incubations utilizing peptides 12, 7, 17, 20 are means of duplicate incubations.

sequence (Table I). These results suggest that the carboxylase recognizes the three-dimensional arrangement of the glutamic acid residues in prothrombin precursor and in the low molecular weight substrates.

We have obtained evidence that substrate conformation affects the extent that model peptides are carboxylated. Peptides 1, 24, 25 (Table V) represent a series of analogs of pentapeptide substrate 1 in which the residue in second position was modified (18). As the size of the substituent is reduced the carboxylation is reduced. Since hydrophobic residues can increase carboxylation of a substrate, the decreased carboxylation observed for 25 could be rationalized in terms of diminished hydrophobic property of the peptide leading to weaker binding at this residue. Some apparent k_m values for these and other substrates are given in Table V. The better substrates have low k_m values but we do not know if this is related to k_s exclusively.

TABLE V. Apparent K_m Values for Modified Pentapeptide Substrates[a]

		Biol. Act.(%)	K_m(mmol)
1	Phe-Leu-Glu-Glu-Leu	100	2-4
24	Phe-Ala-Glu-Glu-Leu	72	1.5
25	Phe-Gly-Glu-Glu-Leu	3.5	14.0
4	CH_3CH_2CO-Phe-Leu-Glu-Glu-Leu	149	1.43
5	Boc-Phe-Leu-Glu-Glu-Leu-OMe	24	6.8 (8.2)
7	Boc-Glu-Glu-Leu-OMe	107	4.4 (4.0)

[a]The method for determination of apparent k_m values of substrates for K-dependent carboxylase has been described for compound 1 (18). The apparent k_m value for the other five substrates was determined in the same manner.

Alternatively the low activity of 25 relative to 1 or 24 could be caused by changes in the conformation of the peptide. Chou and Fasman have developed a method for predicting probable conformations of amino acid sequences in proteins (24,25). In Table VI we have calculated the conformational parameters for several carboxylase substrates. The data suggest that all peptides in Table VI except 25 have a preference for α-helical conformations and that none are likely to form β-structures or β-turns. The calculations reflect the fact that leucyl residues and the anionic form of glutamic acid residues strongly prefer α-helical conformations. In contrast glycine strongly disfavors α-helical structures and is considered an α-helix breaker. These results should not be interpreted to mean that peptides 1, 24, 26, 27 necessarily exist in α-helical structures but rather indicate that the conformation of the glycine containing peptide 25 is likely to have a very different conformation from 1 and 24 and that this may be a contributor to the reduced carboxylation of 25. Extension of this argument to two substrates not closely related structurally to 1, would predict that the peptide with less α-helix character would be carboxylated less. Calculations for 26, 27, two analogs of the β-chain of hemoglobin, indicate that peptide 26 has greater α-helix character. Peptide 26 also is carboxylated to a greater extent by the enzyme (Table VI) even though it is more negatively charged. The lower carboxylation observed for either 26 or 27 relative to 1 may be caused by the additional charged residues which would increase water solubility.

TABLE VI. Calculated Conformational Parameters for Substrates Containing Glu-Glu Sequences.

	Compound	$\langle P_\alpha \rangle^a$	$\langle P_\beta \rangle^a$	% Activity[b]
1	Phe-Leu-Glu-Glu-Leu	3.77	0.319	100
24	Phe-Ala-Glu-Glu-Leu	4.43	0.204	72
25	Phe-Gly-Glu-Glu-Leu	1.77	0.184	3.5
26	Val-His-Leu-Ser-Ala-Glu-Glu-Lys-Glu-Ala	8.05	0.012	26
	(for sequence 5-10)			
		4.4	0.009	
	(for sequence 4-9)			
	1 5 10			
27	Val-His-Leu-Ser-Ala-Glu-Glu-Lys-Gln-Ala	5.84	0.052	17
	(for sequence 5-10)			
		3.18	0.038	
	(for sequence 4-9)			

[a] Calculations were carried out according to the method of Chou and Fasman (24,25).
a. $\langle P_\alpha \rangle$ is defined as α-helical parameter for a polypeptide fragment. $\langle P_\beta \rangle$ is defined as β-sheet parameter for a polypeptide fragment.   b. Per cent activity is defined in other tables.

Synthesis of Conformationally Restricted Substrates

The data we have obtained suggests that both conformational and hydrophobic properties contribute to the specificity of the carboxylase for substrates. In order to further evaluate the effect of conformation on substrate specificity we have initiated the synthesis of cyclic hexapeptide 29 (Scheme I). Peptide 29 corresponds to residues 18-23 in prothrombin precursor (2). Examination of molecular models indicates that cyclic peptide 29 will have an unusually restricted conformation because of the constraint imposed by the 20-membered disulfide ring system and the prolyl residue. Two β-turn conformations are possible with a hydrogen bond between Cys^{18}-CO---HN-Glu^{21} or Glu^{20}-CO---HN-Cys^{23}. Alternatively these β-turn structures could exist without the intramolecular hydrogen bonds.

Calculations suggest the former possibility is preferred. Cyclization of linear hexapeptide 28 has not been completed so that the substrate activity of 29 has not been determined.

More data are needed before it will be known how much conformation influences substrate specificity. The problem is complicated by the fact that two structurally distinct systems are each carboxylated: Boc-Glu-OCH$_2$C$_6$H$_5$ and peptide substrates with adjacent glutamyl residues. The first structure establishes that adjacent glutamyl residues are not essential for carboxylation to occur whereas analogs of 1 and 7 suggest that carboxylation is favored by peptides able to adopt conformations with α-helical character. The situation is further complicated by the fact that dipeptide 8 is not carboxylated under standard conditions while data presented elsewhere indicate that the first glutamyl residue in pentapeptide 1 is preferentially carboxylated (22). These results suggest that relationships between enzyme specificity and substrate conformation and sequence may be subtle, and that additional factors such as multiple binding or carboxylation mechanisms may be involved.

Scheme I. Synthesis of Sequence 18-23 of Prothrombin Precursor.

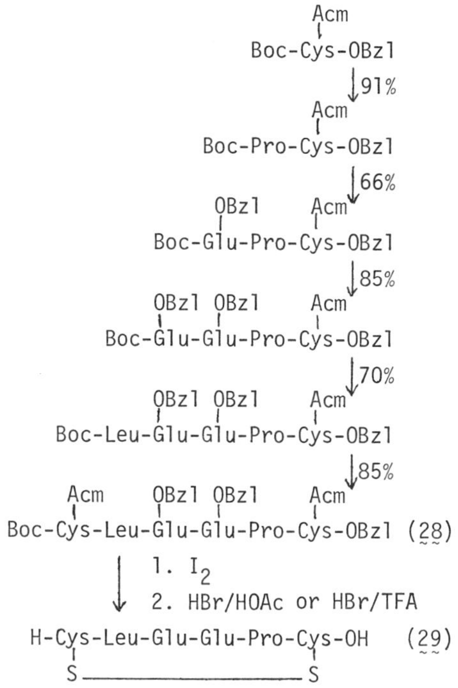

```
                        Acm
                         |
                  Boc-Cys-OBzl
                           ↓91%
                        Acm
                         |
                Boc-Pro-Cys-OBzl
                           ↓66%
                 OBzl    Acm
                   |      |
              Boc-Glu-Pro-Cys-OBzl
                           ↓85%
            OBzl OBzl    Acm
              |    |      |
          Boc-Glu-Glu-Pro-Cys-OBzl
                           ↓70%
            OBzl OBzl    Acm
              |    |      |
      Boc-Leu-Glu-Glu-Pro-Cys-OBzl
                           ↓85%
      Acm   OBzl OBzl    Acm
       |      |    |      |
   Boc-Cys-Leu-Glu-Glu-Pro-Cys-OBzl  (28)
       │ 1. I$_2$
       ↓ 2. HBr/HOAc or HBr/TFA
     H-Cys-Leu-Glu-Glu-Pro-Cys-OH    (29)
         |                      |
         S ──────────────────── S
```

ACKNOWLEDGEMENTS

This work was supported in part by the College of Agriculture and Life Sciences, The School of Pharmacy and by grant AM 14881 from the National Institutes of Health.

REFERENCES

1. Suttie, J. W. and Jackson, C. M. (1977) Physiol. Rev. 57, 1-70.
2. Stenflo, J. and Suttie, J. W. (1977) Ann. Rev. Biochem. 46, 157-172.
3. Uy, R. and Wold, F. (1977) Science 198, 890-896.
4. Esmon, C. T., Sadowski, J. A. and Suttie, J. W. (1975) J. Biol. Chem. 250, 4744-4748.
5. Sadowski, J. A., Esmon, C. T. and Suttie, J. W. (1976) J. Biol. Chem. 251, 2770-2775.
6. Esmon, C. T. and Suttie, J. W. (1976) J. Biol. Chem. 251, 6238-6243.
7. Friedman, P. A. and Shia, M. (1976) Biochem. Biophys. Res. Commun. 70, 647-654.
8. Girardot, J.-M., Mack, D. O., Floyd, R. A. and Johnson, B. C. (1976) Biochem. Biophys. Res. Commun. 70, 655-662.
9. Mack, D. O., Suen, E. T., Girardot, J.-M., Miller, J. A., Delaney, R. and Johnson, B. C. (1976) J. Biol. Chem. 251, 3269-3276.
10. Jones, J. P., Fausto, A., Houser, R. M., Gardner, E. J. and Olson, R. E. (1976) Biochem. Biophys. Res. Commun. 72, 589-597.
11. Friedman, P. A. and Shia, M. A. (1977) Biochem. J. 163, 39-43.
12. Houser, R. M., Carey, D. J., Dus, K. M., Marshall, G. R. and Olson, R. E. (1977) FEBS Letters 75, 226-230.
13. Helgeland, L. (1977) Biochim. Biophys. Acta 499, 181-193.
14. Jones, J. P., Gardner, E. J., Cooper, T. G. and Olson, R. E. (1977) J. Biol. Chem. 252, 7738-7742.
15. Wallin, R., Gebhardt, O. and Prydz, H. (1978) Biochem. J. 169, 95-101.
16. Esnouf, M. P. Green, M. R., Hill, H. A. O., Irvine, G. B. and Walter, S. J. (1978) Biochem. J. 174, 345-348.
17. Suttie, J. W., Hageman, J. M., Lehrman, S. R. and Rich, D. H. (1976) J. Biol. Chem. 251, 5827-5830.
18. Suttie, J. W., Lehrman, S. R., Geweke, L. O., Hageman, J. M. and Rich, D. H. (1979) Biochem. Biophys. Res. Commun. 86, 500-507.
19. Merrifield, R. B. (1963) J. Amer. Chem. Soc. 85, 2149-2151.
20. Erickson, B. W. and Merrifield, R. B. (1976) "Solid Phase Peptide Synthesis" in The Proteins Vol. II, Neurath, H., Hill, R. L. eds. Acad. Press, New York, pp. 257-528.
21. Suttie, J. W., Geweke, L. O., Finnan, J. L. and Goodman, H. L. Abstract #46, This volume pp.
22. Finnan, J. L., Geweke, L. O. and Suttie, J. W. (1979) Abst. 3411 Fed. Proc. 38, 876.
23. Finnan, J. L., Goodman, H. L. and Suttie, J. W. Abstract #14, This volume pp.
24. Chou, P. Y. and Fasman, G. D. (1974) Biochem. 13, 222-244.
25. Chou, P. Y. and Fasman, G. D. (1978) Ann. Rev. Biochem. 47, 251-276.

GLUTAMIC ACID DERIVATIVES AS SUBSTRATES FOR THE VITAMIN K-DEPENDENT CARBOXYLASE

J. L. FINNAN, H. L. GOODMAN, and J. W. SUTTIE

Department of Biochemistry
College of Agricultural and Life Sciences
University of Wisconsin-Madison
Madison, WI 53706

INTRODUCTION

The initial report (1) of vitamin K-dependent carboxylase activity in rat liver microsomes followed the incorporation of radioactive CO_2 into the endogenous microsomal precursors of the vitamin K-dependent proteins which were present in microsomes isolated from vitamin K-deficient rats. Subsequent investigations in various laboratories (2) utilized essentially the same assay. The inability to systematically alter the concentration of the endogenous substrate for the enzyme raises problems in studying the action of this enzyme, and Suttie et al. (3) have described the use of low-molecular-weight peptides containing Glu-Glu sequence substrates for the enzyme. These peptides are being increasingly used (2) as substrates in the study of this enzyme, and the relative properties of the enzyme when studied with a soluble peptide substrate or the endogenous microsomal proteins have been described (4). The difficulty involved in synthesizing these peptides in some laboratories and the high cost of their commercial purchase has prompted a search for readily available low-cost substrate for this enzyme.

METHODS

All compounds assayed as carboxylase substrates (Fig. 1) were obtained from commercial sources and were used without further purification. The conditions of assay were similar to those employed for the substrate Phe-Leu-Glu-Glu-Leu (4), and incubation was at 7° C for 240 min at a concentration of 2 m$\underline{M}$. Following incubation, the incorporation of radioactivity into the TCA supernate was assayed as previously described (4). Activity of the various compounds has been expressed as ρmoles of product formed based on a determination of the specific radioactivity of the CO_2 fixed.

RESULTS

The data in Figure 2A indicate that of the various glutamic acid derivatives assayed, only compound VII, t-BOC-$\underline{L}$-Glu-α-benzyl ester (BOC-Glu-Bz) had sufficient activity to be a useful substrate. The activity of this compound is, however, much less (Fig. 2B) than that of Phe-Leu-Glu-Glu-Leu which has been the standard substrate used in our laboratory. BOC-Glu-Bz is relatively soluble and significantly greater activity can be obtained as the concentration is increased. The apparent K_m for this substrate is 6-7 m$\underline{M}$; and, at 10 m$\underline{M}$, it demonstrates about the same initial rate of $^{14}CO_2$ fixation as 1 m$\underline{M}$ Phe-Leu-Glu-Glu-Leu. The reaction proceeds at a linear rate for a longer time with BOC-Glu-Bz as a substrate. The

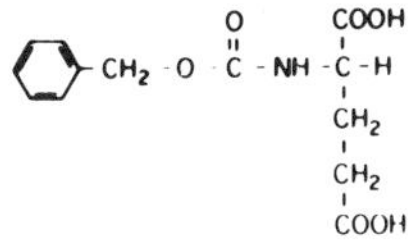

I

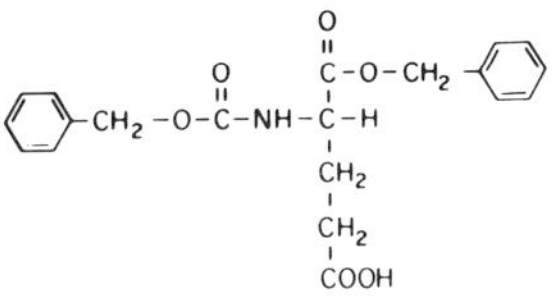

II

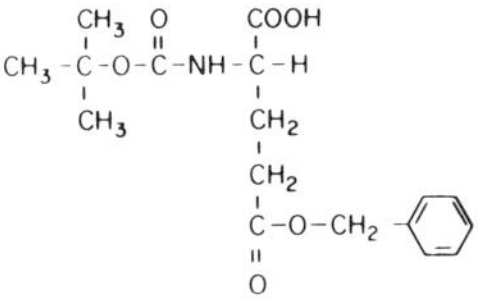

III

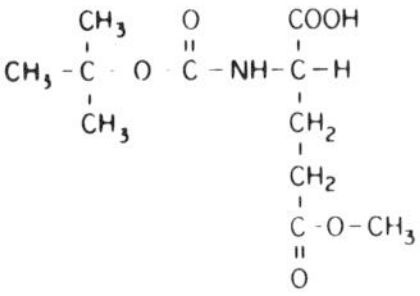

IV

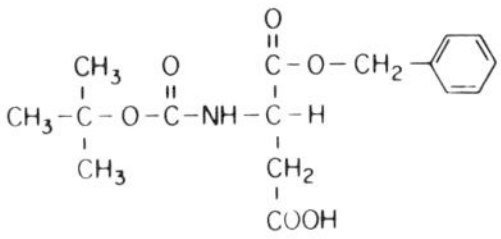

V

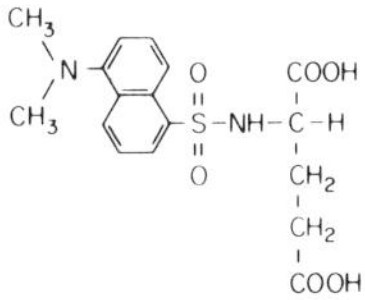

VI

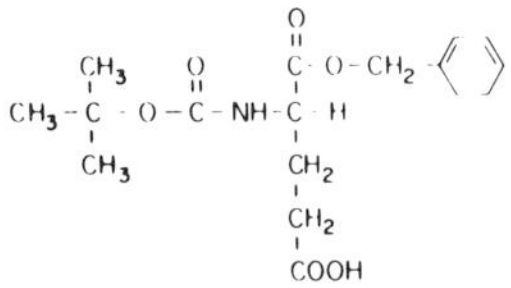

VII

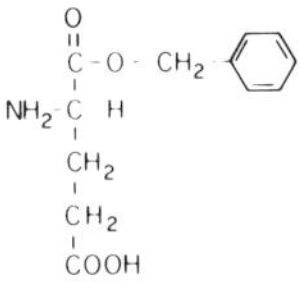

VIII

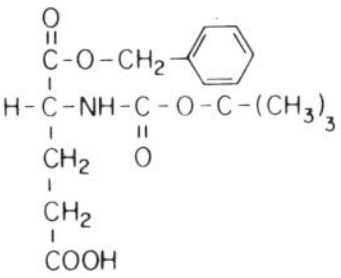

IX

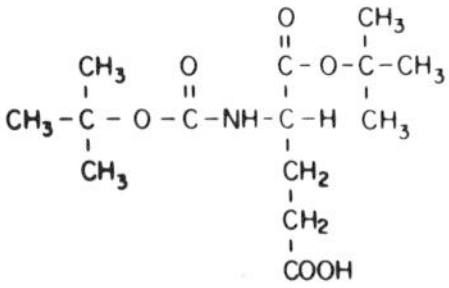

X

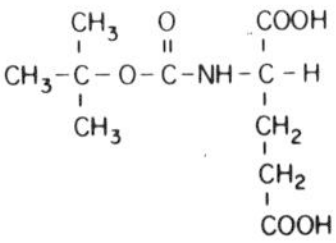

XI

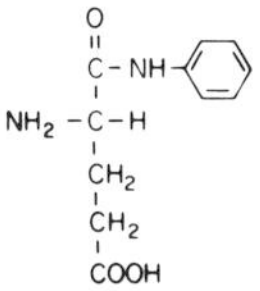

XII

FIGURE 1. Structures of the glutamic acid derivatives assayed for vitamin K-dependent carboxylase activity.

incorporation of $H^{14}CO_3^-$ into BOC-Glu-Bz has been shown to be present in γ-carboxyglutamic acid by its acid lability and co-chromatography with authentic Gla. The similarity between this compound and Phe-Leu-Glu-Glu-Leu as a substrate for the carboxylase is evident from the observation (5) that the carboxylated product of both of these substrates is converted to a more basic form by the microsomal preparation.

DISCUSSION

These studies have demonstrated that a simple, low-cost derivative of glutamic acid, BOC-Glu-Bz, is an effective substrate for the vitamin K-dependent carboxylase. Not only is this a good substrate for routine analysis, but the ease of its synthesis should make it relatively easy to produce potential substrates which are of particular interest in studying the enzyme. Rich _et al._ (6) have shown (see IX and V of Fig. 1)

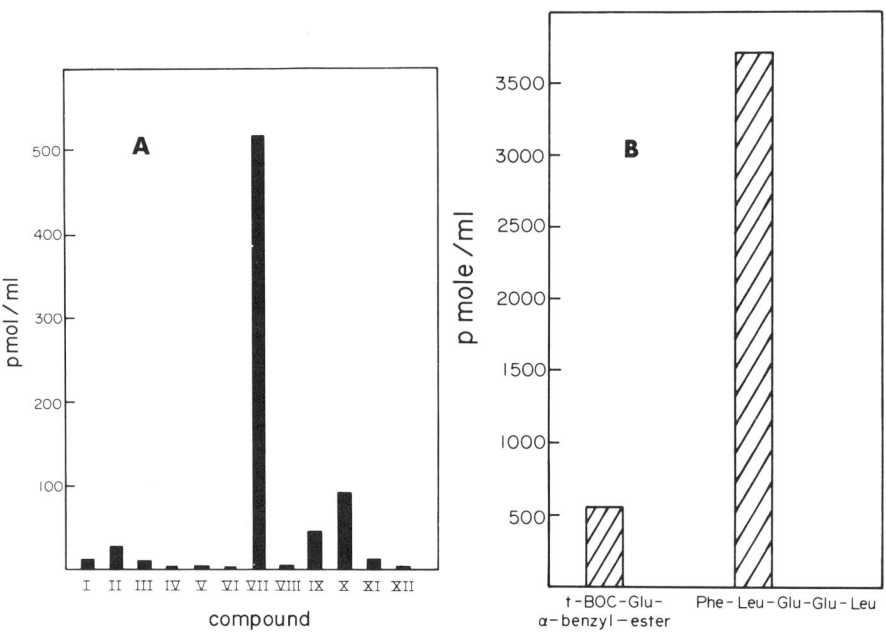

FIGURE 2. (A) Carboxylase activity of a number of glutamic acid derivatives. The numbers correspond to the structures shown in Figure 1. (B) Comparison of the carboxylase activity of 2 mM BOC-Glu-Bz and Phe-Leu-Glu-Glu-Leu.

that D-Glu and L-Asp are not carboxylated when they are incorporated into a pentapeptide substrate and the data presented here on the activity of simple derivatives of these amino acids support this observation. Friedman et al. (7) have incorporated β,γ-^{3}H-Glu into a peptide substrate to study rates of exchange of the hydrogen from the γ-position. Such studies might well be conducted with much less effort by the use of a simple glutamic acid derivative such as BOC-Glu-Bz.

ACKNOWLEDGEMENTS

These studies were supported by the College of Agricultural and Life Sciences, University of Wisconsin-Madison, and in part by grants AM-14881, AM-21472, DE-07031, and HL-05649 from the National Institutes of Health.

REFERENCES

1. Esmon, C. T., Sadowski, J. A., and Suttie, J. W. (1975) J. Biol. Chem. 250, 4744-4748.

2. Suttie, J. W. (1978) Handbook of Lipid Research 2, "The Fat-soluble vitamins" (DeLuca, H. F., ed.) pp. 211-277, Plenum Press, New York.

3. Suttie, J. W., Hageman, J. M., Lehrman, S. R., and Rich, D. H. (1976) J. Biol. Chem. 251, 5827-5830.

4. Suttie, J. W., Lehrman, S. R., Geweke, L. O., Hageman, J. M., and Rich, D. H. (1979) Biochem. Biophys. Res. Commun. 86, 500-507.

5. Finnan, J. L., and Suttie, J. W. (1979) these proceedings.

6. Rich, D. H., Lehrman, S. R., Goodman, H. L., and Suttie, J. W. (1979) these proceedings.

7. Friedman, P. A., Shia, M. A., Gallop, P. M., and Griep, A. E. (1979) Proc. Natl. Acad. Sci. USA, in press.

REGULATION OF VITAMIN K-DEPENDENT CARBOXYLATION

A. DUBIN, E. T. SUEN, R. DELANEY and B. C. JOHNSON

Oklahoma Medical Research Foundation, and
University of Oklahoma Health Sciences Center
Oklahoma City, OK 73104

INTRODUCTION

The activity of vitamin K-dependent carboxylation was found to be consistently higher in hypoprothrombinemic rats than in normal rats (1). This increased activity is correlated to decreased plasma prothrombin levels. The enhanced enzyme activity was also suggested to be due to the de novo synthesis of the carboxylase (2).

The stimulation of pyridoxal-5'-phosphate on peptide carboxylation activity has been demonstrated (3). This stimulation is due to the interaction of microsomal enzyme(s) and pyridoxal-5'-phosphate (4). Activation of vitamin K-dependent carboxylase is observed by adding partially decarboxylated vitamin K-dependent protein(s) to the Triton X-100 soluble microsomal system (5).

In this report, we provide evidence indicating that the increased carboxylation activity observed in the hypoprothrombinemic state is primarily due to the stimulation of enzyme activity by accumulated protein substrates, rather than increased enzyme synthesis.

MATERIALS AND METHODS

Incubation Conditions

The 2% Triton X-100 soluble fractions of rat liver microsomes was prepared by the method of Mack et al. (6) and modified by the use of 50 mM phosphate buffer, pH 7.4, instead of imidazole. Peptide carboxylation activity was determined in the presence of 2.5 mM pyridoxal-5'-phosphate as described earlier (4). Prothrombin precursor activity was assayed using Echis carinatus venom (7).

Preparation of partially decarboxylated vitamin K-dependent plasma protein and antibody against vitamin K-dependent plasma protein

Vitamin K-dependent proteins were isolated from normal rat plasma by barium adsorption and sodium citrate elution. Decarboxylation of these proteins was conducted according to Poser and Price (9). This resulted in 35% decarboxylation. Antibody was raised in rabbits and immunoglobulin was isolated according to to the method of Marboe and Ingild (8).

Purification of Rat Liver Prothrombin Precursor

Prothrombin precursor from warfarin-treated or vitamin K-deficient rats was isolated by a modified method of Grant and Suttie (10). The final product, after 150-fold purification, is 80% pure, judged by SDS-PAGE.

RESULTS AND DISCUSSION

Previous study has shown that pyridoxal-5'-phosphate stimulates pentapeptide carboxylation activity 2- to 3-fold (5). The initial rate study at 0°-1° indicates that an additional stimulatory effect can be obtained by adding partially decarboxylated vitamin K-dependent protein (Fig. 1). However, no significant effect, by either compound, can be observed in protein carboxylation activity (data not shown). These results suggest that the activation of pentapeptide carboxylation activity may be one of the important regulation mechanisms.

Both vitamin K-dependent protein carboxylation and peptide carboxylation activities gradually decrease after vitamin K_1 administration to vitamin K-deficient rats (Fig. 2). Protein carboxylation activity is rapidly reduced to less than 20% after 15 min. Even after 60 min of vitamin K_1 administration, about 50% of the peptide carboxylation activity remains. Measurement of prothrombin and its precursor by Echis carinatus venom, before and after absorption with barium sulfate, indicates that 80% of the precursor has been carboxylated, and up to 40% has been released into the blood within 15 min after in vivo vitamin K_1 administration. After 120 min, the pentapeptide carboxylation activity decreases to about 35% of the original activity. At this point, the addition of partially decarboxylated vitamin K-dependent protein to the same level of Echis carinatus assayable activity as the original solution, totally restores peptide carboxylation activity (Fig. 2-A).

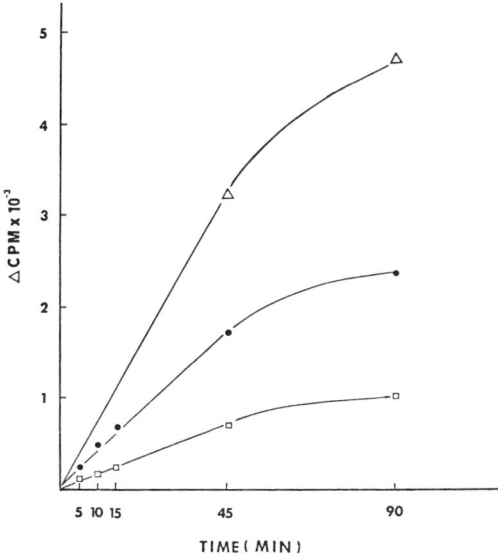

FIGURE 1 The effect of pyridoxal-5'-phosphate and partially decarboxylated vitamin K-dependent protein on the initial rate of peptide carboxylation. The incubation mixture contains Triton X-100 solubilized microsomes isolated from vitamin K-deficient rats. Carboxylation is conducted at 0-1° for various time periods without pyridoxal-5'-phosphate (□), with 2.5 mM pyridoxal-5'-phosphate (●), and with both 2.5 mM pyridoxal-5'-phosphate and 3 μg of partially decarboxylated vitamin K-dependent protein (△).

486   Dubin et al.

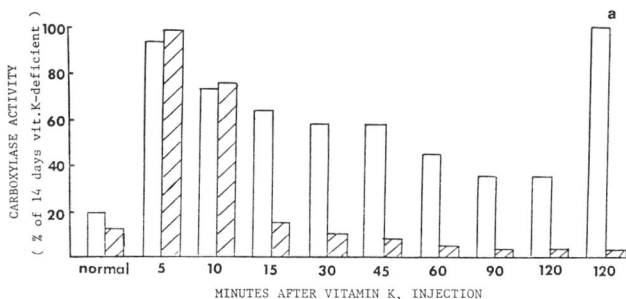

FIGURE 2 Effect of in vivo injection of vitamin K_1 on peptide and protein carboxylation activity. The carboxylation activity in vitamin K-deficient rats is set as 100%. After injection of vitamin K_1 (5 mg/Kg body weight) for various periods of time, the rats were decapitated and the livers removed. Carboxylation activity was measured with 2.5 mM pyridoxal-5'-phosphate. Cross-hatched bars are protein carboxylation activities and non-cross-hatched bars are pentapeptide carboxylation activities. a - the activity is assayed with partially decarboxylated vitamin K-dependent protein, which is added to give the same level of Echis carinatus activity as in the original vitamin K-deficient soluble system. The values are means for three experiments (6 rats in each group).

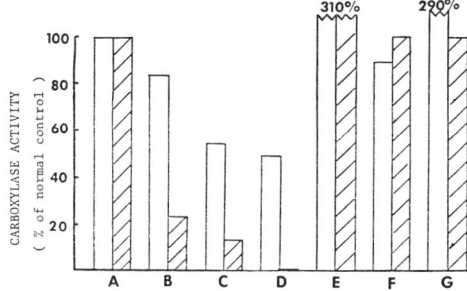

FIGURE 3 Effect of in vivo injection of vitamin K_1, cycloheximide or warfarin on the activities of pentapeptide and protein carboxylation. Carboxylation activity of normal rat liver microsome soluble system is set as 100%. Cross-hatched bars are protein carboxylation activities and non-cross-hatched bars are pentapeptide carboxylation activities. A - normal control, B - 2 h after cycloheximide injection, C - 2 h after vitamin K_1 injection, D - 2 h after cycloheximide and vitamin K_1 injection, E - 5 h after warfarin injection, F - 5 h after warfarin and cycloheximide injection, G - the sample in F is assayed with partially decarboxylated vitamin K-dependent protein, which is added to give the same level of Echis carinatus activity as warfarin-treated rat liver microsome soluble system.

Injection of either vitamin K_1 or cycloheximide results in a similar decrease in both peptide and protein carboxylation activity (Fig. 3-A, B, C). The co-administration of both compounds totally eliminates protein carboxylation, however, 50% of peptide carboxylation remains (Fig. 3-D). While these data indicate that peptide carboxylation does not require the presence of endogenous protein substrates, the 50% decrease in peptide carboxylation activity (D versus A) indicates that the endogenous protein substrate may play a role in peptide carboxylation. While the injection of warfarin into normal rats was followed by a 3-fold increase in both peptide and protein carboxylation (Fig. 3-E), the injection of cycloheximide along with warfarin (Fig. 3-F) abolished both carboxylation increases.

The addition of partially decarboxylated vitamin K-dependent protein from rat plasma, to the same level of Echis carinatus assayable activity in warfarin-treated rats, increases the peptide carboxylation activity 3-fold, i.e., to the level found following warfarin treatment (Fig. 3-G).

In order to further substantiate the activation of the carboxylation system by partially decarboxylated vitamin K-dependent protein, in vitro experiments were carried out in which antibody against vitamin K-dependent plasma protein was added to the Triton X-100 soluble microsomal system from vitamin K-deficient rats. As shown in Figure 4, this antibody inhibits both peptide and protein carboxylation activity. The prothrombin precursor (Echis carinatus assayable activity) decreases sharply to zero

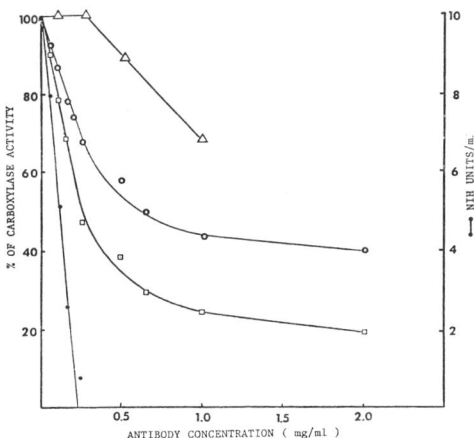

FIGURE 4 Effect of antibody against vitamin K-dependent rat plasma protein on vitamin K-dependent carboxylation activity. Pentapeptide carboxylation activity (O), protein carboxylation activity (□), prothrombin precursor level (●), and pentapeptide carboxylation activity assayed with partially decarboxylated vitamin K-dependent protein which is added to give the same level of Echis carinatus activity as in the original vitamin K-deficient rat liver microsomal system (△). Antibodies were added to the soluble system derived from vitamin K-deficient rat liver microsomes (set as 100%). The antigen-antibody complex was removed by centrifugation at 850 x g for 10 min after standing overnight at 0-4°. The supernatant was collected to assay for carboxylation activity.

488   Dubin et al.

when a small amount of antibody (0.25 mg/ml) is added to Triton X-100 solubilized microsomes. Both peptide and protein carboxylation activities also greatly decrease as the concentration of the antibody increases to 0.5 mg/ml. Addition of partially decarboxylated vitamin K-dependent protein to these antibody-treated samples results in stimulation of peptide carboxylation activity. At low concentrations of antibody (up to 0.25 mg/ml), 100% activation was observed. However, when excess antiobdy was present, the reactivation was reduced. These data indicate that the decrease in enzyme is to to the removal of enodgenous protein substrates, rather than the enzyme. This result also demonstrates that the reactivation of carboxylation can be achieved by adding back partially decarboxylated vitamin K-dependent protein. The addition of partially decarboxylated vitamin K-dependent protein is not adequate above 0.5 mg/ml antibody because of the excess soluble antibody in the system.

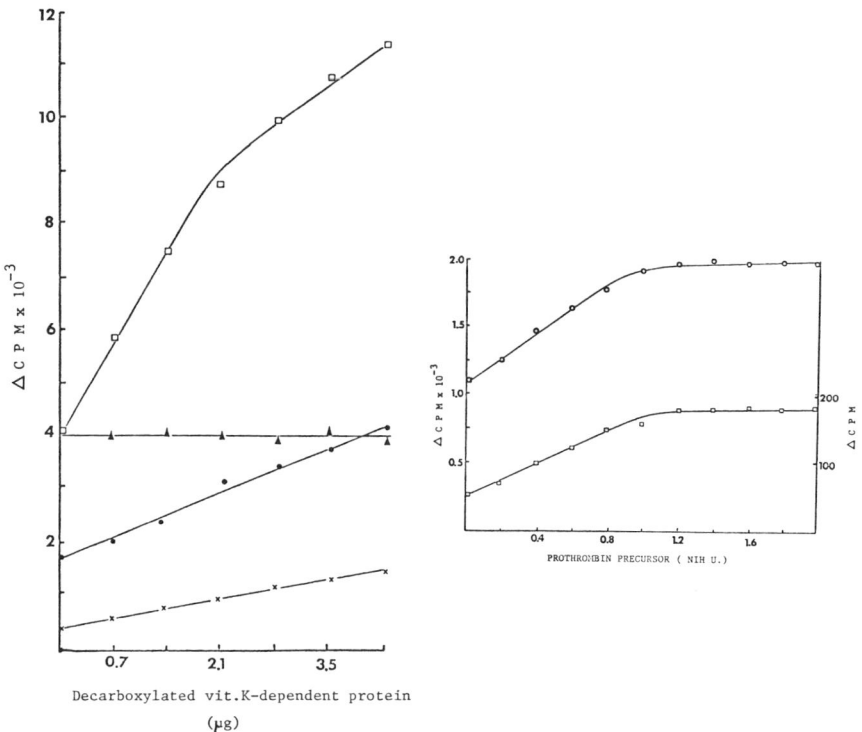

FIGURE 5 (Left) Effect of partially decarboxylated vitamin K-dependent protein on pentapeptide carboxylation activity in the liver microsome soluble system derived from vitamin K-deficient rats (□), warfarin-treated rats (●), and normal rats (×). Control (▲) contains Triton X-100 solubilized microsomal fraction from vitamin K-deficient rats, but unheated vitamin K-dependent rat plasma protein was added.

FIGURE 6 (Right) Effect of purified prothrombin precursor on carboxylation activity of pentapeptide (○) or protein (□). Purified prothrombin precursor is added to the soluble system derived from vitamin K-deficient rats which have been injected with vitamin K_1, 60 min before decapitation.

Figure 5 shows a linear increase in peptide carboxylation activity in three microsomal, Triton X-100 solubilized systems prepared from vitamin K-deficient, warfarin-treated, and normal rats by adding increasing amounts of partially decarboxylated vitamin K-dependent proteins. All three types of microsomes show the same stimulation ratio (about 3-fold). On the other hand, adding unheated vitamin K-dependent protein has no effect on carboxylation activity indicating that prothrombin inhibition of carboxylation does not occur. Although this result suggests that activation of peptide carboxylation by partially decarboxylated vitamin K-dependent protein can occur even when endogenous precursor protein is accumulated in the hypoprothrombinemic state, it appears that much higher levels of partially decarboxylated vitamin K-dependent proteins are needed to reach a plateau.

The stimulation of both peptide and protein carboxylation activity by purified prothrombin precursor is illustrated in Fig. 6. Again, a linear increase was observed by adding prothrombin precursor to the Triton X-100 solubilized microsomal system from vitamin K-deficient rats injected with vitamin K_1 (60 min). The increase in protein carboxylation is interesting, but too small to provide useful information. It is possible that the acceptor protein needs some specific properties which are required for the binding of carboxylating enzyme and that the isolation procedure may have altered these properties.

The data presented above indicate that prothrombin precursor or partially decarboxylated vitamin K-dependent protein can serve as an activator for the vitamin K-dependent carboxylation system. It appears that exogenous addition of carboxyl-acceptor proteins primarily stimulate peptide carboxylation, whereas increases in endogenous carboxyl-acceptor proteins stimulate both peptide and protein carboxylation. The primary effect of warfarin-induced hypoprothrombinemia on carboxylation is through increased levels of precursor (activator) in the liver, rather than by increased synthesis of carboxylating enzyme.

ACKNOWLDEGEMENTS This work was supported in part by NIH grant No.HL17619. We would like to thank Ms. Patricia Ownbey for aid in the preparation of of this manuscript.

REFERENCES

1. Mack, D.O., Suen, E.T., Girardot, J.M., Miller, J.A., Delaney, R. and Johnson, B.C. (1976) 251, 3269-3276.
2. Shah, D.V. and Suttie, J.W. (1978) Arch. Biochem. Biophys. 191, 571-577.
3. Suttie, J.W., Lehman, S.R., Geweke, L.D., Hageman, J.M. and Rich, D.H. (1979) Biochem. Biophys. Res. Commun. 86, 500-507.
4. Dubin, A., Suen, E.T., Delaney, R., Chiu, A. and Johnson, B.C. (1979) Biochem. Biophys. Res. Commun. In Press.
5. Dubin, A., Suen, E.T., Delaney, R. and Johnson, B.C. (1979) Fed. Proc. 38, 2971.
6. Mack, D.O., Wolfensberger, M., Girardot, J.M., Miller, J.A. and Johnson, B.C. (1979) J. Biol. Chem. 254, 2656-2664.
7. Shah, D.V., Suttie, J.S. and Grand, G.A. (1973) Arch. Biochem. Biophys. 159, 483-491.
8. Marboe, N. and Ingild, A. (1976) in Manual of Quantitative Immunoelectrophoresis (Axelson, N.W., Krøu, J., and Weeke, B., eds.), Universitetsforloget, Oslo-Bergen-Tromsø.
9. Poser, J.W. and Price, P.A. (1979) J. Biol. Chem. 254, 431-436.
10. Grant, G.A. and Suttie, J.W. (1976) Biochemistry 15, 5387-5393.

PURIFICATION OF THE RAT LIVER
VITAMIN K-DEPENDENT CARBOXYLASE

R. WALLIN, L. M. CANFIELD, T. A. SINSKY, and J. W. SUTTIE

Department of Biochemistry
Cowlege of Agricultural and Life Sciences
University of Wisconsin-Madison
Madison, WI 53706

INTRODUCTION

The metabolic role of vitamin K is that of an essential cofactor for a microsomal enzyme that converts glutamyl residues of precursor proteins to γ-carboxyglutamyl residues in the completed proteins. This carboxylase has been most extensively studied in rat liver microsomes where it has been shown to require the reduced form of vitamin K, O_2, CO_2, and a peptide-bound glutamyl residue as a substrate. The enzyme can utilize synthetic peptides containing a Glu-Glu sequence as substrate, and this has facilitated studies of the role of the vitamin. The molecular events associated with the action of vitamin K as an essential cofactor for the carboxylase are still unclear. The general properties of this system have been recently reviewed (1-4).

Glutamyl Residues — $\begin{array}{c} CH_2 \\ | \\ CH_2 \\ | \\ COOH \end{array}$ $\xrightarrow[\text{Vitamin K}]{CO_2 \quad O_2}$ $\begin{array}{c} CH_2 \\ | \\ HC-COOH \\ | \\ COOH \end{array}$ — γ-Carboxyglutamyl Residues

All of the available data dealing with the properties of this enzyme have been obtained using a crude rat liver microsomal preparation. Early studies (5,6) demonstrated that the carboxylase activity could be readily solubilized in detergents, but it has proven difficult to purify. A preliminary report of a purification of the detergent-solubilized enzyme from rat liver (7) by various chromatographic procedures indicated that a reasonable increase in specific activity was achieved, but that total yield was only a few percent of the starting activity. Attempts in our laboratory to fractionate the activity from detergent-solubilized microsomes by conventional and affinity chromatography yielded similar results. This report describes a rapid procedure for extracting much of the protein in the crude microsomal pellet away from the carboxylase to yield a reproducible preparation of this enzyme. This preparation, which we have called carboxylase complex A, is greatly increased in both total and specific activity over the solubilized microsomal preparation. This preparation should be useful for more detailed studies of the mechanism of action of the enzyme and has also provided us with a starting point for further purification of this unique carboxylase.

MATERIALS AND METHODS

Hypoprothrombinemia was produced in male 250-300 g Holtzman strain rats by feeding a vitamin K-deficient diet for 7 days in coprophagy-preventing cages. All rats were fasted 18 h prior to killing by decapitation.

Microsomal pellets were obtained as previously described (5) and suspended in two volumes of 0.25 $\underline{M}$ sucrose, 0.025 $\underline{M}$ imidazole HCl, 1 m$\underline{M}$ dithiothreitol (DTT) at pH 7.2 (buffer A) prior to beginning the purification procedure. This and all subsequent preparations during the purification were made 1% in Triton X-100 before carboxylase assays were performed. Incorporation of $H^{14}CO_3^-$ into the peptide substrate Phe-Leu-Glu-Glu-Leu was essentially as previously described (8). For the standard incubation, 10 µl 0.5 mCi/ml $NaH^{14}CO_3^-$, 50 µl 5 m$\underline{M}$ peptide in 0.025 $\underline{M}$ imidazole HCl, pH 7.2, and 10 µl 5 mg/ml vitamin KH_2 in ethanol were added to 0.4 ml of the preparation to be assayed and incubated at 17° C for 30 min with rotary mixing in 13 x 100 glass tubes sealed with parafilm.

Vitamin K-dependent fixation of $^{14}CO_2$ into the added peptide substrate and endogenous microsomal precursors was measured as previously described (8). Vitamin K epoxidase activity was assayed as previously described (15). To assay proteins in Triton X-100-containing buffers, three volumes of cold (4° C) acetone were added; and, after 30 min, the precipitate was collected by centrifugation in the cold for 10 min at 10,000 x g. Pellets were redissolved in 0.025 $\underline{M}$ imidazole-HCl, 1 m$\underline{M}$ DTT at pH 7.2 (buffer B) containing 1% recrystallized deoxycholate to a concentration suitable for a Lowry protein assay. Samples in Triton X-100-free solution were treated with 1% deoxycholate prior to Lowry assay.

RESULTS

Preparation of Complex A

Microsomes obtained from vitamin K-deficient rats were surface-washed twice with 1 ml buffer B and suspended to the original microsomal volume in buffer B containing 0.1% octylglucoside, and 1 m$\underline{M}$ PMSF (added as a 0.2 $\underline{M}$ solution in absolute ethanol) and homogenized with six strokes of a Kontes glass homogenizer (type A). The suspension was shaken gently for 30 min at 4° C prior to centrifugation for 60 min at 100,000 x g. This procedure removed periferal proteins and resulted in the loss of about 35% of the original microsomal protein. For carboxylase assays, the resulting pellet was suspended in buffer B which had been made 1% in Triton X-100.

The pellet obtained after centrifugation was resuspended to the original microsomal volume with gentle homogenization in buffer B containing 0.25 $\underline{M}$ $NaClO_4$ and 2 m$\underline{M}$ DTT. The suspension was frozen rapidly in Corex centrifuge tubes in a slurry of dry ice-methanol for 10 min and thawed in a 30° C water bath for 4 min. This procedure was repeated and the resulting suspension pelleted by centrifugation as before. This fractionation reduced the total amount of protein to a little less than half that originally in the microsomal preparation. Neither freezing and thawing nor fractionation with sodium perchlorate alone was effective in removing protein from the particulate preparation at this stage.

Preparation of Complex A

Rat liver
↓
Postmitochondrial supernate
↓
Crude microsomes
(5.4 U, 0.25 U/mg)
↓
Octylglucoside extraction
(15 U, 1 U/mg)
↓
Sodium perchlorate extraction
(204 U, 20 U/mg)
↓
Cholate extraction
(204 U, 25 U/mg)
↓
$(NH_4)_2SO_4$ precipitation
↓
Complex A
(188 U, 37 U/mg)

FIGURE 1.

The pellet obtained after ClO_4^- treatment was extracted with bile salts. Solid NaCl and 10% recrystallized Na cholate were added to buffer B to a final concentration of 0.75 $\underline{M}$ NaCl and 0.3% Na cholate and the pellet was suspended in the original microsomal volume of this solution by homogenization. This mixture was incubated at 4° C with gentle shaking for 30 min and pelleted by centrifugation as before. This pellet contained about 35% of the original microsomal protein. The pellet obtained from bile salt solubilization was resuspended in 40 times the original microsomal volume of buffer B. Saturated ammonium sulfate was slowly added to this solution over a period of 5 min to give a final concentration of 33% ammonium sulfate and mixing was continued for 30 min at 4° C. The pellet was collected by centrifugation for 10 min at 10,000 x g. Large volumes of buffer were used to remove the cholate. The pellet was resuspended in the original microsomal volume of 0.025 $\underline{M}$ imidazole-HCl, 1% Triton X-100, 10% glycerol, 1 mM DDT, 0.5 $\underline{M}$ KCl at pH 7.2 (buffer D) and dialyzed against 100 volumes of buffer D with one change over night. The resultant preparation (complex A) was used immediately or stored at -70° C until ready for use. For assay of carboxylase activity at the final or any of the intermediate steps of the purification, the pellets were dialyzed against buffer D as described for complex A.

Characterization of Complex A

Results of a typical purification are shown in Figure 1. A unit of carboxylase activity is arbitrarily defined as the fixation of 1000 dpm of $H^{14}CO_3^-$ into 0.5 mM Phe-Leu-Glu-Glu-Leu in 30 min at 17° C, and the activity in each step of the purification is that obtained from 1 ml of the crude microsomal suspension. Numerous preparations of complex A have been obtained over the past year, and the specific activity of the final pellet has usually been increased 100-150-fold over the washed microsomes. In some cases, considerable activity was lost in the final step, apparently due to a loss of lipid, as activity could be restored upon readdition of lipid. A number of inhibitors and stimulators of the carboxylase system have been reported and these were tested on complex A. Qualitatively similar results were obtained to those reported earlier (8) for the carboxylation of peptide substrates by crude microsomes. Complex A was slightly less sensitive to the effects of pyridoxal phosphate, Warfarin, and Chloro-K, but slightly more sensitive to the effects of DTT and PHMB than has been observed for the solubilized microsomal preparation.

As is the case for the solubilized microsomal preparation, the optimal assay temperature for complex A is 17° C, and the preparation is unstable at higher temperatures (Fig. 2A). The temperature stability of complex A is shown in Figure 2B. About half of the activity of the preparation remained after six weeks of storage at -70° C, and this method of preservation of the activity was routinely used during these studies. The requirement for the

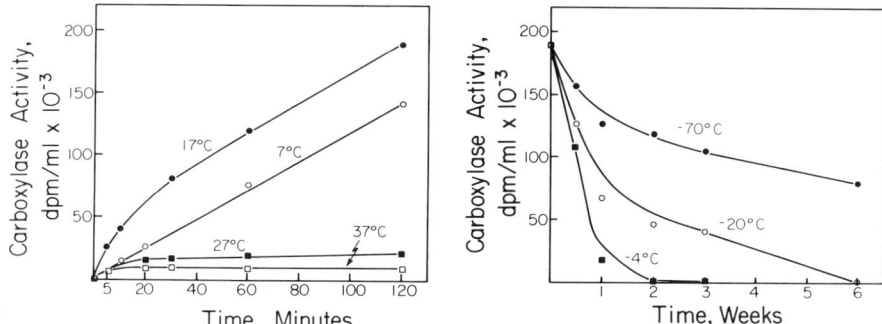

FIGURE 2. (A) Effect of temperature on carboxylation rate. Two ml incubation mixtures were incubated at each temperature, and duplicate aliquots taken for assay at the times indicated. The means of the values are plotted. ● = 17° C; ○ = 7° C; ■ = 27° C; □ = 37° C. (B) Effect of temperature on stability. Two ml aliquots of complex A were prepared and stored at various temperatures for the indicated time intervals. Values are means of duplicate assays. ● = -70° C; ○ = -20° C, ■ = -4° C.

reduced form of vitamin K was found to be absolute, and the vitamin required was greatly increased over that of the solubilized microsomal preparation. About 80 μg vitamin KH_2 per ml were required for half-maximal activity of complex A as compared to 20 μg/ml for solubilized microsomes. The pH optimum for complex A was found to be about 6.5 which was slightly more acidic than that observed for the microsomal preparation. The carboxylase in complex A was not saturated at the 0.5 mM concentrations of Phe-Leu-Glu-Glu-Leu routinely used, and considerably more activity was expressed at higher substrate concentrations. Using the initial linear rates of carboxylation observed for various concentrations of Phe-Leu-Glu-Glu-Leu over the first 20 min of incubation (Fig. 3), an apparent K_m of 1.7 mM was observed. This is less than half that of the soluble system.

The large increase in carboxylase activity observed during the preparation of the complex was compared to alterations in the amount of related enzymes in the preparation (Table 1). The fixation of $H^{14}CO_3^-$ into endogenous microsomal acceptors by complex A was about 75% of that seen with the crude microsomal preparation. The possible relationship between vitamin K epoxidase activity and the carboxylase activity has recently been reviewed (10), and about 40% of the epoxidase activity of the microsomal preparation could be detected in complex A. The enzyme responsible for conversion of the quinone form of the vitamin to the hydroquinone form has apparently been lost during purification, as complex A has an absolute requirement for the reduced form of vitamin K. No activity was observed when [vitamin K + NADH] was used in the reaction. Total P-450 activity of complex A was about 20% of that in the starting microsomal preparation, and the specific activity of P-450 in complex A is essentially unchanged from that of microsomes. It has also been shown (11) that the phospholipid to protein ratio of the original microsomal preparation is not appreciably altered during the purification, and that complex A no longer contains intact membrane structures.

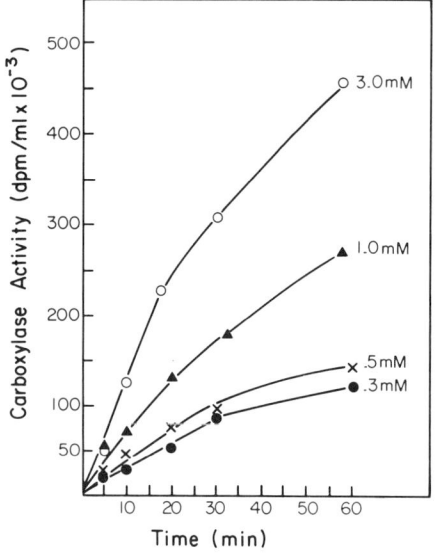

FIGURE 3. Effect of concentration of Phe-Leu-Glu-Glu-Leu on peptide carboxylase activity. A 2 ml assay mixture was incubated at 17° C, and duplicate aliquots removed at the times indicated. The means of the values are plotted.

TABLE 1. Activity of various microsomal membrane proteins.

Microsomal Activity	Enzyme Units	
	Microsomes	Complex A
Peptide carboxylase	5.4	188
Protein carboxylase	27	20
NADH-dependent carboxylase	5.4	0
Vitamin K epoxidase	3.75	1.67
Cytochrome P-450	0.53	0.12

The data represent the activity in a ml of the starting microsomal pellet suspension (25 mg protein/ml) and the amount of complex A obtained from it. All activities were assayed by standard methods.

Endogenous Inhibitors of the Carboxylase

Much of the apparent increase in total carboxylase activity observed (Fig. 1) during the preparation of complex A appears to be due to the presence of an inhibitor of the carboxylase in liver microsomes. This inhibitor could be partially solubilized by treatment of microsomes with buffer A to which 0.5 $\underline{M}$ KCl and 0.1% Triton X-100 or octylglucoside was added. Microsomes treated in this way had 140% the activity of unextracted microsomes (11), and this extract was capable of inhibiting carboxylase activity in the crude microsomal preparations. The effects of the inhibitor fractions were reversed by boiling, and the activity was not retarded by passage of the inhibitory fraction over a Sephadex G-25 column. Presence of the inhibitor decreased both the rate and extent of the carboxylase reaction. Perfusion of the liver with 0.025 $\underline{M}$ imidazole, pH 7.2 caused extensive membrane damage and removed about 25% of the microsomal protein and all of the inhibitor with no loss of carboxylase activity. It is likely that the crude microsomal preparations from unperfused livers are highly contaminated with hemoglobin, and the effect of addition of hemoglobin to the preparation was determined. Relatively low concentrations of hemoglobin (150 μg/ml) were found to inhibit the carboxylase reaction by 50%. A second heme protein, cytochrome C, was without significant effect. The nature of this inhibition was not determined, but it is likely that hemoglobin contamination was a major component of the inhibitory protein fraction which was present in crude microsomes.

Further Fractionation of Complex A

To further fractionate the activity in this particulate preparation, complex A was solubilized by detergent extraction. Of a number of conditions utilized, the most successful procedure was the extraction with 0.5% Triton X-100 in 0.5 $\underline{M}$ KCl. This extraction solubilized about 30% of the carboxylase activity with no change in specific activity from complex A. Initial attempts to fractionate the detergent extract by gradient elution on different chromatographic supports resulted in most cases in a complete loss of activity.

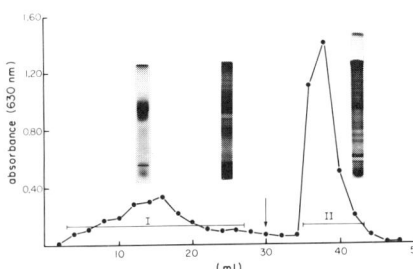

FIGURE 4. Chromatography of complex A on Sepharose-deoxycholate. Complex A was desalted on Sephadex G-25 as described in the text and applied to a Sepharose-deoxycholate column and eluted with the same buffer. At the point marked with an arrow, 0.5 $\underline{M}$ KCl was added to the buffer. Fractions pooled for assay are shown by the bars. SDS-gel-electrophoresis was carried out on unretarded protein in fractions corresponding to the positions of the gels in the figure and on pooled fraction II.

When carboxylase activity was detected, the pooled fractions contained only a small fraction of the total activity applied to the columns, and the specific activity was very low. As a consequence of these observations, subsequent experiments utilized stepwise elution from column supports to avoid dilution of the eluted protein which could have contributed to the loss of activity. Stepwise elution also aided in the successful recombination of components of a multienzyme complex which may have been separated by this procedure.

Chromatography on Sepharose-4B to which the ionic detergent deoxycholate had been chemically coupled proved to be an effective procedure for further purification of the carboxylase. Prior to being subjected to this affinity chromatographic step, the KCl-Triton X-100 extract of complex A was desalted on a column of Sephadex G-25 equilibrated in imidazole buffer (0.025 $\underline{M}$, pH 7.2) containing 0.25% Triton X-100 and 10% glycerol. The carboxylase activity coeluted with the void volume protein peak from this column. Electrophoresis in SDS of the proteins eluted in the void volume

TABLE 2. Purification of vitamin K-dependent carboxylase.

Fractions	Volume (ml)	Protein (mg/ml)	Total Protein (mg)	Activity (U/ml)	Total Activity (U)	Specific Activity (U/mg)	Increase in Specificity (fold)	Recovery (%)
Triton X-100 extract of complex A	13.0	0.54	7.0	19.6	254.8	36.3	145	100
Sephadex G-25	16.0	0.43	6.9	14.4	230.4	33.5	134	90
Sepharose-DOC Fraction I	29.0	0.09	2.6	0	0	0	—	0
Sepharose-DOC Fraction II	9.0	0.33	3.0	25.7	231.3	77.9	312	91
Sepharose-lipid Fraction I	9.3	0.13	1.21	0.6	5.6	4.6	18	2
Sepharose-lipid Fraction II	6.0	0.20	1.20	1.8	10.8	9.0	36	5
Sepharose-heparin Fraction I	9.1	0.17	1.63	2.4	21.8	13.4	57	9
Sepharose-heparin Fraction II	3.7	0.20	0.74	6.5	24.0	32.5	130	10

Fractions from the various modified Sepharose columns are pooled eluates as indicated in Figures 4 and 5. The fold increase in specific activity is based on the increase over the original solubilized microsomal pellet (see Fig. 1) while the yeidl fo enzyme is based on the enzyme activity present in the Triton X-100 extract of complex A. This extract has about half of the total activity of complex A.

revealed protein bands ranging in molecular weights from 7000-8000 to about 150,000 with a predominant band corresponding to a molecular weight of 51,000. This desalted fraction was subsequently loaded on a Sepharose-4B deoxycholate column equilibrated in the same buffer as used for desalting the protein on Sephadex G-25. The column was washed with the equilibration buffer and the retained protein eluted with KCl (Fig. 4). Electrophoresis in SDS revealed a single protein band of molecualr weight 51,000 in the first fractions of the unretarded protein with increasing contamination of other proteins in later fractions. This protein corresponds to the main protein observed in the Triton X-100 extract of complex A. Consequently, the fraction eluted with KCl showed a significant reduction in proteins migrating in the 51,000 position, and contained all of the vitamin K-dependent carboxylase activity. The data in Table 2 indicate that this procedure had achieved a two-fold increase in specific activity of the vitamin K-dependent carboxylase compared to complex A with little loss in total amount of enzyme activity.

Further fractionation of peak II from the Sepharose-deoxycholate column has resulted in a significant fractionation of the proteins present, but has also resulted in a loss of activity. Chromatography on either Sepharose-phosphatidylcholine (Fig. 5A) or Sepharose-heparin (Fig. 5B) was effective in separating the proteins into two peaks; and, on the basis of SDS-gel electrophoresis, it was apparent that a fractionation of the protein in the preparation had occurred. The data in Table 2 indicate that roughly 80% of the applied protein was recovered in both of the procedures, but that the carboxylase activity was greatly reduced. Attempts to restore activity by mixing these fractions or by various methods of reconstitution have not yet been successful.

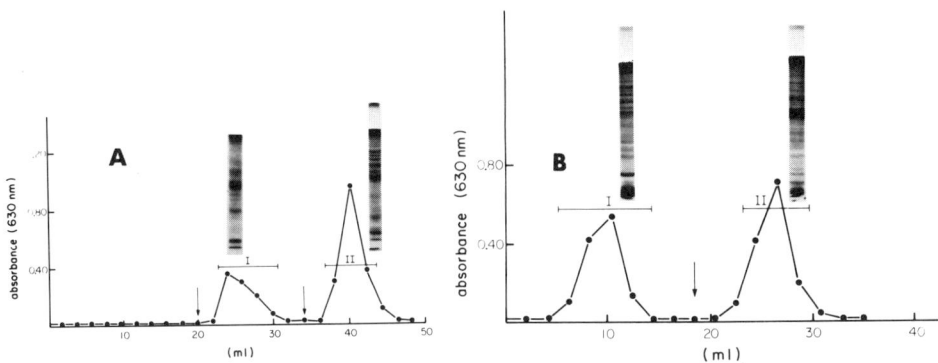

FIGURE 5. Chromatography of fraction II of the Sepharose-deoxycholate column on Sepharose-phosphatidylcholine (A) or Sepharose-heparin (B). Fraction II was dialyzed against 0.025 $\underline{M}$ imidazole buffer (pH 7.2) containing 10% glycerol and 0.25% Triton X-100 and applied to column A or dialyzed against 0.025 $\underline{M}$ potassium phosphate buffer (pH 7.2) containing 10% glycerol and 0.25% Triton X-100 and applied to column B. The columns were eluted with the equilibration buffer and were indicated by the arrows with 0.25 and 1.0 $\underline{M}$ KCl (A) or with 0.5 $\underline{M}$ KCl (B). Fractions were pooled as indicated by the bars, and enzyme assays and SDS-gel-electrophoresis carried out on the pooled fractions.

DISCUSSION

Complex A is a highly active, easily prepared, microsomal preparation which represents an increase in specific activity of the vitamin K-dependent carboxylase activity of over 100-fold compared to microsomes. The complex has the same general sensitivity to various inhibitors and stimulators, and similar temperature and pH optima as the solubilized microsomal carboxylase preparation. It differs from the preparation in that it has a considerably higher requirement for vitamin K than the unfractionated system, and the apparent K_m for a peptide substrate is decreased to less than half of that of the crude microsomal preparation.

The presence of considerable protein carboxylase activity in complex A suggests that at least some of the endogenous substrates for the enzyme are tightly bound to it and follow it through in the purification. Some cytochrome P-450 activity remained in the preparation, and vitamin K epoxidase activity was diminished during the purification procedure, but still detectable. Efficient epoxidation of vitamin K may depend on the presence of additional proteins in the microsomes which were lost during the preparation of complex A. The purification procedure has also removed the various vitamin K reductase activities in the microsomes, and the system is now dependent on the presence of reduced vitamin K. Much of this reductase activity is associated with a peripheral membrane protein form of the largely cytosolic DT-diaphorase that can readily be removed from the membrane (12).

The large (15-fold) increase in total carboxylase activity during the preparation of complex A appears to result from a number of factors. The enzyme is a very tightly bound integral membrane protein, and it is likely that little if any of it is extracted by the procedures used. Removal of hemoglobin and other inhibitors present therefore greatly increases the total activity. The purification procedure utilized may also open up more sites on the enzyme by removing other membrane components or by dissociating the complex into subunits.

Fractionation of detergent-solubilized complex A on a Sepharose-deoxycholate column effectively doubled the specific activity of the carboxylase from that present with essentially complete recovery of activity. The total increase in specific radioactivity at this point is about 300-fold over that of the starting microsomal preparation, and this preparation should be useful in studies of the molecular role of vitamin K in this carboxylation reaction. The different protein patterns observed by SDS-gel-electrophoresis in the two fractions eluted from either a Sepharose-phosphatidylcholine or a Sepharose-heparin column, and the loss of activity on the columns suggests the existence of an enzyme complex which is partially disrupted during chromatography. The possibility that loss of activity was caused by the elution conditions seems unlikely, as the concentration of KCl used has been shown to have no effect on the system. The basis for the failure to reconstitute activity upon mixing of the column fraction is not clear. It may be that the appropriate conditions have not been found, or it may be that there is an essential component which has not been eluted from the columns. About 20% of the total protein was unaccounted for, and it may be that some essential component of the carboxylase is still bound to the column. In any event, the preparation obtained from the Sepharose-deoxycholate column does represent a substantial enrichment of the vitamin K-dependent carboxylase activity, and serves as a basis for further fractionation.

ACKNOWLEDGEMENTS

This work was supported by the College of Agricultural and Life Sciences, University of Wisconsin-Madison, and in part by grants AM-14881, HL-05326, and DE-07031 from the National Institutes of Health, and by a grant from the University of Wisconsin Graduate School.

REFERENCES

1. Suttie, J. W., and Jackson, C. M. (1977) Physiol. Rev. 57, 1-70.
2. Suttie, J. W. (1978) In Handbook of Lipid Research 2, "The Fat-soluble Vitamins" (DeLuca, H. F., ed.) pp. 211-277, Plenum Press, New York.
3. Stenflo, J. (1978) Adv. Enzymol. 46, 1-31.
4. Olson, R. E., and Suttie, J. W. (1978) Vitamins and Hormones 35, 59-108.
5. Esmon, C. T., and Suttie, J. W. (1976) J. Biol. Chem. 251, 6238-6243.
6. Mack, D. O., Suen, E. T., Girardot, J.-M., Miller, J. A., Delaney, R., and Johnson, B. C. (1976) J. Biol. Chem. 251, 3269-3276.
7. Houser, R. M., Hall, A. H., and Olson, R. E. (1978) Fed. Proc. 37, 1588 (abstr.).
8. Suttie, J. W., Hageman, J. M., Lehrman, S. R., and Rich, D. H. (1976) J. Biol. Chem. 251, 5827-5830.
9. Whitlon, D. S., Sadowski, J. A., and Suttie, J. W. (1978) Biochemistry 17, 1371-1377.
10. Suttie, J. W., Larson, A. E., Canfield, L. M., and Carlisle, T. L. (1978) Fed. Proc. 37, 2605-2609.
11. Canfield, L. M., Sinsky, T. A., and Suttie, J. W. (1979) Fed. Proc. 38, 710 (abstr.).
12. Wallin, R., Gebhardt, O., and Prydz, H. (1978) Biochem. J. 169, 95-101.

RECONSTITUTION OF VITAMIN K-DEPENDENT CARBOXYLATION ACTIVITY

JOY A. PRICE and B. CONNOR JOHNSON

Oklahoma Medical Research Foundation, and
University of Oklahoma Health Sciences Center
Oklahoma City, OK 73104

INTRODUCTION

Attempts to purify a vitamin K-dependent "carboxylase" enzyme from rat liver microsomes have met with only limited success (1-3). Our experiences have been similar in that low yields of activity were obtained after relatively mild separation procedures. Recombination of separated fractions resulted in no further recovery of activity. However, when the detergent (Triton X-100) concentration was lowered to 0.33% and ethylene glycol added to 33%, recombination of separated protein fractions results in reconstitution of vitamin K-dependent carboxylation of synthetic pentapeptide (PheLeuGluGluLeu). The demonstration of purification and fractionation of the carboxylation system is more difficult with the rapid carboxylation of endogenous precursor protein substrates. This is not surprising, since the synthetic pentapeptide is a smaller molecule than the endogenous protein substrates and thus may require more extensive orientation in the carboxylation system. This study demonstrates that vitamin K-dependent carboxylation from rat liver microsomes is a multi-component system. The system can be fractionated and reconstituted under appropriate conditions.

MATERIALS AND METHODS

Vitamin K_1 (Aqua-Mephyton) was obtained from Merck, Sharp and Dohme. [^{14}C]-sodium carbonate (58 mCi/mmole) was purchased from Amersham-Searle. The pentapeptide, PheLeuGluGluLeu, was synthesized by Mr. Craig Ferris under the supervision of Dr. Robert Delaney and Dr. Andrew Chiu, using solid phase peptide synthesis (4). Dr. Adam Dubin synthesized the [^{125}I]-Triton X-100 (5). Triton X-100 (scintillation grade) and sodium dithionite were purchased from the Eastman Kodak Co. Scintisol was obtained from Isolab. Affi-Gel 501 (para-chloromercuribenzoate-agarose), an organomercurial agarose, was obtained from Bio-Rad Laboratories. Phenyl Sepharose CL-4B was purchased from Pharmacia Fine Chemicals, Inc. Amberlite XAD-2 was obtained from Rohm and Haas, Ltd. All other chemicals were reagent grade.

Vitamin K deficiency was produced in male, Sprague-Dawley rats by placing them in coprophagy-preventing cages (6) and feeding them a vitamin K-deficient diet (7) for 10 to 14 days. Microsomes were prepared as previously described (8), except that 50 mM sodium phosphate buffer, pH 7.4, was used in place of imidazole. The soluble system was prepared by diluting 1 ml of microsomal suspension with 0.5 ml of a solution of 6% Triton X-100, 800 mM NaCl, and 8 mM benzamidine hydrochloride in 50 mM phosphate buffer, pH 7.4. The suspension was then centrifuged at 100,000 x g for 1 h and the pellet discarded. The resulting soluble system contained 15 to 20 mg per ml protein.

Vitamin K_1 hydroquinone was prepared by adding 0.2 ml vitamin K_1 to a 1 ml hypo vial (Pierce), which was then sealed and alternately evacuated and flushed with oxygen-free nitrogen. Five to 10 μl of an oxygen-free sodium dithionite solution (0.1 g sodium dithionite in 0.5 ml distilled water) was then added to the vitamin K_1 solution using a Hamilton syringe until the solution became clear (vitamin K_1 hydroquinone).

The carboxylation assay system consisted of: 0.06 ml of soluble system (or protein fraction); 0.06 ml of 50 mM phosphate buffer, pH 7.4, (or a second protein fraction); 0.04 ml of peptide (final concentration 1.5 mM) in 0.12 M phosphate buffer, pH 7.2; 0.015 ml of 50 mM phosphate buffer, pH 7.4, containing 2.5 μCi [^{14}C]-sodium carbonate; and 0.0005 ml vitamin K_1 hydroquinone (0.55 mM final concentration). Vitamin K_1 hydroquinone and [^{14}C]-carbonate were added immediately before incubation in a 25°C water bath with constant shaking for 30 min. The reaction was stopped by addition of 1 ml cold 10% trichloroacetic acid. One-tenth ml of bovine serum albumin (10 mg/ml) was added to facilitate protein precipitation. The solution was allowed to stand in ice for 30 min, then centrifuged at 2500 rpm for 10 min. One ml of clear supernate was removed (the precipitate saved) and bubbled with air for 30 min, then added to 4 ml of Scintisol. The radioactivity was measured using either an Inter-technique SL30 or Packard scintillation counter. The radioactivity measured in the supernate was that incorporated into synthetic pentapeptide. The precipitate was washed twice with 2% sodium carbonate as previously described (8), and its radioactivity measured as an indication of endogenous substrate carboxylation activity.

A modified procedure of Holloway (9) was used to remove Triton X-100 from the soluble system. [^{125}I]-Triton X-100 was used to monitor the removal of detergent using Amberlite XAD-2, a neutral porous styrene-divinylbenzene copolymer. After the addition of Amberlite XAD-2, the cloudy supernatant was drawn off with a pipet or filtered through a Whatman No. 1 filter, then centrifuged at 100,000 x g for 1 h. The supernate was removed and the pellet resuspended in 0.5% Triton X-100, 0.5 M NaCl in 50 mM phosphate buffer, pH 7.4, then diluted one-third with ethylene glycol and mixed thoroughly.

Fractionation of the resolubilized pellet was carried out on three 10 ml columns of either phenyl-Sepharose or para-chloromercuribenzoate-agarose (pCMB-agarose). The resolubilized system (2-10 ml) was added (in a 4° C cold room) at a flow rate of 1-2 ml per h. Protein was eluted by adding either 1% Triton X-100 in phosphate buffer (for the phenyl-Sepharose columns) or 5 mM dithiothreitol, 1% Triton X-100 in 50 mM phosphate buffer (for the pCMB-agarose columns). Protein fractions were concentrated using Aquacide II (Calbiochem) and assayed for carboxylation, protein and precursor activity.

RESULTS

In order to solubilize the microsomal proteins involved in vitamin K-dependent carboxylation, high concentrations of the non-ionic detergent, Triton X-100, are required. Optimal activity is obtained using 2% Triton X-100. When this detergent is removed with using Amberlite XAD-2 after solubilization, carboxylation activity precipitates out of solution. This activity can be resolubilized either by adding back the original detergent concentration or by adding lower concentrations of detergent in conjunction with ethylene glycol.

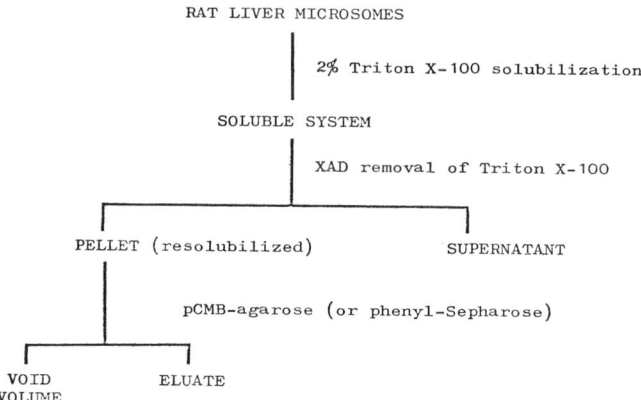

FIGURE 1 Fractionation scheme for separation of the components involved in vitamin K-dependent carboxylation.

The fractionation scheme used in this study is outlined in Figure 1. The pellet, formed after treatment with Amberlite XAD-2, was resolubilized using 0.33% Triton X-100, 0.33 M NaCl and 33% ethylene glycol in 0.33 M phosphate buffer, pH 7.4. This resolubilized system was then added to pCMB-agarose or phenyl-Sepharose in order to fractionate the carboxylation system. The component, which eluted from these columns, contained less than 10% of the original carboxylation activity present using vitamin K-deficient rat liver microsomes. The eluate fractions contained no pentapeptide or endogenous carboxylation activity when microsomes were prepared from normal rats injected with vitamin K. When these eluate fractions were recombined with void volume fractions from either column, 80% to 100% of the original peptide carboxylation activity was recovered (Table I). The void volume fractions alone contained 30 to 40% of the original peptide carboxylation activity. The eluate fraction from either vitamin K-deficient or vitamin K-sufficient microsomal preparations could be used to recover activity when recombined with void volume fractions. In order to obtain maximum carboxylation activity, void volume fractions from vitamin K-deficient microsomes were necessary.

It was also observed that the supernatant fractions remaining after treatment of the soluble system with Amberlite XAD-2, when added to eluate fractions from pCMB-agarose or phenyl-Sepharose, gave increases in the recovery of peptide carboxylation (Table II). After Amberlite XAD-2 treatment, the supernatant fraction, and the void volumes from phenyl-Sepharose and pCMB-agarose appear to behave similarly in giving reconstitution of peptide carboxylation when added to eluate fractions.

Since two separate fractions were identified as being necessary for carboxylation activity, free pCMB was added to each fraction prior to recombination. Unreacted pCMB was removed by gel filtration on Sephadex G-25. The less hydrophobic component (void volume fractions and supernatant fraction) contained the essential free sulfhydryl necessary for carboxylation. It should be noted that the more hydrophobic fraction (eluate from pCMB-agarose or phenyl-Sepharose) also contains a free sulfhydryl, but this sulfhydryl group is not essential for carboxylation activity. Apparently the essential free sulfhydryl residue, located on the less hydrophobic component, is buried within the molecule. It is not accessible to immobilized pCMB, since this component comes through in the void volume after pCMB-agarose. The idea that the free sulfhydryl necessary for vitamin K-dependent carboxylation is buried within the molecule is supported by the observation that the more hydrophobic sulfhydryl reagents are better inhibitors of carboxylation than hydrophilic reagents.

The endogenous precursor activity was detected with the Echis carinatus snake venom assay (10). The precursor activity was detectable in the same fractions containing the less hydrophobic component (void volume fractions and supernatant fraction).

TABLE 1 Fractionation and reconstitution of vitamin K-dependent carboxylation activity

| | Percent Carboxylation Activity | | | | | |
| | Void Volume | | Eluate | | Reconstituted | |
Column	Peptide	Endog.	Peptide	Endog.	Peptide	Endog.
pCMB-agarose^a	42	50	2	4	72	44
phenyl-Sepharose	28	39	4	8	102	48

TABLE 2 Recombination studies using fractions separated by treatment with Amberlite XAD and fractionation on phenyl-Sepharose

| | $\dfrac{\text{Activity Obtained}}{\text{Activity Expected}}$ | |
Fractions Recombined	Ratio for Peptide Carboxylation	Ratio for Endogenous Carboxylation
Void volume + eluate	2.6	1.0
Void volume + supernate	1.2	1.2
Supernate + eluate	2.8	1.3

DISCUSSION

When purification procedures such as gel filtration, affinity chromatography and hydrophobic interaction chromatography, were originally used to fractionate the vitamin K-dependent carboxylation system, from 50 to 90% of the activity was lost. Neither peptide nor endogenous substrate carboxylation activity could be recovered by recombining separated fractions. Not until the detergent concentration was lowered and ethylene glycol added to the system, was reconstitution possible.

The observations that only peptide carboxylation activity can be reconstituted and little (10%) recovery of endogenous substrate carboxylation occurs, are not surprising. The endogenous substrate may undergo steric changes after fractionation and, therefore, cannot recombine efficiently with the "carboxylase" system.

From the results presented here, it is evident that vitamin K-dependent carboxylation is a multi-component reaction. The two components can be separated by at least three methods. One component can be identified in the supernatant fraction of the soluble system after removal of Triton X-100. This is the less hydrophobic factor. This factor can also be seen in the void volume fractions from phenyl-Sepharose and pCMB-agarose columns. This component contains the essential sulfhydryl. Although this fraction contains a free thiol group, it does not bind to pCMB-agarose. The thiol residue is probably buried within the molecule, which would explain why the more hydrophobic SH reagents are better inhibitors of carboxylation. This factor is altered in some manner between the state of vitamin K sufficiency and vitamin K deficiency in rat liver microsomes. Maximum carboxylation activity is obtained, only after isolation from vitamin K-deficient rat liver microsomes, when this component is added to eluate fractions. The eluate fractions, from either vitamin K-deficient or vitamin K-sufficient rat liver microsomes, function equally well.

The second component, identified as necessary for vitamin K-dependent carboxylation, binds to phenyl-Sepharose and pCMB-agarose under appropriate conditions. This factor, therefore, also contains a free sulfhydryl group, but the SH is not essential for vitamin K-dependent carboxylation. This component is also more hydrophobic than the other factor, since it precipitates from solution after removal of Triton X-100 and binds to phenyl-Sepharose (a hydrophobic interaction column). This factor has been further purified 20 to 30 fold from solubilized microsomes.

The two components may have quite different molecular weights, as well, since carboxylation activity is easily lost after gel filtration.

The exact identity of these separated fractions remains unknown. These results may be related to those of Wallin (11) who noted that more than one protein fraction was necessary for optimum vitamin K-dependent carboxylation. The question, as to whether one of the necessary fractions is the epoxidase (2), endogenous substrate (12), or another protein, remains to be answered.

ACKNOWLEDGEMENTS This work was supported in part by NIH grant # HL17619. We would like to thank Ms. Vicki Bartels for her technical assistance and Ms. Patricia Ownbey for aid in the preparation of this manuscript.

REFERENCES

1. Houser, R.M., Hall, A.H., and Olsen, R.E. (1978) Fed. Proc. 37, 1588.
2. Suttie, J.W., Larson, A.E., Canfield, L.M., and Carlisle, T.L. (1978) Fed. Proc. 37, 2605-2609.
3. Canfield, L.M., Sinsky, T.A. and Suttie, J.W. (1979) Fed. Proc. 38, 710.
4. Stewart, J.W. and Young, J.D. in Solid Phase Peptide Synthesis (W.H. Freeman, ed), San Francisco.
5. Greenwood, F.C., Hunter, W.M. and Glover, J.S. (1963) Biochem. J. 89, 114-122.
6. Metta, V.C., Nash, L., and Johnson, B.C. (1961) J. Nutr. 74, 473-476.
7. Mameesh, M.S. and Johnson, B.C. (1959) Proc. Soc. Exp. Biol. Med. 101, 467-468.
8. Price, J.A., Bartels, V.L., Delaney, R., and Johnson, B.C. (1979) Biochem. Biophys. Res. Commun. (Submitted for publication).
9. Holloway, P.W. (1973) Anal. Biochem. 53, 304-308.
10. Nelsestuen, G.L., and Suttie, J.W. (1972) J. Biol. Chem. 247, 8176-8182.
11. Wallin, R. (1979) Biochem. J. 178, 513-519.
12. Dubin, A., Suen, E., Delaney, R. and Johnson, B.C. (1979) Fed. Proc. 38, 792.

HIGH PRESSURE LIQUID CHROMATOGRAPHIC ANALYSIS OF THE VITAMIN K DEPENDENT CARBOXYLASE SYSTEM

LOUISE M. CANFIELD, JANE MA and E. G. SANDER

Department of Biochemistry
West Virginia University Medical Center
Morgantown, WV 26506

INTRODUCTION

Vitamin K dependent carboxylase (K carboxylase) catalyzes a complex, four substrate reaction of undertermined stoichiometry. The assay system currently employed involves measurement of $^{14}CO_2$ into the gamma carboxyglutamic acid (Gla) product. With this assay, it is difficult to determine the stoichiometry of the reaction. Hence the objective of this work is to develop a sensitive assay system which can reproducibly measure both the substrates and the products of the K carboxylase catalyzed reaction.

MATERIALS AND METHODS

High pressure liquid chromatography (HPLC) was accomplished with a Waters Model 244 instrument equipped with a 254 nm ultraviolet detector. Chromatography of the various vitamin K species and the glutamic acid (Glu) substrates was conducted using separate injections all on a Waters µBondapak C_{18} reverse phase column operating under isocratic conditions. Linear relationships between peak height and concentrations of oxidized vitamin K (K_o) and vitamin K epoxide (K_e) were constructed by injection of 50 µl aliquots of the vitamin species dissolved in hexane. In the case of the benzyl ester of t-BOC-glutamic acid (t-BOC-glu-∅) which was used as the Glu substrate (1), the standard curve was determined by injection of 25 µl of the amino acid derivative dissolved in 25 mM imidazole buffer, pH 7.2. Elution of the vitamin species was accomplished with 93% methanol:7% H_2O, room temperature, flow rate 1.5 ml min^{-1}. Elution of t-BOC-Glu-∅ was with 60% methanol:40% H_2O containing 0.1% H_3PO_4, room temperature, 1.5 ml min^{-1}. Enzymatic reaction mixtures were 25 mM imidazole buffer (pH 7.2), 4.0 mM t-BOC-Glu-∅, 0.017 mM reduced vitamin K (K_r), 0.068 mM warfarin, 160 mM sucrose, 322 mM KCl, and microsomes which were solubilized in 0.25% Triton X-100, 0.25 M sucrose, 0.50 M KCl and 25 mM imidazole buffer (pH 7.2), final volume 0.62 ml. After appropriate incubation at 17°C, reaction mixtures were quenched by the addition of two volumes of isopropanol:hexane (3:2, vol:vol), mixed, chilled in ice (5 minutes) remixed and centrifuged at 4°C (5 minutes). The organic phase was aspirated, dried under a stream of oxygen to reoxidize K_r, and redissolved in a known volume of hexane. A 50 µl aliquot was subjected to HPLC analysis using the appropriate solvent and compared to the standard curve. After recentrifugation, 25 µl of the extracted aqueous phase was analyzed on the HPLC for t-BOC-Glu-∅ and for potential Gla products. Enzyme activity in solubilized microsomes was measured using the standard $^{14}CO_2$ incorporation assay (2).

505

RESULTS AND DISCUSSION

The HPLC elution profiles of both the t-BOC-Glu-∅ and the vitamin K species are shown in Fig. 1. In this case, the organic phase was not evaporated with O_2 thus showing that the system can resolve K_o, K_e and K_r. In the latter case, quantitation is not possible due to air reoxidation of K_r. The elution profile of t-BOC-Glu-∅ shows a Warfarin peak which serves as an internal standard, as well as two reproducible peaks, Peaks 1 and 2, which occur upon the incubation of t-BOC-Glu-∅ with solubilized microsomes. Peak 1 appears to be benzyl alcohol, however firm assignment

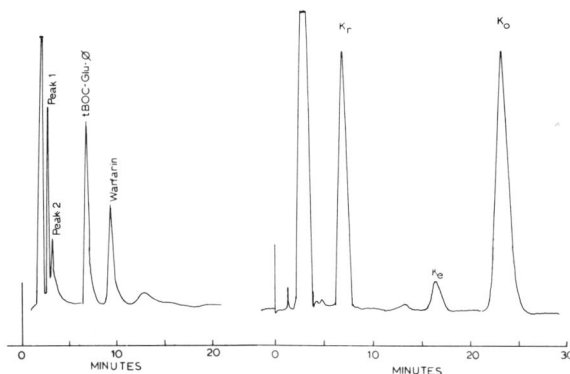

Fig. 1. Elution profiles of t-BOC-Glu-∅ (left), and vitamin K species (right).

of both Peak 1 and Peak 2 must await synthesis of chemically characterized chromatography standards. Fig. 2 shows the quantitative relationship between peak height and known concentrations of t-BOC-Glu-∅ and both K_o and K_e. Fig. 3 shows the direct relationship between the rate of $^{14}CO_2$ incorporation into t-BOC-Glu-∅ and the formation of K_e, the vitamin K species hypothesized to be a product of the K carboxylase catalyzed reaction. These data cannot be used to determine the stiochiometry of Gla and K_e formation, however, they clearly show that at equal enzyme and vitamin concentrations, the two compounds are formed at a kinetically equivalent rate and hence argue that K_e may well be the vitamin K

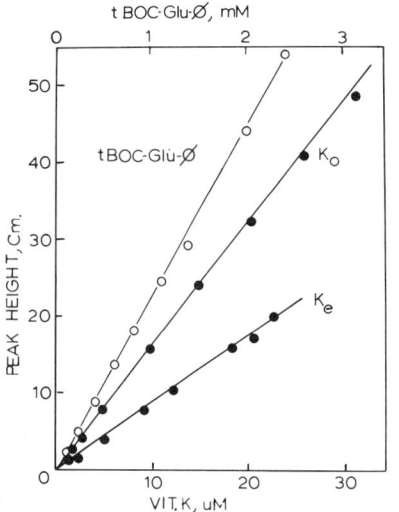

Fig. 2. Quantitative relationship between peak height and concentrations of t-BOC-Glu-∅ (O, upper) and K_o and K_e (●, lower).

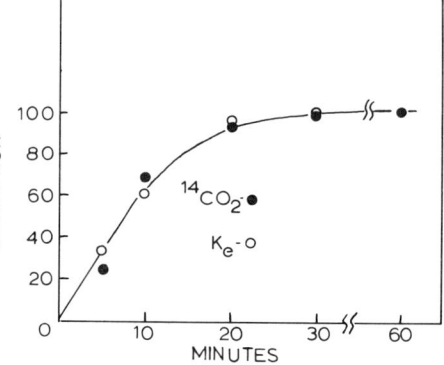

Fig. 3. Relationship between the rate of $^{14}CO_2$ incorporation and rate of K_e formation at 17°, pH 7.2.

product of the K carboxylase catalyzed reaction. This notion is further supported by the data shown in Fig. 4. These data show the stimulation in K_e caused by increasing concentrations of t-BOC-Glu-$\emptyset$, an observation consistent with that previously made by Suttie et al. (3) who measured both the stimulation of $^{14}CO_2$ incorporation and $\overline{K_e}$ formed as a function of increased concentrations of phe-leu-glu-glu-leu. In addition, these data show a correlation between Glu substrate concentration and both the concentrations of K_e as well as the ratio of K_e/K_o which has previously been used in thin layer chromatography systems as an index of K_e formation (4). Of further interest is the fact that some K_e is formed independently of added t-BOC-Glu-$\emptyset$, a result which can be explained either by the carboxylation of endogenous Glu substrates in the microsomal preparation or by the non-Glu substrate dependent collapse of the vitamin K hydroperoxide intermediate proposed by Larson and Suttie (5). In an attempt to use the HPLC system to monitor the formation of Gla products, the time course of the disappearance of t-BOC-Glu-$\emptyset$, and the appearance of Peaks 1 and 2 (Fig. 1) were measured, both in the presence and absence of K_r, using solubilized microsomes as a source of enzyme (Fig. 5). The results show the utility of the HPLC system for kinetically monitoring micromolar quantities of compounds of this type. As evidenced by the rate and extent of $^{14}CO_2$ incorporation, this system has K carboxylase activity. However, the fact that t-BOC-Glu-$\emptyset$ disappearance does not depend on added K_r makes it impossible under these reaction conditions to conclude that the disappearance of t-BOC-Glu-$\emptyset$ is direct evidence for Gla product formation. It is likely that microsomal esterase activity causes the hydrolysis of the carboxyterminal benzyl ester. However, identical incubations in the presence of 1.0 mM PMSF (phenylmethyl sulfonyl fluoride), a known trypsin and chymotrypsin

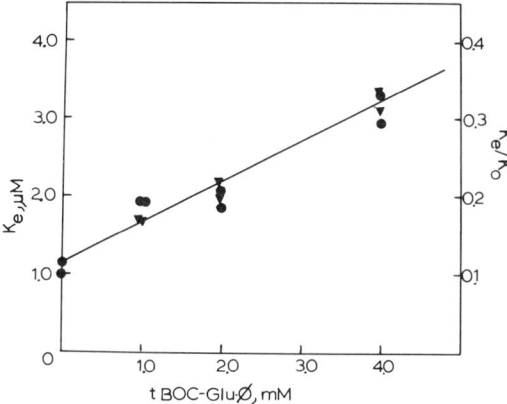

Fig. 4. Stimulation of K_e formation as a function of t-BOC-Glu-$\emptyset$ concentration at 17°C, pH 7.2. K_e concentration ●; K_eK_o, ▼.

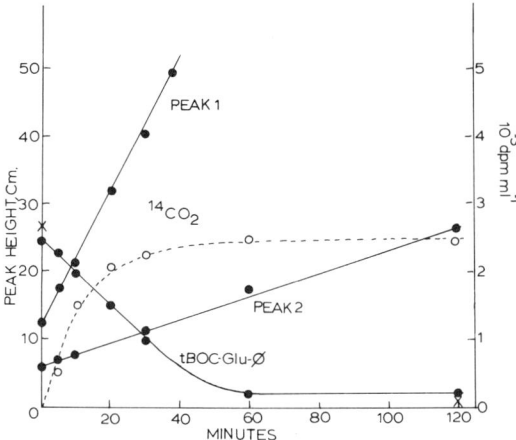

Fig. 5. Kinetics of $^{14}CO_2$ incorporation and t-BOC-Glu-$\emptyset$ disappearance in solubilized microsomes, 17°C, pH 7.2. (X) shows t-BOC-Glu-$\emptyset$ concentration in the absence of K_r.

inhibitor (6) gave similar results. Thus using solubilized microsomes as the enzyme source, it cannot be concluded that t-BOC-Glu-$\emptyset$ disappearance as seen by ultraviolet detection on HPLC is directly related to carboxylation. Unequivocal evidence for the K carboxylase-catalyzed conversion of t-BOC-Glu-$\emptyset$ into the Gla analog will likely require purified K carboxylase (7) and HPLC analysis of Gla product formation rather than Glu product utilization. In one preliminary experiment, incubation of 4 mM t-BOC-Glu-$\emptyset$ with the purified enzyme in the absence of K_r caused no time dependent decay of the t-BOC-Glu-$\emptyset$ peak. Experiments are presently underway to further characterize these products and to determine the stoichoimetry of the K carboxylase catalyzed reaction.

ACKNOWLEDGEMENTS

This work was supported by Grant No. Ca 21167 from the National Institutes of Cancer.

REFERENCES

1. Finnan, J. L., Goodman, H. L. and Suttie, J. W., these proceedings

2. Suttie, J. W., Lehrman, S. R., Geweke, L. O., Hagemen, J. M., and Rich, D. H. (1979) Biochem. Biophys. Res. Commun. 86, 500-507

3. Suttie, J. W., Larson, A. E., Canfield, L. M., and Carlisle, T. L., (1978), Fed. Proc. 37, 2605-2609

4. Sadowski, J. A., Esmon, C. T. and Suttie, J. W., (1976)., J. Biol. Chem. 251, 2770-2775.

5. Larson, A. E. and Suttie, J. W., (1978), Proc. Natl. Acad. Sci. USA 75, 5413-5416.

6. Fahrney, D. E. and Gold, A. M., (1963), J. Am. Chem. Soc. 85 997-1000.

7. Canfield, L. M., Sinsky, T. A. and Suttie, J. W., submitted to J. Biol. Chem.

CARBOXYLATION OF LOW-MOLECULAR-WEIGHT SUBSTRATES BY THE RAT LIVER VITAMIN K-DEPENDENT CARBOXYLASE: CHARACTERIZATION OF PRODUCTS

J. L. FINNAN and J. W. SUTTIE

Department of Biochemistry
College of Agricultural and Life Sciences
University of Wisconsin-Madison
Madison, WI 53706

INTRODUCTION

Vitamin K functions in the postribosomal modification of liver microsomal precursor proteins to form biologically-active prothrombin and the other vitamin K-dependent plasma clotting factors. The vitamin K-dependent modification of these precursors involves the carboxylation of specific glutamyl residues to form γ-carboxyglutamyl residues in the completed proteins, and *in vitro* microsomal systems which carry out this vitamin K-dependent carboxylation have been developed. Progress in this area has recently been reviewed (1-4). Detailed investigations of the mechanism

```
                                                              CH₂
         Precursor                    Prothrombin              |
                                                            HC-COOH
         CH₂          CO₂   O₂         CH₂                     |
Glutamyl  |          ────────────►     |          γ-Carboxy-
Residues  CH₂         Vitamin K        HC-COOH    glutamyl
          |                            |          Residues
          COOH                         COOH
```

of action of this enzyme have been hampered by a dependence on the endogenous microsomal precursor protein(s) as a substrate for the reaction, and we have shown (5-7) that low-molecular-weight peptides containing Glu-Glu sequences will serve as a substrate for this reaction. Although the initial report of the use of these substrates (5) demonstrated the vitamin K-dependent formation of Gla residues in the pentapeptide Phe-Leu-Glu-Glu-Leu, neither the extent of carboxylation (mono- vs. dicarboxylation) nor the specificity of possible monocarboxylated forms (Glu-Gla vs. Gla-Glu formation) was determined. This report presents further details of the action of the vitamin K-dependent carboxylase on a pentapeptide substrate and describes a previously unidentified postcarboxylational modification of the peptide substrate which we have observed (8).

MATERIALS AND METHODS

Male, 250-300 g Holtzman strain rats were used and vitamin K deficiency produced as previously described (9). The animals were routinely fasted overnight before being decapitated. A crude microsomal pellet was obtained from liver homogenates as previously described (10), and this pellet was resuspended in a volume of 0.25 $\underline{M}$ sucrose-0.025 $\underline{M}$ imidazole-

0.5 M KCl - 1.5% Triton X-100 equal to that of the original postmitochondrial supernate. Vitamin K-dependent incorporations of $H^{14}CO_3^-$ into the peptide substrate Phe-Leu-Glu-Glu-Leu or into t-BOC-Glu-α-benzyl ester (11) was measured essentially as previously described (6). The volume of the incubation mixture varied with different experiments but all incubations contained 100 μg/ml vitamin KH_2 and 1 mM DTT. The conditions used to separate products of the carboxylation reaction are described in the appropriate figure legends.

RESULTS

Detection of the Products of Peptide Carboxylation

To insure that the products of peptide carboxylation were not altered by the acidic conditions used to stop the reaction in the normal assay system, carboxylated Phe-Leu-Glu-Glu-Leu was isolated from the incubation mixture by direct gel filtration. The combined presence of the peptide

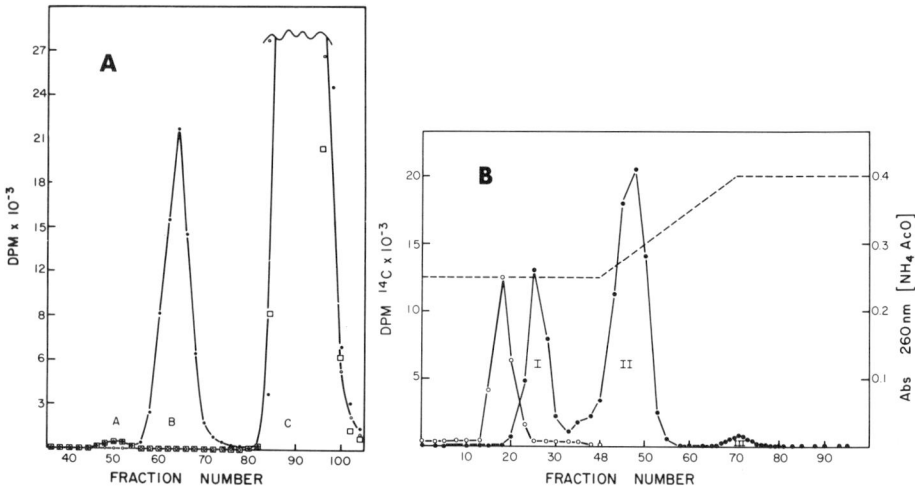

FIGURE 1. Chromatography of solubilized microsomes after incubation with $H^{14}CO_3^-$. (A) Gel filtration: After 7 h at 15°, 5.3 ml of solubilized microsomes were applied to a column (2.1 x 80 cm) of Sephadex G-25 and eluted with 0.10 M NH_4HCO_3. ●—●, 5 mM Phe-Leu-Glu-Glu-Leu + vitamin KH_2 (100 g/ml); O—O, 5 mM peptide minus vitamin KH_2; □—□, minus peptide + vitamin KH_2: (B) Ion exchange: Peak B (Fig. 1A) along with added peptide (10 mg) was applied to a column (1.0 x 20 cm) of DEAE-Sephadex A-25 and eluted with NH_4AcO. ●—●, ^{14}C radioactivity; O—O, absorbance at 260 nm; -----, [NH_4AcO].

substrate Phe-Leu-Glu-Glu-Leu and vitamin KH_2 in the incubation mixture resulted in the incorporation (Fig. 1A) of nonvolatile $H^{14}CO_3^-$ into microsomal endogenous precursor proteins (peak A) and product(s) (peak B) which were of a size within the middle of the fractionation range of Sephadex G-25. Control microsomal preparations incubated in the absence of vitamin K revealed radioactivity only in the HCO_3^- region (peak C), and incubation in the absence of added peptide resulted in the appearance of radioactivity only in peaks A and C. When peak B was pooled and applied to DEAE-Sephadex, it was resolved into three peaks of radioactivity (Fig. 1B). All three peaks eluted after the peptide substrate and were more acidic than the parent peptide. Peak III, the minor and most acidic component, was found (data not shown) to cochromatograph with synthetic Phe-Leu-Gla-Gla-Leu. Efforts were, therefore, directed toward the characterization of the major products, peaks I and II. The influence of various factors on the relative amount of peaks I and II formed in the incubation was investigated. It soon became apparent (Fig. 2) that peak II was formed early in the incubation and that peak I appeared to be formed from peak II. This explanation of the kinetics of formation of these two products was verified when it was demonstrated (data not shown) that isolated peak II could be converted by incubation with rat liver microsomes to peak I. This conversion was not dependent on the vitamin K status of animals which were used to obtain the liver microsomal preparations. Isolated peak I was not altered when it was incubated with similar microsomal preparations.

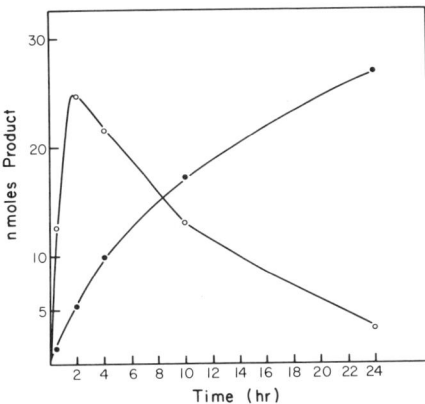

FIGURE 2. Time dependence of the formation of peak I and peak II. Peaks I and II were determined at various times during incubation of Phe-Leu-Glu-Glu-Leu by ion exchange chromatography after gel filtration of the 5.3 ml mixtures as shown in Fig. 1. ●—●, peak I; ○—○, peak II.

Carboxylation of a Glutamic Acid Derivative

A survey of a number of glutamic acid derivatives (11) has demonstrated that the compound t-BOC-Glu-α-benzyl ester will serve as a substrate for the vitamin K-dependent carboxylase. When the products of the incubation of t-BOC-Glu-α-benzyl ester as a substrate for the carboxylase were separated by gel filtration, it was apparent that two products were formed. As in the case of the peptide substrate, Phe-Leu-Glu-Glu-Leu, carboxylation of this glutamic acid derivative resulted in the formation of two products, peaks A and B which could be separated on the basis of molecular weight (Fig. 3A) and could also be resolved on an ion exchange column (Fig. 3B). These data suggested that the two carboxylated products formed during the incubation of Phe-Leu-Glu-Glu-Leu do not represent an artifact introduced by metabolism of the peptide by the crude microsomal preparation. Rather, the alteration appears to be closely associated with the formation of Gla residues. In an attempt to get a better estimation of the possible molecular weight changes associated with this modification, all four products were chromatographed on a calibrated Bio-Gel P-2 column (Fig. 4). Peaks A and B were readily separated on this column, and peak A had a calculated molecular weight 131 mass units larger than peak B. Peaks I and II chromatographed near the void volume of the column; and, although they were both easily separated from the uncarboxylated substrate, they were not resolved.

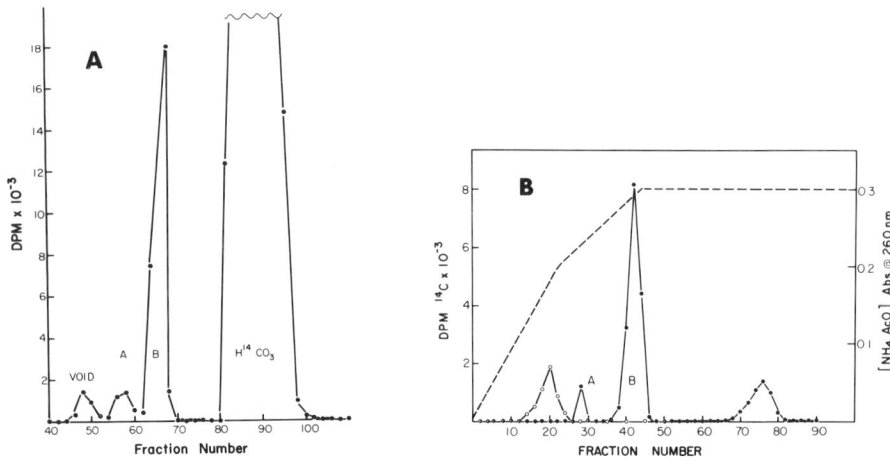

FIGURE 3. Chromatography of solubilized microsomes after incubation with $H^{14}CO_3^-$ and simple substrate. (A) Gel filtration: After 7 h at 7°, 5.3 ml of solubilized microsomes containing 10 mM t-BOC-Glu-α-benzyl ester and vitamin KH_2 (100 μg/ml) were applied to a column (2.1 x 100 cm) of Bio-Gel P-2 and eluted with 0.10 M NH_4HCO_3. (B) Ion exchange: The separate peaks A and B (Fig. 3a) along with 20 mg t-BOC-Glu-α-benzyl ester were applied to DEAE-Sephadex and eluted with NH_4AcO. ●—●, ^{14}C radioactivity; ○—○, absorbance at 260 nm; -----, [NH_4AcO].

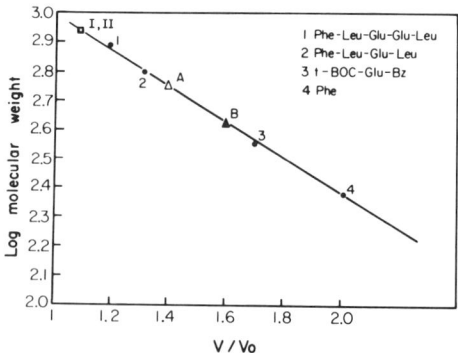

FIGURE 4. Molecular weight determination by gel filtration. The various biosynthetic products (peaks I, II, A, and B) and the indicated standards were applied to a column (1.0 x 200 cm) of Bio-Gel P-2 and were eluted with 0.10 M NH_4HCO_3. The positions of the various species were determined by either their uv absorbance or their radioactivity.

Sequencing of Peak I and Peak II

Thin-layer chromatography following acid and base hydrolysis established that both peaks I and II contained Gla residues but did not reveal the location of this residue. Both products were sequenced by the manual

Edman degradation method and radioactivity released at each step to determine where the Gla residue was positioned in each product. Inconsistent results were initially obtained, and these erratic data suggested that the lability of the Gla carboxyl group during the sequencing procedure may have been a source of the problem. Decarboxylation of the Gla residues to Glu residues before sequencing by a mild decarboxylation procedure was considered as a possible solution. Mild pyridine decarboxylation of malonic acid proceeds 100-fold faster than strong acid decarboxylation (12), and the use of this solvent was investigated as a procedure which would convert Gla to Glu residues with a minimal cleavage of peptide bonds. Refluxing pyridine was found to cause the loss of half of the radioactive label in both peaks I and II in 30 min with no additional loss at the end of 1 h. Ion exchange chromatography (Fig. 5) of the two peaks after a

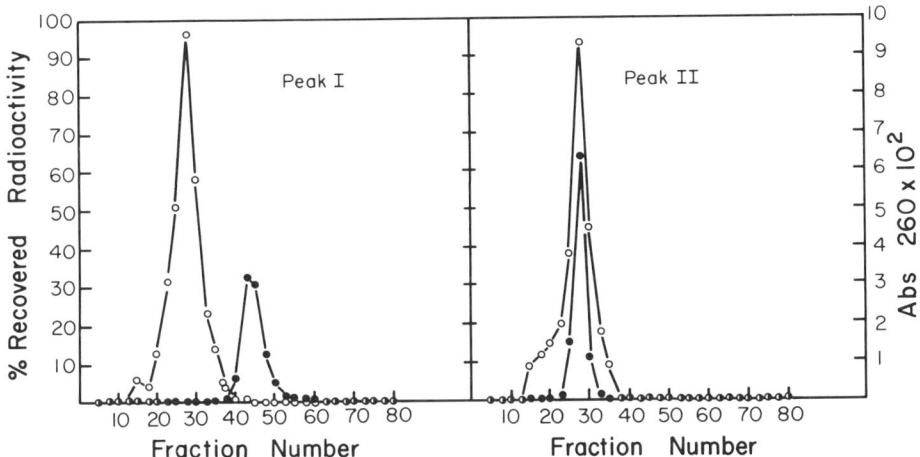

FIGURE 5. Ion exchange chromatography of peaks I and II after pyridine decarboxylation. After refluxing the respective peaks in pyridine and evaporating, their residues were applied to DEAE-Sephadex with added Phe-Leu-Glu-Glu-Leu and eluted with 0.25 $\underline{M}$ NH$_4$AcO. O—O, absorbance at 260 nm; ●—●, ^{14}C radioactivity.

one-hour pyridine decarboxylation demonstrated that the radioactivity remaining eluted as one peak and that any degradation of the peptide had been minimal. The products formed by decarboxylation of peaks I and II did, however, exhibit different elution patterns. The peak II product coeluted with added Phe-Leu-Glu-Glu-Leu indicating that the loss of a carboxyl group transformed it back into the starting product. The product formed when peak I was subjected to pyridine decarboxylation did not co-elute with added substrate again indicating that some type of chemical modification in addition to carboxylation may have occurred. When the decarboxylated and rechromatographed peaks I and II were subjected to Edman degradation, the profile of the radioactivity released during each step of the sequence was essentially identical for the two peaks (Fig. 6) and supported the conclusion that both peaks I and II contained largely Phe-Leu-Gla-Glu-Leu. Thin-layer chromatography of the PTH-derivatives and detection by autoradiography also revealed that the radiolabel in the third residue of decarboxylated peak II was located in PTH-Glu. However, the PTH-derivative from the third residue of the decarboxylated peak I

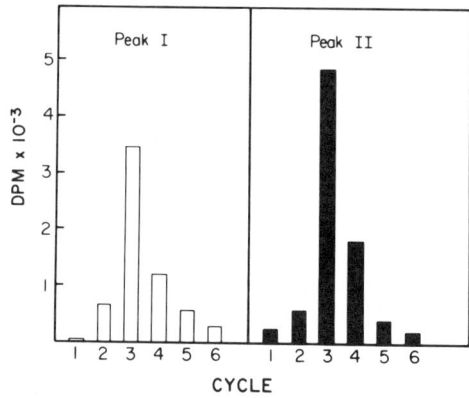

FIGURE 6. Profile of the location of radioactivity in peaks I and II. After chromatography (Fig. 5) of the decarboxylated peaks (10^6 dpm), they were subjected to standard Edman degradation. The cleavage products were sampled at each cycle for their radioactivity.

chromatographed as a species considerably more polar than PTH-Glu, again suggesting that the Gla residue in peak I was modified. As the decarboxylated peak I product contained radioactivity in the same residue of the peptide as the decarboxylated peak II product, modification of the peak I product must have occurred in the side chain of the Gla residue rather than the uncarboxylated Glu residue. The only functional groups in this residue available for modification are the carboxyl groups. The peak I product lost half of its radioactivity when treated with pyridine, and no radioactivity appeared as PTH-Glu. Therefore, if peak I was modified at a Gla carboxyl group, the modification would have had to be equally distributed between the original carboxyl group and the added one. It is also possible that the relatively acidic carbon which is α to the carboxyl groups of the Glu residues has been derivatized. If this were the case, it would explain the lack of modification of uncarboxylated Glu residues.

Mass Spectral Analyses of Peaks A and B

In an attempt to completely characterize the products of this postcarboxylation event, large scale incubations of t-BOC-Glu-α-benzyl ester were employed. The incubations were carried out at 7° in the presence of $H^{14}CO_3^-$ for 4 h (for maximum yield of peak B) and for 36 h (for maximum yield of peak A). The products of the incubation were subjected to chromatography on Bio-Gel P-2 and then on DEAE-Sephadex A-25. The peak material which could be identified by following radioactivity was again chromatographed on Bio-Gel and DEAE-Sephadex and again on Bio-Gel. The material from the final column was methylated by treatment with diazomethane and the methylated products were chromatographed on silica gel plates. The radioactive area on the plate was scraped off and the desired products eluted from the silicic acid. These products were then subjected to mass fragmentation analysis. The fragmentation pattern of authentic chemically-synthesized t-BOC-Gla-α-benzyl ester is shown in Figure 7A and compared to the fragmentation pattern of isolated peak B in Figure 7B. It is apparent that peak B is identical to the presumed product of the carboxylation, t-BOC-Glu-α-benzyl ester. The existence of a large number of peaks in Figure 7B which are two mass units larger than other major peaks is due to the high specific radioactivity of the $H^{14}CO_3^-$ which was used in the incubations. From the known specific activity of the $H^{14}CO_3^-$ added to the incubations, and the relative height of the ^{12}C and ^{14}C mass fragmentation peaks, it is possible to calculate that the added ^{14}C has been diluted to about 30% of its original specific activity by exchange with

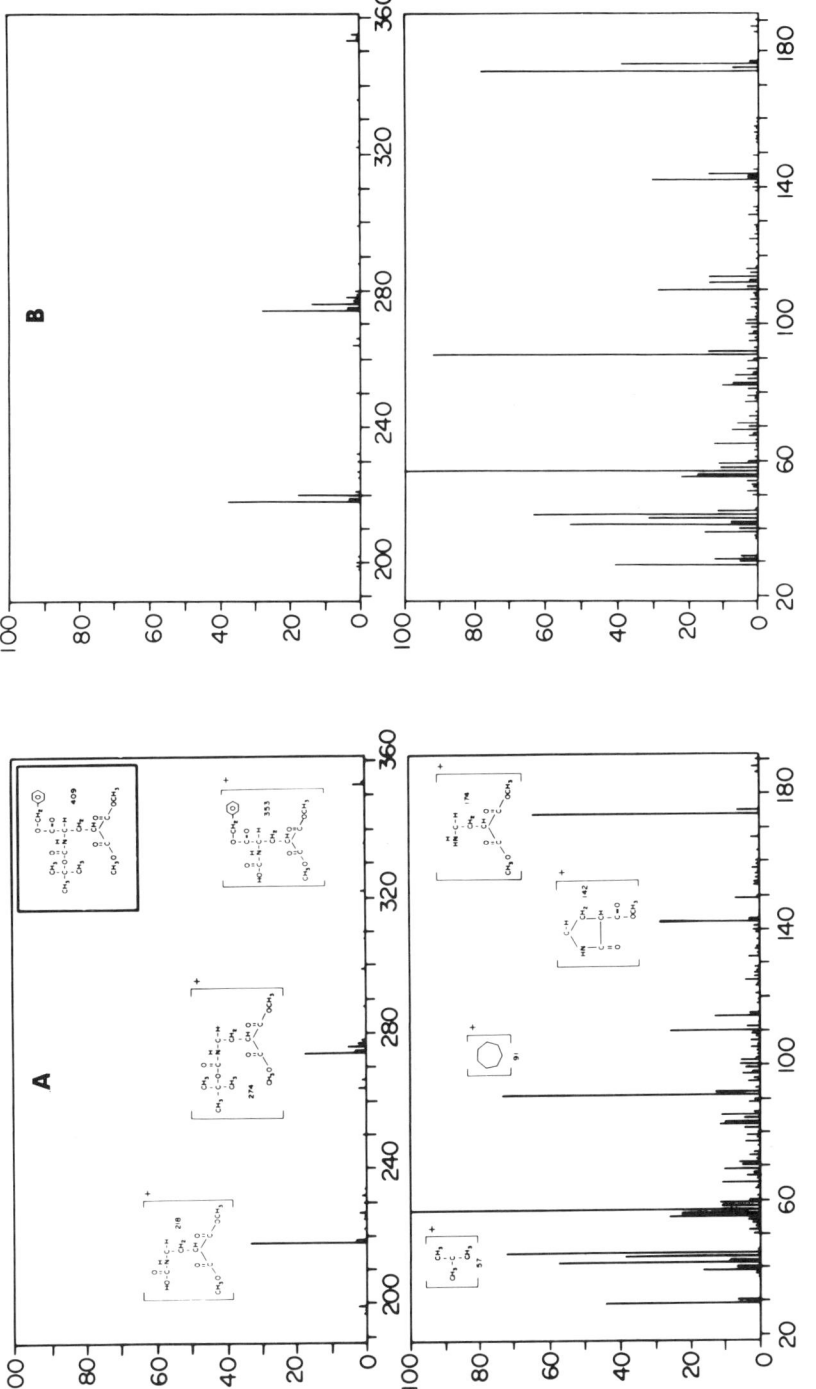

FIGURE 7. Mass spectra of synthetic and isolated peak B. (A) Synthetic t-BOC-Gla-α-benzyl ester after diazomethane treatment was analyzed by direct-probe inlet at 70 eV ionization energy. The molecular ion at m/e 409 is absent due to the lability of the t-butyl linkage. (B) Methylated peak B, after purification as described, was analyzed as above.

$H^{12}CO_3^-$ during the course of the incubation. When methylated peak A was subjected to mass fragmentation analysis, the same peaks which were characteristic of peak B and authentic t-BOC-Gla-α-benzyl ester were observed. In addition, there were distinct peaks which contained ^{12}C, ^{14}C doublets that must have been derived from the t-BOC-Glu-α-benzyl ester substrate following its carboxylation to peak B. These peaks have not been definitely identified at this time, but they do support the general conclusion that the initial carboxylated product is further modified by a microsomal dependent addition of some group to the Gla residue.

DISCUSSION

These data have demonstrated that the predominant actions of the vitamin K-dependent carboxylase on the substrate Phe-Leu-Glu-Glu-Leu is carboxylated at the first of the two Glu residues. The amount of radioactivity found in the third residue of the product (the second Glu of the peptide) was only about 30% of that observed in the first Glu; and, when the incompleteness of yield in each step is considered, it is apparent that very little of the activity is at the second Glu position. A very small amount of the di-Gla product was formed, but it is definitely a minor product. These data also provide evidence that the same microsomal preparation which is able to carry out the vitamin K-dependent carboxylation of peptide-bound glutamyl residues is also able to promote a second posttranslational modification of these substrates. The available evidence strongly suggests that the modifications involve the newly formed Gla residue. The presence of two forms of the carboxylated Phe-Leu-Glu-Glu-Leu could conceivably be due to metabolism of any of the amino acid residues of the peptide, or to cleavage of one or more of the residues from the parent substrate. This seems unlikely, as both of the products peak I and peak II appear to be larger than the substrate, and the PTH-Gla formed from the degradation of peak I does not have the chromatographic properties consistent with this derivative. The observation of two products formed from the incubation of t-BOC-Glu-α-benzyl ester appears to offer final proof that the modification is at the Gla residue. The chemical nature of this derivative is not yet known, nor is it clear if it is of physiological significance. Munns and his coworkers (13) have shown that the form of prothrombin precursor which is the substrate for the vitamin K-dependent carboxylase is a rather acidic species, and that following carboxylation this is converted to a more basic species. The observation that a pentapeptide carboxylated in an _in vitro_ system is subsequently converted to a derivatized species would be consistent with this observation and supports the possibility that the modification observed in this system is related to the physiological process of prothrombin production.

ACKNOWLEDGEMENTS

These studies were supported by the College of Agricultural and Life Sciences, University of Wisconsin-Madison, and in part by grants AM-14881, DE-07031, and HL-05649 from the National Institutes of Health.

REFERENCES

1. Suttie, J. W., and Jackson, C. M. (1977) Physiol. Rev. 57, 1-70.

2. Olson, R. E., and Suttie, J. W. (1978) Vitamins and Hormones 35, 59-108.

3. Stenflo, J. (1978) Adv. in Enzymol. 46, 1-31.

4. Suttie, J. W. (1978) Handbook of Lipid Research 2, "The Fat-soluble Vitamins" (DeLuca, H. F., ed.) pp. 211-277, Plenum Press, New York.

5. Suttie, J. W., Hageman, J. H., Lehrman, S. R., and Rich, D. H. (1976) J. Biol. Chem. 251, 5827-5830.

6. Suttie, J. W., Lehrman, S. R., Geweke, L. O., Hageman, J. M., and Rich, D. H. (1979) Biochem. Biophys. Res. Commun. 86, 500-507.

7. Rich, D. H., Lehrman, S. R., Goodman, H. L., and Suttie, J. W. (1979) In "Synthesis and Function of Vitamin K-dependent Proteins" (Suttie, J. W., ed.) University Park Press, Baltimore.

8. Finnan, J. L., and Suttie, J. W. (1979) Fed. Proc. 38, 876 (abst.).

9. Esmon, C. T., Sadowski, J. A., and Suttie, J. W. (1975) J. Biol. Chem. 250, 4744-4748.

10. Esmon, C. T., and Suttie, J. W. (1976) J. Biol. Chem. 251, 6238-6243.

11. Finnan, J. L., Goodman, H. L., and Suttie, J. W. (1979) In "Synthesis and Function of Vitamin K-dependent Proteins" (Suttie, J. W., ed.) University Park Press, Baltimore.

12. Fraenkel, G., Belford, R. L., and Yankeich, P. E. (1954) J. Am. Chem. Soc. 76, 15-18.

13. Graves, C. B., Grabau, G. G., and Munns, T. W. (1979) In "Synthesis and Function of Vitamin K-dependent Proteins" (Suttie, J. W., ed.) University Park Press, Baltimore.

VITAMIN K-DEPENDENT CARBOXYLATION OF PEPTIDES CONTAINING THE GLU-GLU SEQUENCE: LOCALIZATION OF γ-CARBOXYGLUTAMIC ACID

H. RIKONG-ADIE, P. DECOTTIGNIES-LE MARÉCHAL,
R. AZERAD and A. MARQUET

Institut de Biochimie, Université de Paris-Sud,
Orsay, France and Université Pierre et Marie Curie,
Paris, France

INTRODUCTION

The involvement of vitamin K in the formation of the clotting factors is now well established : vitamin K functions as a cofactor in the postribosomal carboxylation of selected glutamic acid residues in the N-terminal end of liver precursors to form the γ-carboxyglutamic acid residues of prothrombin and the other vitamin K dependent plasma clotting factors, Factors VII, IX and X (1,2). This function was confirmed by the demonstration that a solubilized microsomal preparation from rat liver was able to carboxylate the prothrombin precursor or synthetic peptides containing an adjacent pair of glutamyl residues (3, 4, 5). As synthetic models have shown that two γ-carboxyglutamic acids are necessary to confer Ca^{2+} binding ability (6, 7), an essential property for the Ca^{2+} mediated interaction of prothrombin with phospholipid surfaces, it would be of interest to know which γ-carboxyl groups, perhaps not necessarily adjacent, are functionnally paired in multi-carboxylated proteins. However, until now, no detailed data have been reported about the relative rate of carboxylation of different glutamyl residues in the same substrate molecule. Similarly, when undercarboxylated forms of prothrombin have been isolated, in animals treated with Vitamin K antagonists, it was not possible to determine which particular residues were carboxylated (8).

As an approach to this problem, we have investigated the nature of the carboxylation products of synthetic peptides, formed by the solubilized microsomal preparation from rat liver, in the presence of vitamin K and NADH. On the other hand, the identification of the carboxylated residue(s) was necessary as a preliminary part of a programme devised to determine, via isotope labeling of glutamic acid residue(s), the stereochemistry of the carboxylation process.

MATERIALS AND METHODS

Male Wistar rats (150-200 g) were fed a K-deficient diet (9) with drinking water containing 0.2 % neomycine sulfate, 0.1 % streptomycine sulfate, 0.1 % bacitracine and 0.1 % cephaloridine for 10-15 days, at which time their prothrombin level, measured by a one-stage method, was below 5 %. Liver microsomes were prepared as described by Suttie et al. (10) then suspended in about 0.5 ml/g liver of 0.25 M sucrose, 0.025 M imidazole, 0.08 M KCl buffer pH 7.6 containing 1.5 % Triton X-100, 1 mM NAD^+ and 1 mM DTT. Phylloquinone was used as a solution in 5 % Triton X-100. Peptides were prepared by usual stepwise procedures using benzyl and BOC protected aminoacids and aminoacid activated esters.

Incubations were carried out at 20°C or 28°C in agitated microtubes containing, in a final volume of 280 μl, 100 μl of the microsomal preparation, 6 μCi NaH^{14}CO$_3$ (CEN, Saclay ; 53 μCi/μmole), 1.75 mM NADH, 250 μM phylloquinone and peptide, and completed by addition of trichloroacetic acid. After centrifugation, aliquots of the supernatant were transferred to counting vials, dried in vacuo and counted in 1 ml of water and 10 ml of Instagel (Packard) in a liquid scintillation spectrometer.

Microsomal proteins were measured by the biuret method (11). Isolation and preliminary purification of carboxylated products was carried out by chromatography on Sephadex G-25 and Biogel P-2 (4). Decarboxylation of peptides was obtained by heating in a water solution at 150°C in sealed tubes for 0.5 - 1 hour. Alkaline hydrolysis of peptides and identification of γ-carboxyglutamic acid was performed as described by Tabor and Tabor (12).

Epoxidase activity was determined according to Friedman and Smith (13).

RESULTS AND DISCUSSION

Properties of The Solubilized Carboxylation System

As shown in Table 1, the carboxylation reaction, measured by ^{14}C incorporation in the trichloroacetic supernatant, in the presence of various

TABLE 1. Carboxylation of various peptide substrates[a]

	Vitamin K[b]	PLP[c]	Incorporation cpm/mg protein
No substrate	+	+	200
Phe-Leu-Glu-Glu-Val	-	+	200
Phe-Leu-Glu-Glu-Val	+	+	36,280
Phe-Leu-Glu-Glu-Ile	+	+	36,640
Leu-Glu-Glu-Val	+	+	7,500
Phe-Leu-Glu-Glu-Val	+	-	9,040
" "	+	+	21,180
NaBH$_4$-reduced Schiff base[d] of PLP-Phe-Leu-Glu-Glu-Val	+	-	11,470
" "	+	+	6,110
Phe-Leu-Glu-Glu-Val	+	-	13,460
" "	+	+	23,920
BOC-Phe-Leu-Glu-Glu-Val	+	-	1,760
" "	+	+	2,910

The solubilized microsomal preparation from vitamin K deficient rat liver was incubated at 20°C for 30 min as described in Material and Methods.
[a] Peptide concentration : 0.9 mM ; [b] 0.25 mM ; [c] 1 mM ; [d] prepared from an equimolecular solution of PLP and peptide treated at pH 7.5 during 30 min by excess NaBH$_4$ then purified by gel permeation and ion exchange chromatography.

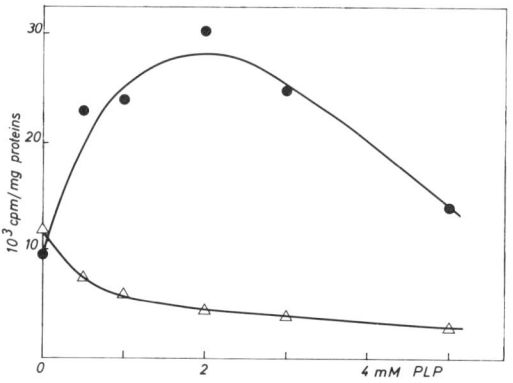

Figure 1. Effect of pyridoxal phosphate concentration on carboxylase activity, with 0.9mM Phe-Leu-Glu-Glu-Val as substrate (●——●), or a 0.9mM solution of $NaBH_4$-reduced Schiff base of PLP-Phe-Leu-Glu-Glu-Val (△——△).

peptide substrates, was strictly vitamin K dependent, even when microsomes from normal (not deficient) rats were used. The Triton X-100 solubilized microsome preparation can use Phe-Leu-Glu-Glu-Val or Phe-Leu-Glu-Glu-Ile at nearly comparable rates, as precedently described (5). The tetrapeptide Leu-Glu-Glu-Val was also used, but at a lower rate. Pyridoxal phosphate (PLP) as recently demonstrated by Suttie et al. (5) increases significantly the extent of incorporation with all peptides used. As PLP concentration necessary for maximal activity was fairly high, a coenzyme function in the carboxylation reaction was difficult to understand. In fact, when a Schiff base of PLP and Val-pentapeptide was reduced with sodium borohydride and the purified aminoderivative tested as substrate, it was found as active as the Val-pentapeptide (in the absence of PLP) ; incorporation was not increased by PLP addition, but rather inhibited in a similar way to that exhibited by the carboxylation of Val-pentapeptide in the presence of excess PLP (Fig. 1). Thus the effect of PLP can probably be ascribed to the formation of a Schiff base with the peptide substrate, making it more available for enzyme binding, as confirmed by a double-reciprocal plot of carboxylase activity versus peptide concentration with and without PLP (Fig. 2). BOC-pentapeptide, an intermediate in the chemical synthesis of the peptide substrate, is not used by the microsome preparation with or without

Figure 2. Double reciprocal plot of carboxylase activity (^{14}C cpm incorporated/ 0.1 ml in 30 min at 20°C) and Val-pentapeptide concentration, with (▲——▲) and without (■——■) 1 mM PLP.

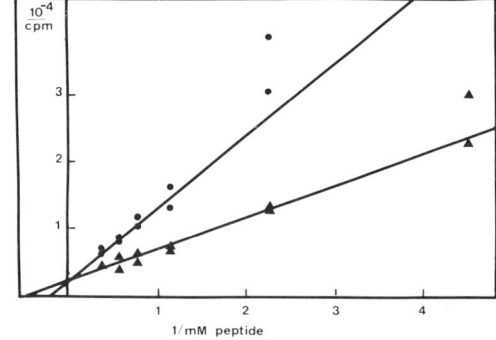

addition of PLP (Table 1) : the small amount of carboxylase activity measured can be ascribed to some elimination of the BOC-group in the incubation conditions.

The apparent Km for phylloquinone was about 20 μM (Fig. 3) and the optimum pH of the carboxylation reaction was in the neighborhood of 7.6 - 7.8 (Fig. 4).

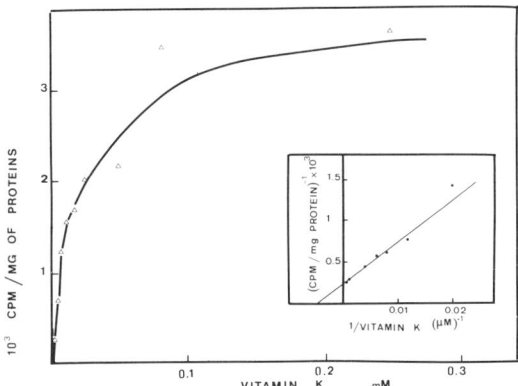

Figure 3. Effect of phylloquinone concentration on the carboxylation of Val-pentapeptide at 28°C.

A four to five-fold increase in the carboxylase activity (and vitamin K epoxidase activity) was noticed when deficient rat microsomes (less than 5 % prothrombin) were compared to normal rat microsomes or to microsomes from deficient rats treated with about 5 μg K/day during one week (Fig. 5). It is remarkable that while normal prothrombin time was restored with 2 μg K/day, carboxylase activity remained still high. This indicates that available preprothrombin is probably the rate limiting factor in the natural vitamin K-dependent carboxylation reaction (14,15).

Isolation of The Carboxylation Products of The Val-Pentapeptide

The trichloroacetic acid supernatant obtained from large scale incubations at 28°C with $NaH^{14}CO_3$ and the Val-pentapeptide as substrate was

Figure 4. Effect of pH on the carboxylation of Val-pentapeptide at 28 °C.

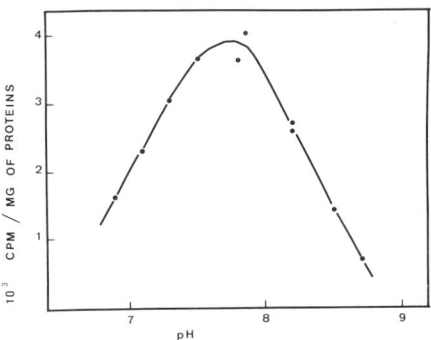

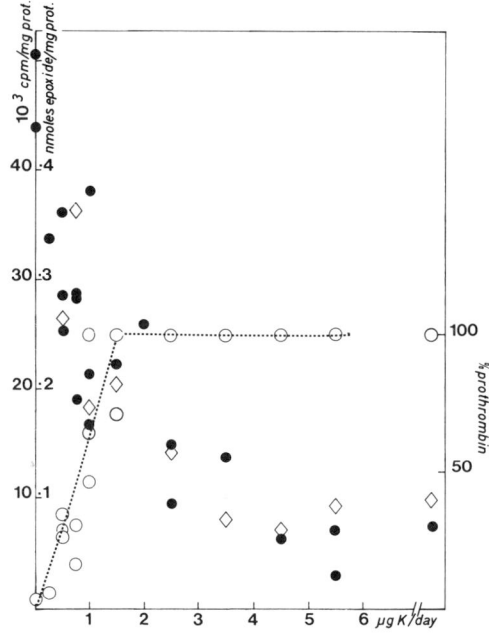

Figure 5. Carboxylase (●) and epoxidase (◊) activities of solubilized liver microsomes prepared from vitamin K deficient rats (see Material and Methods) given orally different doses of phylloquinone during one more week. Prothrombin (o······o) was determined by a one stage method.

fractionated by exclusion chromatography on Sephadex G-25 and BioGel P-2 (4), then chromatographed on a column of DEAE-Sephadex A-25 (acetate form). Two radioactive peaks I and II were consistently obtained by elution with an acetic acid gradient (Fig. 6) ; the slower one (peak II) increased more rapidly with longer incubation times. After acidic hydrolysis of the two peaks with 6 N HCl (110°C, 22 h) 50 % of the initial radioactivity was retained in glutamic acid. ^{14}C γ-Carboxyglutamic acid was also directly identified after alcaline hydrolysis (12) of the two products. When the purified peaks were heated in a water solution (150°C, sealed tube), peak I was quantitatively decarboxylated within 30 min, retaining half of the initial radioactivity, and the decarboxylated product migrated on electrophoresis at pH 2.0 exactly like the substrate pentapeptide. Peak II was decarboxylated more slowly (about 1 h) and the ^{14}C-decarboxylated product migrated faster than the Val-pentapeptide.

Localization of The Carboxylated Residue in Peak I

^{14}C-Peak I, diluted with the Val-pentapeptide (0.2 mg) was decarboxylated, then submitted to extended hydrolysis by Staphylococcus aureus V8 protease , an enzyme which specifically splits Glu-X bonds (16). The resulting hydrolysis products were separated by bidimensional electrophoresis at pH 2.0 and 3.6, then the radioactive products, located by autoradiography, were compared with ninhydrin reactive spots and counted after elution. Fig. 7 shows that the radioactivity migrating with glutamic acid and the dipeptide Glu-Val was negligible, compared to that associated with the tripeptide Phe-Leu-Glu (less than 5 %). As hydrolysis was limited, a large part of the radioactivity remained associated with the Val-pentapeptide.

A limited acidic treatment (1 N HCl, 90°C, 2 h) of peak I caused a limited decarboxylation and hydrolysis of the carboxylated peptide.

Figure 6. DEAE-Sephadex chromatography of ^{14}C-carboxylated products obtained by incubation of Phe-Leu-Glu-Glu-Val with solubilized microsomes at 28°C during 30 min (A), 2h (B) or 5 h (C). The chromatography was carried out on carboxylated products previously filtered on Sephadex G-25 and Bio Gel P-2 (4). Elution with a linear gradient from 0 to 1.5 N acetic acid in water.

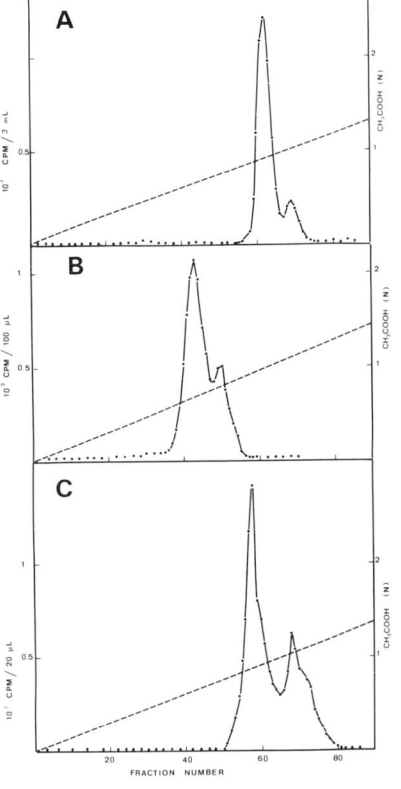

Bidimensional electrophoresis (Fig. 8) showed again a negligible amount of radioactivity (less than 10 %) in Glu-Val, compared to the tripeptide Phe-Leu-Glu. A group of radioactive products, which did not migrate at pH 3.6, probably represents the corresponding carboxylated species.

These results undoubtedly indicate that the vitamine K-dependent carboxylase, obtained by Triton X-100 solubilization of rat liver microsomes, is able to incorporate $^{14}CO_2$ into only one of the two glutamic residues of the Val-pentapeptide, with a high selectivity, leading to the main product Phe-Leu-Gla-Glu-Val.

The Formation And Nature of Peak II

Peak II, which was formed in low amounts during incubations with the Val-pentapeptide, could be obtained quantitatively and rapidly from purified ^{14}C peak I, at pH 7.5 and 28°C, by incubation with Triton X-100 solubilized microsomes, in the absence of added vitamin K and NADH. This conversion was inhibited by the Val-pentapeptide as shown on Fig.9. This inhibition probably explains the limited formation of peak II during incubation with the carboxylase system.

When decarboxylated peak II was treated by <u>S. aureus</u> V8 protease, no significant hydrolysis was detected, indicating, like the slow decarboxylation rate of peak II, that some modification of the γ-carboxyglutamic acid residue has occurred.

When peak II was treated with dansylchloride, its electrophoretic mobility at pH 2.0 was decreased, as expected for a peptide bearing a free amino terminal group, but still remained higher than the mobility of the corresponding derivative of peak I.

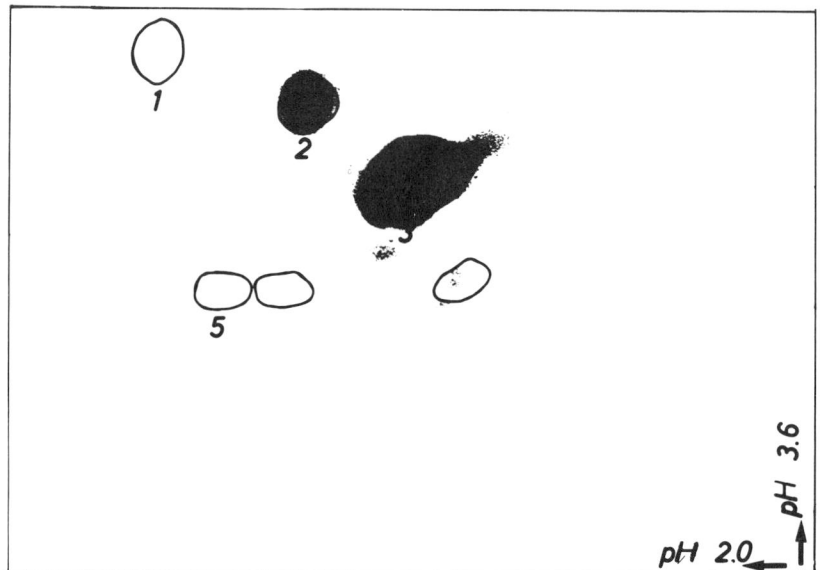

Figure 7. Radioautogram of the bidimensional electrophoresis of the hydrolysis products of decarboxylated ^{14}C peak I (+ Val-pentapeptide) incubated 24 h with S. aureus V8 protease. Circled areas correspond to ninhydrin positive spots (see Fig. 8).

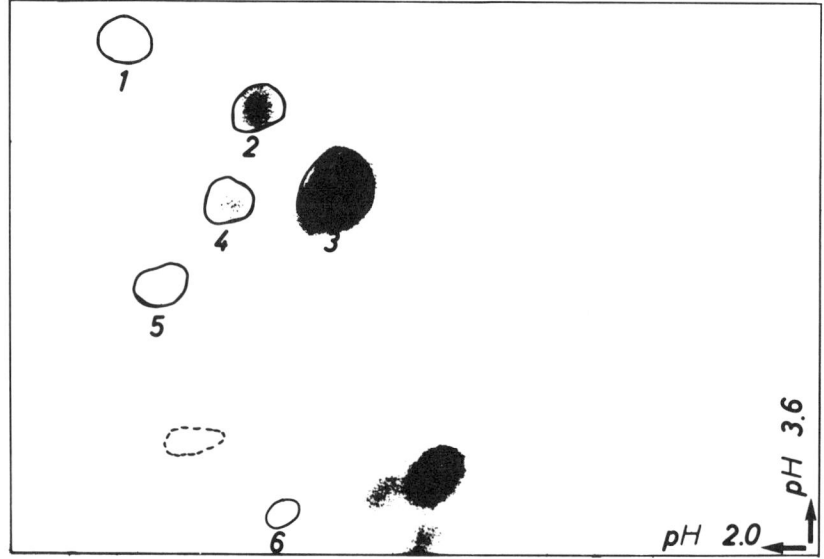

Figure 8. Radioautogram of the bidimensional electrophoresis of ^{14}C peak I (+ Val-pentapeptide) after limited acidic treatment. Circled areas correspond to ninhydrin positive spots : 1 : Glu-Val ; 2 : Phe-Leu-Glu ; 3 : Val-pentapeptide ; 4 : assumed to be Phe-Leu-Glu-Glu ; 5 : Val ; 6 : Glu.

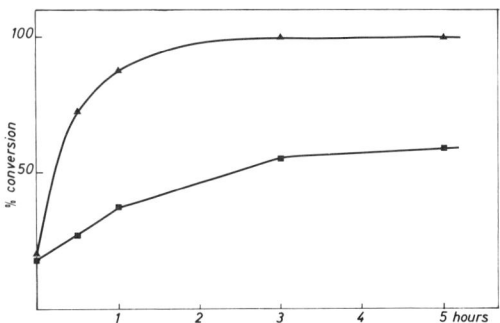

Figure 9. Kinetics of the conversion of peak I into peak II : 90,000 cpm of ^{14}C-carboxylated product (before DEAE Sephadex chromatography) (■——■) were incubated at 28°C in a final volume of 130 μl, pH 7.5, with solubilized microsomes (1.3 mg proteins). Aliquots were treated with 10 % trichloroacetic acid, deposited on a Whatman N° 3 paper and submitted to electrophoresis at pH 4.0 to separate peak I and peak II. The conversion ratios were determined by radioactivity scanning. Same experiment (▲——▲) with a mixture of peaks I and II (80,000 cpm) obtained after DEAE Sephadex chromatography, i.e. free of remaining pentapeptide substrate.

In order to detect any correlation between peak II formation and carboxylating activity, the conversion rate of purified peak I was measured in incubations with solubilized microsomes from normal rats or vitamin K deficient rats (Table 2). No significant difference was recorded, indicating that peak II formation from peak I, a vitamin K independent reaction, is again not dependent on the deficiency status of the animal.

TABLE 2. Conversion of peak I into peak II by incubation with solubilized microsomes from normal or vitamin K deficient rats.

Incubation time[a]	% pic II formed	
	Normal rats	K-Deficient rats[b]
0	0	0
10 min	22	28
30 min	49	54
60 min	66	74

[a] 120,000 cpm of purified peak I in 80 μl of 0.05 M imidazole buffer pH 7.5 were incubated with 30 μl of the solubilized microsome preparation. 25 μl aliquots were treated with 10 % trichloroacetic acid (50 μl) then deposited on a Whatman N°3 paper and submitted to electrophoresis at pH 4.0. The amounts of peak II formed were calculated from radioactivity scanning of the electrophoregram.

[b] Less than 3 % prothrombin compared to normal rats.

AKNOWLEDGEMENTS

This work was supported in part by Grants from the Institut National de la Santé et de la Recherche Médicale, by a Contract 77.7.1132 from the Délégation Générale à la Recherche Scientifique et Technique and by a subvention from the Commissariat à l'Energie Atomique, for radioactive products.

REFERENCES

1. Olson, R.E. and Suttie, J.W. (1977) Vitamins and Hormones 35, 59-108.
2. Stenflo, J. (1978) Adv. Enzymol. 46, 1-31.
3. Esmon, C.T. and Suttie, J.W. (1976) J. Biol. Chem. 251, 6238-6243.
4. Suttie, J.W., Hageman, J.M., Lehrman, S.R. and Rich, D.J. (1976) J. Biol. Chem. 251, 5827-5830.
5. Suttie, J.W., Lehrman, S.R., Geweke, L.O., Hageman, J.M. and Rich, D.J. (1979) Biochem. Biophys. Res. Comm. 86, 500-507.
6. Marki, W., Oppliger, M. and Schwyzer, R. (1977) Helv. Chim. Acta 60, 807-815.
7. Sperling, R., Furie, B.C., Blumenstein, M., Keyt, B. and Furie, B. (1978) J. Biol. Chem. 253, 3898-3906.
8. Esnouf, M.P. and Prowse, C.V. (1977) Biochim. Biophys. Acta 490, 471-476.
9. Mameesh, M.S. and Johnson, B.C. (1959) Proc. Soc. Exp. Biol. Med. 101, 467-469.
10. Sadowski, J.A., Esmon, C.T. and Suttie, J.W. (1976) J. Biol. Chem. 251, 2770-2776.
11. Gornall, A.G., Bardawill. C.J. and David, M.M. (1949) J. Biol. Chem. 177, 751-756.
12. Tabor, H. and White Tabor, C. (1977) Anal. Biochem. 78, 554-556.
13. Friedman, P.A. and Smith, M.W. (1977) Biochem. Pharmacol. 26, 804-805.
14. Shah, D.V. and Suttie, J.W. (1978) Arch. Biochem. Biophys. 191, 571-577.
15. Siegfried, C.M., Knauer, G.R. and Matschiner, J.T. (1979) Arch. Biochem. Biophys. 194, 486-495.
16. Drapeau, J.R., Boily, Y. and Houmard, J. (1972) J. Biol. Chem. 247, 6720-6726.

PROTHROMBIN BIOSYNTHESIS

BIOSYNTHESIS AND PROCESSING OF PRECURSOR PROTHROMBINS

C. BRUCE GRAVES, GARY G. GRABAU, and
THEODORE W. MUNNS

Edward A. Doisy Department of Biochemistry,
St. Louis University School of Medicine,
St. Louis MO 63104

INTRODUCTION

The existence of precursor prothrombins in vitamin K-deficient and anticoagulant-treated animals has been established by a variety of investigations (1-11). Major findings in this regard include the presence and absence of γ-carboxyglutamate residues in the N-terminal portion of mature- and precursor-prothrombin sequences, respectively (1-4), the conversion of precursor prothrombins to thrombin with Echis Carinatus venom (5), and the in vitro vitamin K-dependent carboxylation of precursor prothrombins derived from rat liver microsomal preparations (6-8). In addition, several proteins have been isolated from microsomes of warfarin-treated rats that possess many of the properties assigned to precursor prothrombins (9-11), i.e., molecular weight, amino acid composition, and generation of common polypeptides by specific proteases. Characterization of these latter precursors via isoelectric focusing techniques has revealed the presence of two major proteins possessing pI values of 7.2 and 5.8 (12-14). Whereas the 5.8 isoelectric specie has been tentatively identified as the asialo derivative of mature prothrombin (12,13) the nature of the 7.2 precursor remains to be elucidated. Although these studies have provided sufficient evidence for the existence of precursor prothrombins, no information is available regarding their intracellular processing.

In view of the above, we became interested in examining prothrombin biosynthesis in cultured hepatoma cells and perfused rat livers since these systems offer a variety of technical advantages not present in intact animals (e.g., chemically defined growth media, efficient utilization of radioactive isotopes, reproducible responses to antimetabolites and antibiotics, retention of intact transcriptional and translational systems, etc.). Recently, we have demonstrated that H-35 rat hepatoma cells (Reuber cells) respond to vitamin by rapidly decreasing their intracellular pools of precursor prothrombin and secreting to the culture medium mature prothrombin (15).

Our more recent efforts have been concentrated upon the development of an immunochemical approach for the rapid and quantitative isolation of precursor- and mature-prothrombins. The utility of this approach is provided by the findings presented herein. These findings indicate that the secretion of mature rat prothrombin (pI 5.0) by hepatoma cells or perfused livers is preceded by the appearance of five discrete intracellular precursors of prothrombin possessing pI values of 7.2, 6.7, 6.2, 5.8 and 5.5. As evaluated by pulse-labeling experiments and subcellular fractionation data, the order of processing of these precursors is: 6.7(RER)* → 7.2(SER) → 6.2(SER) → 5.8(GOLGI) → 5.5(GOLGI). Based upon these and other data (16-19), it now appears that the vitamin K-dependent processing step is at the junction between the rough and smooth endoplasmic reticulum, i.e., 6.7(RER) $\overset{K}{\leftrightarrow}$ 7.2(SER).

MATERIALS AND METHODS

Materials: Radioactive supplies including [4,5-^{3}H]leucine (50-60 Ci/mmol), [^{125}I]Iodine, NCS (tissue solubilizer), and spectrofluor were purchased from Amersham Searle. Ampholyte carrier buffers were obtained from LKB and CNBr-activated Sepharose 4B, Sephadex G-25, DEAE-Sephadex, and Cellex-D from Pharmacia. Phylloquinone (vitamin K) as the solubilized preparation "AquaMephyton" and insulin "Iletin" were obtained from Merck, Sharp and Dohme and Eli Lilly, respectively. Phenylmethylsulfonyl fluoride (PMSF), soybean trypsin inhibitor (STI), Echis carinatus snake venom, fatty acid-free bovine serum albumin (BSA), and Triton X-100 were purchased from Sigma Chemical Co., and Nonidet P-40 (NP-40) from Shell Oil Co. All chemicals were of analytical reagent grade.

Culture systems: H-35 rat hepatoma cells (20,21) were grown in monolayer cultures at 37°C in T-75 flasks (growth area, 75 cm^2) in an atmosphere of 95% air and 5% CO_2 in the presence of 15 ml Swim's S-77 media (Gibco) supplemented with 20% horse- and 5% fetal calf-serum. Confluent H-35 cells yielded 2 x 10^7 cells per T-flask with a total cell protein, RNA, and DNA content of 4.2 $\pm$ 0.3, 0.45 $\pm$ 0.04 and 0.17 $\pm$ 0.02 mg/10^7 cells, respectively (15). As evaluated by the Echis carinatus coagulation assay (22), the intracellular prothrombin (precursor) content was 0.5 to 0.6 µg/10^7 cells and represented approximately .012% of the total cell protein.

Confluent cells were maintained for 24 hr with serum-free medium containing 1 µg/ml of insulin. Radioactive pulses were initiated by refeeding cells with leucine-free Swim's S-77 medium containing 1 µg/ml of insulin and 0.2 to 2 mCi of [^{3}H]leucine (some cultures also received 0.1 µg/ml vitamin K). Cells were subsequently harvested and washed by low speed centrifugation in the presence of phosphate-buffered saline (PBS; 150 mM NaCl, 10 mM phosphate, pH 7.4) containing soybean trypsin inhibitor (40 µg/ml) and 1.0 mM PMSF. Medium samples were collected (1.0 ml) and adjusted to contain 40 µg/ml of STI and 1.0 mM PMSF.

Details regarding the rat liver perfusion system have been described in detail by Bartosek et al., (23). Briefly, liver from Sprague-Dawley, adult male rats, (250 to 350 g) were perfused with 125 ml of leucine-free Swim's S-77 medium supplemented with fatty acid-free BSA (30 mg/ml) and 2 to 5 mCi of [^{3}H]leucine for 1 to 2 hr. Viability parameters included the (a) general appearance of the organ, (b) flow rate of the perfusion medium through the liver, (c) rate of accumulation of bile from the canulated bile duct, (d) the uptake of [^{3}H]leucine and (e) rate of secretion of [^{3}H]leucine-labeled protein into the perfusion medium. The latter parameter was linear after a 15 to 20 min lag period indicating that both translational and secretory processes were functional over a 2 hr period.

---

*RER and SER are rough- and smooth-endoplasmic reticulum.

Immunochemistry: The immunochemical approach employed to isolate [^{3}H]leucine-labeled prothrombins will be described in detail elsewhere (24). A brief description of these procedures (resulting in the construction of an anti-prothrombin/ Sepharose adsorbent) are presented in the text as well as diagrammed schematically in Figure 2.

Immunochemical Isolation of [^{3}H]Leucine-Labeled Precursor Prothrombins: Intracellular precursor prothrombins were initially obtained by homogenizing cell pellets or perfused rat livers (0.2 to 1.0 g) in the presence of 5 volumes of 10 mM TRIS, pH 9.5 together with protease inhibitors. Homogenates were adjusted to contain 2% Triton X-100 and incubated with stirring for 30 min at 4°C prior to centrifugation (100,000 xg for 60 min). Supernatant fractions (1.0 to 2.0 ml) were incubated directly with anti-rat prothrombin/Sepharose (wet wt. vol. 0.075 ml) for 30 min at 25°C prior to washing the immunoadsorbent successively with 3.0 ml of PBS, bicarbonate buffer (0.1 M NaHCO$_3$, 0.5 M NaCl, pH 7.5), and phosphate buffer (10 mM PO$_4$, pH 7.4) by repeated low speed centrifugation and resuspension. [^{3}H]leucine-labeled precursor prothrombins (antigens) were eluted from the immunoadsorbent with 0.25 to 0.5 ml of urea-SDS (7 M urea, 2% SDS, 10 mM PO$_4$, pH 7.2). Identical adsorption techniques were performed with aliquots derived from culture medium, purified subcellular fractions, and ^{125}I-prothrombin standards. Eluted antigens were characterized by various gel electrophoretic techniques (see below).

Electrophoretic Techniques: SDS-polyacrylamide gel electrophoretic techniques were conducted according to the procedures of Weber and Osborn (25). Aliquots containing eluted antigens (i.e., in 7 M urea, 2% SDS) were adjusted to 5% β-mercaptoethanol (v/v), heated for 3 min at 100° and applied directly to precast gels (7.5% acrylamide, 0.5 x 10.0 cm). Isoelectric focusing (IEF) acrylamide gels were prepared as outlined by Piperno et al., (26). Appropriate quantities of urea, Nonidet and acrylamide/bisacrylamide were dissolved in H$_2$O (gentle heating) such that their final concentrations were 9.0 M, 2% (w/v) and 4%, respectively. To 20 ml of this solution varying amounts of stock ampholytes were added to construct the desired pH gradients after which riboflavin and TEMED were added. Both SDS- and IEF-gels were sliced into 1.0 or 2.0 mm sections for determination of radioactivity profiles.

Ancillary Methods: The radioimmunoassay for prothrombin was performed as described previously (26) and employed purified rat plasma prothrombin as the competing standard antigen. This same standard was employed for the Echis carinatus coagulation assay (22). Clotting times for this assay in the range of 20 to 100 seconds were considered quantitative.

Subcellular fractionation of perfused rat livers to yield purified rough- and smooth-endoplasmic reticulum (RER, SER) and golgi were performed according to the methods outlined by Fleischer and Kervina (27). These methods consisted of a series of gradient centrifugation steps (flotation, discontinuous and continuous gradients). The criterion for purification was based primarily upon the RNA/protein ratio, i.e., 0.25 and 0.05 for RER and SER, respectively, as well as visualization of various preparations via electron microscopic techniques.

RESULTS

The ability of confluent monolayers of H-35 rat hepatoma cells to respond to vitamin K has been previously documented by Munns et al., (15). Briefly, when H-35 cells were incubated in the presence of vitamin K, the intracellular levels of precursor prothrombins were significantly decreased (50 to 70% of control values) with a concomitant appearance of mature prothrombin in the medium. This type of response is illustrated in Figure 1. Quantitation and identification of precursor- and mature-prothrombins in the above investigation were based upon radioimmunoassays, differential clotting assays and selective barium adsorption. Although these initial studies revealed that H-35 cells respond to vitamin K in a manner analogous to that of K-deficient rats, these types of data did not permit an accurate assessment of rates of synthesis, secretion, and degradation of precursor- and mature-prothrombins. Furthermore, they did not reveal the complexities of precursor prothrombin processing or the actual types of precursors present. To this end, studies were initiated to investigate the potential of an immunochemical approach for the isolation of prothrombin precursors obtained from H-35 cells previously pulse-labeled with [^{3}H]leucine.

This immunochemical approach is illustrated in Figure 2 and consisted of purifying anti-rat prothrombin antibodies by affinity chromatography employing prothrombin (antigen)-coupled Sepharose. Once purified, anti-rat prothrombin antibodies were in turn coupled to Sepharose and this immunoadsorbent tested for its ability to quantitatively and exclusively retain precursor-

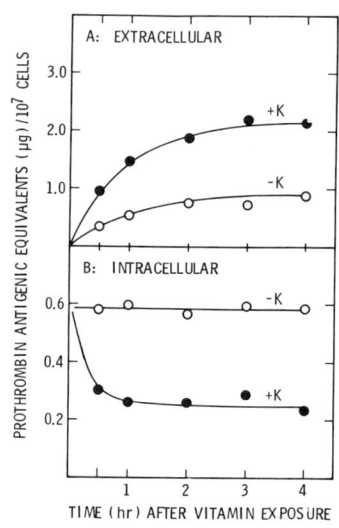

FIGURE 1: The effects of vitamin K on the redistribution of prothrombin antigenic equivalents present in cultured H-35 rat hepatoma cells (15).

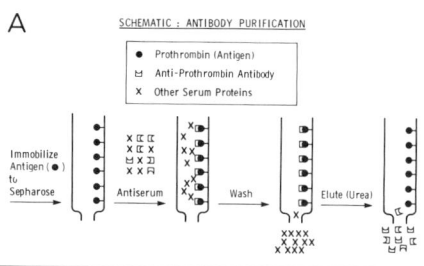

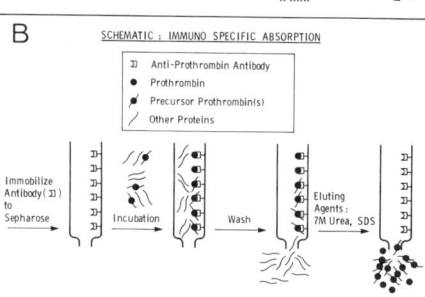

FIGURE 2: Antibody purification and immunoadsorption techniques.

TABLE I. Immunospecific Adsorption of <u>Echis Carinatus</u> - Activatable Protein Protein.[a]

Adsorbent	Echis Carinatus Activatable Protein ($\mu g/10^7$ cells) in 105,000 xg Supernatant		
	Before BaSO$_4$ and Immunospecific Adsorption	After BaSO$_4$ Adsorption	After Immunospecific Adsorption
Anti-prothrombin/Sepharose			
Exp 1	0.53	.48	ND
Exp 2	0.49	.51	ND
Non-immune IgG/Sepharose			
Exp 1	.55	.52	.55
Exp 2	.53	.50	.51

[a] <u>Echis Carinatus</u> assays and barium adsorption studies were performed as previously reported (22). ND, represents no detectable activity.

and mature-prothrombins. These criteria were met by the findings that both ^{125}I-prothrombin (not shown) and precursor prothrombins obtained from cells maintained in the absence of vitamin were quantitatively adsorbed to anti-rat prothrombin/Sepharose. As presented in Table 1, the ability of anti-rat prothrombin/Sepharose to retain prothrombin precursors was provided by the finding that immunospecific adsorption of intracellular fractions possessing precursor prothrombins resulted in complete loss of <u>Echis</u>-activatable material. The inability of pre-immune rabbit IgG/Sepharose adsorbents to remove <u>Echis</u>-activatable material also supported the conclusion that the adsorption of precursor prothrombin was immunospecific.

Although the above studies indicated that anti-rat prothrombin/Sepharose quantitatively retained precursor- and mature-prothrombins, it remained to be demonstrated whether these were the only proteins immunospecifically adsorbed. To test exclusive retention, intracellular fractions (105,000 xg supernatants) obtained from cell cultures previously labeled for 2 hr with [^{3}H]leucine were subjected to the immunospecific adsorption procedures described above. Characterization of the immunospecifically retained, [^{3}H]leucine-labeled protein(s) via electrophoresis in SDS-acrylamide gels revealed a single peak of radioactivity, migrating identically to that of purified prothrombin and possessing an estimated molecular weight of 75,000 daltons (see Figure 3A).

Whereas the above data with SDS-acrylamide gels indicated a molecular weight homogeneity of intracellular precursor prothrombin, previously published data have suggested the presence of multiple precursor forms (8,13,14). In view of these latter observations, aliquots of immunospecifically retained proteins were subjected to isoelectric focusing in acrylamide gels (IEF-gels). Figure 3B illustrates the resulting pH gradients and radioactivity profiles of these [^{3}H]proteins and revealed the presence of 5 distinct [^{3}H]leucine-labeled proteins possessing pI values of 7.2, 6.7, 6.2, 5.8 and 5.5. The identification of these intracellular proteins as precursors of mature prothrombin is based, therefore, upon their (a) immunochemical isolation, (b) inability to be adsorbed by insoluble barium salts, (c) molecular weight in SDS-acrylamide gels, (d) different isoelectric points relative to mature prothrombin and (e) vitamin K-dependency, i.e., the vitamin-dependent reduction of intracellular precursors (see Table II) coupled with the appearance of mature prothrombin in the culture medium (Figure 1).

In view of the above findings which indicated that antiprothrombin/Sepharose adsorbent could rapidly and quantitatively retain precursors of mature prothrombin, additional experiments with H-35 cell cultures were designed to assess the effects of vitamin K on the rates of synthesis, processing and secretion of these precursors. Thus, H-35 cells were labeled with [^{3}H]leucine for various periods of time (5 to 120 min) and the extent of incorporation of isotope into these precursors measured as a function of both pulse time and vitamin status. These results are presented in Table II and Figure 4 and indicate that vitamin K had no effect on the rate of incorporation of [^{3}H]-leucine into prothrombin precursors since equivalent amounts of radioactivity were incorporated into these precursors after a 5- or 10-min pulse period. Also presented

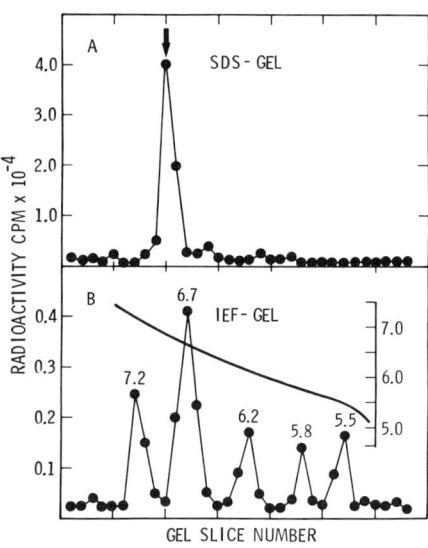

FIGURE 3: Characterization of immunospecifically adsorbed [^{3}H]precursor prothrombin in SDS (A) and IEF(B) acrylamide gels. Arrow in A denotes migration of prothrombin standard.

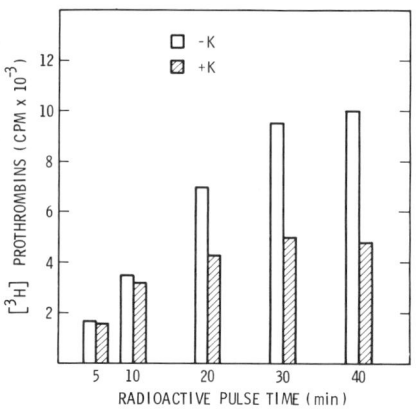

FIGURE 4: The effects of vitamin K on the extent of [^{3}H]leucine incorporation into intracellular prothrombins. CPM/ 6 x 10^6 cells.

TABLE II. Rates of Synthesis and Secretion of [^{3}H]Leucine-Labeled Prothrombins. Effects of Vitamin K.

[^{3}H]Prothrombins: CPM x $10^{-3}/10^7$ Cells (% of "minus" K controls)

Pulse Time (min)	Intracellular		Extracellular	
	-K	+K	-K	+K
5	2.7(100)	2.5(93)	<0.3	<0.3
10	6.3(100)	6.5(103)	<0.3	<0.3
20	14.2(100)	10.2(72)	2.9(100)	5.1(176)
40	21.7(100)	11.4(53)	20.5(100)	43.5(212)
120	26.0(100)	12.2(47)	51.7(100)	125.0(242)

in Table II was the additional finding that significant quantities of [^{3}H]prothrombins appeared in the culture medium only after cells had been labeled with [^{3}H]leucine for 20 to 30 min. Although vitamin K does not appear to be implicated in translation, it does regulate the rate of intracellular processing of these precursors and hence their appearance in the culture medium. This finding is based upon the size of the intracellular and extracellular pools of various [^{3}H]prothrombins when cells were labeled in the presence and absence of vitamin (Table II and Figure 4) and are in excellent agreement with the radioimmunoassay data presented in Figure 1.

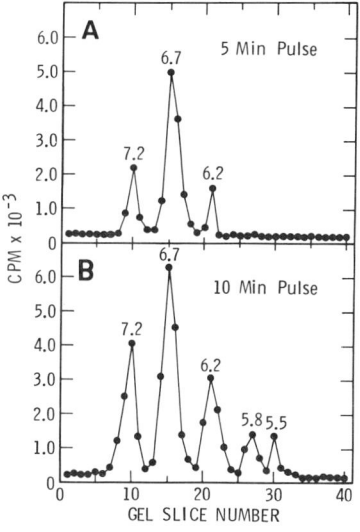

FIGURE 5: Appearance of [^{3}H] leucine into precursor prothrombins present in H-35 cells labeled in the absence of vitamin K.

To establish an apparent order of processing for the 5 individual [^{3}H]prothrombin precursors (Figure 3B), precursors obtained from cells previously pulse-labeled for 5, 10, and 20 min were electrophoresed in IEF gels. The resulting radioactivity profiles of these gels are illustrated in part in Figure 5 and suggest the following order of processing: 6.7 → 7.2 → 6.2 → 5.8 → 5.5. This order is based upon the amount of radioactivity incorporated into each precursor as a function of the pulse-time employed. Thus, as illustrated in Figure 5A, only 3 precursors (7.2, 6.7 and 6.2) were labeled during the initial 5 min pulse period, with the bulk of radioactivity being incorporated into

TABLE III. Distribution of Intracellular [^{3}H]Precursor Prothrombins. Effects of Radioactive Pulse Time and Vitamin K.

	[^{3}H] precursor prothrombins. CPM incorporated/ 10^7 cells (% of "minus" K controls)			
Precursor Prothrombin (pI values)	10 min pulse		120 min pulse	
	-K	+K	-K	+K
7.2	1500 (100)	2300 (153)	6700 (100)	2800 (42)
6.7	3200 (100)	2300 (74)	9700 (100)	3000 (31)
6.2	1000 (100)	1300 (130)	3800 (100)	2500 (66)
5.8	< 300	< 300	2700 (100)	1800 (67)
5.5	< 300	< 300	3000 (100)	1900 (63)
Total	6300 (100)	6500 (103)	25,900 (100)	12,000 (46)

the 6.7 precursors (70% of total). Significant amounts of radioactivity began to appear in the 5.8 and 5.5 species only after the pulse time had been extended to 10 min (Figure 5B).

An analysis of the distribution of radioactivity incorporated into each precursor during a short (10 min) and long (120 min) radioactive pulse of cells maintained in the presence and absence of vitamin provided an insight into the vitamin K-dependent processing step. These data are presented in Table III and indicated that the presence of vitamin significantly altered the percentages of radioactivity incorporated in the 6.7 and 7.2 precursors species. During a 10 min pulse the presence of vitamin increases by 50% the radioactivity associated with the 7.2 precursor while decreasing by 25% the radioactivity incorporated into the 6.7 specie. However, the radioactivity incorporated into both precursors was decreased dramatically (60 to 70%) when cells were labeled in the presence of vitamin for 2 hr. These results reveal that the vitamin K-dependent processing step is associated with the 6.7 and 7.2 precursors and further suggest that the 6.7 specie serves as the substrate for the vitamin-dependent carboxylation reaction resulting in the appearance of a 7.2 product. Of considerable interest was the finding that 6.7 → 7.2 processing step also occurs in the absence of vitamin, yet at a much reduced rate. These findings will be discussed in the following section.

Subsequent studies were undertaken to determine the subcellular localization of these precursors. In anticipation of low yields of precursors during subcellular fractionation, rat livers (ca. 10 gm) previously perfused for 2 hr in the presence of [^{3}H]leucine were employed rather than H-35 hepatoma cells. [^{3}H]leucine-labeled precursors residing in rough endoplasmic reticulum (RER), smooth endoplasmic reticulum

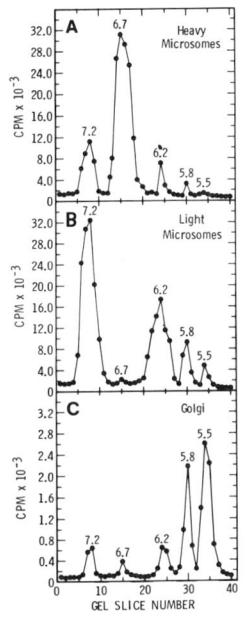
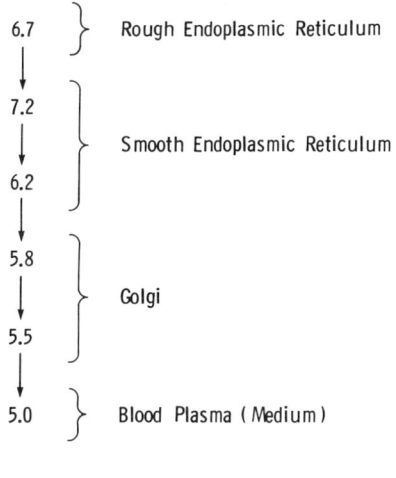

FIGURE 6: Subcellular distribution of [³H]precursor prothrombins obtained from a perfused rat liver labeled with [³H]-leucine.

FIGURE 7: Order of processing of prothrombin precursors as evaluated by pulse kinetic acid subcellular localization data (see Figures 5 and 6).

(SER) and golgi (G) were isolated (immunochemically) and characterized (IEF-gels) as before. The results of these investigations are presented in Figure 6 and indicate that the prominent precursor(s) appearing in the RER, SER, and golgi were 6.7 (RER), 7.2 and 6.2 (SER), and 5.8 and 5.5 (golgi). The appearance of small amounts of radioactive 7.2 and 6.2 in the RER, of 5.8 and 5.5 in the SER, and of 7.2 and 6.2 in the golgi are consistent with previous findings (27) which indicated some cross contamination of SER in the RER, of golgi in the SER, and of SER in the golgi.

In view of the excellent agreement that exists between the kinetic pulse data (Figure 5 and Table III) and the subcellular fractionation data (Figure 6), it is our interpretation that the intracellular processing of prothrombin precursors proceeds in a manner as illustrated in Figure 7. The data presented also imply that vitamin K enhances the rate of processing of the 6.7 (RER) specie resulting in the formation of a 7.2 (SER) precursor. Furthermore, the results from these investigations reveal that additional posttranslational modifications, other than a vitamin K-dependent processing step, are required for the secretion of a mature prothrombin product.

DISCUSSION

Although Esmon et al., (8) and Grant and Suttie (14) have successfully isolated intracellular precursors or rat prothrombin employing conventional purification techniques (e.g., salt fractionation and ion-exchange chromatography), such procedures have resulted in (a) low, non-quantitative yields of precursors, and (b) the loss of some precursor species altogether. Furthermore, relatively large amounts of starting material were required for their isolation, i.e., 20 to 30 rat livers. In view of these findings other approaches were sought that would result in both the rapid and quantitative isolation of small quantities of precursor prothrombins present in cultured hepatoma cells and liver microsomes (31). Since previous reports have indicated that antibodies elicited in response to mature prothrombin immunospecifically recognize precursor prothrombins as well (15,29,30), the feasibility of an immunochemical approach for the isolation of precursor prothrombins was examined.

The results presented herein have established the ability of an anti-prothrombin/Sepharose adsorbent to quantitatively and exclusively retain [^{3}H]leucine-labeled precursor and mature prothrombins obtained from H-35 hepatoma cells previously labeled with [^{3}H]leucine. Subsequent characterization of the immunospecifically retained intracellular proteins revealed the presence of 5 discrete precursor species possessing pI values of 7.2, 6.7, 6.2, 5.8, and 5.5 (Figure 3). When cells were labeled in the presence of vitamin K, there appeared a marked reduction in the intracellular precursors relative to those precursors isolated from cells labeled in the absence of vitamin (Figure 4 and Table II). Additionally, an assessment of the rate of incorporation of [^{3}H]leucine into these precursors indicated that the role of vitamin K is at the posttranslation level. Furthermore, the inability of the vitamin to significantly enhance the incorporation of [^{3}H]leucine into prothrombin precursors during a 5- or 10-min pulse (Table II), provided direct evidence <u>against</u> its involvement at the translational level. This latter data was derived from short pulses of radioactivity to ensure that all labeled precursors were present intracellularly. Only after a 20 min pulse did significant amounts of [^{3}H]prothrombins appear in the culture medium (Table II).

Based upon the data presented herein it is very probable that the 6.7 and 7.2 precursor species serve as the substrate and product, respectively, for the vitamin K-dependent carboxylase reaction. This interpretation is based upon the vitamin-dependent redistribution of radioactivity incorporated into these precursors (Table III), their order or processing (Figure 5), and the subcellular loaction at which they reside (Figure 6). Whereas the results derived from a 2 hr pulse suggested that the 7.2 and/or 6.7 precursors were likely substrates (as a result of their disproportionate decreases in isotope relative to the other precursors), a similar analysis of the data obtained from 10 min pulses implied that the 6.7 precursor was the sole substrate involved in the vitamin K-dependent processing step. This assumption is based upon the vitamin K-dependent decrease and increase in radioactivity associated with the 6.7 and 7.2 precursors, respectively, and is supported by the order of processing of these precursors as well as their subcellular localization, i.e., 6.7(RER) → 7.2(SER) → 6.2(SER) → 5.8(GOLGI) → 5.5(GOLGI). These latter results also exclude the possibility that the 7.2(SER) precursor serves as the substrate for a 6.7(RER) product.

The above interpretations of our data are supported by the finding of Helgeland (19) and Willingham et al., (31). The former established the subcellular site for the conversion of a prothrombin precursor in rat livers by employing clotting assays which distinguish between mature and precursor prothrombins (6,22). Results from these studies revealed that precursor prothrombin was converted (processed) into biologically active prothrombin in the RER and/or at the transition between smooth and rough reticulum. Helgeland (19) further observed that the vitamin K-dependent carboxylase activity was localized in the RER. Most recently, Willingham et al., (31) have isolated (via anti-prothrombin/Sepharose adsorbent) and characterized the [$^{14}CO_2$] product of the vitamin K-dependent carboxylation reaction that occurs in rat liver microsomes (see adjoining chapter). As evaluated by IEF gels, a single [$^{14}CO_2$] protein was observed possessing a pI value of 7.2. The above results are consistent with the concept that vitamin K is required for the carboxylation of a 6.7(RER) precursor, resulting in the formation of a 7.2(SER) precursor. It is suspected that this modification (γ-carboxyglutamate) facilitates the transfer of precursor prothrombin from the RER to the SER.

Since the vitamin K-dependent processing step results in the γ-carboxylation of glutamate residues located near the NH_2-terminus of prothrombin (1-4), it was originally anticipated that vitamin-supplemented cells would possess additional, more acidic precursors not present in control preparations. Yet, as our data indicate, only the <u>amount</u> and not the <u>type</u> of precursors present intracellularly were altered when cells were labeled in the presence of vitamin. Although this apparent inconsistency remains to be resolved, similar observations have been reported by Grant and Suttie (14) and Stenflo (29) with precursor and mature prothrombins obtained from bovine plasma. In the latter investigation both precursor and mature prothrombin preparations possessed three identical protein bands after isoelectric focusing. Also perplexing was the increased basicity (6.7 → 7.2) that accompanied the vitamin K-dependent carboxylation reaction. On the basis that our data has been interpreted correctly, it would seem logical to conclude that additional, uncharacterized modifications participate in the transition of the 6.7 precursor to the 7.2 form, irrespective of the status of the vitamin. Evidence to suggest that such modifications exist are apparent from the findings of Finnan and Suttie (32,33). Their recent investigations have indicated that the vitamin K-dependent carboxylation of a pentapeptide substrate (phe-leu-glu-glu-leu), is immediately followed by an additional modification which increases the basicity of the carboxylated product.

Whereas the exact nature of all of the modifications associated with the 7.2, 6.7, and 6.2 precursor remains to be elucidated, in all likelihood those precursors possessing pI values of 5.8 and 5.5 represent asialo- and/or partially sialated forms of prothrombin, respectively. This identification stems from the observation reported by Grant and Suttie (14) that upon complete removal of sialic acid from mature prothrombin (neuraminidase treatment) the resulting asialo-prothrombin possessed a pI of 5.8. Furthermore, since the addition of sialic acid (glycosyltransferase) reflects terminal glycosylations which appear to be localized within the golgi apparatus (34), it is assumed that these precursors are in the final stages of prothrombin processing. The subcellular data presented in Figure 6 provides additional support for this assumption as does our preliminary findings with tunicamycin. Thus, cells labeled with [^{3}H]leucine in the presence of this inhibitor of glycosylation do not contain the 5.8 or 5.5 precursors.

In conclusion, the application of immunochemical procedures for isolating precursor prothrombins from rat hepatoma cells and perfused livers appears promising. The employment of antibodies elicited in response to a mature protein antigen that immunospecifically recognize precursors of the antigen should serve as useful probes for investigating numerous aspects of protein processing. Studies using these procedures are now in progress to characterize precursor prothrombins with respect to the nature of their post-translational modifications in an attempt to ascertain their functional roles in protein processing, secretion, coagulation, and degradation.

ACKNOWLEDGEMENTS

The authors wish to express their appreciation of Joyce Becker (McArdle Lab, University of Wisconsin) for helpful discussions and advice regarding numerous aspects of cell culture techniques. They thank R.E. Olson (Saint Louis University) for providing rat prothrombin standard, Joyce Becker and Van R. Potter (McArdle Lab) for initial stocks of H-35 rat hepatoma cells and Melody Jennings for her secretarial assistance. This research supported by HL-15619 (NIH).

REFERENCES

1. Stenflo, J. (1974a) J. Biol. Chem. 249, 5527-5535.
2. Stenflo, J., Fernlund, P., Egan, W., and Roepstorff, P. (1974b) Proc. Natl. Acad. Sci. U.S.A. 71, 2730-2733.
3. Nelsestuen, G.L., Zytokovicz, T.H., and Howard, J.B. (1974) J. Biol. Chem. 249, 6347-6350.
4. Magnusson, S., Sottrup-Jensen, L., Peterson, T.E., Morris, H.R., and Dell, A. (1974) FEBS Lett. 44, 189-193.
5. Nelsestuen, G.L., and Suttie, J.W. (1972) Biochemistry 11, 4961-4964.
6. Shah, D.V., and Suttie, J.W. (1974) Biochem. Biophys. Res. Commun. 60, 1397-1402.
7. Esmon, C.T., Sadowski, J.A., and Suttie, J.W. (1975) J. Biol. Chem. 250, 4744-4748.
8. Girardot, J.M., Delaney, R., and Johnson, B.C. (1974) Biochem. Biophys. Res. Commun. 59, 1197-1203.
9. Nelsestuen, G.L., and Suttie, J.W. (1972) J. Biol. Chem. 247, 8176-8182.
10. Stenflo, J., and Ganrot, P.D. (1973) Biochem. Biophys. Res. Commun. 50, 98-104.

11. Morrissey, J.J., Jones, J.P., and Olson, R.E. (1973) Biochem. Biophys. Res. Commun. 54, 1075-1082.
12. Esmon, C.T., Grant, G.A., and Suttie, J.W. (1975) Biochemistry 14, 1595-1600.
13. Grant, G.A. (1975) Ph.D. thesis, University of Wisconsin-Madison.
14. Grant, G.A., and Suttie, J.W. (1976) Biochemistry 15, 5387-5393.
15. Munns, T.W., Johnston, M.F.M., Liszewski, M.K., and Olson, R.E. (1976) Proc. Natl. Acad. Sci. U.S.A. 73, 2803-2807.
16. Graves, C.B., and Grabau, G.G. (1978) Fed. Proc. 37, 1444.
17. Graves, B.C., Grabau, G.G. (1979) Fed. Proc. 38, 620.
18. Willingham, A.K., Martin, S.L., and Graves, C.B. (1979) Fed. Proc. 38, 793.
19. Helgeland, L. (1977) Biochim. Biophys. Acta 499, 181-193.
20. Potter, V.R., Watanabe, M., Becker, J.E., and Pitot, H.C. (1967) Adv. Enzyme Regul. 5, 303-316.
21. Pitot, H.C., Peraino, C., Morse, P.A., and Potter, V.R. (1964) Natl. Can. Inst. Monogr. 13, 229-242.
22. Shah, D.V., and Suttie, J.W. (1971) Proc. Natl. Acad. Sci. U.S.A. 68, 1653-1657.
23. Bartosek, I., Guaitani, A., and Miller, L.L. (1973) Isolated Liver Perfusion and Its Application, Raven Press, New York.
24. Graves, C.B., Grabau, G.G., Olson, R.E., and Munns, T.W. (1979) Submitted to Biochemistry.
25. Piperno, G., Huang, B., and Luck, D.J.L. (1977) Proc. Natl. Acad. Sci. U.S.A 74, 1600-1604.
26. Johnston, M.F.M., Kipfer, R.K., and Olson, R.E. (1972) J. Biol. Chem. 247, 3987-3993.
27. Fleischer, S., and Kervina, M. (1973) Methods in Enzymology 31, 1-26.
28. Munns, T.W., Liszewski, M.K., and Sims, H.F. (1977) Biochemistry 16, 2163-2168.
29. Stenflo, J. (1972) J. Biol. Chem. 247, 8167-8175.
30. Wallin, R., and Prydz, H. (1975) Biochem. Biophys. Res. Commun. 62, 398-406.
31. Willingham, A.K., Martin, S.L., Graves, C.B., Grabau, G.G., and Munns, T.W. (1979) in "Vitamin K Metabolism and Vitamin K-Dependent Proteins" (J.W. Suttie, ed.) University Park Press, Baltimore, in press.
32. Finnan, J.L., and Suttie, J.W. (1979) Fed. Proc. 38, 876.
33. Finnan, J.L., and Suttie, J.W. (1979) in "Vitamin K Metabolism and Vitamin K-Depedent Proteins" (J.W. Suttie, ed.) University Park Press, Baltimore, in press.
34. Schachter, H., Jabbal, I., Roger, L., Pinterie, L., McGuire, E.J., and Roseman, S. (1970) J. Biol. Chem. 245, 1090-1100.

SYNTHESIS OF FACTOR VII IN MORRIS HEPATOMA (MH_1C_1) CELLS

H. PRYDZ and F. HAFFNER

Department of Microbiology, Dental Faculty and
Department of Pharmacology, Medical Faculty
University of Oslo, Norway

INTRODUCTION

Factor VII is synthesized by parenchymal cells in the liver (1). It is a common observation that the level of Factor VII activity in consecutive plasma samples from a healthy person is quite stable over long periods of time (a slight increase with age has been described (2)), but very little is known about the regulatory mechanisms involved. We report here some preliminary experiments towards the establishment of a system for a study of these mechanisms. We have shown previously (3) that a clonal strain of rat hepatoma cells (MH_1C_1) grown in vitro synthesizes Factor VII. These cells were derived from the transplantable Morris hepatoma 7795 and were established as a clonal strain in 1967 (4).

MATERIALS AND METHODS

The cells were grown in 25 cm^2 Falcon or Costar flasks in 3 ml of Dulbecco's modified Eagle medium (DMEM) (GIBCO), supplemented with either 10% pooled rat serum or 15% horse serum and 2.5% fetal calf serum and buffered with either sodium bicarbonate or Hepes. After reaching stationary phase the cells were trypsinized and subcultured (8 · 10^5 cells per flask), using bicarbonate-buffered medium with horse and fetal calf serum. On day 3 or 4 the medium was changed to DMEM with 10% rat serum, 20 mM Hepes and without antibiotics. On day 6 the cultures were washed three times with prewarmed DMEM without serum, and the experimental media added. At the end of incubation the medium was poured off, centrifuged 5000g/20 min and the supernatants frozen. The adherent cells were rinsed 10 times with ice cold saline, drained and scraped off into 1 ml of veronal-buffered saline (5). The cells were frozen and thawed and homogenized using 10 strokes in a manual Potter-Elvehjem teflon-glass homogenizer. The supernatants and homogenates were tested for Factor VII activity in a one stage system (5) using plasma from a patient with a deep congenital deficiency as substrate. Standard curves were prepared using dilutions of rat plasma and serum. Protein (6) and deoxyribose (7) were determined in the cell homogenates, the latter after perchloric acid extraction (8).

Rats were kept in restraining cages to prevent coprophagy and fed a vitamin K-free diet (Teklad, Madison, WI) for 9-10 days to render them vitamin K-deficient. Only serum obtained from plasma with less than 20% of normal Factor VII activity was used. When indicated normal rat serum was treated with $BaSO_4$ as described (9) and subsequently dialysed against 4 shifts of 1000 ml saline before sterilization by Millipore filtration.

RESULTS AND DISCUSSION

MH_1C_1 cells synthesize Factor VII in the presence of serum-free medium (Fig. 1A) and they respond to vitamin K_1 and warfarin as expected (Fig. 1). The addition of vitamin K_1 gave a burst of released activity, but at the beginning as well as at the end of the experiments (usually 20-28 h later) the activity of Factor VII in the homogenates never exceeded 20% of the total activity. The effect of various serum additions to the growth medium was tested. To exclude contributions from the activation of Factor VII present in these sera the activity was determined in cultures with the appropriate serum and cycloheximide (10-33 μg/ml) present in the growth medium. At these concentrations of cycloheximide no increase of Factor VII was observed, showing that neither synthesis nor activation took place. The activity in medium from such cultures was accordingly subtracted as background in each experiment. With $BaSO_4$-treated serum this background was 0.10 - 0.15 units/ml, with serum from vitamin K-deficient rats 1.0 -2.3 units/ml and with normal rat serum 15 - 20 units/ml. The culture medium was then supplemented with 10% serum from vitamin - K deficient rats or serum from which Factor VII had been removed by $BaSO_4$-treatment. The data in figure 2 shows that serum from which Factor VII is almost completely absent has a markedly lower stimulatory activity on Factor VII synthesis than serum from vitamin K - deficient rats where acarboxy-VII is present.

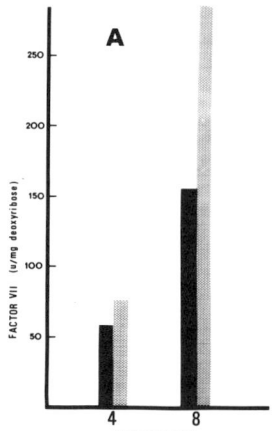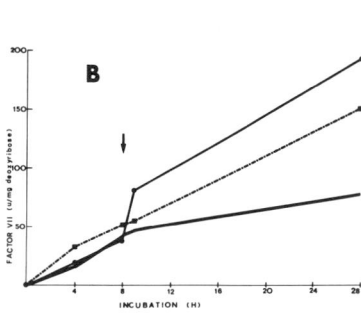

Fig. 1 (A) Effect of vitamin K_1 on the synthesis of Factor VII by MH_1C_1 cells in serum-free medium. The dark bars are controls and the light bars had 0.1 mg/ml Vitamin K_1 added.
(B) Effect of warfarin and vitamin K_1 on Factor VII increase in medium from MH_1C_1 cells cultured in the absence of serum. ---■--- Controls, ——— Warfarin 0.1 mg/ml, —●— Warfarin 0.1 mg/ml from start of experiment, vitamin K_1 0.1 mg/10 ml added at 8 h (arrow).

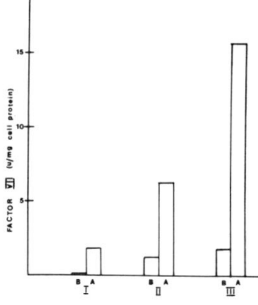

Fig. 2 Effect of $BaSO_4$-treated serum and serum from vitamin K-depleted rats on Factor VII synthesis.

I: Medium without serum
II: Medium with 10% $BaSO_4$-treated serum
III: Medium with 10% serum from vitamin K-deficient rats

A: Without   B: With warfarin (0.1 mg/ml)

The $BaSO_4$-treatment and subsequent dialysis caused a 20% reduction in total protein in the serum. The synthesis of Factor VII was, however, essentially unchanged when this was corrected for by concentration of the serum. In the presence of normal rat serum any synthesis was obscured by the high level of activation observed (data not shown).

Our data may suggest the presence of a coagulopoietin-VII in serum from vitamin K-deficient rats, analogous to the coagulopoietin-II described by the Karpatkins (10). Other explanations are, however, possible and are currently under study. Carboxylation of the added acarboxy-VII (involving uptake, intracellular carboxylation and secretion of Factor VII to the medium) did not take place; in that case a similar increase in the cycloheximide-treated cultures would have been expected, and no such increase was observed. Acarboxy-VII may, however, have a direct positive feed-back effect on its own synthesis. If this is the case, a counteracting regulatory principle must be present in vivo, since the sum of the levels of acarboxy- and normal factor (in the case of Factor X) is reasonably constant when determined immunologically (11). The stimulatory effect of Factor VII-deficient serum ($BaSO_4$-treated) is much less pronounced. Factor VII receptor saturation therefore seems to play essentially no role as an inhibitory signal in Factor VII biosynthesis in the present system.

ACKNOWLEDGEMENT

This work was supported by the Norwegian Research Council for Science and the Humanities through grants to H. P. and F. H.

REFERENCES

1. Prydz, H. (1964) Scand. J. Clin. Lab. Invest. 16, 540-548.
2. Brozović, M. Stirling, Y., Harricks, C., North, W. R. S., and Meade, T. W. (1974) Brit. J. Haematol. 28, 381-391.
3. Rugstad, H. E., Prydz, H., and Johansson, B. (1972) Exp. Cell Res. 71, 41-44.
4. Richardson, U. I., Tashjian, A., and Levine, L. (1969) J. Cell Biol. 40, 236-247.
5. Hjort, P. (1957) Scand. J. Clin. Lab. Invest. 9, suppl. 27.
6. Markwell, M. A. K., Haas, S. M., Bieber, L. L., and Tolbert, N. E. (1978) Anal. Biochem. 87, 206-210.
7. Burton, K. (1956) Biochem. J. 62, 315-322.
8. Munro, H. N., and Fleck, A. (1966) Methods Biochem. Anal. 14, 113-175.
9. Prydz, H. (1964) Scand. J. Clin. Lab. Invest. 16, 409-414.
10. Karpatkin, M., and Karpatkin, S. (1979) Proc. Natl. Acad. Sci. 76, 491-493.
11. Prydz, H., and Gladhaug, A. (1971) Thromb. Diathes. Haemorrhag. 25, 157-165.

BIOSYNTHESIS OF BOVINE PROTHROMBIN IN A CELL-FREE SYSTEM

R. T. A. MACGILLIVRAY, D. W. CHUNG, and E. W. DAVIE

University of Washington,
Seattle, WA 98195

INTRODUCTION

The coagulation of blood is the result of a series of consecutive enzymic conversions of circulating zymogens to form a number of specific enzymes that are primarily serine proteases (1). Four of these zymogens (factors IX, X, VII and prothrombin) require a vitamin K-dependent carboxylation of specific glutamic acid residues in the NH_2-terminal regions of the proteins. The resulting γ-carboxyglutamic acid residues enable the zymogens to bind calcium ions (2). This ultimately facilitates the adsorption of these proteins to negatively charged phospholipid membranes of platelets during fibrin formation.

In the absence of vitamin K, carboxylation does not occur, resulting in the biosynthesis of zymogens which cannot be converted to their corresponding protease. In this situation, blood coagulation is severely impaired. Prothrombin is the most abundant of the four vitamin K-dependent proteins of plasma, and thus this protein has been most extensively studied. Indeed, its complete amino acid sequence has been established by Magnusson and coworkers (3).

The carboxylase enzyme is membrane-bound (4,5) and can be isolated in an active form by solubilizing liver microsomes with a mild detergent such as Triton X-100 (6,7). An <u>in vitro</u> carboxylation system has been developed and carboxylation of several substrates has been demonstrated (6-9). There is also a rat hepatoma cell line that is responsive to vitamin K (10). Little is known, however, of the timing of the carboxylation of prothrombin. Shah and Suttie (11) showed that cycloheximide blocked all protein synthesis in vitamin K-deficient rats, and subsequent administration of vitamin K released a biologically active (i.e., carboxylated) prothrombin into plasma. Accordingly, they suggested that a prothrombin precursor was present in the liver of vitamin K-deficient rats, and its conversion to prothrombin was a post-translational event. However, this does not rule out the possibility that carboxylation may be a co-translational event in healthy rats.

With an <u>in vitro</u> protein synthesizing system, it is possible to study some of the molecular events involved in the biosynthesis and secretion of proteins. Thus, translation of mRNA in a cell-free system that is devoid of membranes has shown that many secreted proteins are synthesized as precursors having an NH_2-terminal extension. This extension, typically 15-30 amino acid residues long, is very rich in hydrophobic residues, and has been termed the signal sequence. Blobel and Dobberstein (12) and Milstein (13) had previously predicted that secretory proteins would contain such an NH_2-terminal extension, which would bind polysomes that were synthesizing secretory proteins on the rough endoplasmic reticulum. The primary translation products of many mRNAs have now been studied, including the sequence analysis of the signal or pre piece (14).

In all but one case, secretory proteins contain an NH_2-terminal signal sequence, whereas non-secreted proteins, such as globin, do not. An exception is ovalbumin (15), but this may have an internal signal sequence (14). Using similar in vitro techniques, Palmiter et al. (16) have shown that the signal peptide for lysozyme is removed after about 60 residues have been initially synthesized. Many workers have also shown that translation of mRNA in a cell-free system containing externally added membranes results in glycosylation of secreted proteins and sequestering of these proteins in vesicles (14). This is accompanied by concomitant processing of the signal peptide by a putative signal peptidase. Several plasma proteins have been synthesized in cell-free systems utilizing liver poly A RNA. These include rat and bovine albumins (17-19), chick transferrin (20) and rat prothrombin (18). Automatic sequence analysis of the preproalbumins (17,19) and pretransferrin (20) has revealed that three proteins contain N-terminal signal sequences. However, the presence of a signal sequence for rat prothrombin was not investigated.

Our laboratory became interested in the use of in vitro protein synthesis to study the events leading to the secretion of plasma proteins, such as prothrombin. A tentative working hypothesis for the transfer of prothrombin through the rough endoplasmic reticulum is illustrated in Figure 1.

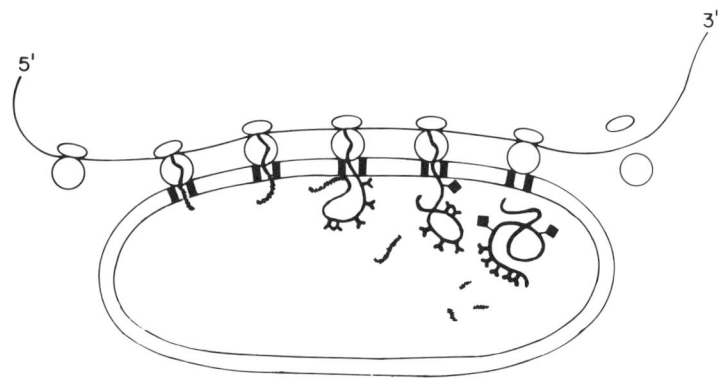

FIGURE 1. Tentative proposal for the transfer of prothrombin through the rough endoplasmic reticulum (modified from ref. 12). ᴡᴡᴡ , signal peptide; ——— , plasma prothrombin sequence; ⋖ , γ-carboxyglutamic acid residues; ◆ , glycosylated residues.

548   MacGillivray, Chung, and Davie

METHODS AND RESULTS

Since prothrombin is a secreted protein, it seemed likely that it would be synthesized on membrane-bound polysomes as a precursor with an NH_2-terminal signal sequence. If vitamin K-dependent carboxylation is a co-translational event, the growing polypeptide chain might be carboxylated by the membrane-bound carboxylase present on the lumen side of the rough endoplasmic reticulum (21). Transfer of the core carbohydrate unit also appears to occur in the rough endoplasmic reticulum (22). Before the prothrombin polypeptide chain is completed, the signal peptide is probably cleaved off and degraded in the membrane or in the lumen of the endoplasmic reticulum.

We chose bovine liver as a source of mRNA, as both bovine plasma and liver are readily available in large quantities, and the various bovine vitamin K-dependent clotting factors have been purified in a homogeneous form in our laboratory. Accordingly, polysomes were prepared from bovine liver by the magnesium precipitation technique (23) and poly A-containing RNA was isolated by chromatography on oligo dT cellulose. Translation of this RNA in a cell-free system derived from rabbit reticulocytes (24) showed that it directed the synthesis of many plasma proteins, including albumin, fibrinogen, prothrombin and antithrombin III (19).

Centrifugation of the poly A RNA on a linear (5-20%) neutral sucrose gradient is shown in Figure 2. The RNA consists of a heterogeneous population sedimenting from ~5S to 28S. When individual fractions of the sucrose gradient were translated in the reticulocyte lysate system,

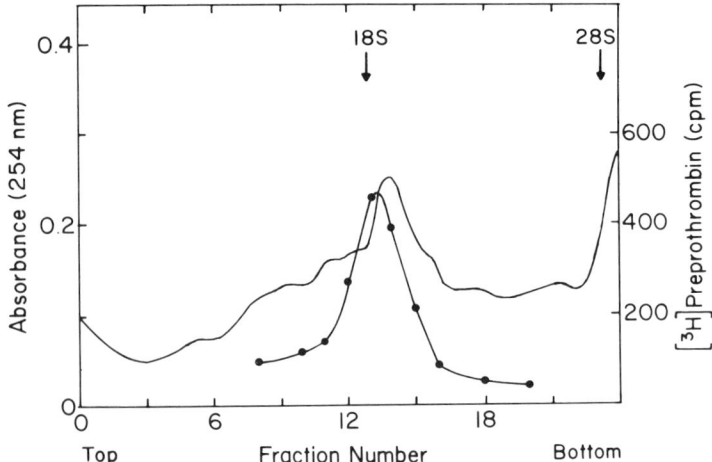

FIGURE 2. Sucrose gradient centrifugation of bovine liver poly A-containing RNA. Poly A-containing RNA was centrifuged on a linear sucrose gradient (5-20%) and fractions were translated in a reticulocyte lysate. ———, absorbance at 254 nm; •——•, [^{3}H]Leucine incorporated into immunoprecipitated bovine prothrombin.

and prothrombin isolated by immunoprecipitation, a single peak of prothrombin mRNA activity was found. This mRNA sedimented with the 18S ribosomal RNA marker. This indicated that prothrombin mRNA was approximately 2200 nucleotides long.

In these experiments, approximately 1% of total liver poly A RNA coded for prothrombin. This level of RNA is too low for many biochemical investigations, and therefore the prothrombin mRNA was enriched using a technique of double antibody immunoprecipitation of polysomes (25). In this way, poly A RNA was enriched 10-15 fold for prothrombin. A sample of this RNA was translated in the reticulocyte lysate system in the presence of [^{3}H]proline, and the radiolabeled prothrombin was isolated by immunoprecipitation. The immunoprecipitate was solubilized in SDS under reducing conditions and subjected to electrophoresis on a 12.5% polyacrylamide gel containing N,N'-diallyltartardiamide as crosslinker in the presence of SDS. The gel was then sliced into 2 mm slices and the radioactivity determined in each slice (Fig. 3). The prothrombin migrated as a single band. Since the prothrombin synthesized in this cell-free system is probably not glycosylated, it was not possible to determine whether or not it contained a short NH$_2$-terminal extension from its apparent molecular weight.

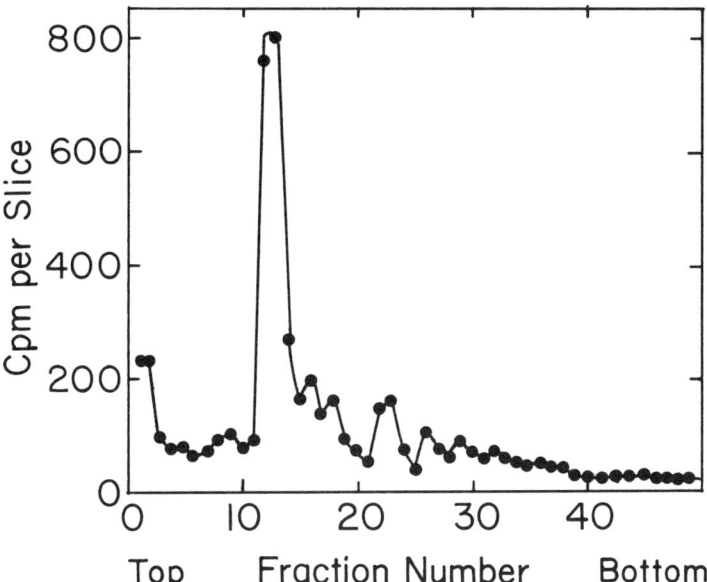

FIGURE 3. SDS-polyacrylamide gel electrophoresis of bovine preprothrombin labeled with [^{3}H]proline.

Thus, the enriched RNA was translated in the presence of [^{3}H]leucine, and the prothrombin was isolated by immunoprecipitation and subjected to automatic Edman degradation. The resulting phenylthiohydantoin derivatives for each cycle were quantitated in a liquid scintillation counter.

Ambiguous results were obtained due to a rapid increase in background radioactivity. Presumably, this resulted from substantial non-specific cleavage of the prothrombin in the automatic sequenator. Thus, the translation and isolation of the immunoprecipitated prothrombin was repeated, and the radiolabeled product was then cleaved by thrombin in the presence of SDS to form Fragment I and Intermediate I (26). Fragment I was isolated by gel electrophoresis and subjected to automatic sequenator analysis. Leucyl residues were released at cycles 8, 12, 14, 17, 20 and 28. As plasma prothrombin has leucine residues at positions 6 and 14 (3), these results indicated that prothrombin is synthesized as a precursor containing an NH_2-terminal extension or signal sequence. In accordance with the nomenclature for other proteins having signal sequences, we have termed this precursor "preprothrombin" and suggest that this term be used to describe only precursors having the signal sequence, rather than prothrombins that are not carboxylated.

Translation of enriched poly A RNA in the presence of other labeled amino acids has shown that the signal sequence of preprothrombin is as follows:

```
    -23              -20              -15              -10
[Met]-Ala- X -Val- X - X -Pro- X -Leu-Pro- X - X -Leu-Ala-Leu-Ala-Ala-
    -5
Leu-Phe- X -Leu-Val- X -
```

X represents an amino acid not yet identified. The residues are numbered backwards from the potential cleavage site by the signal peptidase. As the reticulocyte lysate contains a methionine aminopeptidase which removes methionyl residues in a Met-Ala sequence (27), it is probable that the signal sequence of primary translation product is 23 residues long, and that the methionyl residue at -23 was removed during the translation.

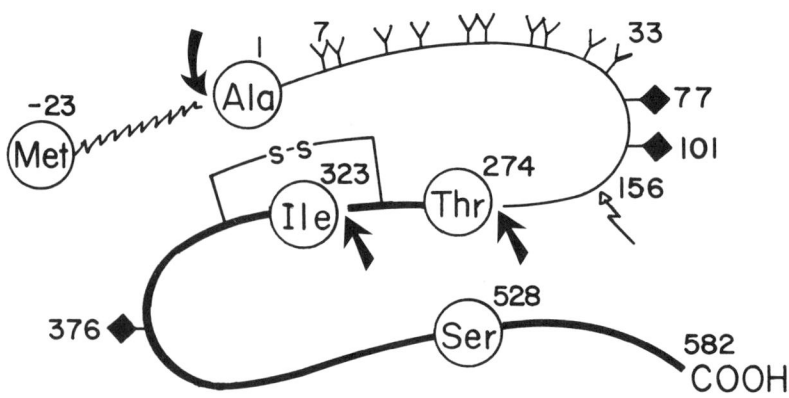

FIGURE 4. Abbreviated structure for bovine preprothrombin. The signal sequence is numbered backwards from the site of cleavage by the signal peptidase (↯). The plasma prothrombin sequence is numbered as in ref. 3. Y, γ-carboxyglutamic acid residues; ◆, glycosylated residues; ↑, sites of cleavage by factor X_a; ⇧, site of cleavage by thrombin. Residue 528 is the active site serine.

Experiments to complete the signal sequence and determine the structure of the primary translation product are currently in progress.

DISCUSSION

An abbreviated structure for bovine preprothrombin is summarized in Figure 4. We have demonstrated that prothrombin is synthesized as a precursor having a signal sequence of 23 amino acids. This signal sequence may be similar for the other vitamin K-dependent proteins of plasma, such that the growing polypeptide chains for these proteins bind to specific receptors on the rough endoplasmic reticulum of liver. The polypeptides may then traverse the membrane through specific channels, such that vitamin K-dependent carboxylation occurs co-translationally. In view of the poor specificity of the carboxylase towards peptide substrates, it is tempting to suggest that the signal peptide may orientate the growing polypeptide chain into a specific conformation. Carboxylation of glutamic acid residues could then occur, the signal peptide proteolytically removed, and vectoral discharge into the lumen could proceed, with co-translational addition of the core carbohydrate unit. Experiments designed to test these and other hypotheses are currently in progress in our laboratory.

ACKNOWLEDGEMENTS

This work was supported in part by Grant HL 16919 from the National Institutes of Health.

REFERENCES

1. Davie, E. W., and Fujikawa, K. (1975) Annu. Rev. Biochem. 44, 799-829.
2. Nelsestuen, G. L., and Lim, T. K. (1977) Biochemistry 16, 4164-4171.
3. Magnusson, S., Petersen, T. E., Sottrup-Jensen, L., and Claeys, H. (1975) Proteases and Biological Control (Reich, E., Rifkin, D. B., and Shaw, E., Eds.), Vol. 2, pp. 123-149, Cold Spring Harbor Laboratory, New York.
4. Jones, J. P., Fausto, A., Houser, R. M., Gardner, E. J., and Olson, R. E. (1976) Biochem. Biophys. Res. Commun. 72, 589-597.
5. Vermeer, C., Soute, B. A. M., and Hemker, H. C. (1978) Biochim. Biophys. Acta 523, 494-505.
6. Suttie, J. W., Lehrman, S. R., Geweke, L. O., Hageman, J. M., and Rich, D. H. (1979) Biochem. Biophys. Res. Commun. 86, 500-507.
7. Jones, J. P., Gardner, E. J., Cooper, T. G., and Olson, R. E. (1977) J. Biol. Chem. 252, 7738-7742.
8. Vermeer, C., Soute, B. A. M., Govers-Riemslag, J., and Hemker, H. C. (1976) Biochim. Biophys. Acta 444, 926-930.
9. Houser, R. M., Carey, D. J., Dus, K. M., Marshall, G. R., and Olson, R. E. (1977) FEBS Lett. 75, 226-230.
10. Munns, T. W., Johnston, M. F. M., Liszewski, M. K., and Olson, R. E. (1976) Proc. Natl. Acad. Sci. U.S.A. 73, 2803-2807.
11. Shah, D. V., and Suttie, J. W. (1971) Proc. Natl. Acad. Sci. U.S.A. 68, 1653-1657.
12. Blobel, G., and Dobberstein, B. (1975) J. Cell. Biol. 67, 835-851.
13. Milstein, C., Brownlee, G. G., Harrison, T. M., and Mathews, M. B. (1972) Nature New Biol. 239, 117-120.
14. Conference on Precursor Processing in the Biosynthesis of Proteins, Ann. N.Y. Acad. Sci., in press.

15. Palmiter, R. D., Gagnon, J., and Walsh, K. A. (1978) Proc. Natl. Acad. Sci. U.S.A. 75, 94-98.
16. Palmiter, R. D., Gagnon, J., Ericsson, L. H., and Walsh, K. A. (1977) J. Biol. Chem. 252, 6386-6393.
17. Strauss, A. W., Bennett, C. D., Donohue, A. M., Rodkey, J. A., and Alberts, A. W. (1977) J. Biol. Chem. 252, 6846-6855.
18. Nardacci, N. J., Jones, J. P., Hall, A. L., and Olson, R. E. (1975) Biochem. Biophys. Res. Commun. 64, 51-58.
19. MacGillivray, R. T. A., Chung, D. W., and Davie, E. W. (1979) Eur. J. Biochem., in press.
20. Thibodeau, S. N., Lee, D. C., and Palmiter, R. D. (1978) J. Biol. Chem. 253, 3771-3774.
21. Helgeland, L. (1977) Biochim. Biophys. Acta 499, 181-193.
22. Czichi, U., and Lennarz, W. J. (1977) J. Biol. Chem. 252, 7901-7904.
23. Palmiter, R. D. (1974) Biochemistry 13, 3606-3615.
24. Palmiter, R. D. (1973) J. Biol. Chem. 248, 2095-2106.
25. Schutz, G., Kieval, S., Groner, G., Sippel, A. E., Kurtz, D. T., and Feigelson, P. (1977) Nucleic Acids Res. 4, 71-84.
26. Owen, W. G., Esmon, C. T., and Jackson, C. M. (1974) J. Biol. Chem. 249, 594-605.
27. Thibodeau, S. N., Palmiter, R. D., and Walsh, K. A. (1978) J. Biol. Chem. 253, 9018-9023.

VITAMIN K-DEPENDENT CARBOXYLATION OF A SPECIFIC PROTHROMBIN PRECURSOR AND OTHER PROTEINS IN RAT LIVER

ALLAN K. WILLINGHAM, SUZANNE L. MARTIN,
C. BRUCE GRAVES, GARY G. GRABAU and
THEODORE W. MUNNS

Departments of Biochemistry, Kirksville College of Osteopathic Medicine, Kirksville, MO 63501 and St. Louis University School of Medicine, St. Louis, MO 63104

INTRODUCTION

Vitamin K catalyzes the post-translational carboxylation of specific glutamic acid (Glu) residues in precursor proteins to form γ-carboxy-glutamic acid (Gla). These residues are present in mature prothrombin, other vitamin K-dependent clotting factors (VII, IX and X) (1,2), plasma proteins C, S and Z (3-5), osteocalcin in bone (6,7) and various proteins in kidney (8,9). A solubilized microsomal system from rat liver has been developed that catalyzes the vitamin K-dependent carboxylation of prothrombin precursor proteins in vitro (10-13). Several proteins possessing the properties of the prothrombin precursors have been isolated from the liver of warfarin-treated rats (14-17). They are glycoproteins similar to prothrombin immunochemically with a molecular weight indistinguishable from rat prothrombin. Characterization via isoelectric focusing initially revealed the presence of two precursor prothrombins possessing pI values of 7.2 and 5.8 (15,16). More recently, five isoelectric forms of precursor prothrombins have been immuno-specifically isolated from rat liver microsomes (pI values of 7.2, 6.7, 6.2, 5.8 and 5.5) (18,19). Although it has been implied that the prothrombin precursor(s) is(are) the major proteins undergoing vitamin K-dependent carboxylation in the liver (2,20) this report demonstrates that there are at least three other classes of proteins, distinct from prothrombin, which participate as substrates in this carboxylation reaction and account for greater than 75% of $H^{14}CO_3^-$ incorporated into rat liver microsomal proteins. We have also found that, of the prothrombin precursors immunospecifically isolated from liver microsomes, only the pI 7.2 form contains ^{14}C as a result of the vitamin K-dependent carboxylation reaction in vitro.

MATERIALS AND METHODS

Vitamin K_1 (Aqua MEPHYTON) was purchased from Merck, Sharp and Dohme (West Point, PA). Sodium warfarin was a gift from Endo Laboratories (Garden City, NY). $NaH^{14}CO_3$ (60 mCi/m mole) and NCS (tissue solubilizer) were purchased from Amersham Searle (Arlington Heights, IL). Ampholyte carrier buffers were purchased from LKB (Chicago, IL). NADH, phenyl-methyl-sulfonyl fluoride (PMSF), soy bean trypsin inhibitor (STI), Echis carinatus venom and Triton X-100 were purchased from Sigma Chemical Co. (St. Louis, MO). Nonidet P-40 was purchased from Particle Data Laboratories, LTD (Elmhurst, IL). Sprague-Dawley derived rats were purchased from Laboratory Supply Co., Inc. (Indianapolis, IN). All other chemicals were analytical reagent grade.

Male rats (250-350 g) were treated with warfarin (5 mg/kg, i.p.) 18 h before they were killed. The rats were fasted during this period. The animals were killed by decapitation and the livers were quickly removed and chilled in homogenizing buffer (0.25 M sucrose, 25 mM imidazole, pH 7.2) containing protease inhibitors PMSF (1 mM) and STI (40 µg/ml). Livers were minced and homogenized in 3 volumes of homogenizing buffer and centrifuged at 10,000 g for 10 min. The resulting postmitochondrial supernatant was centrifuged at 105,000 g for 1 h. The microsomal pellet was surface washed with homogenizing buffer and subsequently homogenized in the same buffer which also contained 2% Triton X-100 and 0.2 M KCl to solubilize the microsomal membranes. These solubilized microsomes (1 ml equivalent to 0.75 g liver) were recentrifuged at 105,000 g for 45 min to remove any insoluble material.

Protein carboxylation by vitamin K was assayed in 1.0 ml incubations containing solubilized microsomes (0.8 ml), NADH (1 mg), $NaH^{14}CO_3$ (50 µCi) and vitamin K_1 (50 µg) which were incubated at 27°C for 30 min. Incorporation of $H^{14}CO_3^-$ into protein was determined by trichloroacetic acid (TCA) precipitation as previously described (10).

Anti-prothrombin/Sepharose was prepared according to the procedure of Graves, et al. (19) and used in these studies to isolate the prothrombin precursor(s) carboxylated by vitamin K. Triplicate incubations were combined (3.0 ml) and treated with 75 µg wet weight of immunoadsorbant for 1-2 h by gentle rotation at room temperature. The immunoadsorbant was collected by low speed centrifugation, washed successively with phosphate buffered saline (10 mM PO_4, pH 7.4), bicarbonate buffer (0.1 M $NaHCO_3$, pH 7.6) and phosphate buffer (10 mM PO_4, pH 7.0) and eluted in 2 ml of 7 M urea, 2% Nonidet P-40 by gentle rotation for 1-2 h at 37°C. Aliquots of immunoadsorbed and eluted protein were analyzed by isoelectric focusing in polyacrylamide gels (19). Sodium dodecyl sulfate (SDS, final concentration 2%) and β-mercaptoethanol (final concentration 5%) were added to samples for analysis by SDS-polyacrylamide gel electrophoresis (21). Proteins that were not immunospecifically adsorbed were chromatographed on Sephadex G-25 equilibrated with 7 M urea to remove small molecular weight ^{14}C-material. Aliquots of the void volume were also analyzed by SDS-gel electrophoresis. After isoelectric focusing or electrophoresis, gels were sliced into uniform 1 mm sections and digested overnight in an aqueous NCS solution (NCS: water, 9:1). Organic scintillation fluid (10 ml) was added and the amount of radioactivity was determined by liquid scintillation spectroscopy. Molecular weights of the ^{14}C-labeled proteins were determined by comparison to standard proteins run in separate gels and stained with Coomassie Blue.

Thrombin activity was determined both before and after immunoadsorption by activation with Echis carinatus venom (22). In order to indicate if the $H^{14}CO_3^-$ incorporated into protein was present in Gla residues, proteins were hydrolyzed in 6 N HCl at 110°C for 24 h. Samples were then evaporated in order to determine the residual radioactivity.

RESULTS

Vitamin K stimulated the incorporation of a significant amount of ^{14}C from $H^{14}CO_3^-$ into TCA precipitable protein in incubations containing solubilized microsomes from livers of warfarin-treated rats (dpm/g liver ± S.D. of triplicate incubations; -K = 5,500 ± 600, +K = 77,000 ± 600). Before using anti-prothrombin/Sepharose to isolate the carboxylated prothrombin precursors produced in these incubations it was necessary to determine if the immunoadsorbant was quantitatively removing the precursor protein. As indicated in Table 1, the lack of prothrombin activity in solubilized microsomes incubated in the presence of anti-prothrombin/Sepharose revealed the effectiveness of the immunoadsorbant to rapidly and quantitatively remove prothrombin from these preparations. A non-immune IgG/Sepharose did not remove any thrombin activity from solubilized microsomes.

TABLE 1. Immunospecific adsorption of prothrombins from solubilized rat liver microsomes

Adsorbant	Echis carinatus activatable protein (thrombin units/g liver)	
	Before Immunoadsorption	After Immunoadsorption
Anti-prothrombin/Sepharose		
Exp. 1	20	N.D.[a] (<3)
Exp. 2	23	N.D.
Non-Immune IgG/ Sepharose		
Exp. 1	19	20
Exp. 2	22	21

[a] N.D. = not detectable

However, similar adsorption studies with microsomal preparations labeled with $H^{14}CO_3^-$ in the presence of vitamin K indicated that the immunoadsorbant was capable of removing only 25% of the ^{14}C-labeled proteins (Table 2). The small amount of $H^{14}CO_3^-$ incorporated into protein in the absence of vitamin K was not adsorbed significantly to the anti-prothrombin/Sepharose. It was concluded from these findings that additional proteins other than prothrombin were participating in the vitamin K-dependent carboxylation reaction.

TABLE 2. Vitamin K-dependent incorporation of $H^{14}CO_3^-$ into microsomal protein of rat liver

	^{14}C-labeled Protein (dpm/g liver x 10^{-3})		
	-K	+K	
	Exp. 1	Exp. 1	Exp. 2
Before Immunoadsorption	4	118	91
After Immunoadsorption	4	94 (80%)	68 (75%)
Amount Adsorbed	< 0.2	24 (20%)	23 (25%)

This conclusion was confirmed by characterizing both the immuno-specifically retained and unadsorbed proteins via SDS-polyacrylamide electrophoresis. These results are presented in Figure 1 and indicate that the protein(s) retained by anti-prothrombin/Sepharose were either prothrombin precursors and/or mature prothrombin. This identification was based upon 1) immunochemical isolation, 2) comparison with mature prothrombin, i.e., approximate molecular weight of 75,000 daltons (17) and 3) activation with E. carinatus venom (Table 1). Similar analysis of the unadsorbed proteins, however, revealed three major peaks of ^{14}C-proteins possessing molecular weight of approximately 60,000 (peak 2), 50,000 (peak 3) and 20,000 (peak 4) daltons. The inability to detect radioactivity in the 70 - 80,000 molecular weight region of the gel again demonstrated the effectiveness of the anti-prothrombin/Sepharose to quantitatively and exclusively retain microsomal prothrombins.

Additional information regarding the rate of carboxylation of these proteins is presented in Figure 2. These data revealed that the vitamin K-dependent incorporation of $H^{14}CO_3^-$ into these proteins paralleled each other and was essentially maximum at 15 min in each case. That the ^{14}C incorporated into prothrombin as well as proteins 2, 3 and 4 was presumably due to the formation of γ-^{14}C-Gla was provided by the findings that about 50% of the radioactivity was removed from these proteins when subjected to acid hydrolysis in 6 N HCl (Table 3).

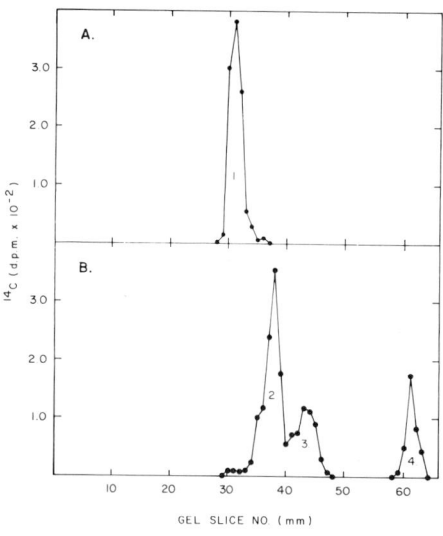
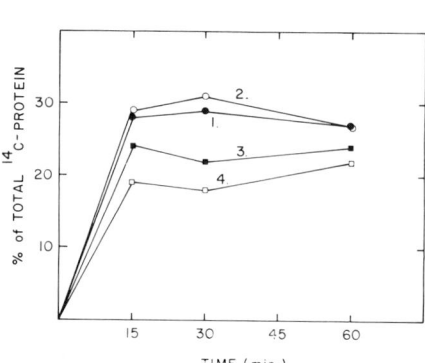

Figure 1. SDS-polyacrylamide gel electrophoresis of immunospecifically adsorbed (A.) and unadsorbed (B.) ^{14}C-labeled proteins carboxylated by vitamin K in vitro. The direction of migration is from left to right towards the anode.

Figure 2. Rates of formation of vitamin K-dependent carboxylated proteins. 1 (●), prothrombin (Fig. 1A.). 2 (o), 3 (■), 4 (□) refer to peaks 2, 3 and 4 Figure 1B.

TABLE 3. Effect of acid hydrolysis in 6 N HCl on ^{14}C-labeled protein

	% of Initial ^{14}C	
	Before Immunoadsorption	After Immunoadsorption
Before acid hydrolysis	100	100
After acid hydrolysis	47	53

The ^{14}C-labeled protein isolated by the anti-prothrombin/Sepharose (peak 1, Fig. 1A.) was further characterized by isoelectric focusing (Fig. 3). The only significant peak of radioactivity migrated with an apparent pI of 7.2. These data indicate that essentially the only product of the vitamin K-dependent carboxylation of the precursor prothrombins is the pI 7.2 form and that little or no further processing of this protein occurs under these experimental conditions (the pI of mature prothrombin in plasma is 5.0).

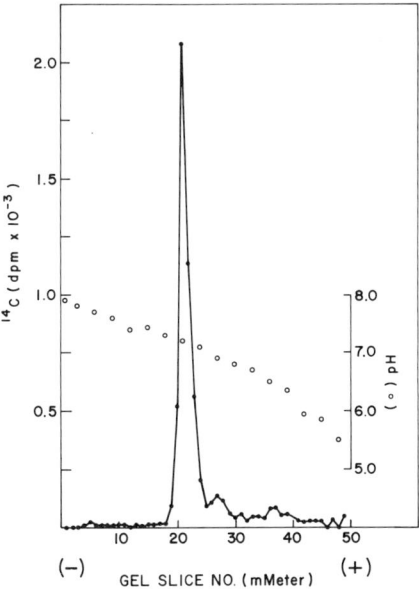

Figure 3. Isoelectric focusing of immunospecifically adsorbed ^{14}C-labeled protein carboxylated by vitamin K in vitro. (●) Radioactivity, (○) pH gradient.

DISCUSSION

The immunochemical techniques used in these studies resulted in the quantitative and exclusive isolation of prothrombin precursors and their vitamin K-dependent carboxylated products produced in liver microsomes. A ^{14}C-labeled protein was obtained that had a molecular weight of 75,000 daltons and a pI of 7.2 (Figs. 1A. and 3). Although the molecular weight is indistinguishable from that of rat prothrombin (17), further processing (i.e. core glycosylation, addition of sialic acid) is required before mature prothrombin (pI 5.0) is produced. The requirements for this transformation were not met in these experiments. An unexpected result obtained in these studies was that the formation of the pI 7.2 prothrombin accounted for such a small amount (25%) of the vitamin K-dependent incorporation of $H^{14}CO_3^-$ into protein with the remaining radioactivity being accounted for in proteins immunochemically and physically different from prothrombin.

It might be assumed that the major portion of the ^{14}C-labeled proteins reported here (peaks 2 and 3, Fig. 1B.) represent carboxylated vitamin K-dependent factors VII, IX and X (23-27). This assumption, however, appears untenable since the concentrations of these clotting factors in blood plasma are considerably less than prothrombin (i.e., <10%) (2). Thus, it would not be expected that their precursors would accumulate to an extent that would allow the synthesis of the high amounts of carboxylated products observed in these experiments. The lowest molecular weight ^{14}C-labeled protein observed in these studies (peak 4, Fig. 1B.) is probably not a breakdown N-terminal fragment of prothrombin or other vitamin K-dependent clotting factor (which could contain Gla residues) due to the following reasons: 1) protease inhibitors (soybean trypsin inhibitor and phenylmethyl-sulfonyl fluoride) were present during homogenization of livers and incubations; 2) there was no lag observed in the formation of peak 4 concomitant with a decrease in radioactivity in any of the other species (Fig. 2); 3) antibodies elicited in response to rat prothrombin have been shown to have binding affinity for N-terminal regions of rat prothrombin (28) which would have resulted in the absorption and subsequent appearance of ^{14}C in the low molecular weight region of Fig. 1A.

The carboxylated proteins that were not immunoadsorbed probably do not represent single proteins, with the possible exception of peak 4, since there are small shoulders accompanying both peaks 2 and 3. Unfortunately we have no data indicating the function of these other proteins (i.e., are they structural or pre-secretory?). However, these studies indicate that prothrombin is only one of many proteins carboxylated by vitamin K in solubilized microsomes from rat liver.

ACKNOWLEDGEMENTS

This work was supported by NIH grants HL-20577 and HL-15619.

REFERENCES

1. Suttie, J.W. and Jackson, C.M. (1977) Physiol. Rev. 57, 1-70.
2. Stenflo, J. and Suttie, J.W. (1977) Ann. Rev. Biochem. 46, 157-172.
3. Stenflo, J. (1976) J. Biol. Chem. 251, 355-363.
4. DiScipio, R.G. and Davie, E.W. (1979) Biochemistry 18, 899-904.
5. Prowse, C.V. and Esnouf, M.P. (1977) Biochem. Soc. Trans. 5, 255-256.
6. Hauschka, P.V., Lian, J.B. and Gallop, P.M. (1975) Proc. Natl. Acad. Sci. USA 72, 3925-3929.
7. Price, P.A., Otsuka, A.S., Poser, J.W., Kristaponis, J. and Raman, N. (1976) Proc. Natl. Acad. Sci. USA 73, 1447-1451.
8. Hauschka, P.V., Friedman, P.A., Traverso, H.P. and Gallop, P.M. (1976) Biochem. Biophys. Res. Commun. 71, 1207-1213.
9. Lian, J.B. and Prien, E.L. (1976) Fed. Proc. 35, 1763 (Abstr.)

10. Esmon, C.T. and Suttie, J.W. (1976) J. Biol. Chem. 251, 6238-6243.
11. Mack, D.O., Suen, E.T., Girardot, J.M., Miller, J.A., Delaney, R. and Johnson, B.C. (1976) J. Biol. Chem. 251, 3269-3276.
12. Jones, J.P., Gardner, E.J., Cooper, T.G. and Olson, R.E. (1977) J. Biol. Chem. 252, 7738-7742.
13. Wallin, R., Gebhardt, O. and Prydz, H. (1978) Biochem. J. 169, 95-101.
14. Morrissey, J.J., Jones, J.P. and Olson, R.E. (1973) Biochem. Biophys. Res. Commun. 54, 1075-1082.
15. Esmon, C.T., Grant, G.A. and Suttie, J.W. (1975) Biochemistry 14, 1595-1600.
16. Grant, G.A. and Suttie, J.W. (1976) Biochemistry 15, 5387-5393.
17. Grant, G.A. and Suttie, J.W. (1976) Arch. Biochem. Biophys. 176, 650-662.
18. Graves, C.B., Grabau, G.G. and Munns, T.W. (1979) Fed. Proc. 38, 620 (Abstr.).
19. Graves, C.B., Grabau, G.G. and Munns, T.W. (1979) in "Vitamin K Metabolism and Vitamin K-Dependent Proteins" (J.W. Suttie, ed.) University Park Press, Baltimore, in press.
20. Esmon, C.T., Sadowski, J.A. and Suttie, J.W. (1975) J. Biol. Chem. 250, 4744-4748.
21. Laemmli, V.K. (1970) Nature (London) 227, 680-685.
22. Shah, D.V., Suttie, J.W. and Grant G.A. (1973) Arch. Biochem. Biophys. 159, 483-491.
23. Fujikawa, K., Legaz, M.E. and Davie, E.W. (1972) Biochemistry 11, 4882-4891.
24. Fujikawa, K., Thompson, A.R., Legaz, M.E., Meyer, R.G. and Davie, E.W. (1973) Biochemistry 12, 4938-4945.
25. Titani, K., Fujikawa, K., Enfield, D.L., Ericsson, L.H., Walsh, K.A. and Neurath, H. (1975) Proc. Natl. Acad. Sci. USA 72, 3082-3086.
26. DiScipio, R.G., Hermodson, M.A., Yates, S.G. and Davie, E.W. (1977) Biochemistry 16, 698-706.
27. Kisiel, W. and Davie, E.W. (1975) Biochemistry 14, 4928-4934.
28. Furie, B., Provost, K.L., Blanchard, R.A. and Furie, B.C. (1978) J. Biol. Chem. 253, 8980-8987.

SOME CHARACTERISTICS OF PURIFIED BOVINE PROTHROMBIN SYNTHASE

M. DE METZ, C. VERMEER, B. A. M. SOUTE, and
H. C. HEMKER

Department of Biochemistry
State University of Limburg, MAASTRICHT
The Netherlands

INTRODUCTION

The synthesis of prothrombin requires a post-ribosomal step, in which 10 glutamic acid residues are converted into γ-carboxyglutamic acid (gla) residues (1,2).
During the last few years several groups have reported the development of a rat-liver cell-free system, that was able to incorporate $^{14}CO_2$ into an endogenous prothrombin precursor, which had accumulated in the microsomal fraction of vitamin K-deficient rats (3-7).
Since in these systems the enzyme and its substrate were present in the same fraction, the purification of the carboxylating enzyme was not taken up before a synthetic pentapeptide had been prepared which could serve as an exogenous substrate because it was analogous to a glu-containing part of the prothrombin precursor, decarboxyprothrombin (3,8).
In the same time we developed and partly purified a similar enzyme system, derived from bovine liver (9,10). The enzyme, which we called prothrombin synthase, was obtained from normal cow livers, and its substrate, decarboxyprothrombin, was obtained and purified from the plasma of coumarin-treated cows.
The amount of newly synthesized prothrombin was used as a measure for the enzyme activity and was routinely assayed with the one-stage coagulation assay. In order to compare the bovine prothrombin-synthesizing system with that obtained from the rat, three questions had to be resolved:
a. is the reaction product really prothrombin?
b. is vitamin K involved in the reaction?
c. is decarboxyprothrombin carboxylated in parallel to its conversion into prothrombin?

In the present communication we wish to report about our efforts to answer these questions.

MATERIALS AND METHODS

Reagents, chemicals, and buffers

Thromboplastin and a reagent for the one-stage determination of prothrombin were prepared as described earlier (11, 12).
Vitamin K_1, warfarin and Triton X-100 were obtained from Sigma, USA. Cl-K (2-Chloro-3-phytyl-1,4-naphtoquinone) was a kind gift of Dr.Suttie. Reduced vitamin K (KH_2) was prepared by adding 0.5 mg of $NaBH_3$ to 1 ml of a solution containing 10 mg of vitamin K_1. Vitamin K epoxide (KO) was prepared as described by Fieser et al. (13).

NaH $^{14}CO_3$ (60 Ci/mol) was obtained from the Radiochemical Centre, Amersham, Great Britain and Aquasol-2 from New England Nuclear, USA. The amidolytic thrombin reagent S 2238 was purchased from AB Kabi Diagnostica, Sweden. All other chemicals were from Merck, GFR.

Buffer A: 50 mM KCl, 200 mM sucrose, 20 mM Tris-HCl.
Buffer B: 50 mM KCl, 0.1 % Triton X-100, 20 mM Tris-HCl.
Buffer C: 250 mM KCl, 0.1 % Triton X-100, 20 mM Tris-HCl.
Buffer D: 50 mM KCl, 20 mM Tris-HCl.
All buffers were adjusted to a pH of 7.8 at $4^{\circ}C$.

Protein determination

The protein concentration in our samples was assessed after removal of the Triton X-100 by extraction with isoamyl alcohol as described by Mather and Tamplin (14).

Coagulation factors, assays and definition of units

Bovine prothrombin was purified according to Owen et al. (15) and decarboxyprothrombin as reported earlier (16). The prothrombin concentration was assessed with the one-stage coagulation assay (12). The amount of prothrombin, present in our reference plasma (11) was assumed to be about 100 µg/ml or 1 U/ml (17).
One unit of prothrombin synthase is defined as the amount of enzyme, that is able to convert decarboxyprothrombin into prothrombin at a rate of 1 µMole per minute at $37^{\circ}C$.

Gel electrophoresis

Crossed immuno-electrophoresis in 1 % agarose gels was performed as described by Stenflo and Ganrot (18) using a buffer system containing 2 mM Ca-lactate and 0.05 M barbital buffer, pH 8.6. Samples containing about 0.5 µg of antigen were applied to each well.

Measurement of prothrombin synthesis

In our routine tests, reaction mixtures of 0.1 ml containing 10^{-6} U/ml prothrombin synthase, 0.6 µM decarboxyprothrombin, 5 % ethanol (v/v) and 1 mM $MnCl_2$ in buffer C were incubated at $37^{\circ}C$ for 1 h and subsequently diluted five fold with cold buffer D. Prothrombin synthase was defined as the activity that is able to increase the prothrombin concentration (measured with the one-stage coagulation assay) in the reaction mixture during the incubation at $37^{\circ}C$.

Preparation and partial purification of prothrombin synthase

Crude microsomes (10) from 500 g bovine liver were supplemented with Triton X-100 to a final concentration of 2 %, incubated at $0^{\circ}C$ for 30 minutes and centrifuged for 1½ h at 150,000 x g. The supernatant was applied to a Sepharose 4 B column (10 x 120 cm) in buffer B (Fig. 1 A). The fractions containing prothrombin synthase activity were pooled, concentrated by batchwise absorption onto DEAE Sephadex (1.5 g/l), followed by elution with buffer C. The eluate was dialyzed against buffer B and applied to a DEAE Sephacel column (1 x 30 cm). Prothrombin synthase was eluted with a linear gradient (2 x 250 ml) from buffer B to buffer C (Fig. 1 B). Two activity peaks were eluted indicating that at least two forms of prothrombin synthase were present in the original preparation. The fractions containing prothrombin synthase with a high specific activity were pooled as indicated, concentrated and applied to a Sephadex G-100 column (2 x 100 cm, Fig. 1 C) in buffer B. The position at which the enzyme was eluted from the column was compared with that of five reference proteins and correspond with a molecular weight of approximately 60,000 D. The active fractions were pooled and frozen at $-70^{\circ}C$ in 0.5 ml portions. When analyzed on polyacrylamide gels in SDS, the preparation still contained three protein bands.

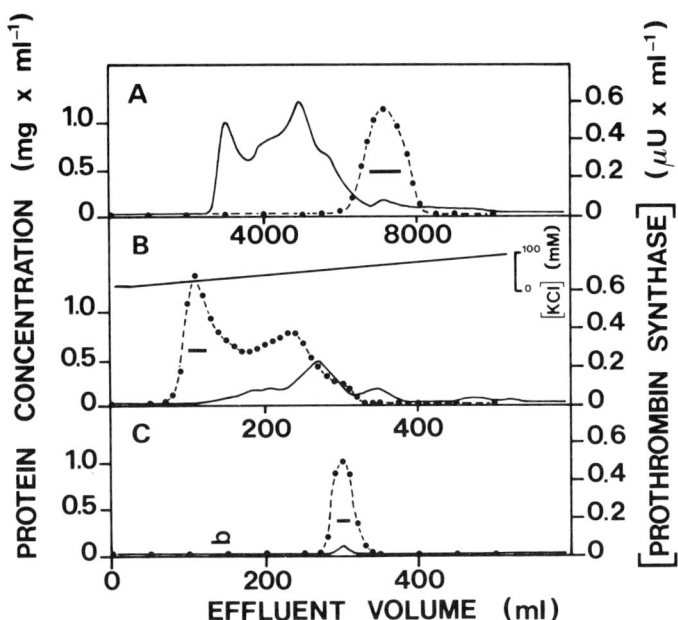

FIGURE 1. Partial purification of prothrombin synthase.
Prothrombin synthase was solubilized from washed microsomes with Triton X-100 and fractionated on Sepharose 4 B (Fig. 1 A), DEAE Sephacel (Fig. 1 B) and Sephadex G-100 (Fig. 1 C). For further details, see text.

Extraction of vitamin K from prothrombin synthase

Warfarin was added to prothrombin synthase to a final concentration of 50 mM and ethanol to a final concentration of 5 % (v/v). The mixture was incubated for 1 h in ice and then extracted once with an equal volume of a mixture containing isopropanol : hexane = 3 : 7 and twice with hexane alone. Subsequently the water phase was supplied with Triton X-100 to a final concentration of 0.1 % and dialyzed against buffer B.

RESULTS

A. Analysis of synthesized prothrombin

The product that was formed during the incubation of decarboxyprothrombin in the presence of prothrombin synthase was compared with normal bovine prothrombin in several ways. The reaction product appeared to be indistinguishable from prothrombin with respect to its behaviour on Sephadex G-100 and DEAE Sephadex columns (see section C), and to its ability to absorb onto $BaSO_4$ (not shown here). No thrombin had been formed during the synthase reaction as the chromogenic substrate S 2238 was not split upon incubation for 4 h at 37°C. Moreover, the reaction product showed no reaction with fibrinogen. An analysis of the reaction product by crossed immunoelectrophoresis is shown in fig. 2.

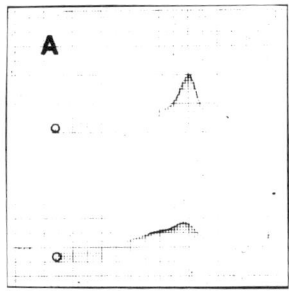 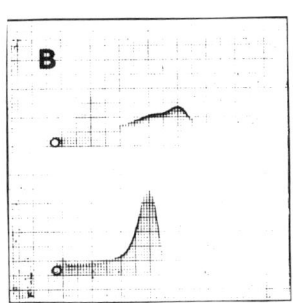 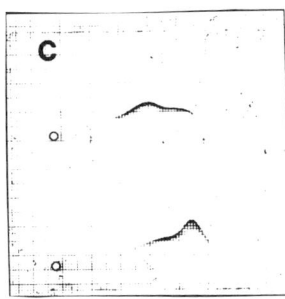

FIGURE 2. Analysis of synthesized prothrombin by crossed immuno electrophoresis.
A: Standard reaction mixture before (upper well) and after (lower well) incubation.
B: Standard reaction mixture after incubation (upper well) and purified prothrombin (lower well, 0.5 μg).
C: Standard reaction mixtures after incubation. Electrophoresis was run in the presence (upper well) and absence (lower well) of purified prothrombin (0.2 μg).

Before incubation only decarboxyprothrombin was present in the reaction mixture and one single peak was observed; after 1 h at 37°C a second peak appeared (Fig. 2 A). This new peak was compared with prothrombin (Fig. 2 B) and with a mixture of prothrombin and the reaction product (Fig. 2 C). It is clear that the in vitro synthesized prothrombin differs from decarboxyprothrombin and is indistinguishable from normal prothrombin in these experiments.

B. Prothrombin synthesis and vitamin K

The in vitro synthesis of prothrombin in our system occurred in the absence of externally added vitamin K. Moreover, additional amounts of the vitamin hardly stimulated the reaction. So we had to assume that endogenous vitamin K was present in our enzyme preparation. This could easily be explained by the fact that prothrombin synthase was obtained from non-anticoagulated cows. The presence of this endogenous vitamin K became more likely when we succeeded in inhibiting the reaction with known inhibitors of vitamin K. Rather high concentrations of warfarin were required to inhibit the reaction (Fig. 3 A), whereas Cl-K inhibited the reaction at about 50 times lower concentrations (Fig. 3 B). It should be noted that even higher concentrations of warfarin were required for an inhibition of the reaction, when ethanol was omitted from the reaction mixture.

After we had ascertained that physiological vitamin K inhibitors also inhibited the in vitro prothrombin synthesis we tried to separate the vitamin from the enzyme by extraction with organic solvents. The best results were obtained after extraction with a mixture of isopropanol and hexane in the presence of warfarin (see Materials and Methods). After this extraction the enzyme became unstable and lost its activity within 48 hours. The extracted enzyme showed a considerably reduced activity, which could only be restored to its normal level by adding reduced vitamin K (KH_2). Neither vitamin K nor vitamin K epoxide (KO) had any effect on the enzyme activity (Fig. 4).

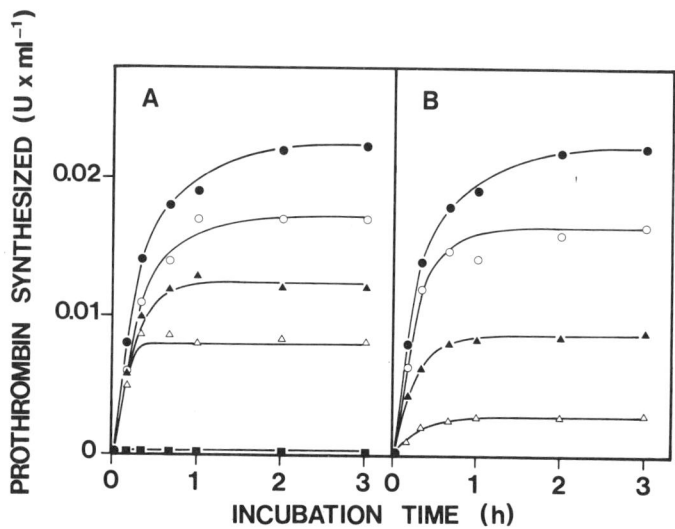

FIGURE 3. Inhibition of in vitro prothrombin synthesis.
A: Prothrombin synthesis in the presence of varying concentrations of warfarin; ● — ●, 0 mM; o — o, 1 mM; ▲—▲, 2 mM; △—△, 5 mM; ■—■, 10 mM.
B: Prothrombin synthesis in the presence of varying concentrations of Cl-K; ● — ●, 0 μM; o — o, 10 μM; ▲—▲, 50 μM; △—△, 200 μM.

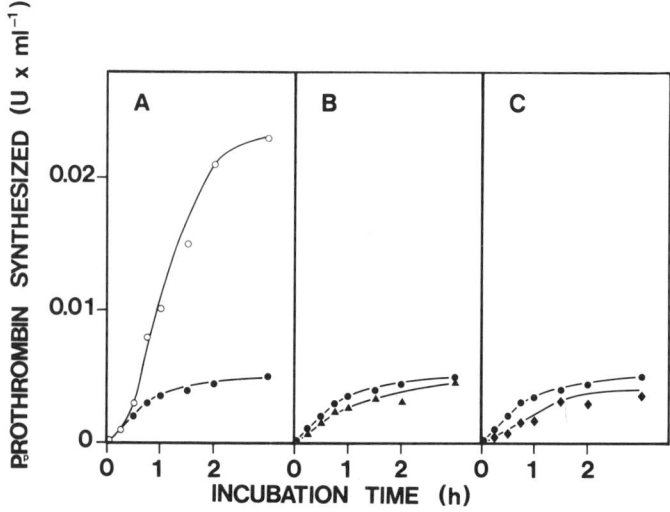

FIGURE 4. Stimulation of prothrombin synthesis by vitamin KH_2.
Endogenous vitamin K was removed from prothrombin synthase by extraction with a mixture of isopropanol and hexane (See Materials and Methods), and the extracted enzyme was assayed for its prothrombin synthesizing ability

in the absence of vitamin K (● — ●) and in the presence of 20 μM of either vitamin KH_2 (o — o), vitamin K (▲—▲) or vitamin K epoxide (◆—◆). The various vitamin K preparations were added to the reaction mixtures as ethanol solutions.

C. Prothrombin synthesis and carboxylation

In order to resolve the question whether carboxylation is involved in the observed generation of prothrombin activity we added 50 μCi $NaH^{14}CO_3$ to 1 ml reaction mixtures. After incubation at 37°C the incubation mixtures were analyzed on Sephadex G-100 columns (Fig. 5). It turned out that some label had been incorporated into high molecular weight material and that this incorporation only took place in the presence of both, prothrombin synthase and decarboxyprothrombin. Furthermore, the incorporated label as well as the newly synthesized prothrombin eluted from the column at the same position as did prothrombin and decarboxyprothrombin. The label could be precipitated quantitatively with TCA and after acid hydrolysis half of the radioactivity was left. Since decarboxyprothrombin was added in a highly purified form, only protein that could have been carboxylated is decarboxyprothrombin itself.

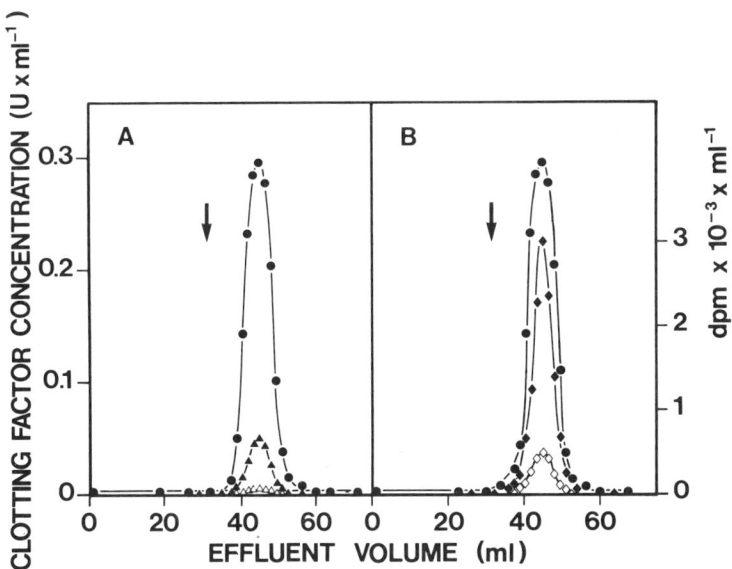

FIGURE 5. Fractionation of protein-bound $NaH^{14}CO_3$ on Sephadex G-100. Reaction mixtures (1 ml) containing 50 μCi $NaH^{14}CO_3$ were incubated at 37°C and the reaction was stopped by adding 10 volumes of cold buffer B. Prothrombin and decarboxyprothrombin were adsorbed to DEAE Sephadex (1 ml slurry) which was brought into a column and unbound $NaH^{14}CO_3$ was removed by washing with at least 2 l of a buffer containing 10 mM $NaHCO_3$ in buffer B. Subsequently the bound proteins were eluted with 0.5 M NaCl in buffer B and applied to a Sephadex G-100 column. Fractions of 1 ml were eluted and assayed for prothrombin activity with the one-stage coagulation assay, with the Echis carinatus assay and for incorporated $NaH^{14}CO_3$ by supplementing 0.5 ml aliquots of each fraction with 10 ml of aquasol and counting them in a Packard Tricarb scintillation counter.

●—●, decarboxyprothrombin + prothrombin tested with Echis carinatus venom;
△—△, prothrombin activity before incubation;
▲—▲, prothrombin activity after incubation
◇—◇, dpm before incubation
◆---◆, dpm after incubation.

When similar $NaH^{14}CO_3$-containing reaction mixtures were analyzed on DEAE Sephadex columns, the newly formed prothrombin was eluted at a slightly higher salt concentration (Fig. 6) than decarboxyprothrombin does. Moreover, the incorporated label eluted from the column in the prothrombin containing fractions only. So it appeared, that the incorporated label could not be separated from the in vitro synthesized prothrombin and we therefore concluded that the latter protein was the product of the observed carboxylation reaction.

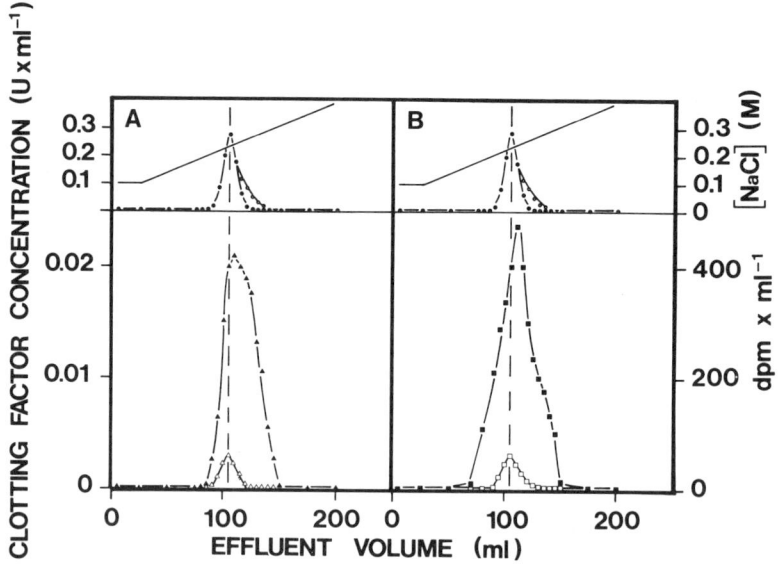

FIGURE 6. Fractionation of protein-bound $NaH^{14}CO_3$ on DEAE Sephadex. Similar reaction mixtures as those described in the legend to Figure 5 were applied to DEAE Sephadex columns (1 x 20 cm) immediately after incubation at 37°C. The columns were washed with at least 2 l of 10 mM $NaHCO_3$ in buffer B and subsequently a linear gradient (2 x 100 ml) was applied from 100 to 400 ml NaCl in 20 mM Tris-HCl, pH 7.4. Fractions of 2 ml were collected and assayed as described in the legend to Figure 5. Decarboxyprothrombin + prothrombin tested with Echis carinatus venom before (●—●), and after (o—o) incubation; prothrombin activity before (△—△), and after (▲—▲) incubation and incorporated label before (□—□), and after (■—■) incubation.

D. Prothrombin synthesis at varying reaction conditions

With the vitamin K-dependent enzyme, its substrate and separately obtained vitamin K, we were able to investigate the reaction kinetics at limiting concentrations of each one of these reaction components. It turned out that the enzyme concentration only determines the initial reaction rate, but not the end point of the reaction (Fig. 7 A). On the other hand, lowering the concentration of either decarboxyprothrombin or vitamin KH_2 hardly decreased the initial reaction rate but caused a substantial reduction of the total amount of synthesized prothrombin (Fig. 7 B and 7 C). In these experiments it is striking that decarboxyprothrombin seems to be a poor substrate for the reaction since at most 3-5 % of it was converted into prothrombin at all conditions measured (see further discussion).

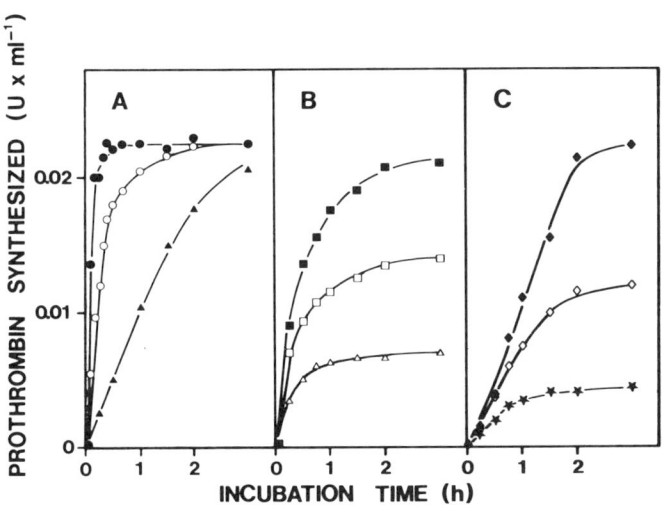

FIGURE 7. Prothrombin synthesis at varying concentrations of prothrombin synthase, decarboxyprothrombin and vitamin KH_2.
A: Decarboxyprothrombin (0.6 μM) and vitamin KH_2 (20 μM) were incubated at standard conditions in the presence of varying concentrations of prothrombin synthase. ▲—▲, 0.1 μU/ml; ○—○, 1.0 μU/ml; ●—●, 2 μU/ml.
B: Prothrombin synthase (1 μU/ml) and vitamin KH_2 (20 μM) were incubated with varying concentrations of decarboxyprothrombin. △—△, 0.15 μM; □—□, 0.3 μM; ■—■, 0.6 μM.
C: Prothrombin synthase (1 μU/ml) and decarboxyprothrombin (0.6 μM) were incubated in the presence of varying concentrations of vitamin KH_2. ✶—✶, 0 μM; ◇—◇, 5 μM; ◆—◆, 20 μM.

Since prothrombin synthesis was inhibited by EDTA, we tried to remove bivalent metal ions by adding 0.1 M EDTA to prothrombin synthase, followed by dialysis against buffer B. The EDTA treated enzyme had lost its activity and this activity could be restored by adding 1 mM $MnCl_2$ to the reaction mixture. Other bivalent ions were far less effective in this respect, and Cu^{2+} turned out to be a potent inhibitor. Although Mn^{2+} is known to play a role in the binding of CO_2 in many carboxylating enzymes, a similar function during prothrombin synthesis cannot yet be concluded from our experiments, however.

DISCUSSION

In the present paper we describe the isolation from bovine liver of an enzyme which is able to generate prothrombin activity from decarboxyprothrombin. The observed increase in the procoagulant activity of decarboxyprothrombin cannot be ascribed to a conversion of the latter into thrombin because:
a. the molecular weight of the reaction product is similar to that of decarboxyprothrombin and is much higher than that of thrombin;
b. the reaction product does not react with the amidolytic substrate S 2238, or with fibrinogen.

The alternative explanation is that decarboxyprothrombin is converted into prothrombin and this explanation was supported by experiments in which the reaction product was analyzed with the aid of twodimensional immunoelectrophoresis. Before incubation at $37^{\circ}C$ the reaction mixture contained only decarboxyprothrombin that precipitated in a symmetrical peak. After 1 h at $37^{\circ}C$ a second peak arose that was indistinguishable from normal prothrombin. Moreover, we showed that
a. vitamin K is involved in prothrombin synthesis, and
b. decarboxyprothrombin is carboxylated during this reaction.

The involvement of vitamin K was demonstrated by the inhibiting effect of known vitamin K-inhibitors. In agreement with the observations of others (3), we found that rather high concentrations (10 mM) of warfarin were required for a complete inhibition of prothrombin synthesis. The vitamin K antagonist Cl-K turned out to be a much more potent inhibitor since 200 µM effectively inhibited the reaction.

The direct proof that vitamin K is present on native prothrombin synthase was furnished by experiments in which we extracted the vitamin from the enzyme with organic solvents. In the water phase about 20% of the residual prothrombin synthase activity was left, which could be stimulated 3-4 fold by adding vitamin KH_2. Neither vitamin K nor its epoxide were effective in this respect. In the organic phase preliminary experiments showed the presence of vitamin K (unpublished results).

The increase in prothrombin procoagulant activity was shown to occur in parallel with the incorporation of $^{14}CO_2$ into protein. The label was demonstrated to elute together with prothrombin activity on DEAE Sephadex and Sephadex G-100 columns and could be precipitated with TCA. Moreover, acid hydrolysis caused half of the radioactivity to disappear which is characteristic for the presence of gla-residues containing one labeled carboxylgroup (19). We concluded that we had an in vitro prothrombin synthesizing system in which the enzyme (prothrombin synthase) converts its substrate (decarboxyprothrombin) into prothrombin in the presence of vitamin KH_2.

An important question which remains to be answered is: why does the reaction stop when about 3-5% of the decarboxyprothrombin is converted into prothrombin? The reason for this may be:
1. A shortage of one of the reaction components.
2. All decarboxyprothrombin is carboxylated, but less than 10 gla residues are introduced in the in vitro system. The procoagulant activity of this intermediate prothrombin is still very low.
3. During the reaction an inhibitor is synthesized.
4. Only a small part of the added decarboxyprothrombin is able to serve as a substrate for the reaction. This implies a heterogeneity of decarboxyprothrombin.

In Figure 7 it is shown that the amount of prothrombin synthesis is independent of the enzyme concentration over a wide range of concentrations. Only the initial reaction rate varied proportional to the prothrombin synthase concentration. Therefore, it is unlikely that a shortage of the enzyme or an enzyme-bound cofactor would determine the end point of the reaction. The possibility that all decarboxyprothrombin is carboxylated only at one site is excluded by the experiments in which the reaction mixtures were analyzed by crossed immunoelectrophoresis (Fig. 2). These experiments showed that most of the decarboxyprothrombin remains unchanged and that a small part of it is transformed into a protein with the same electrophoretic mobility as exhibited by prothrombin. Thus it seems that only some decarboxyprothrombin is carboxylated but that when carboxylation has started the molecule is converted into prothrombin and not into partly carboxylated intermediates.

When the end point of the reaction would be determined by an inhibitor which is formed during incubation at 37°C, we have to conclude that the inhibiting effect can be overcome by adding more decarboxyprothrombin and not by adding prothrombin synthase. This type of inhibition would be expected for a competitive inhibition of the reaction by its own product, prothrombin.

In experiments with less purified prothrombin synthase we indeed observed an inhibitory effect of externally added prothrombin (10), but in more purified enzyme systems prothrombin synthesis was observed even after adding 0.05 U/ml of prothrombin to the reaction mixtures, which is twice the end level of the reaction. Therefore another explanation for the low conversion of decarboxyprothrombin has to be found and we are inclined to think that the bulk of the decarboxyprothrombin is not a suitable substrate for prothrombin synthase and that only 3 - 5 % of it is capable of being transformed into prothrombin. In that case the end point of the reaction is reached because of a lack of substrate, whereas a considerable amount of inactive decarboxyprothrombin is left. Obviously a difference must exist between the active and inactive substrate, but up to now we did not succeed in separating two forms of decarboxyprothrombin.

REFERENCES

1. Stenflo, J., Fernlund, P., Egan, W., and Roepstorff, P. (1974) Proc. Natl.Acad.Sci. USA 71, 2730-2733.
2. Nelsestuen, G.L., Zytkovicz, T.H., and Howard, J.B. (1974) J.Biol. Chem. 249, 6347-6350.
3. Suttie, J.W., Lehrman, S.R., Geweke, L.O., Hageman, J.M., and Rich, D.H. (1979) Biochem.Biophys.Res.Comm. 86, 500-507.
4. Jones, J.P., Gardner, E.J., Cooper, T.G., and Olson, R.E. (1977) J.Biol.Chem. 252, 7738-7742.
5. Friedman, P.A., and Shia, M. (1976) Biochem.Biophys.Res.Comm. 70, 647-654.
6. Mack, D.O., Suen, E.T., Girardot, J.M., Miller, J.A., Delaney, R., and Johnson, B.C. (1976) J.Biol.Chem. 251, 3269-3276.
7. Esnouf, M.P., Green, M.R., Hill, H.A.O., Irvine, G.B., and Walter, S.J. (1978) Biochem.J. 174, 345-348,
8. Suttie, J.W., Hageman, J.M., Lehrman, S.R., and Rich, D.H. (1976) J.Biol.Chem. 251, 5827-5830.
9. Vermeer, C., Soute, B.A.M., Govers-Riemslag, J.W.P., and Hemker, H.C. (1976) Biochim.Biophys.Acta 444, 926-930.
10. Vermeer, C., Soute, B.A.M., and Hemker, H.C. (1978) Biochim.Biophys. Acta 523, 494-505.
11. Vermeer, C., Soute, B.A.M., and Hemker, H.C. (1977) Thrombos.Res. 10, 495-507.
12. Vermeer, C., Soute, B.A.M., and Hemker, H.C. (1978) Thrombos.Res. 12, 713-716.
13. Fieser, L.F., Tishler, M., and Sampson, W.L. (1941) J.Biol.Chem. 137, 659-692.

14. Mather, I.H., and Tamplin, C.B. (1979) Anal.Biochem. 93, 139-142.
15. Owen, W.G., Esmon, C.T., and Jackson, C.M. (1974) J.Biol.Chem. 249, 594-605.
16. Vermeer, C., Govers-Riemslag, J.W.P., Soute, B.A.M., Lindhout, M.J., Kop, J., and Hemker, H.C. (1978) Biochim.Biophys.Acta 538, 521-533.
17. Suttie, J.W., and Jackson, C.M. (1977) Physiol.Rev. 57, 1-70.
18. Stenflo, J., and Ganrot, P.O. (1972) J.Biol.Chem. 247, 8160-8166.
19. Tuan, R.S. (1979) J.Biol.Chem. 254, 1356-1364.

MECHANISM OF WARFARIN INHIBITION OF PROTHROMBIN COMPLEX GLYCOSYLATION

D. COURI and R. G. MEEKS

Ohio State University College of Medicine
Columbus, OH 43210

INTRODUCTION

It is well established that the functional role of vitamin K is to stimulate the post-translational carboxylation of specific glutamic acid residues in the prothrombin molecule (1-4). It has further been shown that the indirect acting coumarin anticoagulants, including warfarin, can block the incorporation of CO_2 into these glutamic acid residues (2-3). However, studies performed in our laboratory suggest that vitamin K and the indirect acting anticoagulants may have an alternative site of action (5-11) which is summarized in this report. Pereira and Couri (5-7) have shown in whole animal studies that warfarin can block the incorporation of glucosamine into prothrombin. Upon administration of vitamin K to warfarin-treated animals, the rate of incorporation of glucosamine into prothrombin increased, and paralleled the rate of return of normal plasma prothrombin activity. The effect of these agents on glycosylation was also demonstrated in rat liver slices (7). Incorporation of glucosamine into prothrombin and in glycolipids was decreased when liver slices were incubated for 3 hr in 2×10^{-5} M dicoumarol.

RESULTS AND DISCUSSION

Subcellular distribution studies (11) of [^{3}H] glucosamine incorporation into liver proteins of warfarin-treated rats demonstrated that warfarin inhibited the incorporation of glucosamine into the rough and smooth microsomal fractions (Table 1). Administration of vitamin K to warfarinized rats reversed this inhibition. Neither warfarin nor vitamin K had an effect on glucosamine incorporation in any of the other subcellular fractions.

TABLE 1

SUBCELLULAR DISTRIBUTION OF [^{3}H]-GLUCOSAMINE IN RAT LIVER[a]

	P_1[b]	S_1[c]	P_2	S_2	P_3 (Rough Microsome)	S_3	P_4 (Smooth Microsome)	S_4
Control	3042	5669	4569	6452	15905	5010	18129	4804
Control + K_1	5952	5099	5807	4590	17765	5962	18350	5339
Warfarin	6610	5127	5354	5165	7102	6002	12129	4254
Warfarin + K_1	5889	4058	4944	4598	18310	5951	18710	4787

[a] Groups of 6-8 rats were administered warfarin (10 mg/kg) or saline 24 hrs prior to sacrifice. Three hours prior to sacrifice each rat was administered 5 μCi [^{3}H] glucosamine as well as saline or vitamin K_1 (5 mg/kg). At time of sacrifice, the livers were removed and fractionated according to the procedure of Lawford and Schacter (19). [b] P = pellet; results expressed as DPM/mg protein. [c] S = supernatant; results expressed as DPM/mg protein.

It has been shown that glycoproteins which have a common core oligosaccharide attached through an N-glycosidic linkage to an asparagine residue may be synthesized through a lipid-saccharide intermediate (12-14). In this synthetic route, a glucosamine residue is attached to the polyisoprenoid dolichol phosphate. This attachment is followed by the sequential addition of glycosyl residues to form an oligosaccharide-lipid. The oligosaccharide chain is then transferred to the asparagine residue of the nascent peptide molecule.

Prothrombin is a glycoprotein and Nelsestuen and Suttie (15) have determined the composition and structure of its oligosaccharide chain. Examination of their results reveal that the composition and structure of the core oligosaccharide is identical to the composition and structure of the core oligosaccharide of the glycoproteins that are synthesized through the lipid-saccharide mediated pathway.

We have shown that warfarin may act at the level of synthesis of the dolichol intermediate (9-11). Rats treated with warfarin showed a time-dependent decrease in the incorporation of glucosamine into liver prothrombin clotting activity as shown in Fig. 1A. Warfarin treatment also caused a time-dependent decrease in the incorporation of glucosamine into dolichol mono- and oligosaccharides (Fig. 1B) in a manner which paralleled the inhibition of glucosamine incorporation into liver prothrombin. The administration of vitamin K to warfarinized rats stimulated the incorporation of glucosamine into dolichol mono- and oligosaccharides. Again, the incorporation rate paralleled the rate of return of prothrombin activity in the plasma.

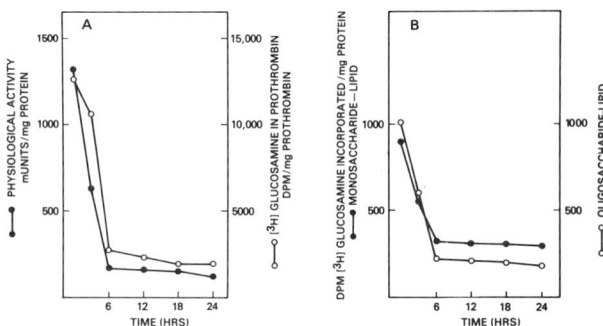

FIGURE 1. Effect of warfarin on prothrombin synthesis and glucosamine incorporation (A) as well as on the incorporation of glucosamine into lipid-saccharides (B).

Also, evidence to support that warfarin and vitamin K may act at the level of glycosylation comes from symptoms of manganese deficiency reported by Doisy (16). Evidence was presented for a coincident deficiency of vitamin K and manganese in man in which a patient was unable to increase his clotting protein levels to normal in response to a challenge of vitamin K. This effect was confirmed further using chickens as the model. Chickens deficient in both manganese and vitamin K exhibited a reduced ability to respond to vitamin K in elevating plasma clotting proteins. These actions were attributed to a probable need for manganese in the synthesis of glycoproteins. It was suggested by Doisy (16) that manganese acts to complete the biosynthesis of the glycoprotein clotting factors. This conclusion was based upon observations by Leach (17) who showed that manganese was necessary for optimal activity of glycosyltransferases in vitro.

Using partially purified enzyme systems, Pereira and Couri (5) showed that the site of action of warfarin and vitamin K was at the level of the glycosyltransferase enzymes. Waller and Couri (8) used ESR studies which yield insight into the immediate environment to examine the possible interactions between the glycosyltransferases, manganese, warfarin, and vitamin K.

Aqueous solutions of manganese gave an ESR signal with six symmetrical peaks. The addition of warfarin to the aqueous solution of manganese showed no change in the shape or the intensity of the ESR signal. Golgi membranes isolated from rats treated with a single dose (100 mg/kg) of warfarin gave a reduced manganese signal (Table 2) compared to animals treated with saline.

TABLE 2

MANGANESE ESR SIGNAL WITH GOLGI MEMBRANE FRACTIONS FROM WARFARIN TREATED RATS

	Signal Height (mm)	% Change
Control	50.8 ± 1.6	--
Warfarin	32.3 ± 2.2	36.5

Golgi membranes were isolated from rats four hours after treatment with warfarin (100 mg/kg) or saline diluent.

Golgi membranes isolated from untreated control rats were dialyzed against warfarin. The dialyzed membranes exhibited reductions in the observed ESR signal height which was dose related and was of the same nature as that observed from Golgi membranes isolated from rats treated with warfarin (Fig. 3). Using [^{14}C] UDP-N-Acetylglucosamine as the substrate in an enzyme assay for glycosyltransferase activity showed that membranes dialyzed against 5×10^{-4} M warfarin lost activity. However, the glycosyltransferase activity could be restored by adding 10 μM manganese, and maximal activity was obtained by the addition of 2 mM manganese. Treatment of Golgi membranes with lysolecithin and EDTA inhibited glycosyltransferase activity. The addition of several cations (Fig. 3) showed little, if any, effect on the enzymatic activity. But the addition of 10 mM manganese to the assay system effectively stimulated the Golgi membrane N-acetylglucosaminyl-transferase activity. Thus, on a molecular level it appears that warfarin may act at a site which directly or indirectly modifies the binding of manganese to glycosyltransferases involved in the synthesis of glycoprotein clotting factors as proposed by Doisy (16).

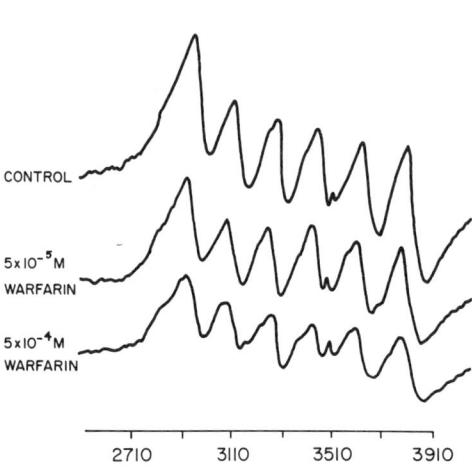

FIGURE 2. Effect of warfarin on manganese ESR signal height in Golgi membranes.

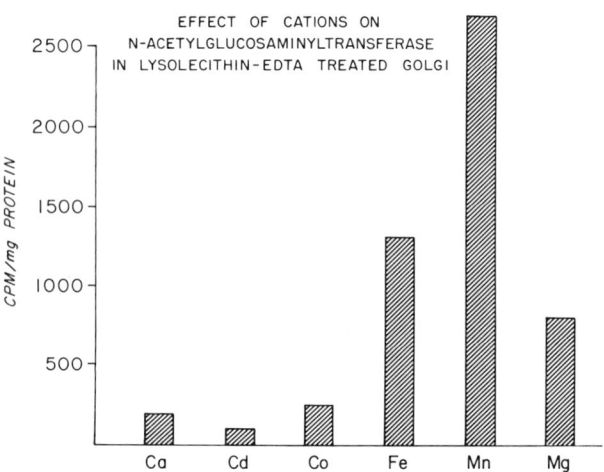

FIGURE 3. Effect of the addition of cations to Golgi membranes treated with lysolecithin and EDTA.

Therefore it appears that warfarin and vitamin K not only control post-translational carboxylation of glutamic acid residues in prothrombin but it also appears to control the post-translational attachment of carbohydrate moieties to the core protein. Our studies also indicate that prothrombin may be synthesized through a lipid-saccharide mediated pathway as shown for other glycoproteins including hen oviduct membranes and thyroglobulin. It is possible that the effect of warfarin and vitamin K on glycosylation of prothrombin is at the site of attachment of glucosamine residues to the lipid intermediate since the effect of warfarin on prothrombin synthesis is similar, if not identical, to the effect of the novel antibiotic tunicamycin on the synthesis of hen oviduct membranes (18). It seems likely that this is the site of action since it has been shown that warfarin can effect the binding of manganese either directly or indirectly to the glycosyl-transferase enzymes. It has been shown by us (8) and by others (16,17) that manganese is necessary for the normal functioning of the glycosyl-transferase enzymes. Based on these studies it is proposed that vitamin K and warfarin may have a dual site of action. It is possible that glycosylation is followed by carboxylation or that the two events occur simultaneously and both processes are under the control of vitamin K and the indirect acting anticoagulants. However, in vivo studies performed by us to test this hypothesis showed that carboxylation seems to occur independent of the vitamin K status of the animal (9).

ACKNOWLEDGMENT

Part of the work presented here was performed by Dr. Michael Pereira and Dr. Donald Waller. The authors would also like to thank Ms. Carolyn Groff for her excellent assistance in the preparation of this manuscript.

REFERENCES

1. Esmon, C.T., Sadowski, J.A., and Suttie, J.W. (1975) J. Biol. Chem. 250, 4744-4748.
2. Sadowski, J.A., Esmon, C.T., and Suttie, J.W. (1976) J. Biol. Chem. 251, 2770-2775.
3. Esmon, C.T., and Suttie, J.W. (1976) J. Biol. Chem. 251, 6238-6243.
4. Suttie, J.W., Hageman, J.M., Leberman, S.R., and Rich, D.H. (1976) J. Biol. Chem. 251, 5827-5830.
5. Pereira, M., and Couri, D. (1971) Biochim. Biophys. Acta 237, 348-355.
6. Pereira, M., and Couri, D. (1972) Biochim. Biophys. Acta 261, 375-378.
7. Pereira, M., and Couri, D. (1972) Experienta 28, 1170-1171.
8. Waller, D.P., and Couri, D. (1973) The Pharmacologist 15, 330.
9. Meeks, R.G., and Couri, D. (1978) Biochim. Biophys. Acta 544, 634-637.
10. Meeks, R.G., and Couri, D. (1979). Biochim. Biophys. Acta, submitted.
11. Meeks, R.G. (1978) Ph.D. Thesis. The Ohio State University.
12. Richards, J.B., Evans, P.J., and Hemming, F.W. (1971) Biochem J. 124, 957-959.
13. Parodi, A.J., Behrens, N.H., Leloir, L.F., and Carminatti, H. (1972) Proc. Natl. Acad. Sci. (USA). 69, 3268-3272.
14. Behrens, N.H., Carminatti, H., Staneloni, R.J., and Leloir, L.F., and Cantoiella, A.I. (1973). Proc. Natl. Acad. Sci. (USA) 70, 3390-3394.
15. Nelsestuen, G.S., and Suttie, J.W. (1972) J. Biol. Chem. 247, 6096-6102.
16. Doisy, E.A., Jr. (1972) In Trace Substances In Environmental Health--VI, Proceedings of University of Missouri's 6th Annual Conference on Trace Substances in Environmental Health. Ed. D. Hemphill, University of Missouri, Columbia, MO.
17. Leach, R.M., Jr. (1971) Fed. Proc. 30, 991-994.
18. Stuck, D.K., and Lennarz, W.J. (1976) J. Biol. Chem. 252, 1007-1013.
19. Lawford, G.R., and Schacter, H. (1966) J. Biol. Chem. 241, 5408-5418.

HUMORAL SUBSTANCES REGULATING THE LEVEL OF COAGULATION FACTORS: COAGULOPOIETINS. EVIDENCE FOR A SPECIFIC COAGULOPOIETIN FOR PROTHROMBIN

M. KARPATKIN and S. KARPATKIN

New York University Medical School,
New York, NY 10016

INTRODUCTION

Levels of coagulation factors remain fairly constant throughout life both for a species and its individual members. The mechanisms that maintain these constant levels have not been elucidated. Studies from our laboratory suggest that humoral factors (coagulopoietins) participate in maintenance of these levels in plasma of coumadin treated rabbits (1,2), rabbits who have undergone disseminated intravascular coagulation (3) and in rabbits who have been specifically depleted of one clotting factor (factor II) (4,5).

COUMADIN TREATED ANIMALS

New Zealand white rabbits (2-3.5 kg) of both sexes were divided into four groups as follows: 1) donor test animals; 2) donor control animals; 3) recipient test animals; 4) recipient control animals.

Donor test animals were given intramuscular coumadin daily until vitamin-K-dependent coagulation factors were <25% of their levels in a pool of normal rabbit plasma. These rabbits were then exsanguinated and their plasma injected into recipient test animals. Levels of the vitamin-K-dependent clotting factors were then measured in the recipient rabbits and compared to their pre-injection levels.

Donor control animals were given physiologic saline and their plasma injected into recipient control animals.

A blood sample was withdrawn from each recipient animal on three separate days (at 3-7 day intervals) and the plasma stored at -30°C (baseline samples). When the three baseline samples had been obtained, the injection schedule was started. Donor plasma was thawed just before use and injected slowly into a lateral ear vein.

A blood sample was withdrawn each morning before injection of the donor plasma 12 hrs after the last donor plasma injection. Further daily blood samples were withdrawn for variable time periods after completion of the injection schedule. Clotting factor assays were performed on stored samples after completion of an experiment. The mean value of the three baseline samples was designated 100% for that animal and the ensuing samples expressed in relation to this value. A 'significant increase' in level was considered to have occurred if a factor rose above the baseline 100% level by 2 standard deviations of the mean for the assay on at least two consecutive days. Factors II, V, VII, and X were assayed by methods based upon the single-stage prothrombin time using deficient plasma and the factor-IX assay was based upon the kaolin activated partial thromboplastin time using plasma from a patient congenitally deficient in this factor.

In the first experiment 2 recipient test rabbits each received 4 ml of test donor plasma twice daily at 8 hourly intervals for 4 1/2 days with daily morning blood withdrawal for 7 days. At the same time, recipient

control rabbits received the same volume of control donor plasma and had
blood withdrawn in an exactly similar manner. Results of this experiment
are shown in Fig 1. All the vitamin-K-dependent coagulation factors rose

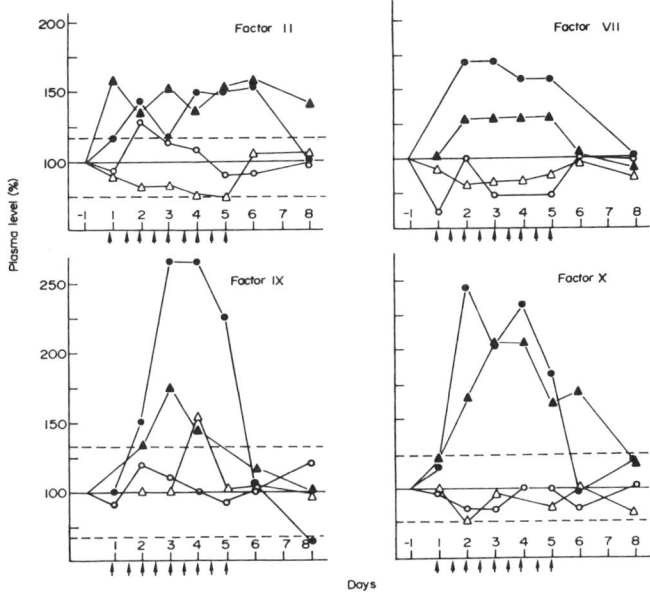

FIG 1. Changes in vitamin-K-dependent coagulation factors in test and control recipient rabbits following injection of donor test and control plasma. Arrows refer to intravenous injections of 4 ml of either test or control donor plasma, twice daily for $4\frac{1}{2}$ days. Horizontal interrupted lines refer to ± 2 S.D. for the assay. The symbols refer to test recipient 1, ●; test recipient 2, ▲; control recipient 1, ○; control recipient 2, △.

to significant levels in the test recipient animals by day 2, reaching
their peak on day 1 for factor II, day 2 for factor VII, day 2-4 for factor X and day 3 for factor IX. Following cessation of injection of test
donor plasma on day 5, coagulation factor levels returned to normal on
the sixth to eighth day. In the control recipient animals there was no
significant increase in any of the coagulation factors measured.

The next experiments were designed to determine the smallest volume of donor plasma required to cause an increase in vitamin-K-dependent coagulation factors in recipient animals. A total of 9 test recipient animals
each received 3 injections ranging from 0.25 to 16 ml each. Two control
animals each received 3 injections of 2 ml and 16 ml respectively of control donor plasma. Factors II, VII, IX, and X rose in animals receiving
0.25 to 4.0 ml of test donor plasma but there was no increase in the animals receiving 8 and 16 ml suggesting the presence of inhibitory factors.
Control donor plasma had no effect on factor levels in recipient animals.

Thirteen animals received between 0.25 and 4 ml of test donor plasma
B.I.D. A significant rise occurred for factor II in 12 of 13 animals;
factor VII in 6 of 8 animals; factor IX in 6 of 9 animals and factor X in
9 of 13 animals.

A total of 10 animals received control donor plasma. No rise occurred in
2, 8 and 7 animals in whom factors VII, IX and X were assayed respectively. There were 2 out of 10 elevations in factor II.

Factor V was assayed in both test and control recipient animals in order to determine the change, if any, of a non-vitamin-K-dependent factor. Factor V rose 4 of 10 times in the test recipient animals and 3 of 9 times in the controls, suggesting a non-specific response, secondary to manipulation and/or injection.

ANIMALS UNDERGOING DISSEMINATED INTRAVASCULAR COAGULATION (D.I.C.)

A goat antiserum (GAS) against rabbit prothrombin was injected into donor rabbits in order to specifically lower prothrombin. Instead, D.I.C. was induced with reduction of platelets and all clotting factors measured (factors II, V, VII, X and fibrinogen) with return to above baseline values 12-36 hours later. A similar response was obtained with normal goat serum (NGS). Donor animals were exsanguinated 48 hours after injection of GAS or NGS and the plasma injected into recipient rabbits using similar techniques to those used in the coumadin study. Results are shown in Figure 2.

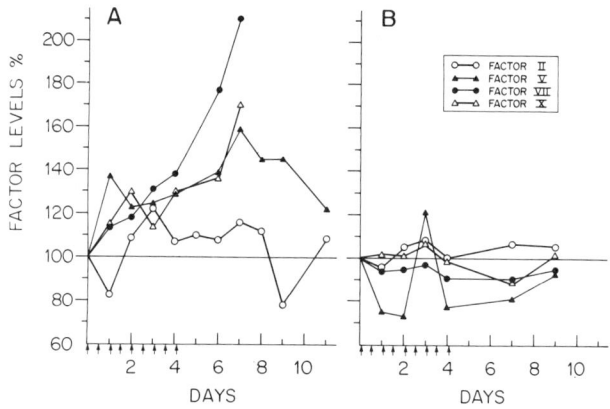

Fig. 2. (A) Response of seven normal recipient rabbits to the intravenous injection of plasma from rabbits given goat serum containing anti-rabbit factor II (five recipients) or normal goat serum (two recipients). The combined mean of seven experiments is given. The arrows refer to the intravenous injection of 1-4 ml plasma. o———o, factor II; ▲——▲, factor V; •——•, factor VII; △——△, factor X. The 100% value refers to the mean of three samples drawn on each animal on three separate days prior to starting the injection schedule. (B) Response of four normal recipient rabbits to the intravenous injection of plasma from normal rabbits. Protocol and symbols are the same as in (A).

All factors measured (II, V, VII, and X) rose in the 7 recipient test animals but did not change in controls that received plasma from normal rabbits.

ANIMALS IN WHICH FACTOR II (PROTHROMBIN) IS SPECIFICALLY LOWERED.

Factor II was prepared from rabbit plasma by the method of Morrison and Esnouf (6). The purified factor had a specific activity of 9,000 units/mg and gave one band on electrophoresis with 5% SDS polyacrylamide gel. It contained less than 1% factors VII and X. The purified material was used to raise an antibody in a goat. The antiserum gave one line on immunodiffusion against normal rabbit plasma diluted 1:512 and one line on immunoelectrophoresis. The ability of the antiserum to remove factor II activity in vitro was demonstrated as follows: antiserum was incubated with an equal volume of normal rabbit plasma at 37° for 30 minutes, and the factor II activity measured. As a control, normal goat serum which had been heated at 56° for 30 minutes was similarly incubated with normal rabbit plasma and the factor II activity measured. Results shown in Table I indicate that factor II activity was reduced by the goat antiserum at an antiserum dilution of 1:16. Levels of factors V, VII, and X were also measured and were unchanged by the antiserum.

COAGULOPOIETIN FOR PROTHROMBIN

TABLE 1. EFFECT OF GOAT ANTISERUM ON RABBIT PLASMA FACTOR II LEVELS IN VITRO°

Mixture	Factor II μ/ml
Goat Serum and Rabbit Plasma	0.5
Goat Antiserum and Rabbit Plasma	<0.01
Goat Antiserum 1:16 and Rabbit Plasma	0.14

°Goat anti-factor II antiserum or serum was incubated with an equal volume of normal rabbit plasma for 30 minutes at 37°C. Factor II activity of the mixture was then measured.

A crude globulin fraction of the antiserum was made by precipitation with 50% saturated ammonium sulfate, resuspension of the precipitate in a volume of phosphate buffered saline pH 7.4 equal to the volume of the original serum, and extensive dialysis against the same buffer. The globulin was centrifuged at 100,000g for 1 hour immediately prior to its use and 13.5 ml/kg infused into the lateral ear vein of a rabbit over a 1 hour period. At the end of that time, factor II was 40% of baseline and 6 hrs later was still 60% of baseline. Fibrinogen, platelets, and other coagulation factors measured (V, VII, and X) were not affected. At the end of 6 hours, the animals were exsanguinated and their plasma stored as described previously (2). Control donor plasma was prepared from rabbits which had been similarly infused with a globulin fraction of normal goat serum.

Normal rabbits were injected with donor plasma as follows: 3 baseline blood samples were collected as described previously and the plasma stored (2). The animals then received a 3 ml intravenous injection of donor plasma at 9 a.m. and 5 p.m. for 4 days. A blood sample was drawn at midday on the second, third, and fourth days, and on the day after completion

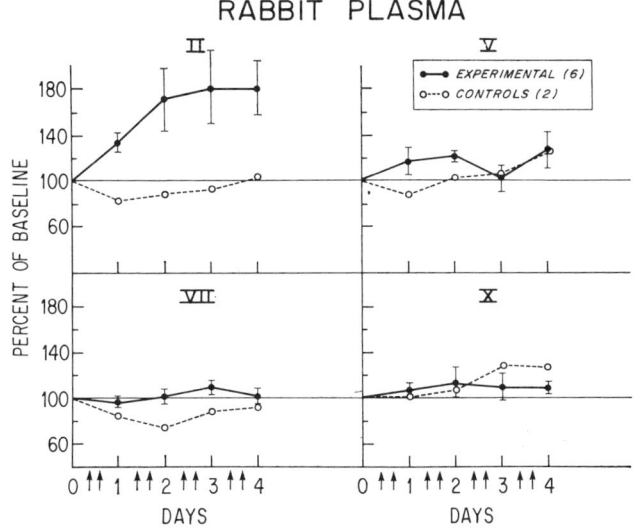

FIG. 3. Coagulation factor response of recipient rabbits to injection of experimental donor plasma and control donor plasma. Three baseline samples were drawn on 3 different days before starting the injection schedule. Arrows indicate intravenous injecton of 3 ml plasma. Samples were drawn on mornings of days 2, 3, 4, and 5. The S.E.M. and number of experiments (n) are given.

of the injection schedule (day 5). Plasma was separated, stored, and assayed for clotting factor activity as described previously (2). In addition prothrombin was also measured by a two-stage technique (7). Five of 6 animals that received test donor plasma showed an increase in factor II levels above baseline (more than 2 S.D. for the assay on at least two consecutive days, P<0.001). In 2 animals that received control donor plasma (prepared by injection of normal goat globulin into 2 donor rabbits), there was no such rise, as had been the case in 12 previously reported controls (2,3). Factors V, VII, and X were assayed in both test and control animals and showed no significant rise in either group (Fig 3).

Samples from 5 experimental animals and 5 controls were measured by an immunoelectrophoresis technique (8). Results are shown in Fig 4 with the values for the biologic assay in the 5 experimental animals. The immunologic assay does display an increase in activity in the test animals but it is far less than the rise in biologic activity.

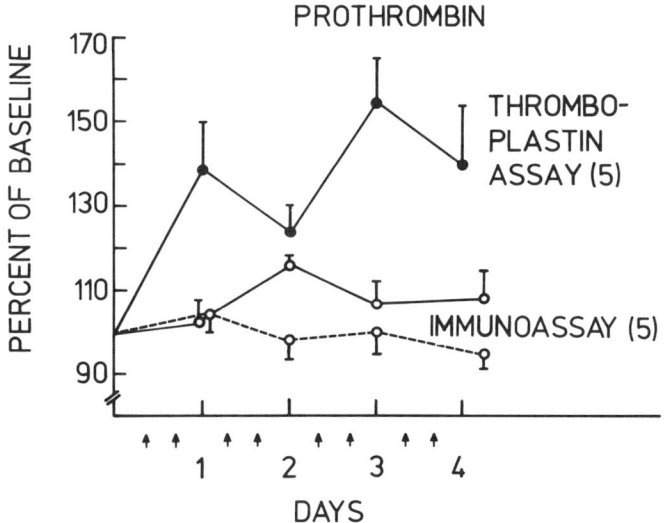

Fig 4. Comparison of biologic and immunologic activity ± SEM of 5 rabbits injected with coagulopoietin II. Biologic activity of experimental samples (●—●), controls not shown; immunologic activity of experimental samples (o—o); control samples (o--o), P<0.01 on day 2.

Donor plasma was boiled for 30 minutes at pH 6.8 and then injected into recipient rabbits according to the above schedule. Factor II rose significantly in animals who received test donor plasma, but did not rise in those who received control plasma (P<0.001). Other factors assayed (V, VII, and X) did not rise in either group of animals (Fig 5).

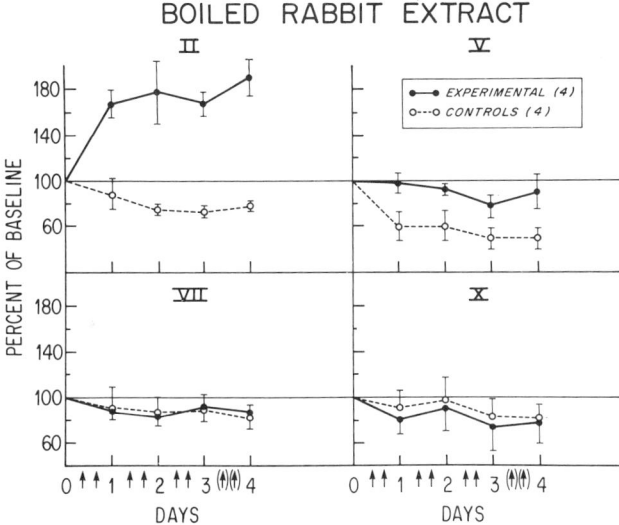

FIG. 5. Coagulation factor response of recipient rabbits to injection of boiled experimental donor plasma and boiled control donor plasma. Three baseline samples were drawn on 3 different days before starting the injection schedule. Arrows indicate intravenous injection of 3 ml plasma. In some experiments, the injections were omitted on day 4. Samples were drawn on mornings of days 2, 3, 4, and 5. The S.E.M. and number of experiments (n) are given.

Boiling resulted in 30-fold purification of coagulopoietin activity. Further purification (60-fold) was achieved by G-50 Sephadex filtration of the boiled plasma. Nine ml of boiled plasma was then placed on the G-50 column and eluted with 100 ml of 0.85% NaCl. Two protein fractions were separated (280 mµ absorbance material); protein eluting in the void volume, and protein remaining in the retained volume. Rabbits were injected with either the retained or the void volume fraction. In 3 experiments (5 rabbits), factor II levels rose significantly in animals that received the retained volume (values ranging from 125-152% of baseline on days 2-5; whereas factors V, VII, and X did not rise above baseline values). No rise in factor II occurred in those given the void volume (Table 2).

TABLE 2. PERCENT OF PRE-INJECTION BASELINE LEVEL FOLLOWING INJECTION OF PLASMA FRACTIONS SEPARATED BY G-50 GEL FILTRATION*

		Days Post Injection			
		2	3	4	5
Factor II	Retained Volume†	147	125	152	137
	Void Volume‡	75	86	66	88
Factor V	Retained Volume	82	82	61	65
	Void Volume	88	82	66	54
Factor VII	Retained Volume	103	109	—	134
	Void Volume	100	133	133	117
Factor X	Retained Volume	109	115	89	79
	Void Volume	89	81	80	80

*Boiled experimental plasma was lyophilized and reconstituted in 0.5 ml of water. This was then placed on a G50 Sephadex column and eluted with 100 ml of 0.85% NaCl. The void volume and retained volume were separately combined and tested for coagulopoietin activity.
†Mean of three experiments.
‡Mean of two experiments.

This suggests that coagulopoietin-II has a molecular weight of less than 30,000.

Boiled donor plasma was evaluated in an in vitro rabbit liver system. Minced liver (35 mg/ml, wet weight) from a freshly killed rabbit was incubated at room temperature on a rotator in 10 ml of Dulbecco's modification of Eagle's medium containing 10% fetal calf serum and 1.6 mg of gentamicin per ml, under 95% O_2/5% CO_2. After 5 hr, the medium was removed and replaced with fresh medium of the same composition. Samples (0.1 ml) from the medium were taken at intervals and prothrombin was measured by the two-stage technique.

No significant difference from control incubations was noted during the first 5 hr of incubation, prior to the change of medium. With the addition of control boiled plasma, prothrombin activity increased to 15 ± 6% and 45 ± 12% (mean + SEM) of baseline activity at 16 and 40 hr, respectively (Fig 6). Addition of cycloheximide at 5 mg/ml almost completely

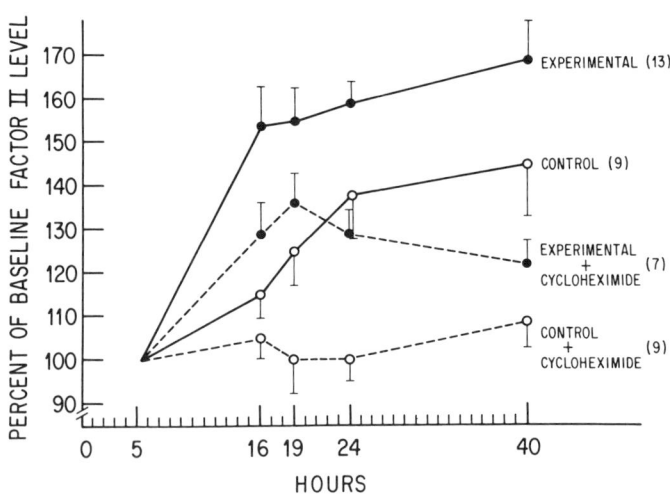

Fig 6. Prothrombin response of an in vitro liver mince system to incubation with boiled experimental plasma (●—●, n = 13); boiled control plasma (o—o); boiled control + 5 mg cycloheximide/ml (o--o); and boiled experimental and 5 mg cycloheximide/ml (●--●). Boiled control or experimental rabbit plasma containing 20 µg of protein per ml was added to the medium with or without cycloheximide.

inhibited prothrombin activity during this time interval (P<0.01), indicating that the in vitro liver system was synthesizing prothrombin protein. Addition of boiled experimental plasma protein (coagulopoietin-II) at 20 µg/ml increased prothrombin activity by 54 ± 9% and 69 ± 9% of baseline values at 16 and 40 hr, respectively (which was 3.6 and 1.5-fold greater than the respective control values). The differences between control and experimental plasma were statistically significant (Student's t test) at 16 and 19 hr (P<0.05). Of particular interest was the observation that cycloheximide did not appear to inhibit the effect of experimental plasma.

DISCUSSION

These data provide evidence for the presence of humoral substances (coagulopoietins) in animals with depleted coagulation factors, which are capable of raising coagulation factors in recipient animals. The data obtained with coumadin first suggested the presence of such humoral factors. Since rabbit plasma does not contain precursor (descarboxy) vitamin K coagulation factors (9), it is unlikely that the enhancement of biologic activity for factors II, VII, IX and X resulted from infusion of precursor.

The data obtained from rabbits subjected to DIC supported our previous observations on the presence of coagulopoietins. The increased activity in the recipient animals could not have been derived from activated coagulation factors generated in the donors during DIC, since activated factors are rapidly removed from the circulation, probably within minutes; and the coagulation factors, in the recipients, were still elevated 3 days after the last injection of donor plasma.

The above 2 studies did not provide evidence for the presence of a specific coagulopoietin for a specific coagulation factor. We therefore designed an experimental protocol which was capable of specifically lowering a single factor (prothrombin). This was accomplished by the slow infusion of a partially-purified specific antibody for prothrombin. Donor plasma obtained from these rabbits, when injected into recipients, elevated prothrombin activity only. The humoral substance is stable to boiling, has a low molecular weight, and stimulates a liver mince system to enhance biologic activity. Although control prothrombin production in this system was inhibited by cycloheximide, the humoral substance-induced prothrombin activity was not inhibited. Thus it is unlikely that this coagulopoietin operates via protein synthesis.

Preliminary studies with an antibody specific for factor X have provided similar data. Donor plasma from rabbits depleted of factor X specifically raised factor X when injected into 10 recipient rabbits. The factor was assayed by one-stage techniques, chromogenic substrate, and Laurell technique. Immunologic activity was elevated, but only to approximately half of biologic activity. Coagulopoietin-X is also stable to boiling.

The mode of action of these coagulopoietins remains to be elucidated. 1) The coagulopoietins may specifically enhance de novo protein synthesis. This is unlikely from the in vitro cycloheximide experiments. 2) They may stimulate a specific carboxylase for the vitamin-K dependent carboxylation of a specific factor. 3) They may enhance release of already-formed biologically active coagulation factor. 4) They may decrease the catabolism of a specific coagulation factor.

ACKNOWLEDGEMENTS:

This work was supported by grants PCM 7918282 and HLBI 13336-10.

REFERENCES:

1. Karpatkin, M.H. and Karpatkin, S.: 1971, J. Clin. Invest. 50:52a.
2. Karpatkin, M.H. and Karpatkin, S.: 1973, Brit. J. Haemat. 24:553.
3. Friedman, E.W., Karpatkin, M.H. and Karpatkin, S.: 1976, Blood 48:949.
4. Karpatkin, S., Karpatkin, M.H. and Altszuler, H.: 1978, Trans. Assoc. Amer. Phys. 91:351.
5. Karpatkin, M.H. and Karpatkin, S.: 1979, Proc. Natl. Acad. Sci. USA, 76:491.
6. Morrison, S.A. and Esnouf, M.P.: 1973, Nature 242:92.
7. Shapiro, S.S. and Waugh, D.F.: 1966, Thromb. Diath. Haemorrh. 16:469.
8. Laurell, C.: 1966, Anal. Biochem. 15:45.
9. Carlisle, T.L., Shah, D.V., Schlegel, R. and Suttie, J.W.: 1975, Proc. Soc. Exp. Biol. Med. 148:140.

STUDIES OF A HUMORAL FACTOR
INFLUENCING PROTHROMBIN LEVELS IN THE RAT

D. V. SHAH, L. J. NYARI, J. C. SWANSON, and J. W. SUTTIE

Department of Biochemistry
College of Agricultural and Life Sciences
University of Wisconsin-Madison
Madison, WI 53706

INTRODUCTION

Plasma prothrombin levels under normal physiological conditions remain constant within a specific range when animals are maintained on a vitamin K-adequate diet. Earlier studies by Karpatkin's group (1,2) presented evidence for the existence of a plasma factor in hypoprothrombinemic rabbits capable of increasing the level of vitamin K-dependent coagulation factors in normal rabbits. The mechanism by which the vitamin K-dependent coagulation factors are increased in normal rabbits upon injection of this postulated humoral agent was not established by this early investigation. This report confirms these observations in a second species and presents some data which relate to the mechanism of the response.

METHODS

Treatment of Animals and Preparation of Plasma

Male 180 to 200 g rats of the Holtzman strain were fed Purina laboratory chow and given menadione (50 µg/100 ml) in their drinking water for 8 to 10 days before they were used as either donor or plasma recipient rats. A recipient experimental group received donor test plasma, and a recipient control group received donor control plasma. Donor plasmas were obtained from groups of 6 to 8 rats. Donor control plasma was prepared from 5.0 ml blood per donor control rat whose prothrombin levels were 250 ± 3.4 µ/ml (SEM). Donor test plasma was similarly prepared from vitamin K-deficient male rats whose prothrombin levels were 14.5 ± 3.7 U/ml (SEM). The blood was drawn by cardiac puncture from rats anesthetized with ether into 0.1 $\underline{M}$ potassium oxalate (9:1) and centrifuged at 2000 g for 20 min in a refrigerated centrifuge. Pooled oxalated donor (control/test) plasma was stored in aliquots at -20° C.

Prothrombin and Total Clotting Activity

Blood (0.5 ml) for prothrombin assay was obtained by cardiac puncture into 0.1 $\underline{M}$ potassium oxalate (9:1) at each time point. Plasma prothrombin was assayed by the two-stage method of Ware and Seegers as modified by Shapiro and Waugh (3), and total clotting activity (prothrombin and any circulating precursor forms) by activation with E. carinatus venom (4). The plasma prothrombin and total clotting activity at zero time for individual recipient rats was set at 100% to study the prothrombin and total clotting levels at various times after administering donor (control/test) plasma. Rat prothrombin antigen was assayed by the methods of Laurell (5). Antisera from rabbits injected with purified rat prothrombin was harvested and precipitated with $(NH_4)_2SO_4$ to obtain the IgG fraction. The antibody titre was checked by quantitative precipitation. A 1.5 mm thick gel was prepared by pouring 30-45 ml of a 1% agarose/barbital (w/v) solution containing .15% antibody onto a glass plate (260 x 125 x 1.5 mm) fitted with a mold. The glass plate was placed on a LKB Multiphor apparatus and connected to the buffer (.075 $\underline{M}$ barbital pH 8.6, 2 m$\underline{M}$ calcium) using paper wicks. Plasma samples (5 µl) diluted 1:2 in barbital buffer were applied to 3 mm punched wells and electrophoresed at 8 volts/cm of gel for 5 h using a circulating water bath to maintain a 12° C temperature under the plate. After electrophoresis, the gel was pressed, washed, dried, and stained in .5% Coomassie Blue R-250. Peak heights were measured and compared to standard control donor plasma to determine prothrombin units. Plasma prothrombin antigen activity at zero time for individual recipient rats was set at 100% to study alterations in antigen levels after administration of donor (control/test) plasma.

RESULTS

Plasma prothrombin was assayed in plasma of recipient rats at various periods after the injection of donor (control/test) plasma. Plasma prothrombin levels in the experimental group were increased about 27% after 24 h compared to a 3% increase in the control group (Fig. 1A). The maximum increase in plasma prothrombin in the experimental group was seen at

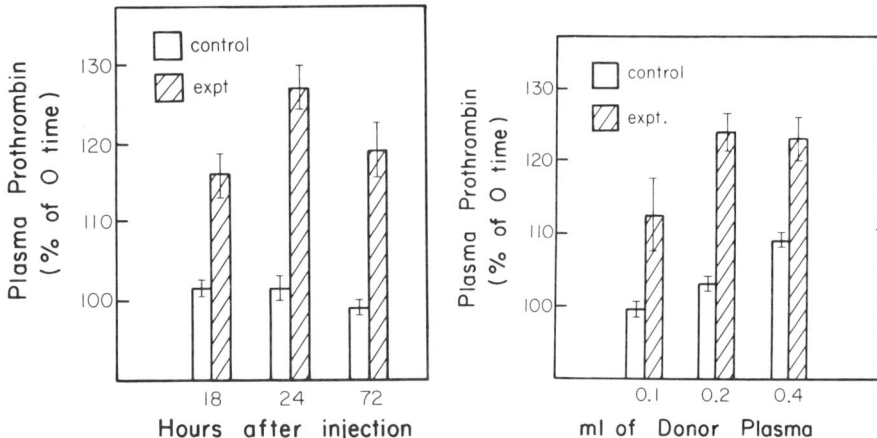

FIGURE 1. (A) Effect of plasma injection on prothrombin concentration of recipient rats. Rats were administered intracardially 0.2 ml/rat of control of experimental (vitamin K-deficient) plasma at zero time, and blood drawn at the times indicated. Two-stage prothrombin activity of each rat before donor plasma administration was set at 100%. Values are mean ± SEM for 12 to 16 recipient rats in each group. (B) Effect of donor plasma volume on prothrombin levels of recipient rats. Rats were administered either control or experimental plasma intracardially at zero time. Blood was drawn before injection (zero time) and 24 h after the administration of donor plasma and assayed as in 1A. Values are mean ± SEM for 6 to 12 recipient rats in each group.

24 h. When three 0.2 ml injections of donor plasma were given during a 24-hour period, the response remained the same at 48 h and showed a slight decline at 72 h. The data in Figure 1B indicate that the response seen after injecting 0.2 ml donor plasma was enhanced over that observed with 0.1 ml. Doubling the amount of injected plasma to 0.4 ml did not result in an increased response in plasma prothrombin levels in recipient rats. When donor test plasma was obtained from Warfarin-treated rats (5 mg/kg body weight, 18 h prior) rather than vitamin K-deficient rats, plasma prothrombin levels in recipient rats did not increase.

These observations are in agreement with the earlier reports (1,2) presenting evidence for a humoral agent capable of raising vitamin K-dependent coagulation factors in rabbits and extend them to a second species. An increase in the steady-state levels of plasma prothrombin could be due either to an increased rate of formation or a decreased rate of distraction of prothrombin. The rate of decay of plasma prothrombin was studied by injecting sufficient Warfarin to block prothrombin synthesis (5 mg/kg) along with donor (control/test) plasma to recipient rats. Both groups showed a similar decline in plasma prothrombin levels suggesting that humoral factor is not affecting prothrombin decay, and the observed increase in plasma prothrombin levels is not due to any effect on degradation of prothrombin levels.

Two ways in which a humoral factor could increase plasma prothrombin levels in the experimental group would be to increase the level of the vitamin K-dependent carboxylase activity or the rate of synthesis of and possibly the concentration of prothrombin precursors in the liver. Efforts to correlate such changes in the liver with the observed response in the plasma prothrombin have yielded variable results. Studies have been carried out at 18, 24, and 48 h after the donor plasma injections. The response in both liver carboxylase activity and prothrombin precursor levels has been variable, and no consistent effect has been observed. It is possible that the time after injection might be an important variable and that there is a significant alteration in these parameters which has not been detected.

This apparent increase in plasma prothrombin could be due to an increase in the amount of prothrombin or to some alteration in the plasma which increased the apparent two-stage activity of the same amount of prothrombin. Preliminary studies indicate that when prothrombin was assayed by an immunochemical technique (Fig. 2), there appeared to be an increase in total prothrombin antigen in both the control and experimental groups. These data suggested that the immunochemical assay was detecting an antigenically active form of prothrombin that did not assay by the two-stage assay. If there was a significant amount of a circulating descarboxy (abnormal) prothrombin form, this should also be detected by an assay which uses E. carinatus venom to generate thrombin. The data (Table 1) from the three different methods that have been used suggest that a clear difference in response of animals to the control or test plasma can be detected only with the two-stage assay, and that venom activation or an immunochemical assay detect a significant increase in plasma prothrombin in both groups.

DISCUSSION

The studies have confirmed the observation that the injection of plasma from a hypoprothrombinemic animal into the normal animal can cause an increase in plasma prothrombin (two-stage activity) in the recipient

TABLE 1. Plasma prothrombin levels of rats receiving 0.2 ml plasma.

Plasma Injected	Two-stage Prothrombin	Venom Generated Activity	Immunologic Response
Control	103 ± 2	111 ± 4	131 ± 1
Vitamin K-deficient plasma	124 ± 5	119 ± 6	119 ± 2

All values are expressed as % of zero time at 24 h and are mean ± SEM for 3-4 recipient rats in each group.

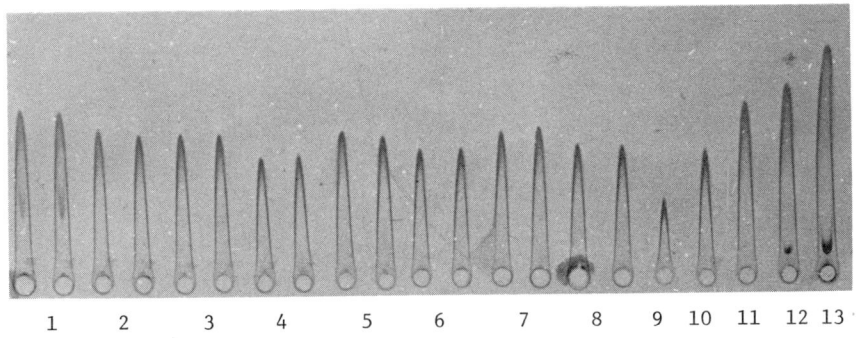

FIGURE 2. Quantitation of rat plasma prothrombin by immunoelectrophoresis. The data are for individual rats run in duplicate: Wells # 1 and 5 -- 24 h experimental; 2 and 6 -- 0 h experimental; 3 and 7 -- 24 h control; 4 and 8 -- 0 h control; 9-13 -- control donor plasma at dilutions of 20%, 40%, 60%, 80%, 100%.

animal. This increase does not appear to be due to an alteration in the turnover rate of plasma prothrombin, nor has it been possible to correlate it with changes in liver prothrombin precursor concentrations or vitamin K-dependent carboxylase activity.

When prothrombin is assayed by methods that detect total prothrombin antigen or total thrombin-generating capacity, a significant increase in prothrombin was found in the plasma of rats injected with either experimental (hypoprothrombinemic) or control plasma. A satisfactory explanation of this response is not yet available. However, until this response of the control animals is understood, the role of this proposed humoral factor in regulating prothrombin concentrations will remain uncertain.

ACKNOWLEDGEMENTS

This study was supported by the College of Agricultural and Life Sciences, University of Wisconsin-Madison, and in part by grant AM-14881 from the National Institutes of Health.

REFERENCES

1. Karpatkin, M., and Karpatkin, S. (1973) Brit. J. Haematol. 24, 553-562.
2. Friedman, E. W., Karpatkin, M., and Karpatkin, S. (1976) Blood 48, 949-954.
3. Shapiro, S. S., and Waugh, D. F. (1966) Thrombos. Diathes. haemorrh. 16, 469-490.
4. Carlisle, T. L., Shah, D. V., Schlegel, R., and Suttie, J. W. (1975) Proc. Soc. Exp. Biol. Med. 148, 140-144.
5. Laurell, C. B. (1966) Anal. Biochem. 15, 45-52.

INDEX

A-Fragment, 8
Absorption difference spectroscopy, 49, 54, 58, 123
Acenocoumarol, 349
Active transport, 183, 193
Alanine hydroxylation, 13
Apolipoproteins, 15
Atherocalcin, 269
Bernardi reaction, 401
t-Boc-L-Glu-α-benzylester, 480, 505, 509
Bone disease, 225, 237, 375
Bone, Gla protein in,
  acid decarboyxlation of, 231
  antibodies toward, 224
  biosynthesis, 226, 227, 245
  concentration in bone, 219, 227, 237
  function of, 219, 227, 237, 245
  in cartilage, 260
  in elasmobranches, 263
  in organ culture, 219, 245
  in plasma, 224
  in vitro synthesis, 245
  thermal decarboyxlation of, 221
Brodifacoum, 349, 393
Bromadiolone, 393
t-butyl-OOH, 413, 422, 433
β-carboxyglutamic acid, 166
γ-carboxyglutamic acid (Gla),
  acid decarboxylation of, 231
  assay for, 150, 153, 166
  chemical synthesis of, 137, 157
  identification of, 161, 171
  in abnormal prothrombins, 62
  in atherosclerotic plaque, 269
  in bone, 219, 227, 237, 259
  in elasmobranches, 263
  in invertebrates, 207
  in kidney, 303, 307
  in plasma proteins, 3, 13, 28, 58, 62, 129
  in ribosomes, 150, 274, 279
  in urine, 153, 166, 375
  peptide synthesis utilizing, 137, 157

pyridine decarboxylation of, 512
thermal decarboxylation of, 171, 221, 484
Cell and organ culture, 219, 245, 311, 340, 529, 542
Chloro-K,
  effect on cis/trans vitamin, 333,
  effect on vitamin K metabolism, 338, 348
  HPLC standard, 326, 362
Chromogenic assays, 384
Chorioallantoic membranes, 294
Circular dichroism, 45, 140
Coagulopoietin, 576, 584
Collagen, 219, 227
C reactive protein, 129
Difenacoum, 349
Disseminated intravascular coagulation, 579
Dansylation of Gla, 150
E. carinatus assay, 384, 533
Elasmobranches, 263
Electron paramagnetic resonance spectra, 422, 573
Factor Xa inhibitor, 380
Factor V(Va), 75, 110
Factor VII,
  biosynthesis in cell culture, 542
  regulation of plasma level, 577
  response to vitamin K, 345
  structure of, 5, 30
Factor IX
  Gla residues in, 4
  regulation of plasma levels, 577
  response to vitamin K, 345
  structure of, 14, 30
Factor X
  activation peptides, 120
  comparison of X_1 and X_2, 120
  effect of warfarin on, 381
  Gla domain-less, 124
  metal binding properties, 16, 58
  regulation of plasma levels, 577
  response to vitamin K, 345
  structure of, 5, 14, 16, 30, 58, 120

Fluorescence quench,
 31, 39, 137
Fragment F-1,
 antigenic properties of, 68
 conformational alterations of,
  39, 49, 54, 58
 crystallographic investigations
  of, 8
 metal binding to, 16, 28, 39,
  49, 54, 58, 137
 membrane interactions of, 28
 modification of, 28
Fragment-3, 116
Gla peptides,
 carboxylase products, 509, 518
 metal binding to, 137
Glutathione peroxidase, 413, 422
Glycosylation reactions, 571
α-Helix structures,
 in fragment-1, 58
 in peptide substrates, 471
 in plasma proteins, 30
High voltage paper electrophoresis,
 171
HPLC,
 of t-BOC-Glu-α-benzylester,
  505
 of osteocalcin, 233
 of vitamin K and K oxide, 318,
  368, 505
Hummel-Dreyer column technique, 23
Incisor, effect of warfarin on, 255
Kidney Gla protein,
 in chicken, 303
 in bovine, 307
Kinetic analysis,
 of carboxylase products, 505
 of epoxide reductase inhibition,
  368
 of plasma clotting factors, 345
 of plasma vitamin K, 317, 328
 of prothrombin activation, 106,
  110
Laser-induced luminescence, 144
Microorganisms,
 biosynthesis of vitamin K in,
  174, 188
 γ-carboxyglutomic acid in, 274
 vitamin K function in, 177, 193,
  203
Mineralization, 219, 227, 237,
 255, 259, 263, 269, 375
Nuclear magnetic resonance, 141
Osteocalcin, 36, 237, 245, 255
Oxidative phosphorylation, 193
Peptide substrates,
 identification of products, 509,
  518

 in specificity studies, 471, 520
 mass fragmentation spectra of,
  417, 509
 synthesis of, 41, 450, 471
 tritiated form of, 401
 pyridoxal phosphate relationship,
  450, 484, 519
Perfused rat liver, 529
Phenylbutazone, 370
Phenylthiohydantoin derivative of
 Gla, 161
Protein C
 amino acid composition, 173
 amino acid sequence, 84
 effect on clot lysis, 79
 function of, 72, 89
 inactivation of factor Va, 75
 interaction with factor X, 89
 structure of, 5, 14, 30, 84
Protein M, 96
Protein S,
 amino acid composition, 104, 173
 purification, 102
 structure of, 5, 30, 104
Protein Z, 171
Prothrombin,
 activation of, 62, 72, 89, 96
  106, 110, 116, 124
 abnormal (decarboxy) forms, 62,
  66, 92, 342, 384, 388, 529
 antibodies toward, 66, 116, 282,
  342, 388, 484, 529, 553, 560,
  577, 584
 biosynthesis of, 13, 529, 546,
  553, 560, 571
 Ca^{++} interaction, 17, 28, 39, 79,
  54, 58, 66
 carbohydrate modification of, 33
 γ-carboxyglutamic acid in, 4, 13,
  28, 84
 conformational changes in, 16, 28,
  49
 crystallographic studies of, 8
 effect of warfarin on, 343, 249,
  370, 380, 388, 529, 571
 Fragment-1 from 16, 28, 39, 49,
  54, 58
 helical properties of, 30, 58
 metal binding to, 17, 28, 39, 49,
  54, 58
 phospholipid association, 28, 102,
  106
 physical properties of, 16, 28, 39,
  49, 54, 58
 plasma regulation of, 577, 584
 precursor forms of, 384, 388, 529,
  546, 553, 560
 proteolytic cleavage of, 35, 58,
  62

m-RNA translation, 546
signal peptide for, 546
structure of, 5, 8, 14, 16, 30, 49, 66
Prothrombin synthase, 560
Prothrombinase complex, 96, 110
Pyridoxal phosphate, 205, 450, 484, 519
Rachitic bone, 241
Ribosomal Gla, 150, 171, 274, 279
Sequenator analysis of Gla, 161
Sphingolipid biosynthesis, 177, 203
Spin trapping agents, 413, 422
Superoxide, 424
Superoxide dismutase, 413, 422
Vitamin D deficiency, 237
Vitamin K
analogs, activity of, 455
biosynthesis of, 182, 188, 208
bacterial function, 177, 193, 203, 274
cis/trans forms of, 333
cytochrome interaction, 179, 193
food content of, 324
in active transport, 183, 193
in electron transport, 177, 193
in invertebrates, 208
in plasma, 326, 328, 349
in sphingolipid synthesis, 177, 203
nutritional aspects of, 317, 328, 343
semiquinone generation, 419
tissue distribution, 286
Vitamin K dependent carboxylase,
activity of analogs, 456
effect of drugs on, 373
effect of metabolic inhibitors, 458
indogenous inhibitors of, 494
endogenous substrates for, 484, 553
Glu derivatives as substrates, 480
HPLC assay of products, 505
hydroperoxide intermediates, 408, 413, 422, 433
in bone, 345, 340
in bovine liver, 422, 557
in chick embryo, 245, 294
in choriollantoic membrane, 294
in fibroblasts, 311
in kidney, 292, 299, 303, 311
in lung, 286
in pancrease, 311
in rat liver, 279, 286, 354, 370, 401, 413, 422, 433, 443, 450, 455, 467, 471, 480, 484, 490, 500, 505, 509, 518, 553
in spleen, 292, 299
in various species, 446
induction of, 443, 484
oxygen involvement in, 408, 413, 422, 433
peptide substrates for, 401, 413, 453, 471, 509, 518
purification of, 433, 490, 504, 560
radical involvement in, 408, 413, 422
reaction mechanism, 354, 401, 408, 413, 422, 433, 471, 509
relationship to epoxidase, 505
specificity of sulfhydryl poisons, 465
stimulation by 1,4-naphthoquinones, 467
stimulations by precursor, 484
stimulation by pyridoxal phosphate, 450, 465, 484, 518
subcellular distribution, 339, 447, 534
Vitamin K epoxidase
effect of hormones, 337
fetal/maternal activity, 339
in bone cells, 340
in various tissues, 292
relationships to carboxylase, 505
subcellular distribution, 338, 447
Vitamin K epoxide,
analysis of, 318, 362, 505
in invertebrates, 208
in plasma, 328, 349
Vitamin K epoxide reductase
assay by HPLC, 361
effect of R/S warfarin, 366
effect of warfarin metabolites, 368
in various species, 361
in various tissues, 292
subcellular distribution, 447
stimulation by ERSA, 355
Warfarin,
action in rabbits, 348, 380
effect on bone, 222, 227, 237, 245, 255
effect on epoxide reductase, 354, 361, 366
effect on Gla excretion, 375
effect on glycosylation reactions, 571
effect on factor X_a inhibitor, 380
effect on plasma clotting factors, 342, 349, 370, 380, 388
effect on teeth, 255

effect on vitamin K metabolism,
  329, 349
enantiomers of, 366
in invertebrates, 208
metabolism of, 366
phenylbutazone interaction with,
  370
plasma turnover of, 371
Mn deficiency relationship, 573
resistant rat population, 392